CLINICAL
SPORTS
NUTRITION

Second Edition

Edited by
Louise Burke
and
Vicki Deakin

The McGraw-Hill Companies, Inc.

Beijing Bogotà Boston Burr Ridge IL Caracas
Dubuque IA Lisbon London Madison WI
Madrid Mexico City Milan Montreal New Delhi
New York San Francisco Santiago Seoul
Singapore St Louis Sydney Taipei Toronto

McGraw·Hill Australia

A Division of The McGraw·Hill Companies

Reprinted 2002, 2003
Text © 2000 Louise Burke and Vicki Deakin
Illustrations and design © 2000 McGraw-Hill Book Company Australia Pty Limited
Additional owners of copyright material are credited on the Acknowledgments page.

National Library of Australia Cataloguing-in-Publication data:

Clinical sports nutrition.

2nd ed.
Includes index.
ISBN 0 074 70828 7.

1. Athletes—Nutrition. 2. Physical fitness—Nutritional aspects. 3. Exercise—Physiological aspects. I. Burke, Louise. II. Deakin, Vicki.

613.2088796

Published in Australia by
McGraw-Hill Australia Pty Limited
Level 2, 82 Waterloo Road, North Ryde, NSW 2113
Acquisitions Editor: Meiling Voon
Production Editor: Sybil Kesteven
Editor: Emma Hardman
Illustrator: Alan Laver, Shelly Communications
Designer: Kim Webber, Southern Star Design
Cover image: Stockmarket/Chris Hamilton
Typeset in 11/13 pt Goudy by Post Pre-press Group
Printed on 80gsm woodfree by Pantech Limited, Hong Kong

CONTENTS

When the first edition of this book was published in 1994, it marked the work of a special interest group in Sports Nutrition, supported by the Australian Sports Medicine Federation and the Dietitians Association of Australia. We developed the text from the material produced for a Continuing Education Course in Sports Nutrition for Dietitians, hoping that dietitians experienced in sports nutrition in Australia could provide their knowledge and experience to younger colleagues or colleagues experienced in other fields of nutrition. This four-day course has been held annually at the Australian Institute of Sport in Canberra since 1992 and continues to draw strong interest within Australia and internationally.

Since those early days, our special interest group has evolved into a vibrant professional organisation, Sports Dietitians Australia (SDA). Full membership of this group is open to dietitians who have completed our own course, or other accredited sports nutrition programs. Our mission statement is to promote healthy eating to enhance the performance of Australians, whatever their level of physical activity. Our vision includes a commitment to professional excellence and recognition of the special expertise of sports dietitians. SDA is grateful for the energy of its members and the support of its foundation sponsors in assisting it to accomplish numerous achievements. The publication of the second edition of this textbook has been nominated as a key activity of SDA.

Over the last decade research in sports nutrition and performance has grown exponentially. This second edition of *Clinical Sports Nutrition* provides an updated and expanded collection of chapters on special issues of sports nutrition. New areas include an historical overview of sports nutrition, post-exercise recovery, sports nutrition for the older athlete, and the nutritional considerations for exercise in the extreme environments of heat or altitude. The section on sports foods and dietary supplements has been expanded to take into account the continuing explosion of new products marketed to athletes. Practical advice on feeding athletes has been arranged into two new chapters on the travelling athlete, and catering for athletic groups. As in the first edition we have provided a unique blend of state-of-the-art knowledge in sports nutrition principles, an appeciation of the unique lifestyles and practical needs of athletes, and specialised expertise in nutrition assessment, education and counselling. Each chapter includes a comprehensive review of the current theoretical aspects of sports nutrition, and a separate discussion of the issues underpinning the implementation of this information into real-life practice. In this edition we have expanded our group of authors to include international experts. Many of them have already been part of SDA activities, for instance by lecturing on our course, or being supported as a keynote speaker at the annual Sports Medicine Australia Conferences on sports medicine and science. We hope to increase our opportunities for international collaboration and information exchange.

This new textbook addresses the latest research findings, relevant to both the elite and recreational athlete. It also includes information that is important for the understanding of the role of physical activity in many areas of health.

We hope that this book will continue to inform and inspire students in sports nutrition courses, and assist practitioners to make optimal nutrition a strength of the athletes with whom they work.

ACKNOWLEDGMENTS

Thank you to the sports dietitians and other exercise science and medicine experts who contributed chapters to this book, for providing us with your knowledge and expertise within our tight deadlines. We knew that in choosing the best people to work with, we would be competing with the million other activities and people who make demands on your time, and we are grateful that you made this book a priority.

We thank Meiling Voon, Sybil Kesteven and Emma Hardman from McGraw-Hill who produced this book in various roles. Email and couriers make modern communications much easier, but we tested your patience by spreading ourselves all around the world. Special appreciation must also go to Kim Horne, administrative assistant to the Department of Sports Nutrition at the Australian Institute of Sport (AIS), who kept a finger on the pulse at all times, to organise us or to solve the emergencies.

The dietitians in the Department of Sports Nutrition at the AIS were generous in allowing this book to become an integral part of our team activities. Thank you Greg Cox, Nikki Cummings, Ben Desbrow, Michelle Minehan and Kelly Meredith for contributing your own chapters, and for proofreading to fatigue in order to find the last typos and errors.

Karen Cashel from the GADI Research Centre at the University of Canberra has been invaluable in providing scholarly input, personal support, motivation and encouragement. Louise Catanzarita, a post-graduate student, also contributed to proofing the final edits.

Finally, we thank all the coaches and athletes who have enriched our experiences, and inspired our interest in, and love of, sports nutrition.

Louise Burke, PhD, BSc, Grad Dip Diet, FSMA, FACSM

Louise has been the Head of the Department of Sports Nutrition at the Australian Institute of Sport since 1990 and has over 20 years of experience in counselling and educating athletes. She has been appointed as an Adjunct Professor at Deakin University in Melbourne where she is involved in the development and delivery of undergraduate and post-graduate education in Sports Nutrition. Her research interests include post-exercise recovery, nutritional ergogenic aids, carbohydrate and fat metabolism during exercise, and fluid needs in sport. She has produced a number of education resources for athletes, coaches, students and practitioners, including best-selling books. She was appointed as the Dietitian to the Australian Olympic Team for the 1996 and 2000 Olympic Games.

Vicki Deakin, BSc, Dip T, Grad Dip Nutr Diet

Vicki is a lecturer and researcher at the University of Canberra and convenes the undergraduate course in Human Nutrition. She is a member of the Population Health Research team at the GADI Research Centre at the University of Canberra and also a Consultant Dietitian with the ACT Academy of Sport. Her interest and involvement with elite athletes dates back to her initiation of the nutrition services at the Australian Institute of Sport in 1985. She is actively involved in the professional nutrition education of coaches and athletes throughout Australia and has developed a distance course for the Australian Coaching Council to facilitate this process. She is involved in teaching, research and consultancy in numerous areas including sports nutrition, dietary survey methods, cardiovascular disease, factors affecting dietary behaviour and has published in the lay and professional literature.

EDITORS

Professor Louise Burke, PhD, BSc,
Grad Dip Diet, FSMA, FACSM
Head, Department of Sports Nutrition
Australian Institute of Sport
P.O. Box 176
BELCONNEN   ACT   2616
AUSTRALIA

Vicki Deakin, BSc, Dip T, Grad Dip
Nutr
Sports Dietitian
Lecturer
Faculty of Applied Science
University of Canberra
ACT 2601
AUSTRALIA

CONTRIBUTORS

Dr Tim Ackland, BPE (Hons), MPE,
PhD, FASMF, MAAESS, MESA
Associate Professor
Dept of Human Movement and
Exercise Science
The University of Western Australia
NEDLANDS   WA   6907
AUSTRALIA

Kylie Andrew, MND
Consulting Dietitian
McKinnon Sports Centre
227 McKinnon Rd
McKINNON   VIC   3204
AUSTRALIA

Dr Shona Bass, PhD, MSc, BAppSci
Senior Lecturer
School of Health Sciences
Deakin University
221 Burwood Highway
BURWOOD   VIC   3125
AUSTRALIA

Dr Kim Bennell, BAppSci (Physio), PhD
Senior Lecturer
Centre for Sports Medicine Research
and Education
School of Physiotherapy
University of Melbourne
PARKVILLE   VIC   3052
AUSTRALIA

Liz Broad, BSc, Dip Nutr Diet,
MAppSc (Sports Studies)
Sports Dietitian
Sports Science Co-ordinator—
Australian Canoeing
44 Tallebudgera Ck Rd
ANDREWS   QLD   4220
AUSTRALIA

Lyn Brown, MDAA
Director, Nutrition Services
ACT Community Care
The Canberra Hospital
P.O. Box 11
WODEN   ACT   2605
AUSTRALIA

Professor Louise Burke, PhD, Grad Dip
Diet, FSMA, FACSM
Head, Department of Sports Nutrition
Australian Institute of Sport
P.O. Box 176
BELCONNEN ACT 2616
AUSTRALIA

Glenn Cardwell, BSc, Grad Dip Diet,
Grad Dip App Sc, APD
Sports Dietitian
P.O. Box 1035
BENTLEY DC WA 6983
AUSTRALIA

Professor Ian Caterson, MB BS, BSc
(Med), PhD, FRACP
Boden Professor of Human Nutrition
Dept of Biochemistry
University of Sydney
NSW 2006
AUSTRALIA

Greg Cox, BHMS, Grad Dip Nutr &
Diet
Senior Sports Dietitian
Department of Sports Nutrition
Australian Institute of Sport
P.O. Box 176
BELCONNEN ACT 2616
AUSTRALIA

Nicola K Cummings, BSc, Grad Dip
Diet
Food Service/Sports Dietitian
Department of Sports Nutrition
Australian Institute of Sport
P.O. Box 176
BELCONNEN ACT 2616
AUSTRALIA

Belinda Dalton, B App Sci, Grad Dip
(Nutr & Diet), Grad Cert (Sports
Nutrition)
Sports Dietitian
2A Disraeli St
KEW VIC 3101
AUSTRALIA

Vicki Deakin, BSc, Dip T, Grad Dip
Nutr
Sports Dietitian
Lecturer
Faculty of Applied Science
University of Canberra
ACT 2601
AUSTRALIA

Ben Desbrow, BSc, Grad Dip Nut &
Diet, Grad Dip Sc (HMS)
Nutrition Consultant/Sports Dietitian
Wesley Hospital
PO Box 820
CAPALABA QLD 4157
AUSTRALIA

Associate Professor Kieran Fallon,
MB BS (Hons), MSpExSc, FRACGP,
FACSP
Acting Head
Medical Services
Department of Sports Medicine
Australian Institute of Sport
PO Box 176
BELCONNEN ACT 2616
AUSTRALIA

Dr Mark A Febbraio, PhD
Director
Exercise Physiology & Metabolism
Laboratory
Department of Physiology
The University of Melbourne
PARKVILLE VIC 3010
AUSTRALIA

Dr Mikael Fogelholm, DSc (Nutrition)
Director
Research & Development
University of Helsinki
Palmenia Centre for Research and
Continuing Education
Saimaankatu 11, 15140 Lahti
FINLAND

Professor Peter Fricker, OAM, MBBS,
FACSM, FASMF, FACSP
Head, Sports Science and Sports
Medicine, Australian Institute of Sport
Chair of Sports Medicine
University of Canberra
P.O. Box 176
BELCONNEN ACT 2616
AUSTRALIA

Lorna Garden, BSc, Dip Diet, APD
Consultant and Sports Dietitian
P.O. Box 365
NOOSAVILLE QLD 4566
AUSTRALIA

Professor Mark Hargreaves, PhD
Professor of Exercise Physiology
Head, School of Health Sciences
Deakin University
BURWOOD VIC 3125
AUSTRALIA

Professor John Hawley, PhD, MA,
Cert Ed, BSc (Hons), FACSM
Exercise Metabolism Group
Department of Human Biology and
Movement Science
RMIT University
Bundoora Campus
P.O. Box 71
BUNDOORA VIC 3083
AUSTRALIA

Dr Karim Khan, MD, PhD, FACSP,
FACSM
Assistant Professor
Dept of Family Practice and School of
Human Kinetics
James Mather Building
University of British Columbia
5084 Fairview Ave
VANCOUVER V6T 1Z3
CANADA

Linda Houtkooper PhD, RD
Dept of Nutritional Science
University of Arizona
312A FCR #33
TUCSON AZ 85721
USA

Karen Inge, BSc, Dip Diet, FSMA,
APD
Co-ordinator Nutrition Services
Victorian Institute of Sport
PO Box 148
CANTERBURY VIC 3126
AUSTRALIA

Dr Deborah Kerr, BSc, Grad Dip Diet, MSc, PhD
Lecturer
School of Public Health
Curtin University of Technology
GPO Box U1987
PERTH WA 6845
AUSTRALIA

Melinda M. Manore, PhD, RD
Professor
Department of Nutrition
Arizona State University—East Campus
7001 E. Williams Field Rd
MESA   AZ   85212
USA

Professor Ron Maughan, BSc, PhD
Professor of Human Physiology
Department of Biomedical Sciences
University Medical School
University of Aberdeen
Foresterhill
ABERDEEN   AB25 2ZD
SCOTLAND

Michelle Minehan, BAppSc, MND
Sports Dietitian
Sports Services Officer
Australian Sports Drug Agency
3/4 Stroud Pl
FLOREY   ACT   2615
AUSTRALIA

Dr Helen O'Connor, BSc, Dip ND, PhD, APD
Lecturer
Dept of Exercise and Sport Science
University of Sydney
Cumberland Campus
East St
LIDCOMBE   NSW   2141
AUSTRALIA

Fiona Pelly, BSc, Grad Dip Nut Diet
Sports Dietitian
NSW Institute of Sports Medicine
Hospital Rd
CONCORD NSW 2139
AUSTRALIA

Peter Reaburn, BHMS (Ed) (Hons), PhD
Head of School
School of Health and Human Performance
Central Queensland University
ROCKHAMPTON   QLD   4702
AUSTRALIA

Gary Slater, BSc, Grad Dip Nutr & Diet
Sports Dietitian
Sports Medicine & Sports Science Division
Singapore Sports Council
15 Stadium Rd
National Stadium
SINGAPORE   397718

Ms Terri Sullivan, BSc, PG Dip Nutr
& Diet, APD
Consultant Dietitian
120 Beck St
PADDINGTON   QLD   4064
AUSTRALIA

Mark Tarnopolsky, MD, PhD,
FRCP(C)
Associate Professor, Medicine
(Neurology & Rehabilitation) and
Kinesiology
Neuromuscular Disease Unit
4U4 Neurology
McMaster University Medical Center
HAMILTON   ONTARIO   L8N 3Z5
CANADA

Ms Julie Tatnell, BSc (Nutr), Grad
Dip Diet
Sports and Clinical Dietitian,
22 Primrose St
MOONEE PONDS   VIC   3039
AUSTRALIA

Dr Janice Thompson, PhD, FACSM
Associate Professor, Research Scientist
Dept of Paediatrics
Center for Health Promotion and
Disease Prevention
The University of New Mexico Health
Sciences Center
Surge Building
Albuquerque NM 87131-5311
USA

Professor Janet Walberg-Rankin, PhD
Dept of Human Nutrition, Foods and
Exercise
215 War Memorial Hall
Virginia Tech
BLACKSBURG VA 24061-0430
USA

Clinical Associate Professor J. Dennis
Wilson, BSc (Hons), MB BAO, BCh
(Hons), MD, FRCP, FRACP
Director, Endocrinology
The Canberra Hospital
P.O. Box 11
WODEN   ACT   2606
AUSTRALIA

Nick Wray, MND, BAppSc (Exercise
& Sports Science), Grad Dip Hum
Nutr
Senior Dietitian
Nutrition and Dietetics Dept
Level 4
Flinders Medical Centre
BEDFORD PARK   SA   5042
AUSTRALIA

Dr Mark Young, MB BS, DRCOG,
FACSP
Sports Physician
Wesley Orthopaedic & Sports Injury
Clinic
Level 3
Fanford Jackson Bldg
30 Chasely St
AUCHENFLOWER   QLD   4066
AUSTRALIA

CHAPTER 1

Sports nutrition: an historical perspective

Ron Maughan and Louise Burke

1.1 INTRODUCTION

Of all the sciences, nutrition may have more to offer the athlete than any other. Choosing appropriate foods in suitable amounts at the correct time will not compensate for a lack of natural ability, a reluctance to undertake the required training, nor an absence of tactical awareness. It is equally clear that a poor diet will prevent the athlete from achieving their potential. It is worth remembering that most of the experimental evidence for the beneficial effects of nutritional strategies on exercise performance is derived from studies on relatively untrained individuals. This means that all athletes, not just those few competing at an elite level, should pay attention to this aspect of their preparation.

As with other areas of nutritional science, sports nutrition is in a process of constant change and evolution. As new information emerges, our concept of what constitutes an appropriate diet changes. The recommendations given to athletes today are very different from those of even a decade ago. A good example of this can be seen in the sequence of recommendations for fluid intake in endurance events made by the American College of Sports Medicine (ACSM). The evolution of this series of recommendations is detailed in the time line below.

The process of evolution is further shown by the differences between countries in the recommended daily allowances for various nutrients. The recommended intake for vitamin C, for example, varies between 30 mg/d in Canada to 80 mg/d in France (Truswell et al. 1983). Both cannot be correct, but the discrepancy illustrates the different interpretations put on the available evidence by different expert committees; harmonisation will surely occur as further information emerges.

Until comparatively recently, malnutrition was widespread. Compulsory military service was introduced in the United Kingdom in 1916: in some of the large industrial urban districts of England, as many as 60% of potential recruits were classified as unfit. This finding was responsible for an expansion of research on the links between diet and health, as well as a variety of nutritional measures such as the fortification of certain foods with a range of vitamins, and with iron. Improvements in the diet of the general population have greatly reduced the risk of nutritional deficiencies in most countries of the modern world.

The performances of today's athletes are far superior to those achieved in earlier times, and as with improvements in the health of the general population, nutritional advances have played a role. The increased percentage of the total gene pool which now participates in sport is a major factor in the continuing improvement of world records. For the individual, however, training, diet and the avoidance of illness and injury will remain the most important elements. This book provides a summary of the considerable knowledge of sports nutrition that is available to athletes in the new millennium. It describes the rigorous science behind the principles of sports nutrition and offers guidelines for best practice in the sporting arena. Before starting our contemporary understanding of sports nutrition, it is interesting to consider how its science and practice have evolved over the past decades and centuries. An awareness of the history of sport, and of the evolution of training and nutritional practices, is not only of interest in itself, but can help the understanding of current practice. Following are some of the key steps that have led us to where we are today.

1.2 THE PROGRESS OF THE SCIENCE AND PRACTICE OF SPORTS NUTRITION

6th century BC Milos, a Cretan wrestler, won gold medals at five Olympic Games. According to legend, he carried a calf over his head each day as training—her growth meant gradual training overload! When the calf turned four, Milos carried her the length of the stadium before killing and eating her. His typical daily meat intake was reported to be 10 kg/d.

2nd century BC Galen, the famous Greek philosopher and physician, reported that 'pork contains more real nutriment than the flesh of any other animal: this fact is proved by the example of the athlete who, if they lived for only one day on any other kind of food, find their vigour manifestly impaired the next' (Thom 1813).

1750– Pedestrianism—long distance walking events usually carried out alone and sometimes for substantial wagers—became popular in England. Even allowing for exaggeration, these feats (usually between major cities on poorly constructed public roads) were remarkable. Little information on nutritional preparation prior to the 1800s has survived. In 1804, Lieutenant Fairman ran 60 miles, on a one mile course marked out on Ipswich racecourse (and therefore on rough grass), in a time of 13 h 59 min. He stopped at about halfway to change clothes and take a breakfast of tea and toast, and took bread steeped in madeira at intervals in the later stages of the race. Thom (1813) reported that Fairman was a vegetarian, unlike most other pedestrians of the time.

A Mr Canning of Hampshire walked 300 miles in less than five days: in the process he lost 26 pounds in weight. A Mr Rimmington walked 560 miles in seven days in the same year: 'he was much emaciated by this extraordinary exertion' (Thom 1813). These reports suggest that food intake during these events was inadequate.

1809–

The most famous pedestrian of the time was Captain Barclay Allardyce, who performed many remarkable feats. Perhaps his most famous achievement, in 1809, was to walk 1000 miles in 1000 hours, covering one mile in each successive hour: this meant that he never had more than about 40 minutes of rest for a period of 42 days. During the walk, his weight fell from 176 pounds to 154 pounds. He seems to have favoured a high meat intake, eating five to six pounds of meat per day. His breakfast (at 5 am) consisted of roast chicken and a pint of strong beer followed by tea with bread and butter. Lunch (at 12 noon) consisted of steak or mutton chops, with more beer and two to three glasses of wine. Supper at 11 pm was cold chicken. Unspecified vegetables were also taken. A full description of the training diet recommended by Captain Barclay is given by Thom (1813), of which the following is only a brief excerpt:

> Animal diet is alone prescribed, and beef and mutton are preferred. Biscuit and stale bread are the only preparations of vegetable matter, which are permitted. Vegetables are never given as they are watery and of difficult digestion. Fish must be avoided. Salt, spices, and all kind of seasonings, with the exception of vinegar, are prohibited. Liquors must always be taken cold, and home brewed beer, old but not bottled, is best. Water is never given alone. It is an established rule to avoid liquids as much as possible. (Thom 1813)

It was a strong man who could survive this regimen, to which was added emetics, purgatives and 'sweating liquors': to be able to run after submitting to this treatment is nothing short of remarkable.

1860 Australian sprinter Tom Cusack was noted to eat a bowl of soup, stewed mutton, eggs, toast and drink three cups of tea before racing (Snell 1997).

1902 EC Bredin, a 19th century middle distance runner, provided the following training notes for runners in the 1902 autobiography of champion sprinter, A Downer:

> As regards food, most men can eat as much as they feel inclined, but one had better make a rule to take no liquid whatever between meals unless feeling unduly thirsty . . . The meat should be varied as much as possible, and poultry is a great aid in this direction; toast is better to eat than bread, and all sorts of milk pudding with fruit, stewed or uncooked, according to the time of the year . . . On the day of a race, a light and frugal meal should be partaken of some three hours at least before running: the inside of a chop and one glass of port is quite sufficient for most men, and cannot be beaten. (Bredin 1902)

1909 JE Sullivan provided the following advice for marathon running in his book:

> Don't take any nourishment before going 17 or 18 miles. If you do you will not go the distance. Don't get into the habit of eating or drinking in a marathon race: some prominent runners do, but it is not beneficial. (Sullivan 1909)

1909 Frijtof Nansen conducted extensive studies on the nutrient requirement of men (and of dogs) in preparation for polar exploration. He recognised that in spite of the weight advantage of a high-fat diet, which was an important consideration when all food had to be hauled on sleds, a certain minimum amount of carbohydrate was essential when hard physical work was required on a daily basis.

1911 Physiologist Nathan Zuntz reported that fat and carbohydrate were both used as fuels by exercising muscles and that the relative contribution of fat was increased if dietary carbohydrate intake was restricted in the days prior to exercise.

1920	Krogh and Lindhard confirmed and extended the work of Zuntz, which was not widely accepted at the time.
1923–24	Researchers at the Boston marathon found that some runners finished the race with blood glucose levels regarded as hypoglycaemic. The following year they reported that feeding candy to runners during the marathon improved their blood glucose levels and performances.
1928	A study of ten marathon runners from the 1928 Olympic Games in Amsterdam was conducted. Three of the runners finished with low blood glucose levels. The race day food and fluid intake of runners was noted. Race intake included special sports drinks manufactured by the Japanese runners (extra sugar added to lemonade), tea, cocoa, milk and grapefruit. One runner ate an egg en route. The winning time was 2 h 32 min.
1928	Bock and colleagues reported that the contribution of carbohydrate to energy metabolism was proportional to the exercise intensity.
1930s	Australian rowers were not allowed to drink with their meals and were not allowed to consume 'soups, pastry cream and other fattening foods'. However, they ate a dozen apples a day each. (Snell 1997)
1932	The Harvard Fatigue Laboratory published evidence from dog studies that carbohydrate intake dramatically improved endurance during prolonged moderate intensity exercise.
1936	A textbook on exercise by Grace Eggleton included the following advice:

> If the eating of candy during a race was encouraged by Athletic Organisations, it seems possible that new records might be achieved in very long-distance running. (Grace Eggleton 1936)

1939	A series of papers by Christensen and Hansen demonstrated the critical role of carbohydrate in endurance exercise. They found that endurance time was increased after a high-carbohydrate diet and reduced after a low-carbohydrate diet (relative to their subjects' normal diets). They also found that ingestion of glucose at the point of exhaustion allowed exercise to continue past that point.
1939–45	Interest in war rations for soldiers stimulated research into vitamin status and exercise tolerance.

1948	Olympic teams faced post-war rations during the London Games. The daily ration was 170 g meat, 1 L milk, 680 g potatoes, 450 g bread, 30 g cheese and 55 g sugar.
1948	British Ministry of Health studied the eating practices of athletes at the Olympic Games. Dietary intake was measured for ↘ four days in 28 male athletes from a variety of sports. This was achieved by having dietitians follow each athlete in the central café and collect a duplicate sample of food. These food samples were homogenised and chemically analysed for energy, protein, fat and carbohydrate. The athletes' mean daily intakes were estimated to be 3350 kcal, ranging from 2110 to 4740 kcal/d in individual athletes. Individual food practices noted in a questionnaire include pre-exercise meals of high protein and high-fat foods. A few athletes reported use of vitamin and mineral supplements.
1950s	Oral rehydration solutions (ORS) were developed for the treatment of infectious diarrhoeal disease, a major killer of children. The addition of small amounts of sugar and salt were found to stimulate intestinal water transport. This research was not immediately applied to sport, but was later to form the basis of the formulation of commercial sports drinks.
1950s	Champion Australian sprinter Shirley Strickland was advised by her coach to cut out all soft foods from her diet, and not drink any fluids on the day before a race or on race day itself. He noted that she often drank as much as a gallon of water after the race. (Snell 1997)
1950s	Australian Olympic gold medal swimmer Murray Rose was a vegetarian, an anomaly for these times. He ate fruit, vegetables, eggs, dairy foods and a variety of grains and legumes. (Snell 1997)
1953	According to the International Amateur Athletic Federation (IAAF) guidelines for distance running events, aid stations were allowed in distance running events only after 15 km, and water was the only provision permitted.
1960s	Herb Elliot, champion middle distance runner and world mile record holder, trained on the sand dunes of Portsea with coach Percy Cerutty. His breakfast consisted of raw oats, wheat germ, dried fruit and sliced banana (consumed dry—without milk) followed by french fries. (Snell 1997)

1960s	Australian Olympic swimmers and world record holders Ilsa and Jon Konrads were noted to exclude starchy foods from their diet and concentrate on protein foods. (Snell 1997)
1960s	Australian boxer Lionel Rose took his own food to Japan before his famous bout with Japanese boxer Fighter Harada. He fasted to make weight for the bout before the morning 'weigh in' then ate a steak, a whole chicken and more steak before his evening fight. He won the world boxing bantamweight title. (Snell 1997)
1962	Use of the needle biopsy technique was revived by Jonas Bergstrom, opening the way for direct measurement of the metabolic response of muscles to exercise.
1964	Australian Olympic swimmer Nan Duncan was told by coach Don Talbot (current Australian national head coach) to eat ice-cream, cakes and other high-calorie foods. Being too light (67 kg) was considered a risk for tiredness and illness. Her mother piled up her meals and added lashings of cream. (Snell 1997)
1965	Jonas Bergstrom and Eric Hultman published in the journal *Nature* the results of an ingenious study they conducted on themselves. Each cycled to fatigue using one leg only, followed by muscle biopsy sampling from both legs. Glycogen levels were low in the exercised legs, but normal in the rested leg. Sampling continued for three days during which a high-carbohydrate diet was eaten. Glycogen supercompensation was observed in the exercised leg, with little change in the rested leg.
1967	The Miami Orange Bowl playoff in American College Football saw the Florida Gators in competition against Georgia Tech. The Gators were being badly beaten, and at half-time used a new drink designed for them by Dr Robert Cade of the University of Florida. The drink, containing electrolytes and carbohydrate, was designed to 'replace what the game was taking out of them'. The Florida Gators played well in the second half to overcome their opponents and win their first Orange Bowl. Their drink, called Gatorade, was released commercially. It took another 20 years for sports scientists to embrace the performance benefits of consuming carbohydrate–electrolyte drinks during a wide range of sports. By this time, sports drinks would be a widely accepted sports supplement, and a commercial success.
1968	The decision to hold the Olympic Games in Mexico City focused attention on problems of endurance exercise at altitude.

This stimulated research on the haematological status of athletes, and drew attention to the problems that iron-deficiency anaemia causes for the athlete. This research indirectly led to blood doping and the use of erythropoietin.

1969
The carbohydrate-loading diet was first used in a competitive situation by Ron Hill at the European Championship marathon in Athens in 1969. He was well behind the race leader, Gaston Roelants of Belgium, at 20 miles, but ran strongly in the later stages to win comfortably in a time of 2 h 16 min 48 s. He ran without drinking at all, in spite of the high temperature, and wrote that he gained confidence when he realised that Roelants, far ahead, had begun to drink in the later stages. Hill was a dominant figure in marathon running and was perhaps favourite to win at the Munich Olympics of 1972. However, he believed in a strict form of the diet, with a long hard run followed by three days of training on a diet that was almost carbohydrate-free followed by three days of reduced training on a very high carbohydrate diet. His preparations for the race were disrupted by terrorist activities, which caused the race to be delayed by a day after he had begun his diet. He finished sixth.

1970s
The fitness boom encouraged recreational athletes to take to the streets to complete fun runs and marathons. Carbohydrate loading was practised by some elite distance runners and was then adopted by the running and sports community.

1970s
Sports nutrition experts declared that the protein needs of athletes are no greater than sedentary people.

1971
A field study was published showing that carbohydrate loading enhanced the athlete's performance during a 30 km run, by sustaining the time the athlete could continue at their race pace.

1974
Professors Dave Costill and Bengt Saltin published a paper reporting that fluids containing carbohydrate, even in small concentrations, have reduced gastric emptying characteristics and are not ideal rehydration beverages.

1975
The ACSM published a position statement on thermal injuries during distance running and promoted water as the ideal fluid for ingestion during prolonged exercise. They warned against the consumption of carbohydrate solutions in concentrations greater than 2.5%.

> Rules prohibiting the administration of fluids during the first 10 kilometers of a marathon race should be amended to permit fluid ingestion at frequent intervals along the race course . . . It is the responsibility of the race sponsors to provide fluids which contain small amounts of sugar (less than 2.5%) and electrolytes . . . The addition of even small amounts of sugar can drastically impair the rate of gastric emptying. During exercise in the heat, carbohydrate supplementation is of secondary importance and the sugar content of oral feedings should be minimised. (American College of Sports Medicine 1975)

1979 Papers from Professor Dave Costill's laboratory reported that caffeine ingestion prior to endurance exercise could increase time to exhaustion. Marathon runners started to consume black coffee prior to events.

1979 A paper from Costill's laboratory reported that ingestion of carbohydrate during the hour prior to exercise may reduce endurance, by increasing the rate of muscle glycogen oxidation, or by causing a rebound hypoglycaemia. This fear has persisted despite more than 20 subsequent papers that show that pre-exercise carbohydrate feedings have a neutral or positive impact on exercise performance.

1980s Sports drink companies made new products and provided major funding for research. Numerous studies showed that carbohydrate ingestion improved performance during prolonged moderate intensity events (> 90 min). The new research showed also that gastric emptying and fluid balance did not appear to be compromised until carbohydrate-containing beverages reach concentrations > 8%.

1980 Professor Mike Sherman published a paper showing that well trained athletes can supercompensate their muscle glycogen stores by a simpler carbohydrate-loading protocol, which removed the need for a depletion phase. The 'modified carbohydrate-loading regimen' was launched.

1985 Nathan Pritikin provided the following simplified advice for athletes in his 1985 book *Diet for runners*:

> A special high-performance diet plan is required to meet the special nutritional needs of runners. The Pritikin diet obtains approximately 80% of its total calories from

complex carbohydrate, 10–15% from protein and about 5–10% from fat . . . The Seven Survival Staples (brown rice, cooked beans, simmered chicken, tomato-vegetable stew, frozen bananas, berry-apple compote and 'mock cream' of cottage cheese and buttermilk) are the core of your food plan. (Pritikin 1985)

1987 The ACSM position statement on thermal injuries during distance running updated its views on fluid intake during prolonged events. However, it continued to show a conservative approach to the use of carbohydrate-containing drinks during exercise:

> An adequate supply of water should be available before the race and every 2–3 km during the race . . . Aid stations should be stocked with enough fluid (cool water is the optimum) for each runner to have 300–360 ml at each aid station. (American College of Sports Medicine 1987)

1988 Professor Tim Noakes from the University of Cape Town produced studies and reviews warning athletes that they do not need to consume large amounts of fluid during exercise. He stated that over-drinking could cause the potentially fatal problem of hyponatraemia in some athletes.

1990s Sports drinks became a commercial success. Other tailor-made sports products followed, such as sports bars and sports gels.

1990s Tracer techniques allowed carbohydrate metabolism and the oxidation of ingested carbohydrate to be tracked during exercise. Scientists from a number of laboratories produced studies showing that ingested carbohydrates could supply up to 30% of the muscle's fuel needs in the latter stages of prolonged exercise, and that they were being oxidised at approximately 1 g/min.

1990 Professor Peter Lemon summarised evidence that the protein requirements of both endurance athletes and strength-training athletes are increased by 50–100% above the recommended daily intake (RDI) for sedentary people.

1992 July: Linford Christie won the 100 m sprint at the Barcelona Olympic Games at the age of 31. He announced that his success was in part due to the use of creatine supplements.

November: The journal *Clinical Science* published a study by Roger Harris and Eric Hultman (from carbohydrate-loading fame), which reported that high oral intakes of creatine increase muscle crea-tine and creatine phosphate levels, thus boosting the fuel supply for sprint events.

1992 Professor Ed Coyle's laboratory at the University of Texas showed that dehydration at even minor levels causes an impair-ment of work output and an increased perception of effort when exercising in the heat.

1994 FIFA, the world governing body of soccer, hosted an interna-tional scientific congress on 'Food, nutrition and soccer performance' and issued the following consensus statement:

> Soccer is a worldwide game. Participants include young and old, male and female, amateur and professional, healthy and less healthy, who all play with the common purpose of doing well at the game they hold in such high regard. It is recognised that different cultural, tactical and other factors may influence individual nutritional recom-mendations. (Ekblom & Williams 1994)

1995 The IAAF, the world governing body of athletics, hosted an international scientific consensus conference on 'Current issues in nutrition in athletics' and released a consensus statement:

> Track and field athletics embraces a diversity of events in all of which the genetic potential can only be realised by intensive and consistent training. The inherited charac-teristics and training programs are very different in the various events, but all require adequate nutritional support if success is to be achieved. (Maughan & Horton 1995)

1995–96 Research from the August Krogh Institute in Copenhagen, and from the universities of Cape Town and Maastricht explored the use of high-fat diets and fat supplementation to improve endurance performance.

1996 An American supplement company declared a profit of $195 million dollars from the previous year's sales of creatine.

1996 The ACSM updated its recommendations on the type and pro-vision of fluids during prolonged exercise:

> During intense exercise lasting longer than 1 hour, it is recommended that carbohydrates be ingested at a rate of

30–60 g/h to maintain oxidation of carbohydrates and delay fatigue. This rate of carbohydrate intake can be achieved without compromising fluid delivery by drinking 600–1200 mL/h of solutions containing 4–8% carbohydrate. (American College of Sports Medicine 1996)

1997 Steve Moneghetti, 1980s and 1990s elite distance runner, described the experience of undertaking a 'depletion' phase before carbohydrate loading for marathons:

> The diet makes you feel like death warmed up. You have no energy at all, you're really in heaps of trouble . . . I could feel myself getting more tired and exhausted and run down. I was absolutely gone . . . It's the toughest thing about a marathon. I've enjoyed marathons a lot more since I've stopped doing it. (Moneghetti & Howley 1997)

1997 The Centre for Disease Control in Atlanta recognised the deaths of three college wrestlers within a one-month period. These athletes had undertaken severe practices of sweat- and exercise-induced dehydration, together with restriction of food and fluid in order to make weight for their competitive bouts. An inquiry into these deaths called for strategies to be implemented to ensure safer practices in making weight.

1998 A number of studies reported that the performance of high-intensity exercise of approximately one-hour duration could be enhanced by carbohydrate intake during the event. These findings suggested that carbohydrate supplementation had a number of beneficial outcomes for performance, since depletion of body carbohydrate stores was not expected to occur in events of such short duration.

1999 A number of athletes from different countries tested positive for the banned steroid Nandrolone. It was speculated that some of these cases involved inadvertent doping from the use of dietary supplements containing the pro-hormones 19-norandrostenedione and 19-norandrostenediol. These supplements can be bought over the Internet.

REFERENCES

American College of Sports Medicine. Position statement on prevention of heat injuries during distance running. Med Sci Sports Exerc 1975;7:vii–ix.

American College of Sports Medicine. Position statement on prevention of thermal injuries during distance running. Med Sci Sports Exerc 1987;19:529–33.

American College of Sports Medicine. Position stand: exercise and fluid replacement. Med Sci Sports Exerc 1996;28:i–vii.

Bredin EC. Training notes. In: Downer AR. Running recollections and how to train. Aberdeen: Balgownie Books, 1902, Reprinted 1982.

Ekblom BE, Williams C, eds. Foods, nutrition and soccer performance: final consensus statement. J Sport Sci 1994;12:S3.

Grace Eggleton M. Muscular Exercise. London: Kegan Paul Trench Trubner and Company Limited, 1936.

Maughan RJ, Horton ES, eds. Current issues in nutrition in athletics: final consensus statement. J Sports Sci 1995;13:Si.

Moneghetti S, Howley P. In the long run. Melbourne: Penguin Books, 1997.

Pritikin N. Diet for runners. New York: Simon and Schuster, 1985.

Snell M. Sports Fuel website. www.ausport.gov.au/sportex.

Sullivan JE. Marathon running. New York: American Sports Publishing Company, 1909.

Thom W. Pedestrianism, or an account of the performance of celebrated pedestrians. Aberdeen: Chalmers, 1813.

Truswell AS, Irwin T, Beaton GH, et al. Recommended dietary intakes around the world: A report by Committee 21/5 of the International Union of Nutritional Sciences. Nutr Abst Rev 1983;53:939–1015, 1075–119.

CHAPTER 2

Exercise physiology and metabolism

Mark Hargreaves

2.1 INTRODUCTION

Physical exercise requires a coordinated physiological response involving the interplay between systems responsible for increased energy metabolism, supply of oxygen and substrates to contracting skeletal muscle, removal of metabolic waste products and heat, and the maintenance of fluid and electrolyte status. Knowledge of these responses is important for an understanding of the potential mechanisms by which nutrition can influence exercise and sports performance. It is beyond the scope of this chapter to summarise all of these responses in great detail, and readers are referred to the cited review papers for a more thorough discussion. Nevertheless, this chapter attempts to identify some important aspects of the physiological and metabolic responses to exercise.

2.2 SKELETAL MUSCLE

Skeletal muscle can account for as much as 45% of the total body mass. It is the tissue responsible for the generation of the forces required for joint movement during exercise. Factors influencing the ability of muscle to produce force include total cross-sectional area, fibre type, number of active motor units, motor neuron firing frequency, muscle length and velocity of contraction. The sequence of events involved in muscle contraction is summarised as follows:

1. Motor cortical activation and excitation of alpha motor neuron.
2. Arrival of electrical impulse at neuromuscular junction.
3. Propagation of muscle action potential across sarcolemma.

4. Excitation-contraction (EC) coupling:
   (a) conduction of excitation in t-tubules
   (b) release of calcium from sarcoplasmic reticulum
   (c) action of calcium on actin myofilament.
5. Actin-myosin cross-bridge formation and tension development (sliding filament theory).
6. Re-uptake of calcium by sarcoplasmic reticulum and muscle relaxation.

The chemical energy required for skeletal muscle to undertake mechanical work is provided by the hydrolysis of adenosine triphosphate (ATP), and this reaction is catalysed by myosin ATPase. Since the intramuscular stores of ATP are relatively small (approximately 5 mmol/kg wet weight (ww)), other metabolic pathways responsible for the resynthesis of ATP must be activated in order to maintain contractile activity. These energy pathways are summarised in Figure 2.1. Creatine phosphate (CP) is a high-energy compound, stored in greater amounts (approximately 20 mmol/kg) in skeletal muscle, which can be broken down quickly during

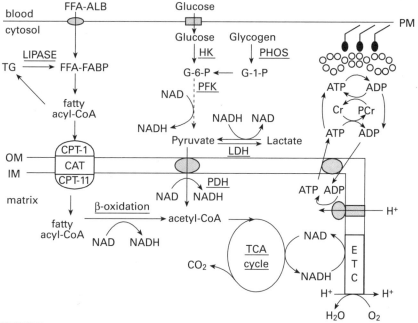

| **Figure 2.1** | *Schematic overview of energy metabolism in skeletal muscle (from Spriet & Howlett 1999, with permission)* |

Abbreviations: PM—plasma membrane; OM, IM—outer and inner mitochondrial membranes; FFA—free fatty acid; ALB—albumin; FABP—fatty acid binding protein; CoA—coenzyme A; CPT 1, 11—carnitine palmitoyltransferase 1 and 11; CAT—carnitine-acylcarnitine translocase; NAD, NADH—oxidised and reduced nicotinamide adenine dinucleotide; HK—hexokinase; PFK—phosphofructokinase; PHOS—glycogen phosphorylase; LDH—lactate dehydrogenase; PDH—pyruvate dehydrogenase; G-6-P, G-1-P—glucose 6- and 1-phosphate; ATP, ADP—adenosine triphosphate and adenosine diphosphate; PCr—phosphocreatine; Cr—creatine; TCA—tricarboxylic acid; ETC—electron transport chain.

intense exercise to provide energy for ATP resynthesis. In addition, ATP can be formed from adenosine diphosphate (ADP) in a reaction catalysed by adenylate kinase. These reactions form what is called the alactic or phosphagen system. The other anaerobic energy system is the lactacid system or anaerobic glycolysis, in which glucose units, derived primarily from intramuscular glycogen reserves, are broken down to lactic acid. These anaerobic energy systems are maximally active during high-intensity exercise of short duration. During prolonged exercise, the aerobic system becomes the predominant provider of energy for contracting skeletal muscle, the major oxidative substrates being carbohydrate (CHO) and lipid.

One aspect of muscle physiology that has received great interest over the years is the potential link between skeletal muscle fibre composition and exercise performance. Human skeletal muscle is composed of two main fibre types: slow twitch (ST) and fast twitch (FT). The FT fibres have been further divided into FTa and FTb on the basis of differences in their glycolytic and oxidative potential. The fibre types differ in their contractile, morphological and metabolic characteristics, and are usually differentiated using histochemical staining for myosin ATPase (Saltin & Gollnick 1983). The ST fibres rely primarily on oxidative metabolism, are well supplied by capillaries and are fatigue resistant. Not surprisingly, they are well suited to prolonged, low-intensity activity. In contrast, FT fibres have a higher glycolytic capacity (FTb > FTa), a lower oxidative capacity (FTb < FTa) and are more fatiguable. They are more suited to high-intensity exercise. During progressive exercise, ST fibres are involved at the lower intensities and as exercise intensity increases, there is progressive recruitment of more ST fibres and the FT fibre populations.

This general pattern of muscle fibre recruitment during exercise has been confirmed in humans using histochemically determined glycogen depletion patterns as an index of fibre involvement. During prolonged, sub-maximal exercise, the ST fibres are preferentially recruited, although there may be involvement of FTa fibres in the latter stages (Vøllestad et al. 1984). As exercise intensity increases, the FT fibres are recruited so that during maximal exercise, all fibre types are involved (Vøllestad & Blom 1985; Vøllestad et al. 1992). These patterns of recruitment have resulted in interest in the link between muscle fibre composition and exercise performance in specially trained athletes. Indeed, elite endurance athletes possess a high percentage of ST muscle fibres (70–90%), while sprint and explosive athletes possess relatively more FT fibres (Costill et al. 1975; Saltin & Gollnick 1983). This appears to be due to a combination of genetic factors and possible training-induced alterations in muscle fibre composition (Saltin & Gollnick 1983; Schantz 1986).

2.3 EXERCISE METABOLISM

During high-intensity, dynamic exercise (e.g. sprinting, track cycling, interval training), the breakdown of ATP and CP, and the degradation of glycogen to lactic acid are the major sources of energy. These substrates are also important during static exercise, particularly above 30–40% maximum voluntary contraction (MVC), since an increase in intramuscular pressure will impair muscle blood flow, thereby reducing oxygen and substrate delivery to contracting skeletal muscle. Activation of muscle phosphagen and glycogen degradation occurs with the onset of exercise. Although the capacity for ATP generation is greater for the glycolytic system (190–300 mmol ATP/kg dry muscle (dm)) than for the phosphagen system (55–95 mmol ATP/kg dm), the power output is lower (4.5 mmol ATP/kg dm/sec compared with 9 mmol/kg dm/sec). For this reason, when the levels of CP decline with maximal exercise the rate of anaerobic turnover cannot be sustained (see Figure 2.2) and this contributes to the decline in power output that is observed during all-out exercise.

During prolonged exercise, the oxidative metabolism of CHOs and lipids provides the vast majority of ATP for muscle contraction. Although amino acid oxidation occurs to a limited extent during exercise (Hood & Terjung 1990), CHOs and lipids are the most important oxidative substrates. The relative contribution of CHOs and lipids is influenced by exercise intensity and duration, preceding diet and substrate availability, training status and environmental factors.

Muscle glycogen is the important substrate during both intense, short-duration exercise and prolonged exercise. Its rate of utilisation is most rapid during the early part of exercise and is related to exercise intensity (Vøllestad et al. 1984; Vøllestad & Blom 1985; Vøllestad et al. 1992). As muscle glycogen declines with continued exercise, blood glucose becomes more important as a CHO fuel source. Muscle

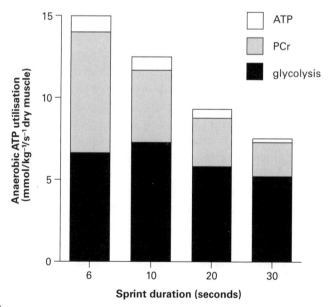

Figure 2.2 *Anaerobic ATP utilisation during maximal cycling exercise of varying duration (from Nevill et al. 1996, with permission)*

glucose uptake increases in both an exercise intensity and duration dependent manner. This is a consequence of increased sarcolemmal glucose transport, due to translocation of the GLUT-4 glucose transporter isoform to the plasma membrane, activation of the metabolic pathways responsible for glucose metabolism and enhanced glucose delivery due to increased skeletal muscle blood flow (Hargreaves 2000). Accompanying the increased muscle glucose uptake is an increase in liver glucose output, so that blood glucose levels usually remain at, or slightly above, resting levels. Liver glycogenolysis supplies the majority of liver glucose output; however, during the latter stages of prolonged exercise, when liver glycogen levels are low, gluconeogenesis is an important source of glucose. Under such circumstances, liver glucose output may fall behind muscle glucose uptake, resulting in hypoglycaemia. Fatigue during prolonged exercise is often, but not always, associated with muscle glycogen depletion and/or hypoglycaemia (Hargreaves 1999). Thus, considerable attention has focused on CHO nutrition and exercise performance, and athletes are encouraged to adopt nutritional strategies that maximise CHO availability before, during and after exercise (Hargreaves 1999; Hawley et al. 1997). These strategies are reviewed in Chapter 13 (Pre-event nutrition), Chapter 14 (Fluid and carbohydrate intake during exercise) and Chapter 15 (Nutrition for recovery after training and competition). There is increasing evidence that lactate, derived from contracting and inactive muscle, is an important oxidative and gluconeogenic precursor and is a valuable metabolic intermediary, rather than simply being a waste product of anaerobic glycolysis (Brooks 1986).

Contracting skeletal muscle also derives energy from the β-oxidation of plasma free fatty acids (FFA), derived from adipose tissue lipolysis. Plasma FFA levels usually peak after 2–4 hours of exercise, at which time they are a major substrate for muscle (Coyle 1995). The muscle uptake and utilisation of FFA is determined, in part, by the arterial FFA concentration and the ability of the muscle to oxidise FFA. Increasing plasma FFA availability and utilisation may reduce the reliance on muscle glycogen and blood glucose, and this has resulted in interest in strategies designed to enhance FFA oxidation (e.g. high-fat diets, caffeine and lipid ingestion and carnitine supplementation), although results in the literature remain equivocal (Hawley et al. 1998). These strategies are reviewed in greater detail in Chapter 16 (Nutritional strategies to enhance fat oxidation during aerobic exercise). It should be noted that a major metabolic adaptation to endurance training is an increased capacity for lipid oxidation. Muscle triglycerides can also be used by contracting muscle and are believed to be more important early in exercise and during exercise at higher intensities where mobilisation of FFA from adipose tissue is inhibited (see Figure 2.3) (Coyle 1995). During high-intensity exercise, mitochondrial oxidation of FFA derived from both adipose tissue and muscle triglycerides is reduced and CHO, predominantly muscle glycogen, is the major fuel.

As mentioned earlier, amino acids, particularly the branched-chain amino acids, can be oxidised during prolonged exercise. The contribution from amino acids is

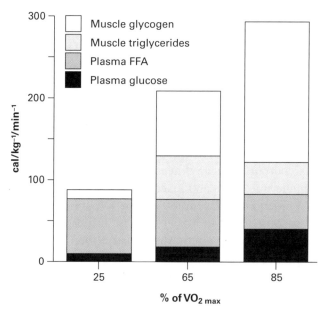

Figure 2.3 *Relative contributions of the various CHO and lipid substrates for oxidative metabolism during exercise of increasing intensity in trained men (from Romijn et al. 1993, with permission)*

enhanced when CHO reserves are low. This is particularly important for athletes in heavy training who are likely to place a large stress on their endogenous CHO reserves and in whom the training-based adaptations (e.g. increased metabolic enzymes, myofibrillar mass and buffer capacity) are protein dependent. Protein requirements for exercise are reviewed in Chapter 5 (Protein and amino acid needs for training and bulking up).

2.4 OXYGEN TRANSPORT SYSTEM

The increased oxidative metabolism during exercise is dependent upon the adequate delivery of oxygen to active muscle and, thus, upon the functional capacities of the cardiovascular and respiratory systems. The most widely accepted measure of aerobic fitness is maximal oxygen uptake ($VO_{2\,max}$) and over the years there has been considerable interest in the physiological determinants of $VO_{2\,max}$.

The cardiovascular system has three important functions during exercise:

1. to increase oxygen delivery to contracting skeletal and cardiac muscle;
2. to transport heat to the skin to facilitate evaporative heat loss; and
3. to maintain mean arterial blood pressure so that cerebral blood flow is maintained.

Skeletal muscle vasodilation occurs due to the release from active muscle of vasoactive metabolites (including hydrogen ion (H^+), potassium (K^+), lactate, adenosine) together with local hypercapnia, hypoxia and hyperosmolality. A recent hypothesis proposes that acetylcholine, released from the neuromuscular junction, causes hyperpolarisation along the endothelial cell layer and vasodilation in the arteriolar network (conducted vasodilation). Furthermore, there has been interest in the potential role of endothelium-derived nitric oxide (NO) in mediating exercise hyperemia, with conflicting results. Mean arterial pressure (MAP) is maintained, despite the decrease in skeletal muscle vascular resistance, due to an increase in cardiac output (increased heart rate and stroke volume) and vasoconstriction in the splanchnic, renal and inactive muscle vascular beds. The cutaneous circulation receives increased flow for the dissipation of heat, although it is a target of sympathetic vasoconstriction at higher exercise intensities. Active skeletal muscle may also be a target for sympathetic vasoconstriction in order to maintain MAP as maximal cardiac output approaches (Saltin et al. 1998). The regulation of the cardiovascular response to exercise involves a number of neurohumoural factors. The general pattern of cardiovascular effector activity is set by descending neural activity from the cardiovascular centre (central command), increased in parallel with motor cortical activation of skeletal muscle (Mitchell 1990). This activity is likely to be influenced by muscle and arterial chemoreflexes, arterial baroreflexes, hypovolemia and hyperthermia (Rowell 1986).

An increase in pulmonary ventilation is essential for maintaining arterial oxygenation and eliminating carbon dioxide, produced by oxidative metabolism in contracting muscle. During incremental exercise, ventilation increases in proportion to the increases in oxygen consumption and carbon dioxide production; however, at higher intensities a point is reached where there is an abrupt increase in ventilation. This is often referred to as the ventilatory or anaerobic threshold, and it has been suggested that it is due to stimulation of the peripheral chemoreceptors by increased carbon dioxide, arising from the bicarbonate buffering of lactic acid produced by contracting skeletal muscle (Wasserman et al. 1986). There is considerable debate and controversy in the literature regarding the mechanisms of lactate production during exercise, and the link between hyperventilation and blood lactate accumulation (Brooks 1986; Wasserman et al. 1986; Katz & Sahlin 1988; Walsh & Banister 1988). The ventilatory responses to exercise are regulated by a number of neural and humoural factors. These include carbon dioxide flux to the lung, descending activity from respiratory neurons in the hindbrain, increased body temperature, alterations in arterial H^+, K^+ and adrenaline levels and feedback from muscle chemoreceptors and proprioceptors (Forster & Pan 1991).

The ability of the muscles to consume oxygen in metabolism, and the combined abilities of the cardiovascular and respiratory systems to deliver oxygen to the muscle mitochondria, are reflected in $VO_{2\,max}$, the most widely accepted measure of aerobic fitness. Values for $VO_{2\,max}$ range from 30–40 mL/kg/min in inactive sedentary individuals to as high as 80–90 mL/kg/min in highly trained endurance athletes. Such high values reflect a combination of genetic endowment and vigorous physical training. The measurement of $VO_{2\,max}$ is useful in the assessment of endurance athletes and, together with the ventilatory/lactate threshold, is a strong predictor of endurance exercise performance (Williams 1990). There has been much interest in the physiological factors that limit $VO_{2\,max}$ (see Figure 2.4), with reasonably general agreement that it is oxygen supply to muscle that represents the major limiting factor (Saltin & Rowell 1980; Wagner 1991). It is likely that all components of the oxygen transport system, by influencing either oxygen delivery to muscle or tissue diffusion of oxygen, will play a role in determining $VO_{2\,max}$ (Wagner 1991). Strategies (e.g. blood doping and erythropoietin supplementation) designed to increase red blood cell mass and arterial haemoglobin, and therefore arterial oxygen-carrying capacity have received attention from

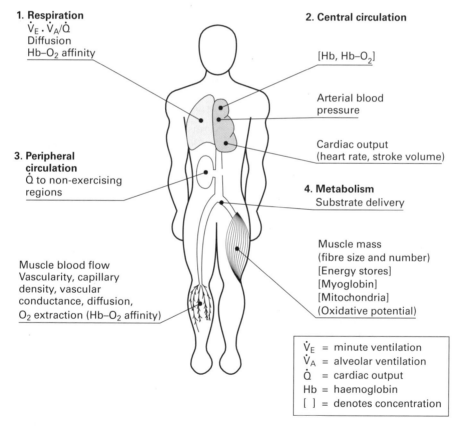

Figure 2.4 *Physiological determinants of maximal oxygen uptake (from Saltin & Rowell 1980, with permission)*

endurance athletes over the years. Furthermore, since iron is an important component of haemoglobin, myoglobin and the cytochromes within the respiratory chain, there has been much interest in the iron status of endurance athletes and the potential effects of iron deficiency, and subsequent supplementation, on endurance exercise performance. Iron requirements for training are reviewed in Chapter 11, Section 11.7.1.

2.5 TEMPERATURE REGULATION AND FLUID BALANCE

The metabolic heat that is produced during exercise must be dissipated so as to avoid hyperthermia. During exercise in air, as much as 75% of this heat loss is achieved by the evaporation of sweat, with approximately 580 kcal of heat being dissipated for each litre of sweat evaporated. Sweat rates can be as high as 1–2 L/h during prolonged exercise and under extreme conditions may reach 2–3 L/h for short periods. The transfer of heat to the skin is achieved by vasodilation of the cutaneous circulation, thereby displacing blood to the periphery (Fortney & Vroman 1985). A fall in central blood volume is thought to result in a decrease in stroke volume and concomitant increase in heart rate during prolonged exercise or exercise in the heat (Rowell 1986). Furthermore, there is the possibility that blood flow to active muscle is reduced due to this 'circulatory conflict' (Rowell 1986), which is exacerbated by the hypovolemia that develops as a result of the sweating-induced fluid losses (Gonzalez-Alonso et al. 1998). Core temperature stabilises at a new, elevated level, depending upon the exercise intensity; however, if the rate of metabolic heat production is maintained, or if heat loss is impaired due to extreme environmental conditions, hyperthermia can develop. Hyperthermia not only impairs exercise performance (Gonzalez-Alonso et al. 1999; Parkin et al. 1999), but can also have potentially life-threatening consequences. Exercise in the heat is also associated with an accelerated liver and muscle glycogenolysis and muscle and blood lactate accumulation (Febbraio et al. 1994; Hargreaves et al. 1996). Although CHO depletion is not thought to contribute to the premature fatigue observed with heat stress (Parkin et al. 1999), the greater CHO use during exercise in the heat has nutritional implications for athletes who regularly train and compete in hot environments (see Chapter 25).

In order to minimise the risk of hyperthermia, athletes are encouraged to become acclimatised to hot environments and to ingest fluids during exercise. Acclimatisation can be achieved, in part, by passive exposure to heat and through exercise training; however, most benefit is gained from exercising in the heat. The physiological adaptations to acclimatisation include an expanded plasma volume, reduced heart rate and body temperature during exercise, increased volume of dilute sweat, earlier onset of sweating and reduced glycogenolysis (Febbraio et al. 1994). Precooling, resulting in a lower body core temperature, has also been shown to enhance exercise tolerance in the heat (Gonzalez-Alonso et al. 1999). The ingestion of fluids during exercise attenuates the increases in heart rate and body temperature that are observed during prolonged exercise (Hamilton et al. 1991). This seems to be due, in part, to the maintenance of a higher blood volume and lower plasma osmolality during exercise, thereby facilitating skin blood flow and heat dissipation (Coyle & Montain 1992).

There has been debate on the optimal volume and composition of rehydration solutions during exercise (Hargreaves 1996). Since sweat is hypotonic, replacement of fluid is a priority; however, during prolonged exercise the inclusion of CHO and a small amount of electrolyte is recommended (Coyle & Montain 1992; Gisolfi & Duchman 1992). The effects of fluid ingestion appear to be graded in proportion to the volume of fluid ingested (Coyle & Montain 1992). Thus, athletes should be encouraged to drink as much as is required to minimise exercise-induced body weight loss; however, this is often a difficult task since fluid is not always readily available and ingestion of large fluid volumes can result in gastrointestinal distress. Although the body has hormonal mechanisms for restoring water and electrolyte levels following exercise, fluid ingestion during recovery should be encouraged to facilitate rehydration. Solutions containing a small amount of CHO and electrolyte appear to provide an advantage over plain water (Maughan et al. 1997). Fluid and CHO intake during exercise is reviewed in detail in Chapter 14.

2.6 FATIGUE

Fatigue is defined as a reduction in the force or power-generating capacity of muscle. The sites of fatigue include the central nervous system and motor outflow, and peripheral sites such as the sarcolemma, t-tubule system, sarcoplasmic reticulum (SR) and myofilaments (Fitts 1994). These peripheral sites reflect the processes of membrane excitation, excitation-contraction coupling and uncoupling, cross-bridge formation and metabolic energy supply. While central fatigue occurs during exercise, most attention has focused on peripheral mechanisms of fatigue. It is unlikely that a single mechanism can explain fatigue under all circumstances, but possible mechanisms include ionic disturbances, impaired excitation-contraction coupling, accumulation of metabolites, and substrate depletion.

Loss of potassium from contracting skeletal muscle has been implicated in fatigue during both intense and prolonged exercise (McKenna 1992). Potassium efflux, most pronounced during intense, short-duration exercise, results in reduced membrane excitability and contributes to intracellular acidosis. Intense exercise is also associated with accumulation of H^+, ADP and inorganic phosphate. Acidosis has been linked to fatigue via a number of mechanisms. These include depression of maximal calcium-activated force and calcium sensitivity, impaired actin-myosin binding, reduced muscle fibre shortening velocity and inhibition of ATP production. Ingestion of oral alkalising agents (e.g. bicarbonate) has been employed to minimise these effects of acidosis and is associated with improved high-intensity exercise performance in many investigations (Linderman & Fahey 1991) (see Chapter 17, Section 17.6.3). Increases in inorganic phosphate and ADP are also believed to inhibit muscle force generation.

A failure of excitation-contraction coupling is also likely to be involved in the fatigue process (Allen et al. 1992; Favero 1999). Possible mechanisms include reduced calcium release from the SR and impaired myofibrillar calcium sensitivity (Allen et al. 1992). Impaired SR calcium release could be due to a reduction in ATP supply in the region of the calcium release channel (Chin & Allen 1997), increased metabolite/ion (e.g. Ca^{2+}, Mg^{2+}, H^+, lactate, inorganic phosphate) accumulation or modification by free radicals (Favero 1999). In addition, reduced SR calcium uptake and calcium ATPase activity following both intense and prolonged exercise (Byrd 1992) suggest impairment of SR function.

Alterations in energy supply may also be an important factor in fatigue during exercise (Sahlin et al. 1998). Muscle ATP levels usually only fall about 30–50% during intense exercise; in contrast, CP levels can be totally depleted following intense exercise (Söderlund & Hultman 1991) and this could account for the reduced power output associated with fatigue during such exercise. Dietary creatine supplementation is a potential intervention to increase skeletal muscle CP availability and enhance high-intensity exercise performance (Greenhaff 1997) (see Section 17.6.1). During prolonged exercise, muscle glycogen depletion and/or hypoglycaemia are often associated with fatigue (Hargreaves 1999). Increased CHO availability, either by muscle glycogen loading prior to exercise (Section 13.3) or CHO ingestion before (Section 13.4) and during exercise (Section 14.3), is associated with enhanced endurance exercise performance (Hargreaves 1999; Hawley et al. 1997). Other factors contributing to fatigue during prolonged, strenuous exercise include dehydration and hyperthermia (Section 14.4), and impaired SR and mitochondrial function (possibly as a consequence of oxidative damage due to increased free radical activity). Thus, in recent years, interest has focused on the potential relationship between antioxidant (vitamins C and E) supplementation and endurance performance, although definitive evidence of their ergogenic benefits is still required (see Sections 12.5.1.6, 12.6.2 and 17.7.1).

2.7　SUMMARY

This chapter provides only a brief overview of the physiological and metabolic responses to exercise. Nevertheless, it should be apparent that nutrition can have a major impact on many physiological aspects of exercise. The specific nutritional strategies designed to optimise exercise and sports performance are described in detail in the following chapters.

2.8 *PRACTICE TIPS*

Nick Wray

- A sound knowledge of the physiology of exercise is critical to the under-standing of the nutritional strategies which can enhance exercise performance. A good comprehension of the specific energy systems used in a sport, and the factors limiting performance, are essential before appropriate nutritional advice can be given.

- To determine this information, it is necessary to establish the characteristics of the athlete's training and competition schedule. Important information for the dietitian to collect to assess the nutritional demands of athletes' training and competition includes:
  1. Training details
     (a) detailed history of type, duration, intensity and frequency of sessions
     (b) timetable of training sessions, e.g. time of day, location
     (c) environmental issues, e.g. will the athlete be training in the heat, indoors or in the cold?
  2. Competition details
     (a) if a team sport, what role does the athlete play? e.g. position, style of play
     (b) duration of competition
     (c) intensity of competition
     (d) frequency/timetable of competition
     (e) environmental conditions of competition
     (f) travel frequency and requirements
     Collection of this information enables a better understanding of the spe-cific physiological requirements of each individual athlete, facilitating more specific dietary advice.

- A good understanding of the physiological characteristics of an athlete's train-ing and competition schedule highlights special nutritional needs, or strategies that can promote optimal performance by addressing the factors that would otherwise cause fatigue. The following examples illustrate how this knowledge of energy systems and training needs can assist a dietitian.
  1. If the athlete is involved in an endurance sport which requires prolonged training sessions (e.g. > 90 minutes), then an understanding of the limi-tations of the aerobic system is essential. Such an athlete needs to be made aware of the importance of adequate carbohydrate intake (see Chapter 13), additional CHO intake during training and competition and adequate hydration (see Chapters 13 and 14), as well as post-exercise muscle glyco-gen replenishment (see Chapter 15).

2. A sprint athlete may be interested in the potential benefits of nutritional ergogenic aids. Once the dietitian determines that a large percentage of the athlete's training is high-intensity, short duration exercise which depends on the phosphagen and lactic acid systems, then it may be useful to consider creatine as a potentially beneficial supplement (see Chapter 17, Section 17.6.1).

3. An ultra-endurance triathlete may request some advice on what CHO foods are best to consume during their race. Once the dietitian identifies that this athlete will spend the first 90 minutes of the event swimming without access to additional CHO or fluid, then appropriate advice as to the nutritional strategies for the remainder of the race can be planned. The timing and glycaemic index of the pre-event meal (see Chapter 13) as well as suitable foods and fluids during the remainder of the event (see Chapter 14) can all be appropriately planned.

- There are a number of ways to learn more about the physiological requirements of specific sports. Many books have been written about individual sports, including texts that may specifically address physiological and training issues. Encyclopaedia of sports are very useful in providing a brief summary of the main rules and features of the vast array of competitive and recreational sports. The Internet may provide websites prepared by the governing bodies of various sports which provide background information about the sport as well as current competition results and items of interest. In Australia, a directory of National Sporting Organisations can be obtained from the Australian Sports Commission. Direct contact with the executive or coaching directors of a sport will allow information exchange, as well as provide contacts for sports nutrition, medicine or science professionals who are closely involved with the sport.

- The applied physiology of individual sports has been addressed in a number of reviews, textbooks and conference proceedings. The resources listed at the end of the chapter provide a useful source of information about the physiological and nutritional considerations of selected sports.

REFERENCES

Allen DG, Westerblad H, Lee A, Lannergren J. Role of excitation-contraction coupling in muscle fatigue. Sports Med 1992;13:116–26.

Brooks GA. The lactate shuttle during exercise and recovery. Med Sci Sports Exerc 1986;18:360–8.

Byrd SK. Alterations in the sarcoplasmic reticulum: a possible link to exercise-induced muscle damage. Med Sci Sports Exerc 1992;24:531–6.

Chin E, Allen DG. Effects of reduced muscle glycogen concentration on force, Ca^{2+} release and contractile protein function in intact mouse skeletal muscle. J Physiol 1997;498:17–29.

Costill DL, Daniels J, Evans W, Fink WJ, Krahenbuhl G, Saltin B. Skeletal muscle enzymes and fibre composition in male and female track athletes. J Appl Physiol 1975;40:149–54.

Coyle EF. Substrate utilisation during exercise in active people. Am J Clin Nutr 1995;61:S968–S979.

Coyle EF, Montain SJ. Benefits of fluid replacement with carbohydrate during exercise. Med Sci Sport Exerc 1992;24(S):324–30.

Favero TG. Sarcoplasmic reticulum Ca^{2+} release and muscle fatigue. J Appl Physiol 1999;87:471–83.

Febbraio M, Snow RJ, Hargreaves M, Stathis CG, Martin IK, Carey MF. Muscle metabolism during exercise and heat stress in trained men: effect of acclimation. J Appl Physiol 1994;76:589–97.

Fitts RH. Cellular mechanisms of muscle fatigue. Physiol Rev 1994;74:49–94.

Forster HV, Pan LG. Exercise hyperpnea: its characteristics and control. In: Crystal RG, West JB, eds. The lung: scientific foundations. New York: Raven Press, 1991:1553–64.

Fortney S, Vroman NB. Exercise, performance and temperature control: temperature regulation during exercise and implications for sports performance and training. Sports Med 1985;2:8–29.

Gisolfi CV, Duchman SM. Guidelines for optimal replacement beverages for different athletic events. Med Sci Sports Exerc 1992;24:679–87.

Gonzalez-Alonso J, Calbet JAL, Nielsen B. Muscle blood flow is reduced with dehydration during prolonged exercise in humans. J Physiol 1998;513:895–905.

Gonzalez-Alonso J, Teller C, Andersen SL, Jensen F, Hyldig T, Nielsen B. Influence of body temperature on the development of fatigue during prolonged exercise in the heat. J Appl Physiol 1999;86:1032–9.

Greenhaff PL. The nutritional biochemistry of creatine. Nutr Biochem 1997;8:610–18.

Hamilton MT, Gonzalez-Alonso J, Montain SJ, Coyle EF. Fluid replacement and glucose infusion during exercise prevents cardiovascular drift. J Appl Physiol 1991;71:871–7.

Hargreaves M. Physiological benefits of fluid and energy replacement during exercise. Aust J Nutr Diet 1996;53(suppl 4):S3–S7.

Hargreaves M. Metabolic responses to carbohydrate ingestion: effects on exercise performance. In: Lamb DR, Murray R, eds. Perspectives in exercise science and sports medicine. Vol 12: The metabolic bases of performance in sport and exercise. Carmel: Cooper Publishing Group, 1999:93–119.

Hargreaves M. Carbohydrate metabolism and exercise. In: Garrett WE, Kirkendall DT, eds. Exercise and Sport Science. New York: Lippincott Williams & Wilkins, 2000:3–8.

Hargreaves M, Angus D, Howlett K, Marmy-Conus N, Febbraio M. Effect of heat stress on glucose kinetics during exercise. J Appl Physiol 1996;81:1594–7.

Hawley JA, Brouns F, Jeukendrup AE. Strategies to enhance fat utilisation during exercise. Sports Med 1998;25:241–57.

Hawley JA, Schabort EJ, Noakes TD, Dennis SC. Carbohydrate-loading and exercise performance: an update. Sports Med 1997;24:73–81.

Hood DA, Terjung RL. Amino acid metabolism during exercise and following endurance training. Sports Med 1990;9:23–35.

Katz A, Sahlin K. Regulation of lactic acid production during exercise. J Appl Physiol 1988;65:509–18.

Linderman J, Fahey TD. Sodium bicarbonate ingestion and exercise performance: an update. Sports Med 1991;11:71–7.

Maughan RJ, Leiper JB, Shirreffs SM. Factors influencing the restoration of fluid and electrolyte balance after exercise in the heat. Br J Sports Med 1997;31:175–82.

McKenna MJ. The role of ionic processes in muscular fatigue during intensive exercise. Sports Med 1992;13:134–45.

Mitchell JH. Neural control of the circulation during exercise. Med Sci Sports Exerc 1990;22:141–54.

Nevill ME, Bogdanis GC, Boobis LH, Lakomy HKA, Williams C. Muscle metabolism and performance during sprinting. In: Maughan RJ, Shirreffs S, eds. Biochemistry of exercise IX. Champaign: Human Kinetics, 1996:243–59.

Parkin JM, Carey MF, Zhao S, Febbraio MA. Effect of ambient temperature on human skeletal muscle metabolism during fatiguing submaximal exercise. J Appl Physiol 1999;86:902–8.

Romijn JA, Coyle EF, Sidossis LS, et al. Regulation of endogenous fat and carbohydrate metabolism in relation to exercise intensity and duration. Am J Physiol 1993;265:E380–E391.

Rowell LB. Human circulation: regulation during physical stress. Oxford: Oxford University Press, 1986.

Sahlin K, Tonkonogi M, Söderlund K. Energy supply and muscle fatigue in humans. Acta Physiol Scand 1998;162:261–6.

Saltin B, Gollnick PD. Skeletal muscle adaptability: significance for metabolism and performance. In: Peachy LD, Adrian RH, Geiger SR, eds. Handbook of physiology, skeletal muscle. Bethesda: American Physiological Society, 1983:555–631.

Saltin B, Rådegran G, Koskolou MD, Roach R. Skeletal muscle blood flow in humans and its regulation during exercise. Acta Physiol Scand 1998;162:421–36.

Saltin B, Rowell LB. Functional adaptations to physical activity and inactivity. Fed Proc 1980;39:1506–13.

Schantz P. Plasticity of human skeletal muscle. Acta Physiol Scand 1986;128(S):558.

Söderlund K, Hultman E. ATP and phosphocreatine changes in single human skeletal muscle fibres after intense electrical stimulation. Am J Physiol 1991;261(E):737–41.

Spriet LL, Howlett RA. Metabolic control of energy production during physical activity. In: Lamb DR, Murray R, eds. Perspectives in exercise science and sports medicine. Vol 12: The metabolic bases of performance in sport and exercise. Carmel: Cooper Publishing Group, 1999:1–44.

Vøllestad NK, Blom PCS. Effect of varying intensity on glycogen depletion in human muscle fibres. Acta Physiol Scand 1985;125:395–405.

Vøllestad NK, Sejersted OM. Biochemical correlates of fatigue. Eur J Appl Physiol 1988;57:336–47.

Vøllestad NK, Tabata I, Medbo JI. Glycogen depletion in different human muscle fibre types during exhaustive exercise of short duration. Acta Physiol Scand 1992;144:135–41.

Vøllestad NK, Vaage O, Hermansen L. Muscle glycogen depletion patterns in type I and subgroups of type II fibres during prolonged severe exercise in man. Acta Physiol Scand 1984;122:433–41.

Wagner PD. Central and peripheral aspects of oxygen transport and adaptations with exercise.

Sports Med 1991;11:133–42.

Walsh ML, Banister EW. Possible mechanisms of the anaerobic threshold: a review. Sports Med 1988;5:269–302.

Wasserman K, Beaver WL, Whipp BJ. Mechanisms and patterns of blood lactate increase during exercise in man. Med Sci Sports Exerc 1986;18:344–52.

Williams C. Value of physiological measurement in sport. J Royal Coll Surg Edin 1990;35(S):7–13.

PRACTICE TIPS' REFERENCES

Anderson RE, Montgomery DL. Physiology of alpine skiing. Sports Med 1988;6:210–21.

Burke LM. The complete guide to food for sports performance, 2nd edn. Sydney: Allen and Unwin, 1995.

Eisenman PA, Johnson SC, Bainbridge CN, Zupan MF. Applied physiology of cross-country skiing. Sports Med 1989;8:67–79.

Ekblom B. Applied physiology of soccer. Sports Med 1986;3:50–60.

Ekblom B, Williams C, eds. Foods, nutrition and soccer performance. J Sports Sci 1994;12(special issue).

Faria IE. Applied physiology of cycling. Sports Med 1984;1:187–204.

Groppel JL, Robert EP. Applied physiology of tennis. Sports Med 1992;14:260–8.

Hagerman FC. Applied physiology of rowing. Sports Med 1984;1:303–26.

Horswill CA. Applied physiology of amateur wrestling. Sports Med 1992;14:114–43.

Lamb DR, Knuttgen HG, Murray R. Perspectives in exercise science and sports medicine. Vol 7: Physiology and nutrition for competitive sport. Carmel: Cooper Publishing Group, 1994.

Lavoie J, Montpetit R. Applied physiology of swimming. Sports Med 1986;3:165–89.

Lin YC. Applied physiology of diving. Sports Med 1988;5:74–98.

Maughan RJ, Horton ES, eds. Current issues in nutrition in athletics. J Sports Sci 1995;13(special issue).

Montgomery DL. Physiology of ice hockey. Sports Med 1988;5:99–126.

Montpetit RR. Physiology of squash. Sports Med 1990;10:31–41.

O'Toole ML, Douglas PS. Applied physiology of triathlon. Sports Med 1995;19:251–67.

O'Toole ML, Douglas PS, Hiller WBD. Applied physiology of triathlon. Sports Med 1989;8:201–25.

Reilly T, Borrie A. Physiology applied to field hockey. Sports Med 1992;14:10–26.

Reilly T, Secher N, Snell P, Williams C, eds. Physiology of sports. London: e & FN Spon, 1990.

Shephard RJ. Science and medicine of canoeing and kayaking. Sports Med 1987;4:19–33.

Smith HK. Applied physiology of water polo. Sports Med 1998:26:317–34.

Sparling RB, Nieman DC, O'Connor PJ. Selected scientific aspects of marathon racing. Sports Med 1993;15:116–32.

Tumilty D. Physiological characteristics of elite soccer players. Sports Med 1993;16:80–96.

White AT, Johnson SC. Physiological aspects and injury in elite alpine skiers. Sports Med 1993;15:170–78.

Measuring nutritional status of athletes: clinical and research perspectives

Vicki Deakin

3.1 INTRODUCTION

Nutritional status measurements provide an indicator of health and a benchmark to monitor athletes' responses to training from a dietary perspective. A nutritional status assessment (or checkup) of an individual athlete by a sports dietitian, in combination with a medical checkup by a sports physician, a musculo-skeletal assessment by a physiotherapist, and a psychological assessment have now become routine for most serious athletes at the start of a training season. Each of these professionals plays a crucial and integrated role in screening athletes and detecting potential short- and long-term problems, preventing injury and promoting the best performance capacity. Many national and professional sporting groups now provide such a team of sports science and medicine professionals to provide screening assessment and ongoing monitoring, treatment and education of athletes in their areas. Clearly, the emphasis in sporting groups has moved from a therapeutic to a preventative approach.

The purpose of a nutritional assessment is to identify athletes at risk or suspected to be at nutrition risk. Coaches and athletes now recognise that an unbalanced diet or a diet inadequate in nutrients can lead to lethargy, early fatigue, irritability, and poor training and competitive performance. Increased incidence of injury and infection, excessive gains or losses in body mass (BM) are also nutrition-related. The development of many of these problems can be prevented through early detection of symptoms and early dietary intervention.

The goals of nutrition assessment are to:

- identify athletes who require nutritional support to restore or maintain nutritional status;
- to provide appropriate nutrition therapy (e.g. dietary intervention, education, behavioural change); and
- to monitor the progress and efficacy of the dietary therapy.

The process of measuring nutritional status is not just an evaluation of what a person eats and drinks. Measurement involves a combination of a number of diagnostic or assessment procedures from social, medical and psychological influences on food intake, dietary evaluation, physique and fatness assessment, to interpretation of biochemical measures of blood and urine. An interpretation of each finding relative to the others is used to determine the total picture. Four assessment procedures are used, as shown in Table 3.1.

Table 3.1 *Components of the nutritional assessment*

Dietary evaluation
Clinical observations/medical history
Biochemical analyses for tissues, such as blood and urine
Anthropometric assessment

The more information gathered about a person, the more accurate the nutrition assessment. For example, an individual may have a history of an inadequate intake of dietary iron but is not necessarily anaemic. Iron deficiency is only confirmed in individuals if biochemical indices of iron status have decreased from that individual's usual level and/or symptoms of iron deficiency such as fatigue or lethargy (clinical observations) are present. The combination of three of the assessment components listed in Table 3.1 (dietary evaluation, biochemical tests and clinical observation) confirm a diagnosis of iron depletion or deficiency.

This chapter focuses on the main techniques of measuring nutritional status in clinical practice and in research studies of individual and groups of athletes and includes the strengths and limitations of these techniques and practical suggestions to improve data collection procedures and interpret these data in an athletic population.

3.2 MEASUREMENT OF DIET

Dietary evaluation involves collecting information on dietary intake and evaluating and interpreting dietary intake using the 'common' reference guidelines or standards available. This is not an easy or simple process (as it may appear to the untrained observer) but one that requires care, precision and a high degree of skill and knowledge at all stages of the process. The limitations of the methods of dietary evaluation and their reliability are not always fully appreciated or described in both clinical practice and in journals. Collection of reliable and accurate dietary intakes of individuals and groups is difficult because of the influence of confounding effects and errors inherent in all dietary survey methods. The focus of this section is not to consider in detail which method of measuring dietary intake is best suited to a clinical or research situation but rather to focus on some of the key pitfalls and issues that should be considered when:

- collecting dietary data from individuals or groups of individuals with particular emphasis on an athletic population; and
- interpreting or analysing dietary data by using the 'common' reference measures.

The athletic population may have different eating habits to the general population—in terms of food choices, serve sizes, frequency of consumption, food preparation and even language about food, however, athletes, particularly adolescents, and those involved in endurance training, have higher nutrient requirements and turnover of nutrients than the sedentary population. Nutrient requirements depend on age, level of maturation, type of physical activity undertaken and intensity and duration of training.

Therefore, the traditional techniques and nutrient references used by dietitians for measuring and interpreting food intake may need to be modified and tested in an athletic population. For example, standard serve sizes listed on commercial foods, commercial food models, and those predetermined on food frequency questionnaires (FFQs) are likely to be too small for many athletes. An athlete (or adolescent) may consume three to five times the volume of breakfast cereal than an adult at one sitting. An awareness of eating habits, food quantities consumed, food attitudes and beliefs of different groups of athletes is important to work successfully with athletes in a clinical setting and crucial to conduct quality research on dietary intakes, dietary attitudes and beliefs.

3.2.1 *Why measure dietary intake?*

Table 3.2 defines the broad uses and applications of measuring dietary intakes in athletes. In most research and clinical situations, nutrients rather than food intakes are the basis for evaluation of dietary assessment and intakes of individual athletes or small groups of athletes. For example, a dietary assessment is used to estimate daily or usual carbohydrate (CHO) intake of an individual athlete or group, an important determinant in recovery for the next training session.

In dietetic practice

Determining dietary intakes and linking this information with other nutritional status measurements of individual athletes is important in a clinical situation to assess nutrient adequacy and dietary balance and the need for, or effects of, dietary intervention (see Table 3.2). Of interest to dietitians in clinical practice is collection of food intake data on individuals for the purpose of assessment of nutrients/food choice, intervention of risk-related dietary behaviours, monitoring of food choices and evaluation of dietary intervention programs. The outcome of dietary assessment is for dietitians to provide a benchmark from which to target appropriate food choice and dietary habits to achieve the desired change.

Table 3.2 *Uses and application of measuring dietary intakes*

Use	Application
Determining nutritional status	Calculating average nutrient intakes in population groups of athletes
	Comparing adequacy of group nutrient intake with population standards (e.g. Recommended Dietary Intakes (RDIs))
	Combination of dietary intake assessment with other parameters (e.g. biochemical, anthropometric, medical) to assess nutritional status of individuals and groups
Assessing the links with performance, diet and health status	Comparing and contrasting indices of nutritional status with the incidence and prevalence of health problems or performance measures in groups
Evaluating nutrition education and intervention	Providing feedback on the efficacy of dietary intervention programs in individuals or groups of athletes
Assessing the effect of different dietary regimens on performance measures or metabolic responses	Determining potential ergogenic effects of diets, components of diets or supplements
Assessing the effect of different training periods or intensities on dietary intake	Determining the turnover of nutrient requirements at different training intensities and duration in combination with other parameters

Adapted from: Sabry (1988)

In research

For research purposes, accurate and reliable measures of food consumption are important for estimating or measuring intakes of nutrients and other food components for individual athletes or groups of athletes. For assessment of group intake, qualitative measures of food consumption are used where ranking of food, meals or nutrient intake is the objective. Qualitative assessments (e.g. less fat, more CHO, more meat, more fruit) may also be used to rank the difference in beliefs and attitudes about foods and food choices of groups of athletes. Most of the published studies of dietary intakes of elite athletes use data collection methods that derive quantitative estimates of nutrient intake rather than qualitative intakes. The main methods used are food records using household measures, which are conducted on small numbers of athletes (Burke et al. 2001). Few studies have undertaken dietary surveys on large numbers of athletes (Short & Short 1983; van Erp-Baart et al. 1989; Fogelholm et al. 1992).

3.2.2 *How many days are needed to measure nutrient intakes with reliability?*

The number of days needed to measure nutrient intakes reliably varies for different subjects and different nutrients. Basiotis et al. (1987) and others (Nelson et al. 1989) have provided estimates of the number of days required to measure true average intake of a range of nutrients with given statistical confidence (i.e. with 95% confidence) for individuals and groups. Estimates from Basiotis et al. (1987) were derived from 26 subjects (13 males, 4 females) who completed diet records for one year. From these data, a minimum of three days was required to capture usual intake of energy from the group, compared with an average of 27 days for individuals within that group. Clearly, these data showed that fewer days of data collection were required to estimate (or rank) usual intakes in the group than in individuals. Intakes of protein, fat and CHO required four, six and five to six days, respectively, to estimate true average intake in both males and females. Micronutrient intakes required much longer. As few as four days of diet records are required to measure phosphorus intake in males and as long as 44 days to measure vitamin A in females (Basiotis et al. 1987). Approaches for calculating the number of days required to determine specific nutrient intakes in the usual diet are beyond the scope of this chapter and vary for different populations (for reviews see Basiotis et al. 1987; Nelson et al. 1989; Beaton et al. 1983; Lee & Nieman 1993, p. 67–8).

3.2.3 *Techniques in measuring food intake*

Techniques for measuring food consumption are categorised into two major types: current dietary intakes (i.e. food records) and past dietary intakes (retrospective short- or long-term recall of foods consumed). Methods for measuring current diet include weighed diet records (sometimes including computerised scales), estimated diet records, and duplicate diets. These methods record food intake at the time of consumption. Retrospective methods include the 24-hour recall, diet history and food frequency questionnaire (FFQ).

Techniques for measuring dietary intakes have been reviewed extensively (Marr 1971; Block 1982; Kranztler et al. 1982; Roberge et al. 1984; Daniels 1984; Bingham et al. 1988, p. 53–106; Lee & Nieman 1993, p. 49–62; Bingham et al. 1994). The main methods and their applications, strengths and limitations are summarised in Table 3.3 opposite.

Table 3.3 Overview of the main applications, strengths and limitations of dietary intake methods for measuring dietary intakes in groups and individuals

Data collection method	Application	Strengths	Limitations
Food records			
Current food consumption			
Weighed method using scales or computerised approaches	Assess food choices and eating habits mostly from 1 to 7 days [1,2]	Weighing is considered an accurate method [4,5]	• Time-consuming to conduct and analyse • Requires trained personnel • Requires literate and co-operative respondents • Distortion of food choice [2,11]
Estimated method using household measures	Acceptable for research because of better compliance than weighed method [7,8]	• Provides information about eating habits • Fairly valid up to 5 days [8] • Provides detailed information	• Poor compliance after 4 days [9,10] • Not representative of usual diet, unless repeated [12,13] • Under-estimates energy intake from 20–50% [6,11]
Duplicate food collections	Uses duplicate meals/foods for direct chemical analysis	Most accurate method	• High respondent burden • Expensive to analyse • Distorts food choice • Under-reporting [14] • Other biases poorly documented
Food consumption in the past (recall methods)			
24-hour recall	Used mainly to rank food or nutrient intakes of groups of people	• Minimal distortion of food intake • Low respondent burden	• Not representative of usual intake of individuals unless repeated at random [15]

(continues)

(continued)

Data collection method	Application	Strengths	Limitations
	Can be used to rank food and nutrient intakes of individuals, if repeated at random [15]	• Good response rate • Low administration cost	• Memory / recall bias • Under-estimates total energy intakes [19]
Food frequency questionnaires (FFQs)	• Mainly for ranking usual food or nutrient intakes of groups of people in qualitative or semi-quantitative terms • As screening tools to detect, measure or rank specific nutrients or food intakes in groups or individuals • As an adjunct to educating, documenting and modifying dietary behaviour of individuals in clinics	• Similar advantages to the 24-hour recall • Measures usual diet and may be more representative of 'usual' intake than repeated diet records [7] • Quick to administer • Cost effective	• Similar limitations to the 24-hour recall • Less accurate than record methods • List of foods may not fully represent foods consumed by respondents • Difficulty quantifying portion sizes • Over-estimates at low energy intake and in long-term studies [20,21] and under-estimates at high energy intakes [10,16,17,18]
Dietary history	• Combines a 24-hour diet recall and a FFQ • Assessment of usual intakes of individuals in clinical practice	• Comprehensive assessment of the usual nutrient intake, including seasonal changes	• Time-consuming to conduct • Dependent on a highly trained interviewer • Dependent on memory and co-operation of the respondent • Tend to over-estimate nutrient intakes [8]

[1]Block 1989, [2]Pekkarinen 1970, [3]Willett et al. 1987, [4]Marr 1971, [5]Bingham 1985, [6]Rutishaser 1988, [7]Lee & Neiman 1993, p. 53-4, 58-9, [8]Bingham et al. 1988, p. 67, [9]Daniels 1984, [10]Gersovitz et al. 1978, [11]Stockley 1985, [12]Willett 1990, p. 63, [13]Block 1989, [14]Lee-han et al. 1989, [15]Sempos et al. 1985, [16]Stunkard & Waxman 1981, [17]Carter et al. 1981, [18]Faggiano et al. 1992, [19]Krall & Dwyer, [20]Sorenson et al. 1985, [21]Larkin et al. 1985.

3.2.3.1 *Dietary intakes in the present (current methods)*

For assessment of dietary intake of individuals where current diet is of interest, diet records (either weighed or estimates using household measures) are usually used (Kristal et al. 1990c; Eck et al. 1991; Buzzard et al. 1994; Munro et al. 1995). However, a 24-hour recall (previous 24 hours) or other recall techniques adapted for assessment of recent dietary intake including diet histories (past week) and food questionnaires or FFQs are used for cross-checking the accuracy of food records in research and in clinical practice.

Diet records

In research

Although there is no truly accurate measure of current dietary intake in free-living people, the diet record is considered the most 'accurate' and feasible method for research (Pekkarinen 1970; Marr 1971; Bingham 1985). The weighed diet record is considered the 'gold' standard against which other or new methods for measuring dietary intake are compared or validated (Marr 1971; Bingham 1987). In a recent review of dietary surveys of athletes by Burke and colleagues (2000), three- or four-day diet records using household measures were predominantly the method of choice. However, dietary records are not representative of measuring usual diet (see Table 2.2) unless repeated several times, two to three months apart (Willett 1990, p. 63; Block 1989). The number of days of dietary records required for 80% reliable classification of individual intake varies from two to three days for some nutrients like sugar or total CHO to two to three weeks for other nutrients, such as dietary cholesterol and fat (Marr & Heady 1986).

Self-reported diet records involve weighing all foods and beverages consumed (including wastage) or estimating weights using standard household measures. One- to seven-day periods are used (Pekkarinen 1970; Block 1989), although up to 12 months of continuous diet recording has been reported (Willett et al. 1987). Computerised approaches for improving the accuracy of weighing food have been developed in the UK (Stockley et al. 1986a; 1986b) and the United States (Kretsch & Fong 1990) but have not been used in Australia. In this approach, food scales are modified to select food group categories and record weights within these categories. Data records are then transferred to a computer for nutrient analysis. The costs of such scales preclude their use in large studies.

The number of days of data collection affects accuracy of responses. Guthrie (1984) and Bingham (1987) suggested that seven days of continuous recording was the most accurate method, although other researchers reported considerable loss of compliance after four days of weighing foods (Daniels 1984; Gersovitz et al. 1978). Periods longer than three- to four-days of food records have shown reduced accuracy and are considered impractical and associated with memory interference, incomplete records and a high drop-out rate (Gersovitz et al. 1978; Krall & Dwyer 1987).

A short-term dietary record, although not considered representative of usual eating habits, does provide a reasonable estimate of the general quality of the diet (Stuff et al. 1983). Numerous researchers recommend, and use, repeated three- to four-day records to measure usual intakes using non-consecutive random days (including weekends) conducted over different seasons (Block 1989; Willett 1990, p. 63). Diet records, however, are time-consuming for both researcher and respondent, and require a literate and co-operative respondent (Marr 1971). Kristal et al. (1990a) suggest that four-day food records, for instance, require a one-hour respondent training session, 30 minutes every day to complete and then an additional 20 minute interview to review the record for accuracy.

Weighed records, although considered the most accurate in quantitative determination of foods (Pekkarinen 1970; Marr 1971; Bingham 1985), have poor compliance and distort food choice (Stockley 1985; Dennis & Shifflett 1985). Although estimated records are less accurate, they have been accepted for most research purposes (Larkin et al. 1989; Kemppainen et al. 1993; Lee & Nieman 1993, p. 53). Providing standard measures and/or calibrated scales rather than relying on 'household' measures and using grids, photographs of foods or food models helps to improve accuracy and decreases respondent error (Rutishauser 1988).

In clinical practice

For assessment of food choices and eating patterns in dietetic practice and the quality of the diet, three- or four-days of diet records (estimated measures) taken over consecutive days are traditionally used. Estimated measures, in most circumstances, are simpler, less demanding for respondents than the weighing method and are associated with good compliance and adherence to usual eating patterns (Nelson & Nettleton 1980; Bingham et al. 1988, p. 67). However, reports in the literature indicate errors of between 20–50% in estimating food portion weights (Rutishauser 1988).

The major advantages of using diet records in clinical practice are to:

- raise awareness of eating habits;
- form the basis for an education resource and evaluation tool for follow-up counselling sessions; and
- provide a self-monitoring and feedback service.

The outcome of food records is detailed information on food intake data that are not reliant on memory (Lee & Nieman 1993, p. 54).

3.2.3.2 *Dietary intakes in the past (recall methods)*
24-hour recall

A 24-hour recall asks respondents to remember foods, beverages and quantities consumed in the previous 24 hours (i.e. yesterday) and may include information on timing of meals and snacks, eating environment and food preparation. Usually a

24-hour recall is administered directly by personal or telephone interview, or the respondent records the information in an open-ended format.

In research

Short-term recalls are not representative of usual intakes because of the day-to-day variation in food and nutrient intakes (especially micronutrients) (Beaton et al. 1983; Sempos et al. 1985) and are used primarily to determine intakes of groups not individuals. Twenty-four hour recalls (24-hour records), repeated a number of times at random, have been recommended to measure usual nutrient intake in individuals. Repeated application over multiple days of data collection also adjusts for individual variation in day-to-day intake and has a place in epidemiological research to measure the links between diet and disease (Sempos et al. 1985, 1992). Presumably, the same technique would provide a more reliable measure of usual intake of micronutrients in individual athletes and groups than the short-term food records favoured in dietary surveys of athletes. The consensus of evidence suggests that repeated 24-hour recalls are valuable aids in classifying dietary intake in groups of people and may provide an accurate assessment of an individual's food intake, if sufficient numbers of recalls are obtained.

In clinical practice

Where usual dietary intakes are erratic or inconsistent, which is not uncommon in adolescents and young adults (Abrahams et al. 1988; Wilkins et al. 1991), a 24-hour recall is used in place of a diet history to elicit information. It forms the foundation for pursuing a broader or more detailed picture of usual intakes.

Food frequency questionnaires (FFQs)

FFQs incorporate a predetermined food list, with or without portion sizes, plus a frequency response option for respondents to report how often (i.e. per day, week, month) each food was eaten. The food list is often supplemented by questions on other foods eaten by the respondent but not on the list, questions about food preparation, supplement use and other food-related behaviours. In its early form, the FFQ was designed as a qualitative method, seeking information on the frequency of consumption of specific food items without specification of the actual serve or portion sizes usually consumed. More recent versions of this approach use portion sizes (Baghurst & Baghurst 1981; Willett et al. 1988; Pietinen et al. 1988a; Fogelholm & Lahti-Koski 1991). Some FFQs provide options for modifying foods and portion sizes (Baghurst & Baghurst 1981; Willett 1990, p. 79) although the effect of this on improving accuracy is still equivocal.

In research

FFQs have been designed and validated to assess foods or nutrients consumed in the past seven days (Bazarre & Myers 1979; Eck et al. 1991; Curtis et al. 1992) or even the preceding month (Lee-Han et al. 1989; Fogelholm & Lahti-Koski 1991; Fogelholm et al. 1992; Welten et al. 1995), but most FFQs are used to measure usual diet of groups in the preceding six to 12 months (Willett et al. 1987; Pietinen et al. 1988a; Goldbohm et al. 1994; Wheeler et al. 1995). FFQs, however, have shown acceptable validity for assessing group rather than individual intakes of food or nutrients.

FFQs have been adapted and validated for new and different uses other than to gain a picture of usual dietary intakes. These uses include screening tools to detect, measure or rank one or several nutrients, e.g. fat (Block et al. 1989; van Assema et al. 1992; Dobson et al. 1993), iron (Hertzler et al. 1986), calcium (Nelson et al. 1988; Angus et al. 1989; Musgrave et al. 1989; Wilson & Horwath 1996), and vitamin A, C, E, selenium, fibre (Pietinen et al. 1988b).

Only one FFQ has been validated and used to measure dietary intakes in sportspeople. Fogelholm et al. (1992) modified the FFQ of Pietinen et al. (1988a) for measuring intakes of specific nutrients (thiamin, vitamin C, magnesium, calcium, zinc and iron) consumed in the previous month by 427 physically active young Finnish men. The modified version which contained 122 food items showed good agreement at the group level when validated against a seven-day food record in another 84 male athletes, but poor agreement in individuals (Fogelholm & Lahti-Koski 1991).

In clinical practice

Several examples of FFQs developed for clinical practice involving short-term retrospective measurement are described below. There are no known FFQs developed or validated for use in athletes for these purposes. The documented purposes of FFQs designed for use in clinical practice are:

- to evaluate the impact of dietary intervention counselling or intervention programs (Strohmeyer et al. 1984; Vailas et al. 1987; Millar & Beard 1988);
- as an education resource, for self-help intervention (Musgrave et al. 1989; Kristal et al. 1990c);
- to document and monitor adherence to diet intervention (Vailas et al. 1987; Lee-Han et al. 1989; Curtis et al. 1992);
- as a rapid screening device (Strohmeyer et al. 1984);
- for a variety of situations (e.g. pregnancy, loss of BM, smoking cessation), where there is a need to gather dietary information over a short period of time (Greeley et al. 1992; Eck et al. 1996); and
- to generate inexpensive and rapid behavioural feedback to the individual on dietary intake (Kristal et al. 1990b).

There is a real need to develop and validate FFQs specifically for use in individual athletes and athletic groups for both clinical practice and research. In dietary research, modifications of previously validated FFQs to target the food supply and food consumption practices of the research population are usually used rather than developing new FFQs. The difficulties inherent in collecting accurate information on food intake in human subjects and the logistics and cost associated with the design, sampling and implementation of any validity study probably precludes the development and validation of new FFQs in athletes. A large sample size is needed.

In Australia, a well-recognised, semi-quantitative FFQ that measures usual diet (Baghurst & Record 1984) has been partially validated (Rohan et al. 1987). Modifications of this FFQ for measuring usual diet in the general population (Wheeler et al. 1995) and in the elderly (Horwath & Worsley 1990), and fat intake in adults (Dobson et al. 1993) have since been validated. Developing and validating similar tools specific to athletes' eating patterns would be invaluable for research purposes.

Diet history

A diet history, originally described by Burke in 1947, includes a combination of techniques including a 24-hour recall and a FFQ to determine usual eating patterns (Burke 1947). The original method also included a three-day record, which Burke suggested was the least valuable component of the diet history (Burke 1947).

In research

Although diet histories provide a comprehensive assessment of food or nutrient intakes in the usual diet including seasonal influences, they are time-consuming, and they are dependent on a skilled interviewer, and the memory and co-operation of the respondent (Block 1989). These factors limit their use in dietary surveys and research.

In clinical practice

A modified diet history, which takes about 20 minutes to complete (Munro et al. 1995), is routinely used in dietetic practice to assess usual dietary intake in the distant or recent past. It includes a combination of dietary survey methods including a 24-hour recall of foods eaten and an assessment of usual eating patterns including a crosscheck using a food-frequency checklist. Further information about social, behavioural and medical influences on eating behaviour is also obtained. Due to their busy training schedules, many athletes have little time to spend buying and preparing food and often rely on easily accessible foods that are either quick to prepare or readily available from local take-away shops. The main factors which determine food intake are training and work schedules, food budget, living arrangements, restrictive or fad diets, expertise in food preparation and, of course, the likes and dislikes of the individual.

As part of a diet history, it is important to determine athletes' knowledge, attitudes and beliefs about nutrition and whether these beliefs reflect actual food choices. How an athlete prioritises nutrition as a component of their training program will influence the success of nutrition education and intervention. Many athletes have no formal nutrition training and obtain nutrition information from a variety of sources. The most frequently cited sources of nutrition information have been coaches and magazines, doctors and other athletes (Hamilton et al. 1994). Both athletes and coaches have demonstrated poor nutrition knowledge on nutrition questionnaires in relation to the nutrient content of foods, methods to lose and gain BM, and vitamin supplements (Jacobsen & Gemmel 1991; Baer et al. 1994; Sossin et al. 1997). In a New Zealand study of 53 female runners, those with a high score for nutrition knowledge were more likely to report nutritionally sound diets (Hamilton et al. 1994). Concerns for weight or BM are suggested to also influence athletes' food choice (Perron & Endres 1985).

3.3 SOURCES OF ERROR IN DIETARY MEASUREMENT

Collection of reliable and accurate dietary intake data of individuals and groups is difficult because of the influence of confounding effects and errors inherent in all dietary survey methods. A number of errors are introduced at each stage of dietary assessment; from collection of food intake data to analysis and interpretation of these data. The magnitude of these errors should be addressed when interpreting research studies of dietary intakes (for review, see Beaton et al. 1997). Obtaining accurate results from dietary intake methods requires a willing athlete, and a high degree of skill, care and dedication on the part of the investigator (Bingham 1991).

3.3.1 Errors in collecting food intake data

The largest error in dietary surveys in the collection of dietary intake data is the inaccuracy in recalling or reporting actual food intake by subjects (Block 1989). The ability of athletes to provide reliable dietary data depends on their motivation, literacy, memory and communication skills, and awareness of food intake. The perception of foods eaten, both in type and quantity, is crucial to the success of data collection. Many athletes give biased responses either in fear of revealing inappropriate dietary behaviour to the coach or investigator, or to impress. Reported intakes can be biased as certain foods (fresh fruits, vegetables) are thought to be socially desirable while sweet foods are undesirable (Worsley et al. 1984). The process of collecting dietary data may itself affect eating behaviour (Marr 1971). Errors can also be introduced by the investigator because of behaviour or personality factors such as the manner of asking questions, gestures, poor communication skills and failure to develop rapport or gain the confidence of the athlete.

Most dietary survey methods (except the dietary history), however, tend to under-estimate food and nutrient intakes (see Table 3.2). Methods to check the magnitude of under-reporting that can be applied to a research or clinical situation are discussed in Section 3.3.2.

3.3.1.1 Errors in collecting information using food records

Few people are experts at recording food intake and providing accurate food records. Motivated and educated volunteers provide the most accurate and reliable food intake data (Black et al. 1991). Athletes may not be motivated or see the relevance of recording food intakes especially if a concerned coach or parent has sent them to see a dietitian. Self-recording food intake changes an individual's eating behaviour by discouraging snacking, inhibiting spontaneous food selection and consumption of mixed meals (because of difficulties weighing or estimating individual ingredients). Self-recording food intake consequently distorts the true food intake (Pekkarinen 1970; Dennis & Shifflett 1985; Stockley 1985). In one study, half of the subjects completing weighed food records admitted altering their intake in some way because of inconvenience, being self-conscious or being ashamed (Macdiarmid & Blundell 1997). Athletes are usually far too busy to collect weighed records, especially if they perceive nutrition as a low priority.

Estimates of dietary intakes using household measures may be more appropriate for the busy athlete than weighed diet records. The major limitations in using estimates are the large variability in serve sizes consumed by athletes and poor reporting of household measures. Males reported lower intakes using household measures than weighed measures (Cade 1988).

Although dietary records are appropriate and considered accurate if the respondents are adequately trained, under-reporting of actual intake either intentionally or unintentionally is higher than other methods. Food records consistently underestimate energy intakes in young non-obese well-educated adults (de Vries et al. 1994) and endurance female athletes (Schoeller 1995), based on doubly-labelled water (DLW) as a criterion measurement for checking under-reporting (see Section 3.2.1 and Chapter 6, Section 6.4.2.2). At the population level, under-reporting is highest in adolescents, women and people who are overweight or trying to lose BM (Briefel et al. 1997; Klesges et al. 1995; Prentice et al. 1996; Pryer et al. 1997). Under-reporting is also associated with diets that are lower in fat (Briefel et al. 1997) and highest among those who are less well educated and heavier (Klesges et al. 1995).

Only a few studies have investigated under-reporting in athletes using the DLW method as an external marker of energy expenditure. Westerterp et al. (1986) found that cyclists competing in the Tour de France kept incomplete diet records for 23 days. Their energy intakes were much less than measured expenditures. Haggarty et al. (1988) has also observed under-reporting in elite female endurance athletes.

3.3.1.2 *Errors in recall methods*

All recall methods depend on the memory, co-operation and communication ability of the athlete and on the skill of the interviewer. Recall methods tend to overestimate the intakes of those with low energy intakes and under-estimate intakes of those with high energy intakes compared with the more accurate food records in the general population (Gersovitz et al. 1978). Barr (1987) suggests that error could be a problem in athletes who have either habitually low or high levels of food intake (e.g. ballet dancers and triathletes). However, validity studies of recall methods to confirm or refute this claim in athletes have not been undertaken.

When using a diet history to collect information about usual intake, a consistent eating pattern and awareness of eating behaviour of the athlete being interviewed is important. If an athlete has difficulty remembering usual daily food consumption patterns, this method may be all that is needed to reveal the existence of an irregular eating pattern and a general dietary imbalance.

The long-term FFQs that measure most nutrients in the usual diet have been criticised for their lower accuracy compared with diet records and the 24-hour recall. Recall bias (Marr 1971; Dwyer & Krall 1988) and varying abilities of respondents to quantify foods accurately (Guthrie 1984; Willett 1990, p. 80; Fogelholm & Lahti-Koski 1991; Tjonneland et al. 1992) are the major reasons for this.

People consistently have difficulty quantifying foods that are not presented in packaged serves like meat, poultry and fish (Willett 1990, p. 80; Faggiano et al. 1992; Tjonneland et al. 1992) and athletes are reported to be no different than the general population in this respect (Fogelholm & Lahti-Koski 1991). There are large discrepancies in perceptions of weight or volume of food consumed and actual weight, particularly meat and cereals, in athletes.

3.3.1.3 *Errors and limitations in converting foods into nutrients using food composition data*

The conversion of food into nutrients is a major source of error in dietary surveys and is a reflection of the skills and knowledge of the researcher, the method of data collection and the available food composition database (for review see Paul & Southgate 1988; Kohlmeier 1992). Translating foods into nutrients, in many instances, is not simply multiplying the amount of food eaten by the nutrient content for that food. A sound knowledge of food composition and skill in data collection is essential to undertake this task. Lack of specificity in the description of food or quantities consumed, together with insufficient knowledge about common preparation methods, edible portions, weight for volume or measure, and how to handle situations which are not instantly matched by the food composition database, compounds the error.

Food composition databases do not contain the large number of foods that are consumed in real life, so inappropriate food substitutes, omission of foods and guesswork may be used. The importance of defining a coding and food substitute protocol to address these issues is crucial for minimising error when analysing food data.

Although researchers usually report the food composition database and coding protocols used in a study, few acknowledge the factors that might influence the accuracy of the nutrient analysis. When interpreting nutrient data derived from food composition tables, the following limitations should be recognised.

(a) Food composition data are only estimates of nutrient composition

Food composition tables or databases can only approximate the nutrient content of foods that are consumed (Murphy et al. 1973; English & Lewis 1992). Nutrient composition of any given food varies considerably within the same country of origin. Firstly natural, biological, geographical and agricultural factors will affect variability in raw foods (Cashel 1990) while cooking and processing are likely to lead to wider differences in composition (Paul & Southgate 1991). In the United States, the variation of nutrient content of individual foods ranges from 10–45% (Life Sciences Research Office 1989). However, English and Lewis (1992) suggest that if this is applied to the nutrient content of a one-day diet, the variation drops to 5–15%. This assumes the variations are random across all food items and therefore tend to cancel each other out.

(b) Food composition data are specific to the country of origin

Nutrient values documented in the Australian food tables or Australian food composition database (NUTTAB), for example, are not appropriate for use in other countries because of the large biological, agricultural and commercial variability in nutrient content of foods between and within countries of origin (Greenfield & Southgate 1992). Based on the sampling procedure (Cunningham 1990), the variability in composition (English & Lewis 1992) and the weighting that may be applied to the food when represented in the Australian food tables (Cashel 1990), nutrient intakes calculated from food tables, irrespective of the country of origin, are estimates only.

(c) Food composition data may require substitute foods

Information on many commercial food and miscellaneous items such as seasoning and spice are limited on NUTTAB95 (the current version of the Australian Food Composition database). Where a specific food or ingredient is unavailable in the food composition tables, substitutions have to be made. If numerous substitutions are made, inaccurate information results. Adding nutrient information from food labels to a food composition database is unacceptable because labels do not have a complete representation of the nutrient composition of a food. For research purposes, nutrient data of a food can only be added to the database if a quality control laboratory recognised in food composition analysis has conducted a comprehensive nutrient analysis of the food.

(d) Serve sizes can be difficult to standardise

Generally, athletes do not eat the serve sizes documented on commercial foods or in software programs containing food composition databases.

(e) Incomplete information on nutrients

The Australian food tables do not contain a comprehensive list of nutrients (e.g. vitamins E, B6, and folate; and minerals, zinc and copper). The recently introduced food standard allowing fortification of folate in specified foods in Australia is not yet reflected in these food tables or in the latest version of NUTTAB95 (Lewis et al. 1995). Food tables do not contain many commercial foods that are modified in salt, fat, sugar or CHO content.

(f) Errors in coding

Inexperienced and untrained people can introduce many errors when coding and entering foods for nutrient analysis. This task takes time, accuracy and frequent checking to avoid errors.

3.3.2 *Techniques used to measure under-reporting of dietary intakes*

The validity of dietary assessment methods is questioned when self-reported energy intakes are compared with more direct and accurate measures of energy expenditures. When such comparisons are made, subjects frequently under-report energy intakes (see Section 3.3.1.1 and Section 3.3.1.2). A number of objective or external criteria are used to determine the extent of under-reporting of actual dietary intakes. These include biochemical indices and the ratio of reported energy intakes (EI) to predicted basal metabolic rates (PBMR). Methods using biochemical indices are best suited to research studies. However, the technique of comparing the ratio EI:PBMR, although a relatively crude measure, is useful to describe under-estimates of energy intakes from food records for both individuals and groups.

3.3.2.1 *The doubly-labelled water method for validating total energy intakes*

The development of the doubly-labelled water ($^2H_2^{18}O$) (DLW) method for use in humans has become a valuable tool in determining energy expenditure in free-living people and for validating methods for assessing dietary intake (Speakman 1998; Schoeller 1999) (see Chapter 6, Section 6.4.2.2). Subjects drink a dose of water containing stable isotopes and provide periodic urine and blood samples to measure the rate of elimination of these isotopes. The use and limitations of this technique are described in detail in Chapter 6, Section 6.4.2.2. This method is expensive for routine use and has been used mainly as a validation tool. A 24-hour urine nitrogen test to validate protein intakes may be a useful alternative in a research or clinical situation.

3.3.2.2 *Validation of protein*

The 24-hour urinary nitrogen test, a measure of nitrogen balance and hence protein balance, is well accepted for external evaluation of the validity of habitual food intake against the more accurate DLW method (Black et al. 1991). Originally proposed by Isaksson in 1980, the 24-hour urine nitrogen method has been used extensively in clinical studies to verify protein intake (Bingham & Cummings 1985). If acceptable agreement exists between urinary nitrogen excretion and estimated protein intake, it can be assumed that intake of other nutrients is fairly well represented (Lee & Nieman 1993, p. 65). Its validity in athletes has not been established and may be distorted in subjects in positive or negative nitrogen balance.

3.3.2.3 *The ratio of energy intake to basal metabolic rate*

A less expensive method than DLW to validate energy intakes is that described by Goldberg and colleagues in 1991 using reported EI divided by EBMR. The final EI : EBMR ratio determines whether reported energy intakes using a food record method are consistent with energy intakes required for a person to live a normal (not bed-bound) lifestyle (McLennan & Podger 1998, p. 140). This ratio is represented by minimum cut-off values derived from whole body calorimetry and DLW measurements for determining energy expenditure (Goldberg et al. 1991). The cut-off limits for the EI:EBMR ratio are adjusted for sample size and duration of measurement of dietary intakes (Goldberg et al. 1991). These researchers defined two categories for cut-off values: those based on habitual intake (cut-off 1) and those based on actual intake over specified measurement period as used in food records (cut-off 2). For example, a sample size of one individual using a three-day diet record can be assessed using cut-off 2. EBMR is calculated using the equations of Schofield et al. (1985) (see Chapter 6, Table 6.1). In contrast, Manore and Thompson in Chapter 6 suggest that the Benedict or Cunningham equations are a better estimate of BMR for athletes than the equations by Schofield and colleagues (see Section 6.4.2.3). These equations are found in Table 6.1.

A review of a number of dietary surveys of selected populations using Goldberg's cut-offs showed 88% of diet recalls, 64% of diet records and 25% of diet histories presented dietary intakes that were below those needed for maintaining a sedentary lifestyle (Black et al. 1991). Although this ratio is crude and dependent on estimates of BMR, which are themselves inaccurate, this method is useful for checking under-reporting of dietary intakes in individuals.

In summary, the EI:EBMR ratio can be applied in both a research and clinical situation when diet records are used to measure intake.

3.4 *CRITERIA FOR INTERPRETING DIETARY INTAKES*

3.4.1 *Dietary goals for athletes*

Dietary goals for athletes are quantitative values for macronutrient intakes relative to total energy intakes. These are similar to those developed for the general population (Table 3.4).

| Table 3.4 | Dietary goals for athletes involved in endurance and non-endurance sports (% of total energy in the diet) |

Nutrient	% of total energy/day
Protein	10–15
Total fat	< 30
Total CHO	60–70 (for endurance sports)
	> 55 (for non-endurance sports)

These goals are recommendations directed at the average daily diet of groups of athletes rather than specific individuals. Therefore, interpretation of nutrient intakes of individuals in relation to these figures should be cautious. There is considerable distortion in relative energy values of macronutrients at high and low energy intakes using these goals. In research publications, the use of absolute measures of macronutrient intakes to interpret daily intakes of individuals and groups are better accepted. Absolute measures can be adjusted for BM, type, intensity and duration of physical activity and can be used as reference standards for individuals as well as groups.

In dietary surveys of athletes, for example CHO intake, data have been reported in numerous ways: from absolute amounts (usually grams per day), per cent of energy from CHO to total energy in the diet, and more recently in g/kg (grams of CHO per kilogram of BM) or in nutrient density terms (grams of CHO/1000 kJ). Adjusting for energy and BM standardises these data and makes comparison between athletes and controls more meaningful. As we now have recommended amounts for CHO and protein intake in athletes, it would be prudent to interpret macronutrient intake adjusted for the BM of an individual or mean BM of the group of athletes measured.

Recommendations for CHO and protein in adult athletes involved in different sporting situations range from 7–12 g CHO/kg BM/d (see Chapter 15, Section 15.2.1) and between 1.2–1.4 g protein per kg BM/d in endurance-trained athletes and up to a maximum of 1.7 g protein per kg BM/d for strength-trained athletes (Lemon 1998; see also Chapter 5, Section 5.5). Estimating energy requirements for athletes is described in Chapter 6 and favours the Benedict's equation for estimating BMR in athletic populations.

3.4.2 *Dietary guidelines for Australian adults, adolescents and children*

Dietary guidelines are a set of qualitative, individual components of the diet that describe the major components of dietary change needed to achieve the dietary goals (e.g. eat more cereals, reduce the intake of fats, particularly saturated fats). The dietary guidelines for Australian adults, children and adolescents are listed in Table 3.5. Dietary guidelines for older Australians have recently been released (National Health & Medical Research Council 1999; see also Chapter 19, Table 19.4).

Table 3.5 *Dietary guidelines for Australian adults, children and adolescents*

Dietary guidelines for adults[1]	Dietary guidelines for children and adolescents[2]
Enjoy a wide variety of nutritious foods	Encourage and support breastfeeding
Eat plenty of breads and cereals (preferably wholegrain), vegetables (including legumes) and fruits	Children need appropriate food and physical activity to grow and develop normally. Growth should be checked regularly
Eat a diet low in fat and, in particular, low in saturated fat	Enjoy a wide variety of nutritious foods
Maintain a healthy body weight by balancing physical activity and food intake	Eat plenty of breads, cereals, vegetables (including legumes) and fruits
If you drink alcohol, limit your intake	Low-fat diets are not suitable for young children. For older children, a diet low in fat and, in particular, saturated fat, is appropriate
Eat only a moderate amount of sugars and foods containing added sugars	Eat only a moderate amount of sugars and foods containing added sugars
Choose low-salt foods and use salt sparingly	Choose low-salt foods
Encourage and support breastfeeding	
Guidelines on specific nutrients	**Guidelines on specific nutrients**
Eat foods containing calcium. This is particularly important for girls and women.	Eat foods containing calcium
Eat foods containing iron. This applies particularly to girls, women, vegetarians and athletes	Eat foods containing iron

Source: [1]NHMRC (1992); [2]NHMRC (1995)

Dietary guidelines for Australians and for other countries provide a baseline for consistent qualitative education messages to the consumer. These same messages are appropriate for nutrition education of athletes and are used by dietitians in combination with *The core food groups* (see Table 3.6) when assessing and advising athletes about food choice.

3.4.3 *Food guides*

Food guides are nutrition education tools to assist schoolchildren and adults to plan and select a nutritionally desirable diet consistent with the dietary guidelines. Most countries have devised food selection guides specific to the food supply of their country and the nutrient recommendations and cultural needs of their population. These food guides translate dietary standards and recommendations into suggested servings of foods from groups that can be easily understood, and used by people who have little formal training in nutrition. Examples of food guides used in Australia are *The five food groups* (Commonwealth Department of Health (c 1980)), the Australian Nutrition Foundation's *Food pyramid* (ANF 1992), the *CSIRO 12345+ Food and nutrition plan* (CSIRO 1991), and *Target on healthy eating* (Smith et al. 1989). Similar food guides are used in other countries, for example, *Food guide pyramid* (United States), *Four food groups guide* (United States) and *Food guide for healthy eating* (Canada) (for reviews see Welsh et al. 1992 (United States); Baghurst et al. 1994a, 1994b (Australian versus 18 overseas food guides)).

Food guides categorise food into groups usually based on similar nutrient content. If the designated serves from each group are consumed daily, a balanced and adequate everyday diet is likely to be the outcome (Lee & Nieman 1993, p. 32).

3.4.3.1 *The core food groups in Australia*

In Australia, *The core food groups* replaced the *Five food groups* in 1995 as the new food guide (see Table 3.6). *The core food groups* was developed using a population approach based on food availability in Australia (i.e. apparent consumption data), RDIs and food consumption from surveys of the Australian population (Cashel & Jeffreson 1995, p. 1–3). They were devised to meet approximately 70% of the RDIs for most nutrients except energy.

A quick way to assess nutrient intakes is to check if the core foods are represented in a day's dietary intake. Diets providing the recommended number of servings from each of the core food groups a day will probably provide adequate nutrients for most individuals. However, this guide will not meet energy requirements for most people, especially athletes. Most athletes need to increase the number of serves to meet their energy and nutrient requirements.

Although the core food groups provide a scientific basis for determining nutrient adequacy, inappropriate food choices that are high in fat, sugar or salt within these groups can lead to dietary imbalance. *The core food groups* should be assessed in conjunction with *Dietary guidelines for Australians*. The recently introduced *Australian guide for healthy eating* provides a food selection guide that incorporates the message of the dietary guidelines for Australian adults, children and adolescents (Smith et al. 1998). Suggested quantities for the core food groups for children, adolescents, and pregnant and lactating women have also been proposed (Cashel & Jeffreson, 1995, p. 64).

3.4.4 *Food composition data*

The Australia food tables as discussed in *Composition of foods, Australia (COFA)*, provide the nutrient composition of Australian foods (Cashel et al. 1989; Commonwealth Department of Community Services & Health 1990a, 1990b, 1990c, 1990d). The latest release of the database version of COFA called NUTTAB95 contains 1805 foods and includes all food published in volumes one to seven of COFA (Lewis et al. 1995).

Table 3.6 *The core food groups for adults*

Core food	Number of serves*	Suggested serves
Cereals Includes breakfast cereals, all breads, pancakes, rice, other grains, spaghetti and other pasta *(B group vitamins [ie ribo-flavin, thiamin, niacin], iron, protein, magnesium, folate, fibre, no cholesterol)*	7	1 slice bread 1 bowl ready-to-eat cereal ¾ cup rice or pasta
Fruit All varieties and their juices; fresh, cooked, frozen and canned *(vitamin C, magnesium, potassium, no cholesterol)*	2	1 piece fruit ½ cup fruit juice ¾ cup stewed fruit
Vegetables All varieties *(folic acid, vitamin A, iron, potassium, no cholesterol)*	5 (cooked weight or volume)	½ cup starchy vegetables (e.g. potato, corn) 1 cup leafy vegetables
Dairy group Includes whole (full-cream), low-fat or skimmed milk drinks, cheese (all varieties), custard, ice-cream *(calcium, riboflavin, protein, phosphorus, vitamin B12)* *(contains cholesterol if a high-fat product)*	450 mL milk or equivalent 550 mL milk or equivalent for adolescents and children (proposed value)	100 mL milk = ½ carton yoghurt (100 g) or 20 g cheese (hard) or ½ cup cottage cheese or 1 scoop of cream or small serve custard
Meat group Includes red meat, chicken or poultry, fish, nuts, beans and lentils (legumes) *(protein, phosphorus, vitamin B6, vitamin B12, zinc, iron, magnesium, niacin, thiamin, contains cholesterol)*	85 g (cooked weight/ volume)	¾ cup cooked beans (e.g. soy beans, baked beans) 4 tablespoons peanut butter 1 small lamb chump chop 100 g raw steak 1 chicken leg 2 eggs 89–90 g nuts

*Serve = minimum number of daily serves needed to achieve at least 70% of the requirements for protein, vitamins and minerals for adults
Adapted from: Cashel and Jeffreson (1995)

The limitations of food composition data are discussed earlier in Section 3.3.1.3 and are important to consider when interpreting dietary intake data. For example, lack of specificity in the description of food and quantities, and the limitation of nutrient databases to contain data on every food, decrease accuracy of the analysis. Considerable nutrition and food knowledge by users of food composition data is important for entering the most representative food on the database. Dietary analysis is not for amateurs.

3.4.5 *Nutrient standards (RDIs/RDAs): relevance to athletes*

Nutrient standards such as Recommended Dietary Intakes (RDIs) (Australia) or Recommended Dietary Allowances (RDAs) (United States) can be used for most athletes because of the wide safety margins for nutrient recommendations (National Research Council 1989; National Health & Medical Research Council 1991). Dietary Reference Intakes (DRIs) is a newly introduced term in the United States which encompasses multiple levels of nutrient intakes including Estimated Average Requirements (EAR), Recommended Dietary Intakes (RDIs) and Tolerable Upper Intake Levels (UL) (see www.nas.edu for new releases of the DRIs). In Australia similar multiple reference values for nutrients for different purposes have also been proposed but are not yet available (Cobiac et al. 1998). DRIs are broader in scope and application than RDAs. Irrespective of these multiple levels of nutrient standards and differences in terminology between countries, the use of the current and former United States RDA and the Australian RDI is similar. Nutrient intakes that meet the RDIs/RDAs are likely to meet the nutrient requirements of nearly all individuals (97.5% of the population) in a life stage or gender group.

However, comparing nutrient intakes of individuals to RDIs/RDAs is open to criticism since these standards 'are recommendations for the average daily amounts of nutrients that population groups should consume over a period of time' (National Research Council 1989). The Council stated that these recommendations 'should not be confused with requirements for a specific individual. Differences in the nutrient requirements of individuals are unknown'. The RDIs/RDAs, despite the limitations of their use, still remain the most frequently used standards when evaluating the adequacy of an individual's diet (National Research Council 1989). They have been used extensively for evaluating the nutrient status of athletes. By convention, nutrient intakes that are below two-thirds of the RDI/RDA are considered inadequate (Stuff et al. 1983). The level of adequacy for nutrients will be clearly specified by the new United States' DRIs when they become available and also in the proposed revision of the Australian RDIs.

Nevertheless, some elite athletes may not fit within the range of these 'average' population values on which nutrient standards are based. Evidence for a slightly higher requirement for protein and CHO than the general population is well documented in some groups of athletes (see Chapters 5 and 15). Recent evidence supports a slight increase in micronutrient recommendations than RDIs/RDAs in physically active people to compensate for losses in sweat, urine and perhaps faeces and for an increase in free radical formation (Chapter 12, Section 12.3). However, this evidence is based on biochemical and physiological indices of micronutrients, which are highly variable among athletes, and difficult to interpret. Of the vitamins and minerals investigated, the nutrient requirements (not recommendations) for antioxidant vitamins (C, E and β-carotene), B group vitamins, magnesium, zinc and iron may need to be slightly higher in athletes than non-athletes (Chapter 12, Section 12.3).

Athletes involved in strenuous endurance training programs or with a large BM are likely to need higher intakes of micronutrients than RDIs/RDAs, although such recommendations have not yet been established and are likely to be highly variable. More research is needed on large groups of athletes participating in different sports to allow micronutrient recommendations to be quantified. In summary, the RDIs/RDAs for micronutrients are satisfactory for use in the majority of athletes.

3.5 CLINICAL OBSERVATION AND MEDICAL HISTORY

The purpose of the clinical examination is to uncover any medical condition or physiological factors that interfere with food intake, digestion and metabolism. Recent or chronic illness, anxiety, depression and some drugs can interfere with absorption of nutrients and thus affect nutritional status. Diarrhoea, loss of appetite, gastrointestinal disturbances and BM loss may be associated with an underlying illness. Loss of appetite for up to one to two hours after exercise is frequently associated with hard workouts. Many athletes also experience GI tract discomfort or nausea if food is consumed before hard exercise, and may avoid eating anything for two to three hours before training.

3.6 BIOCHEMICAL ANALYSIS

Although biochemical tests are objective and often used as external criteria for validating dietary intake methods, they are not necessarily diagnostic of nutrient depletion (for review see Hunter 1990, p. 143–216; Kohlmeier 1991; Lee & Nieman 1993, p. 223–52).

Low blood levels of some nutrients may reflect low dietary intake, defective absorption, increased utilisation or excretion. As well, some nutrient values in the biochemical tests have sufficient diurnal variations, or are under such strict homeostatic control (e.g. calcium) that interpretation is misleading (Fogelholm 1995). Biochemical indices and their interpretation in an athletic population are discussed in detail in other chapters: vitamins and minerals (Chapter 12, Section 12.4.1), iron (Chapter 11, Section 11.6.1) and protein (Chapter 5, Section 5.4).

As reference standards for evaluating biochemical data in athletes is limited, population reference standards are still used in clinical practice and research studies of athletes. These standards may be inapplicable for athletes involved in strenuous training with high turnover or losses of some nutrients but serve as the only available reference guideline until more specific and controlled research is available.

It is generally recommended that several criteria be investigated to establish the micronutrient status of an individual in a clinical situation. A single biochemical analysis representing a nutrient imbalance may not necessarily be diagnostic of a clinical or even sub-clinical condition. Use of several blood tests rather than one blood test gives more reliable information about individuals and may reveal trends. Nutrient depletion or deficiency can only be confirmed on the basis of changes observed from repeated biochemical tests in combination with long-term dietary deprivation of the specific nutrient, and associated clinical symptoms.

3.7 ANTHROPOMETRIC ASSESSMENT

Anthropometry involves the application of physical measurements to appraise human size, shape, proportion, body composition, maturation and gross function. These measurements are useful to reflect both growth and development of children and adolescents and give some indication of body composition in adults. They are also useful as an indication of moderate to severe under-nutrition or overweight or obesity.

Physical measurements including height, BM, skinfolds, mid-arm muscle circumference, girth and frame size are well-recognised measures used by nutritionists and kinanthropometrists. These are used indirectly to estimate body composition and predict estimates of energy requirements. Comparison of height and BM parameters with 'ideal' or reference standards such as the Body Mass Index (BMI) weight (kg)/(height (m)^2) is inappropriate for many athletes. Athletes with a large muscle bulk are categorised by these standards as overweight or, in some cases, obese, despite having low body fat. The BMI and height–weight charts are useful for showing very lean athletes that they are not overweight, but provide no true or reliable indication of body composition.

The sum of skinfold measures is a practical, inexpensive and reliable method to determine body fat or to monitor changes in body composition of athletes over time, so it is particularly useful in a clinical situation. Other methods for measuring body composition are described in Chapter 4 (see Section 4.3). Using absolute values for skinfolds, such as the sum of six to eight skinfold sites on the body, is preferable to using the numerous equations that calculate body fat percentage used extensively in the past (see Chapter 4, Section 4.3.3.2). Because the equations used to determine body fat percentage are derived from cadavers and assume that the fat mass (FM) has the same density as the fat-free mass (FFM), which is an invalid assumption, they are no longer favoured.

The O-scale or Ozscale techniques for measuring skinfolds are recommended for use in athletes (Ross & Marfell-Jones 1991; Norton et al. 1996). Software for comparing these results with normative data is also available (Olds et al. 1994). In Chapter 4, Table 4.1 and Table 4.2 provide normative skinfold data on elite athletes for comparison.

3.8 SUMMARY

The collection of nutritional status measures in sports people is critical to our understanding of the association between nutrition, health and sports performance. Data collection of such measures requires highly trained people who are familiar with the process of data collection, and limitation and bias in collecting and interpreting these data.

In dietary assessment of groups or individuals, only estimates of food or nutrient intakes of athletes are possible. Therefore, techniques chosen for evaluating food or nutrient intakes are related to the intended purpose of the dietary assessment and the data collection method used.

To improve accuracy of food intake data, researchers and clinicians need to have an awareness of the dietary habits of athletes so that appropriate serves and quantities of food likely to be consumed can be made. Despite the use of food models and other techniques for improving accuracy of data collection (e.g. training and standardised household measures), under-reporting or misreporting is a major problem in all dietary survey methods, although under-reporting can quickly be checked against the ratio of EI:EBMR (see Section 3.3.2.3). External techniques to measure error in reporting or recalling food intakes should be an integral part of the research design in all dietary intakes, even those with control groups (see Section 3.3.2).

Population reference standards and guidelines for interpreting dietary intakes and biochemical indices can be applied to athletes, with caution, and with few exceptions. Because of the extensive research on CHO and protein intakes in athletes, specific values for daily intakes of these nutrients are available to assist in devising menu plans and for interpretation in research studies (see Section 3.4.1). More research is needed in varying groups of athletes before such recommendations can be made for micronutrient intakes, except perhaps iron (see Chapter 11). The recommended nutrient values for CHO and protein represent the upper limits as they are derived from laboratory or field studies of mostly elite or semi-elite athletes involved in regular training programs. Recreational athletes, or those involved in intermittent training in team sports, are unlikely to need these upper limits. For such athletes, the RDIs/RDAs are satisfactory.

Normative data on physique and skinfold measures in elite international and national level athletes involved in different sports are available elsewhere for comparative purposes (see Chapter 4, Tables 4.1–4.4). Again, comparison of these data with similar measurements of individuals needs to be interpreted with caution because of the large standard deviations observed. Clearly a large standard deviation between and within sports indicates a high variability in individual differences. Individuals may not fit within these normative data or have optimum physiques for their chosen sport but can still become world champions. Normative data should be used as guidelines only in individuals and should not be the basis for prescriptive values which are impossible for many individuals to attain.

Population reference values for biochemical indices are still applied to athletic populations. Further research is needed in large groups of athletes to compare the distribution of biochemical indices with matched controls. The outcome of this research will determine if micronutrient needs in people undergoing strenuous physical activity need to be higher than in non-athletic groups.

Finally, the use of nutritional assessment measures in athletes, in combination with recent advances in medical technology and performance measures, has enhanced our understanding of the responses of the human system to the stressors of hard physical activity. The importance of collecting measurements on athletes that are standardised around the world is essential for improving our understanding of exercise, health and sports performance.

3.9 PRACTICE TIPS

Vicki Deakin

Overview

- Nutritional assessment involves the collection and interpretation of data to evaluate an individual's nutritional status and identify nutritional needs. The process of nutritional consultation should begin with assessment, followed by planning, implementation and then evaluation. Planning decides the actions necessary to meet needs and who should carry out the actions; implementation involves putting the plan into action; and evaluation determines the effectiveness of the plan and its revision, if needed.

Collecting information

- Obviously, the more information obtained from various sources (e.g. anthropometric, biochemical, medical, client and family interview), the more accurate and reliable the assessment will be. However, comprehensive nutritional assessments are not always appropriate, necessary or feasible. Assessment levels range from minimal screening to comprehensive, and can be tailor-made for an individual athlete or team.

Dietary assessment

- Identify the athlete's reasons for dietary consultation early in the interview.

- Find out the athlete's attitude and beliefs about nutrition (for example, have they been sent by the coach? Do they consider nutrition important in their training program?). Often their beliefs are based on testimony from other athletes or convictions of their coaches.

- Make a preliminary assessment of expected outcomes of the dietary assessment—knowing what they expect to gain by seeing a dietitian is always helpful.

- Enquire about the type, intensity and duration of their training program and determine: the influence of training on eating habits, timing of meals and food preparation (for example, early-morning training sessions may mean that the athlete skips breakfast; late afternoon or early evening sessions may encourage reliance on take-away foods). Allocating a scheduled time for shopping and cooking to fit in with the training program is a worthwhile strategy.

- Assessment of daily fluid intake is a critical factor and requires investigation. It is likely that many athletes are not consuming sufficient fluid to meet the demands of training. Cramps, for instance, are associated with low fluid intakes. Many athletes, especially schoolchildren, drink inadequate fluid at school and before training.

- The use of vitamin and mineral supplements, protein supplements and food replacement drinks is common in athletes (see Chapters 12 and 17) and should be investigated during the interview. Often they are unnecessary and used inappropriately.

- Specific nutritional assessment forms (for example, diet record sheets, food frequency questionnaires, self-assessment checklists for specific nutrients) facilitate the interview process. In clinical practice, dietary histories are the most frequently used method for assessing diet. On occasion, a three- to seven-day diet record using household measures, accompanied by a training diary, is often necessary to gain a full understanding of training commitments, timing of meals and dietary practices. Comprehensive instruction and a data collection protocol are needed to make the diet record worthwhile, especially if dietary analysis is expected. Compliance in reporting intake accurately for as long as seven days needs to be encouraged. Although the intake is likely to be distorted or under-reported (see Section 3.3.1.1), it is useful for providing a window into eating habits, especially in the erratic eater.

- Athletes need specific training and instructions on how to handle a range of issues when recording food intakes, for example, weighing or estimating serve size of individual foods, quantifying components of mixed dishes and recipes, and reporting wastage and foods eaten away from home. The necessity for precision in all aspects of recording needs to be explained clearly. Including instructions about cooked or uncooked foods, type of cooking (grilled, baked), level of fat trimming, use of added sugar, brand name, food descriptor (reduced or modified fat), type and quantity of oil/fat in cooking and beverages are important for improving accuracy of data collection. Determining the day of the week and the number of days of data collection should also be clearly specified.

- Serve sizes on commercial foods are useless for athletes. A standard bowl of breakfast cereal could be a pudding basin for an athlete! It is not uncommon for athletes to have three or more serve sizes of breakfast cereal at one sitting. When collecting information using household measures, distribute standardised measuring devices rather than relying on an athlete's perceived version of a cup or tablespoon.

- Concurrent interaction with computer software for dietary analysis during an interview can be a powerful education tool for helping athletes understand food composition and the effects of modifications to usual eating patterns. This is especially useful for follow-up consultations.

- An assortment of food supplements, vitamin and mineral supplements, protein supplements and commercial ergogenic aids is useful as an education tool to be used where relevant. It is inadvisable to display these items openly in the interview area. They may attract athletes who are looking for that 'extra edge' and detract from the interview.

- For an estimation of energy intake, daily energy expenditure can be estimated using the factorial method (see Chapter 6). This involves estimating BMR assigning and using an activity factor represented as a multiple of BMR. Benedict's equation is considered the most reliable for estimating BMR in athletes (see Table 6.1). As this calculation is a crude estimate, it should be used only as a guideline. The dietitian should always inform the athlete of the limitations of this estimate.

- RDIs/RDAs should be used with caution, as some may be inapplicable to athletes involved in strenuous training. Protein, calcium and iron may need some adjustment (see Chapters 5, 10 and 11).

Clinical observation and medical history

- Despite availability of medical records for some dietitians, further investigation and confirmation of associated or potential clinical factors may be important and overlooked by the medical practitioner. Many athletes fail to mention some of their low-grade symptoms to doctors. It is not uncommon for athletes to experience chronic gastrointestinal symptoms, post-training loss of appetite, recurring infections, nausea, headache, fatigue, flatulence, bladder, bowel, or menstrual problems that may be associated with exercise. Many of these problems can be detected at the dietetic interview.

Biochemical measurements

- Interpretations of nutrient status from one blood test can be misleading, especially if the athlete is dehydrated when tested, and the nutrient tested is under homeostatic control (e.g. calcium). Dehydration can lead to haemoconcentration of blood parameters resulting in falsely high readings.

Anthropometric measures

- The techniques and standards for assessing athletes' body compositions are outlined in Chapter 4. Anthropometric assessment in clinical practice usually includes height, BM, body frame measures and sometimes skinfold. Skinfold measures are usually discouraged in young or adolescent athletes who are rapidly growing as body shape is changing rapidly, especially in girls prior to menstruation. A sudden increase in fat measurement can have devastating effects on the adolescent female athlete; she may think she is suddenly getting very fat—when in fact it is natural for girls to increase skinfold measures at this time. Skinfold measures, however, if used appropriately and conducted by a trained kinanthropometrist, are more reliable than weight measurement for setting BM targets. These targets vary according to the demands of the sport and what is realistic for the individual. Therefore, published average skinfold values for elite national and international athletes are not necessarily applicable to individuals. They are better suited as skinfold targets for teams.

- Most athletes are preoccupied with their BM and body composition. Having a BMI chart prominently displayed can be unnecessarily stressful for large-framed muscular athletes, who should be reassured that many athletes do not fit into usual population reference standards. The BMI chart can, however, be useful for showing very lean athletes of slight build, who are often concerned about being overfat or overweight, that they are not overweight.

- One technique that is useful for discouraging a preoccupation with daily weighing, a pastime often practised by athletes, is to ask athletes to record their weight before and after each training session for one or two weeks. It is not unusual to see fluctuations of one or more kilograms before and after training sessions and large fluctuations between continuous training days and rest days. Athletes soon realise that large diurnal and weekly weight fluctuations occur and that interpretation of changes in weight are difficult and may not be due to food ingestion alone.

Summary

- If dietitians in both clinical practice and in research use standardised methods for anthropometry (i.e. O-scale or Ozscale) and for biochemical indices as well as rigorous protocols for collecting and analysing food intake data, then data can be compared more reliably across studies. There is a real need to collect and analyse dietary data on sufficient numbers of athletes in different sports at varying levels to allow micronutrient recommendations for athletes to be quantified. Also, a dietitian in clinical practice is in an ideal situation to collect and publish longitudinal data on athletes. Tracking studies of nutritional status of athletes, particularly children and adolescents, and even retiring athletes, are scarce to non-existent. Such studies will provide us with a better insight into the association between physical activity, diet and health outcomes.

REFERENCES

Abrahams SF, Mira M, Beumont PJV, Sowerbutts TD, Llewellyn-Jones D. Eating behaviours among young women. Med J Aust 1988;2:225–8.

Angus RM, Sambrook PNM, Pocock NA, Eisman JA. A simple method for assessing calcium intake in Caucasian women. J Am Diet Assoc 1989;89:209–14.

Baer JT, Dean DJ, Lambidindes T. How high school football coaches recommend their players gain lean body mass. J Strength Cond Res 1994;8:72–5.

Baghurst KI, Baghurst PA. The measurement of usual dietary intake in individuals and groups. Trans Menz Found 1981;3:139–60.

Baghurst K, Cobiac L, Record S, Powis G, Pender K. Major food selection guides currently in use in Australia. Published as part of the Review of food selection guides in Australia. Adelaide: CSIRO Division of Human Nutrition, 1994a.

Baghurst K, Cobiac L, Record S, Powis G, Pender K. Review of overseas food guides. Published as part of the Review of Food Selection Guides in Australia. Adelaide: CSIRO Division of Human Nutrition, 1994b.

Baghurst KI, Record SJ. A community dietary analysis system for use with diet diaries or food frequency questionnaires. Comm Health Stud 1984;VII:11–17.

Barr SI. Women, nutrition and exercise: A review of athletes' intakes and a discussion of energy balance in active women. Prog Food Nutr Sci 1987;11:307–61.

Basiotis PP, Welsh SO, Cronin FJ, Kelsay JL, Mertz W. Number of days of food intake records required to estimate individual and group nutrient intakes with defined confidence. J Nutr 1987;117:1638–41.

Bazarre TL, Myers MP. The collection of food intake data in cancer epidemiological studies. Nutr Canc 1979;1:22–45.

Beaton GH, Milner J, McGuire V, Feather TE, Little JA. Source of variance in the 24-hour dietary recall: Implications for nutrition study design and interpretation, carbohydrate sources, vitamins and minerals. Am J Clin Nutr 1983;37:986–95.

Beaton GH, Burema J, Ritenbaugh C. Errors in interpretation of dietary assessments. Am J Clin Nutr 1997;65:1100S–7S.

Bingham SA. Aspects of dietary survey methodology. British Nutrition Foundation, Nutrition Bulletin 44. 1985;10:90–103.

Bingham SA. Limitations of the various methods for collecting dietary intake data. Ann Nutr Metab 1991;35:117–27.

Bingham SA, Cummings JH. Urine nitrogen as an independent validatory measure of dietary intake: a study of nitrogen balance in individuals consuming their normal diet. Am J Clin Nutr 1985;42:1276–89.

Bingham SA. The dietary assessment of individuals' methods, accuracy, new techniques and recommendations. Nutr Abst Rev 1987;57:705–43.

Bingham SA, Nelson M, Paul AA, Haraldsdottir J, Bjorge-Loken E, van Staveren WA. Methods for data collection at an individual level. In: Cameron ME, Van Staveren WA, eds. Manual on methodology of food consumption studies. NY: Oxford University Press, 1988:53–106.

Bingham SA, Gill C, Welch A, et al. Comparison of dietary assessment methods in nutritional epidemiology: weighed records versus 24-hour recalls, food-frequency questionnaires and estimated diet records. Br J Nutr 1994;72:619–43.

Black AE, Goldberg GR, Jebb S, Livingstone MBE, Cole TJ, Prentice AM. Critical evaluation of energy intake data using fundamental principles of energy physiology: 2. Evaluating the results of published surveys. Eur J Clin Nutr 1991;45:583–99.

Block G. A review of validations of dietary assessment methods. Am J Epidemiol 1982;115:492–505.

Block G. Human dietary assessment: methods and issues. Prev Med 1989;18:653–60.

Block G, Clifford C, Naughton MD, Henderson M, McAdams M. A brief dietary screen for high fat intake. J Nutr Educ 1989;21:199–207.

Briefel R, Sempos C, McDowell MA, Chien S, Alaimo K. Dietary methods research in the national Health and Nutrition Examination Survey: underreporting of energy intake. Am J Clin Nutr 1997;65(suppl):1203S–08S.

Burke BS. The dietary history as a tool in research. J Am Diet Assoc 1947;23:1041–6.

Burke LM, Cummings NK, Desbrow B. Guidelines for daily carbohydrate intake: Do athletes achieve them? Sport Med 2001;31:267–99.

Buzzard IM, Sievert YA. Research priorities and recommendations for dietary assessment methodology. Am J Clin Nutr 1994;59(suppl):275–80.

Cade JE. Are diet records using household measures comparable to weighed intakes? J Hum Nutr Diet 1988;1:171–8.

Carter RL, Sharbough CO, Stapell CA. Reliability and validity of the 24-hour recall. J Am Diet Assoc 1981;79:5472–7.

Cashel K. Compilation and scrutiny of food composition data. In: Greenfield H, ed. Uses and abuses of food composition data. Food Aust 1990;42(suppl):S21–S4.

Cashel K, English R, Lewis J. Composition of foods, Australia. Canberra: Australian Government Publishing Service, 1989.

Cashel K, Jeffreson S. The core food groups: the scientific basis for developing nutrition education tools. Canberra: Australian Government Publishing Service, 1995.

Cobiac L, Derosti I, Baghurst K. Recommended Dietary Intakes—is it time for a change? Canberra: Commonwealth Department of Health & Family Services, 1998.

Commonwealth Department of Community Services and Health. Composition of Foods, Australia. Vol 2: Cereal and Cereal Products. Canberra: Australian Government Publishing Service, 1990a.

Commonwealth Department of Community Services and Health. Composition of Foods, Australia. Vol 3: Dairy Products, Eggs and Fish. Canberra: Australian Government Publishing Service, 1990b.

Commonwealth Department of Community Services and Health. Composition of Foods, Australia. Vol 4: Fats and Oils, Processed Meat, Fruit and Vegetables. Canberra: Australian Government Publishing Service, 1990c.

Commonwealth Department of Community Services and Health. Composition of Foods, Australia. Vol 5: Nuts and Legumes, Beverages and Miscellaneous Foods. Canberra: Australian Government Publishing Service, 1990d.

Commonwealth Department of Health. The five food groups (poster). Canberra: Australian Government Publishing Service, 1980s.

CSIRO. The 12345+ food and nutrition plan: a simple guide to healthy eating and weight control. Adelaide: CSIRO, 1991.

Cunningham JH. Sampling of foods for nutrient composition studies. In: Greenfield H, ed. Uses and abuses of food composition data. Food Aust 1990;42(suppl):S16–S17,28.

Curtis AE, Musgrave KO, Klimis-Tavantis D. A food frequency questionnaire that rapidly assesses intake of fat, saturated fat, cholesterol and energy. J Am Diet Assoc 1992;92:1517–19.

Daniels L. Collection of dietary data from children with cystic fibrosis: some problems and practicalities. Hum Nutr: Appl Nutr 1984;38A:110–18.

Dennis B, Shifflett PA. A conceptual and methodological model for studying dietary habits in the community. Ecol Food and Nutr 1985;17:253–62.

de Vries JH, Zock PL, Mensink RP, Katan MB. Underestimations of energy intake by 3-d records compared with energy intake to maintain body weight in 269 non-obese adults. Am J Clin Nutr 1994;60:855–60.

Dobson AJ, Bilijlevens R, Alexander HM, et al. A short fat questionnaire: a self-administered measure of fat-intake behaviour. Aust J Public Health 1993;17:144–9.

Dwyer JT, Krall EA. The problem of memory in nutritional epidemiological research. J Am Diet Assoc 1988;88:1250–7.

Eck LH, Klesges RC, Hanson CL, Slawson D, Portis L, Lavasque ME. Measuring short-term dietary intake: development and testing of a 1-week food frequency questionnaire. J Am Diet Assoc 1991;91:940–5.

Eck LH, Klesges LM, Klesges RC. Precision and estimated accuracy of two short-term food frequency questionnaires compared with recalls and records. J Clin Epidemiol 1996;49:1196–200.

English R, Lewis J. Nutritional values of Australian foods. Department of Community Services and Health. Canberra: Australian Government Publishing Service, 1992.

Faggiano F, Vineis P, Cravanzola D, et al. Validation of a method for the estimation of food portion size. Epidemiol 1992;3:379–83.

Ferro-Luzzi A. Social and public health issues in adaptation to low energy intakes. Am J Clin Nutr 1990;51:309–15.

Fogelholm M. Indicators of vitamin and mineral status in athletes' blood: a review. Int J Sport Nutr 1995;5:267–86.

Fogelholm MG, Juhani-Himberg J, Alopaeus K, et al. Dietary and biochemical indices of nutritional status in male athletes and controls. J Am Coll Nutr 1992;11:181–91.

Fogelholm M, Lahti-Koski M. The validity of a food use questionnaire in assessing the nutrient intake of physically active young men. Eur J Clin Nutr 1991;45:267–72.

Gersovitz M, Madden JP, Smiciklas-Wright H. Validity of the 24-hour dietary recall and a seven-day record for group comparisons. J Am Diet Assoc 1978;73:48–55.

Goldberg GB, Black AE, Jebb SA, et al. Critical evaluation of energy intake data using fundamental principles of energy physiology; 1. Derivation of cut-off limits to identify under-recording. Eur J Clin Nutr 1991;45:569–81.

Goldbohm RA, van den Brandt PA, Brants HA, et al. Validation of a dietary questionnaire used in a large-scale prospective cohort study on diet and cancer. Eur J Clin Nutr 1994;48:253–65.

Greeley S, Storbakken L, Magel R. Use of a modified food frequency questionnaire during pregnancy. J Am Coll Nutr 1992;11:728–34.

Greenfield H, Southgate DAT. Food composition data, production, management: experiences in food composition studies at the national and international level. Proc Nutr Soc Aust 1992;16:96–103.

Guthrie HA. Selection and quantification of typical food portions by young adults. J Am Diet Assoc 1984;84:1440–4.

Haggarty P, McGraw BA, Maughan RJ, Fenn C. Energy expenditure of elite female athletes measured by the doubly-labelled water method. Proc Nutr Soc 1988;47:35A.

Hamilton GJ, Thomson CD, Hopkins WG. Nutrition knowledge of elite distance runners. NZ J Sports Med 1994;Winter:26–9.

Hertzler AA, McAnge TR, Engr M. Development of an iron checklist to guide food intake. J Am Diet Assoc 1986;86:782–6.

Horwath CC, Worsley A. Assessment of the validity of a food frequency questionnaire as a measure of food use by comparison with direct observation of domestic food stores. Am J Epidemiol 1990;131:1059–67.

Hunter D. Biochemical indicators of dietary intake. In: Willett WC, ed. Nutritional epidemiology. New York: Oxford University Press, 1990:143–216.

Institute of Medicine, Food and Nutrition Board. Dietary reference intakes for thiamine, riboflavin, niacin, vitamin B6, folate, vitamin B12, pantothenic acid, biotin, and choline. Washington, DC: National Academy Press, 1998.

Isaksson B. Urinary nitrogen output as a validity test in dietary surveys (letter). Am J Clin Nutr 1980;33:4–5.

Jacobsen BH, Gemmel HA. Nutrition information sources of college varsity athletes. J Appl Sport Sc Res 1991;5:204–7.

Kemppainen T, Rosendahl A, Nuutinen O, Ebeling T, Pietinen P, Uusitupa M. Validation of a short dietary questionnaire and a qualitative fat index for the assessment of fat intake. Eur J Clin Nutr 1993;47:765–75.

Klesges RC, Eck LH, Ray JW, et al. Who underreports dietary intake in a dietary recall? Evidence from the Second National Health and Nutrition Examination Survey. J Consult Clin Psychol 1995;63:438–44.

Kohlmeier L. What you should know about your marker. In: Kok FJ, van't Veer P, eds. Biomarkers of dietary exposure, Proceedings of the 3rd meeting on nutritional epidemiology. London: Smith Gordon, 1991:15–16.

Kohlmeier L. Problems and pitfalls of food-to-nutrient conversions. In: WHO Regional Publications, European series, No. 34. Food and health data: their use in nutrition policy making. Copenhagen: WHO, 1992:73–84.

Krall EA, Dwyer JT. Validity of a food frequency questionnaire and a food diary in a short term recall situation. J Am Diet Assoc 1987;87:1374–7.

Kranztler NJ, Mullen BJ, Comstock EM, et al. Methods of food intake assessment—an annotated bibliography. J Nutr Educ 1982;14:108–17.

Kretsch MJ, Fong AKH. Validation of a new computerized technique for quantifying individual dietary intake: the Nutrition Evaluation Scale System (NESSy) vs the weighed food record. Am J Clin Nutr 1990;51:477–84.

Kristal AR, Abrams BF, Thornquist MD, et al. Development and validation of a food use checklist for evaluation of community nutrition intervention. Am J Publ Health 1990c;80:318–22.

Kristal AR, Shattuck AL, Henry HJ, Fowler AS. Rapid assessment of dietary intake of fat, fiber and saturated fat: validity of an instrument suitable for community intervention research and nutritional surveillance. Am J Health Prom 1990a;4:288–95.

Kristal AR, Shattuck AL, Henry HJ. Patterns of dietary behaviour associated with selecting diets low in fat: reliability and validity of a behavioral approach to dietary assessment. J Am Diet Assoc 1990b;90:214–20.

Larkin FA, Metzner HL, Thompson FE, Flegal KM, Guire KE. Comparison of estimated intakes by food frequency and dietary records in adults. J Am Diet Assoc 1989;89:215–23.

Lee RD, Nieman DC. Measurement of diet. In: Nutritional Assessment. Iowa: WC Brown Comm Inc, 1993:49–76, 103–20.

Lee-Han H, McGuire V, Boyd NF. A review of the methods used by studies of dietary measurement. J Clin Epidemiol 1989;42:269–79.

Lewis J, Milligan G, Hunt A. NUTTAB95 nutrient data table for use in Australia. Canberra: National Food Authority, 1995.

Life Sciences Research Office and Federation of American Societies for Experimental Biology. Nutrition monitoring in the United States: an update report on nutrition monitoring. Prepared for the United States Department of Agriculture and the United States Department of Health and Human Services. DHHS Publication No. 89–1255. Public Health Service. Washington: United States Government Printing Office, 1989.

Macdiarmid JI, Blundell JE. Dietary under-reporting: what people say about recording their food intake. Eur J Clin Nutr 1997;51:199–200.

Marr JW. Individual dietary surveys: purposes and methods. World Rev Nutr Diet 1971;13:105–64.

Marr JW, Heady JA. Within- and between-person variation in dietary surveys: number of days needed to classify individuals. Hum Nutr Appl Nutr 1986;40A:347–64.

McArdle WD, Katch FI, Katch VL. Sports and exercise nutrition. Philadelphia: Lippincott, Williams and Wilkins, 1999:372–425.

McLennan W, Podger A. Australian Bureau of Statistics (ABS) / Commonwealth Department of Health and Family Services (CDHFS), National Nutrition Survey: Selected Highlights Australia, 1995. Canberra: Australian Bureau of Statistics, Cat No. 4802, 1998.

Millar BD, Beard TC. Avoidance of dietary sodium—a simple questionnaire. Med J Aust 1988;149:190–2.

Munro S, Birze I, Samman S. Evaluation of dietary assessment methods used in Australian lipid clinics: a pilot study. Aust J Nutr Diet 1995;52:25–8.

Murphy EW, Watt BK, Rizek RL. Tables of food composition: availability, uses and limitations. Food Tech 1973;27:40–51.

Musgrave KO, Giambalvo L, Leclerc HL, Cook RA. Validation of a quantitative food frequency questionnaire for rapid assessment of dietary calcium intake. Am J Clin Nutr 1989;89:1484–8.

National Health & Medical Research Council. Recommended Dietary Intakes for use in Australia. Canberra: Australian Government Publishing Service, 1991.

National Health & Medical Research Council. Dietary guidelines for Australians. Canberra: Australian Government Publishing Service, 1992.

National Health & Medical Research Council. Dietary guidelines for children and adolescents. Canberra: Australian Government Publishing Service, 1995.

National Health & Medical Research Council. Binns C, ed. Dietary guidelines for older Australians. Canberra: National Health and Medical Research Council, 1999.

National Research Council. Recommended Dietary Allowances, 10th edn. Washington DC: National Academy Press, 1989.

Nelson M, Black AE, Morris JA, Cole TJ. Between- and within-subject variation in nutrient intake form infancy to old age: estimating the number of days required to rank dietary intakes with desired precision. Am J Clin Nutr 1989;50:155–67.

Nelson M, Hague GF, Cooper C, Bunker VW. Calcium intake in the elderly: validation of a dietary questionnaire. J Hum Nutr Diet 1988;1:115–27.

Nelson M, Nettleton PA. Dietary survey methods 1: a semi-weighed technique for measuring dietary intake within families. J Hum Nutr 1980;34:325–48.

Norton K, Whittingham N, Carter L, Kerr D, Gore C, Marfell-Jones M. Measurement techniques in anthropometry. In: Norton K, Olds T, eds. Anthropometrica. Sydney: University of New South Wales Press, 1996:25–75.

Olds TS, Ly SV, Norton KI. LifeSize computer software. Sydney: Nolds Sports Scientific, 1994.

Paul A, Southgate DAT. Conversion into nutrients. In: Cameron ME, van Staveren WA, eds. Manual on methodology of food consumption surveys. London: Oxford University Press, 1988:121–43.

Paul AA, Southgate DAT. McCance and Widdowsons' The composition of foods. London: Holland Biomedical Press, 1991.

Pekkarinen M. Methodology in the collection of food consumption data. World Rev Nutr Diet 1970;12:145–71.

Perron M, Endres J. Knowledge, attitudes and dietary practices of female athletes. J Am Diet Assoc 1985;85:573–6.

Pietinen P, Hartman AM, Haapa E, et al. Reproducibility and validity of dietary assessment instruments. I. A self-administered food use questionnaire with a portion size picture booklet. Am J Epidemiol 1988a;128:655–66.

Pietinen P, Hartman AM, Haapa E, et al. Reproducibility and validity of dietary assessment instruments: II. A qualitative food frequency questionnaire. Am J Epidemiol 1988b;128:667–76.

Prentice AM, Black AE, Coward WA, Cole TJ. Energy intake in overweight and obese adults in affluent societies: an analysis of 319 doubly labelled water measurements. Eur J Clin Nutr 1996;50:93–97.

Pryer JA, Vrijheid M, Nicholls R, Kiggins M, Elliot P. Who are the 'low energy reporters' in the Dietary and Nutritional Survey of British adults? Int J Epidemiol 1997;26:146–54.

Roberge AG, Sevigny J, Seoane N, Richard L. Dietary intake data: usefulness and limitations. Prog Food Nutr Sci 1984;8:27–42.

Rohan TE, Record SJ, Cook MD. Repeatability of estimates of nutrient and energy intake: the quantitative food frequency approach. Nutr Res 1987;7:125–37.

Ross WD, Marfell-Jones MJ. Kinanthropometry. In: MacDougall JD, Wenger HA, Green HJ, eds. The physiological assessment of high performance athletes. Champaign, Illinois: Human Kinetics, 1991.

Rutishauser I. Making measurements: diet. Melbourne: Menzies Technical Report no. 3, 1988;89–120.

Sabry JH. Purposes of food consumption studies. In: Cameron ME, van Staveren, eds. Manual on methodology of food consumption surveys. London: Oxford University Press, 1988.

Schoeller DA. Limitations in the assessment of dietary energy intake by self-report. Metab 1995;44(suppl):18–22.

Schoeller DA. Recent advances from application of doubly labelled water to measurement of human energy expenditure. J Nutr 1999;129:1765–8.

Schofield WN, Schofield C, James WPT. Basal metabolic rate—review and prediction, together with an annotated bibliography of source material. Hum Nutr Appl Nutr 1985;39(C Suppl):1–96.

Sempos CT, Briefel RR, Flegal KM, Johnson CL, Murphy RS, Woteki CE. Factors involved in selecting a dietary survey methodology for national nutrition surveys. Aust J Nutr Diet 1992;49:96–100.

Sempos CT, Johnson NE, Smith EL, Gilligan C. Effects of intraindividual and interindividual variation in repeated dietary records. Am J Epidemiol 1985;121:120–30.

Shekelle RB, MacMillan-Shryock A, et al. Diet, serum cholesterol, and death from coronary heart disease. New Eng J Med 1981;304:65–70.

Short SH, Short WR. Four year study of university athletes' dietary intake. J Am Diet Assoc 1983;82:632–45.

Smith A, Kellett E, Schmerlaib Y. The Australian guide to healthy eating. Adelaide: Children's Health Development Foundation, 1998.

Sorenson AW, Caulkins BM, Connolly MA, Diamond E. Comparison of nutrient intake determined by four dietary instruments. J Nutr Educ 1985;17:92–8.

Sossin K, Gizis F, Marquart LF, Sobal J. Nutrition beliefs, attitudes and resource use of high school wrestling coaches. Int J Sport Nutr 1997;7:219–28.

Speakman JR. The history and theory of the doubly labelled water technique. Am J Clin Nutr 1998;68(suppl):932S–938S.

Stockley L. Changes in habitual food intake during weighed inventory surveys and duplicate diet collections: a short review. Ecol Food Nutr 1985;17:263–9.

Stockley L, Chapman RI, Holley ML, Jones FA, Prescott EHA, Broadhurst AJ. Description of a food recording electronic device for use in dietary surveys. Hum Nutr App Nutr 1986a;40A:13–18.

Stockley L, Hurren CA, Chapman RI, Broadhurst AJ, Jones FA. Energy, protein and fat intake estimated using a food recording electronic device compared with a weighed diary. Hum Nutr App Nutr 1986b;40A:19–23.

Strohmeyer SL, Massey LK, Davison MA. A rapid dietary screening device for clinics. J Am Diet Assoc 1984;84:428–32.

Stuff JE, Garza C, Smith EO, Nichols BL, Montandon CM. A comparison of dietary methods in nutritional studies. Am J Clin Nutr 1983;37:300–7.

Stunkard AJ, Waxman M. Accuracy of self-reports of food intake. J Am Diet Assoc 1981;79:547–51.

Telford R, Tumilty D, Damm G. Skinfold measurements in well performed Australian athletes. Sports Sc Med Quart 1984;1:13–16.

Telford RD, Egerton WJ, Hahn AG, Pang PM. Skinfold measurements and weight controls in elite athletes. Excel 1988;5:21–5.

Tjonneland AT, Haraldsdottir J, Overvad K, Stripp C, Ewertz M, Moller-Jensen O. Influence of individually estimated portion size data on the validity of a semiquantitative food frequency questionnaire. Int J Epidemiol 1992;21:770–7.

Vailas LI, Blankenhorn DH, Selzer RH, Johnson RL. A computerized quantitative food frequency analysis for the clinical setting: use in documentation and counselling. J Am Diet Assoc 1987;87:1539–43.

van Assema P, Brug J, Kok G, Brants H. The reliability and validity of a Dutch questionnaire on fat consumption as a means to rank subjects according to individual fat intake. Eur J Canc Prev 1992;1:375–80.

van Erp-Baart AMJ, Saris WHM, Binkhorst RA, Voos JA, Elvers JWH. Nationwide survey on nutritional habits in elite athletes: parts I and II. Int J Sports Med 1989;10:S3–S16.

Welsh S, Davis C, Shaw A. A brief history of food guides in the United States. Nutr Today 1992;27:6–11.

Welten DC, Kempner HC, Post GB, Van Staveren WA. Comparison of a quantitative dairy questionnaire with a dietary history in young adults. Int J Epidemiol 1995;24:764–70.

Werblow JA, Fox HM, Henneman A. Nutrition knowledge, attitudes and food patterns of women athletes. J Am Diet Assoc 1978;73:242–5.

Westerterp KR, Saris WH, van Es M, ten Hoor F. Use of the doubly labelled water technique in humans during heavy sustained exercise. J Appl Physiol 1986;61:2162–7.

Wheeler CE, Rutishauser IHE, O'Dea K. Comparison of nutrient intake data from two food frequency questionnaires and weighed records. Aust J Nutr Diet 1995;52:140–8.

Wilkins JA, Boland FJ, Albinson J. A comparison of male and female university athletes and non-athletes on eating disorder indices. Are athletes protected? Int J Sport Behav 1991;14:129–43.

Willett WC. Reproducibility and validity of food-frequency questionnaires. Nutritional Epidemiology. New York: Oxford University Press, 1990:92–126.

Willett WC, Reynolds RD, Cottrell-Hoehner MS, Sampson L, Browne MS. Validation of a semi-quantitative food frequency questionnaire: comparison with a 1-year diet record. J Am Diet Assoc 1987;87:43–7.

Willett WC, Sampson L, Browne ML, et al. The use of a self-administered questionnaire to assess diet four years in the past. Am J Epidemiol 1988;127:188–99.

Willett WC, Sampson LS, Stampfer MJ, et al. Reproducibility and validity of a semi-quantitative food frequency questionnaire. Am J Epidemiol 1985;122:51–65.

Wilson P, Horwath C. Validation of a short food frequency questionnaire for assessment of dietary calcium intake in women. Eur J Clin Nutr 1996;50:220–28.

Worsley A, Baghurst KI, Leitch DR. Social desirability response bias and dietary inventory responses. Hum Nutr Appl Nutr 1984;38A:29–35.

CHAPTER 4

Kinanthropometry: physique assessment of the athlete

Deborah Kerr and Tim Ackland

4.1 INTRODUCTION

Kinanthropometry is a term used to describe the appraisal of human physique, which includes the size, shape and proportion, and body composition of the individual (Ross 1991). This appraisal allows the interpretation and monitoring of sports performance and growth. Studies of world class and Olympic athletes indicate there are specific physique requirements for certain sports (DeRose et al. 1989; Carter & Ackland 1994; Ackland et al. 1997a; Ackland et al. 1997b; Ackland et al. 1998). Even within a sport, the position of the player may require unique physique characteristics. Changes in rules or technique can alter the anthropometric characteristics required for successful performance.

In sports where the body mass (BM) must be transported a distance, a lean physique can offer a competitive advantage (Tittel 1978). These sports include gymnastics, distance running or jumping types of sports where the assessment of body composition and body fat is of primary interest. The same assessment is also important for weight category and aesthetic sports (e.g. ballet) where a low level of body fat is also desirable (Wilmore & Costill 1988). An understanding of kinanthropometry is necessary to be able to interpret anthropometric data in relation to performance. A co-operative relationship between the sports dietitian, exercise scientist and coach is essential (Ross et al. 1988a). But physique is only one of many factors that will determine sports performance. Athletes can still achieve competence in their chosen sports without having the optimal physique for this sport.

4.2 PHYSIQUE ASSESSMENT IN ATHLETES

The choice of method for assessing physique depends largely on available resources, testing conditions and the application of the results as a clinical and research outcome. On most occasions, an estimation of the subcutaneous adipose tissue mass, or body fat as it is commonly known, is all that is required. The assessment of physique in sports science has four fundamental applications, as follows:

1. identifying physique characteristics of elite performers;
2. assessing and monitoring growth;
3. monitoring training programs; and
4. determining optimal body composition for weight category sports.

4.2.1 Identifying physique characteristics

Athletes who reach Olympic or world-class standard represent the optimum combination of ethnicity, heredity and environment to produce peak performance (Carter 1984). Kinanthropometry can relate the structure of the athletic body to the specialised function needed for various tasks and can help us to understand the limitations of such relationships (Carter 1984). For example, world championship swimmers were found to have a larger arm span than their height (Carter & Ackland 1994). This information is of interest to the exercise scientist and coach and can be used in the identification of athletic potential (Ross et al. 1991). The methods used to identify physique differences are somatotyping (Carter & Honeyman Heath 1990) and proportionality assessment (Ross & Wilson 1974).

Somatotyping is a combined shape–body composition method, which provides a description of the physique by means of a three-number rating representing the components of endomorphy (adiposity), mesomorphy (muscularity) and ectomorphy (linearity) (Carter et al. 1982). Somatotyping has been used extensively to describe the shape characteristics of athletes. Some sports are less tolerant of size and shape variance (e.g. gymnastics), whereas others display a wider distribution. In the latter group of sports, factors other than physique are dominant (Ross & Marfell-Jones 1991). A detailed description of the method of somatotyping is given by Carter and Honeyman Heath (1990).

Proportionality is described as the relationship of body parts to one another or to the whole body (Ross & Marfell-Jones 1991). The methodology proposed by Ross and Wilson (1974) makes use of a unisex reference human, or 'phantom', as a calculation device. It is not a normative system but enables proportional differences in anthropometric characteristics within and between athletes to be quantified (Ross & Ward 1984). Using this method, which scales anthropometric data to a common stature, proportional differences can be assessed between athletes in different sports and events, and between males and females.

4.2.2 *Assessing and monitoring growth*

Involvement in competitive sport can begin at or prior to puberty. This is a time of rapid changes in size, shape and body composition for both sexes. The onset of puberty, however, can vary considerably between individuals. For example, the difference in age between an early-maturing girl and a late-maturing boy may be as much as six years (Ross & Marfell-Jones 1991). This difference in maturation has important implications for sporting ability, as the late-maturing boy will not be as strong as early-maturing boys, as the spurt in strength will follow the spurt in height (Ackland et al. 1994). In girls, late maturation is an advantage in sports where low BM and narrow hips assist movement such as in gymnastics, ballet and distance running (Ross et al. 1988a).

4.2.2.1 *Changes in adipose tissue during growth*

During pubertal growth, the relative gain in adipose tissue drops markedly for both males and females. This is a response to an increase in energy requirements at this time. The absolute amount of adipose tissue may even decline for adolescent males (Marshall 1978). Following puberty, the increased deposition of fat is much more marked in females than in males. It is important that coaches and young female athletes understand that increased fat deposition may occur with maturation.

4.2.2.2 *Changes in muscle tissue during growth*

A growth spurt in muscle mass occurs during the adolescent growth period. Males under the influence of testosterone show a more marked increase in muscle mass than females. Muscle mass reaches a level greater than 40% of total body mass in adult males, compared with a maximum of 39% in females (Bloomfield et al. 1994).

4.2.2.3 *Assessing peak height velocity*

Monitoring height and the peak height velocity (PHV) can provide important information on maturation (Ross & Marfell-Jones 1991; Faulkner & Tanner 1978). Ideally, height should be measured every three months, prior to and during adolescence. For girls, the PHV usually occurs at 12 years of age. Breast-budding occurs prior to the PHV and the menarche occurs when the height velocity is falling. Therefore menarche is an important indicator of when the height velocity is falling in females. In boys, the adolescent growth spurt usually peaks around 14 years, which is two years later than girls. The peak strength spurt will occur after the spurt in height. This means that males will get stronger after the peak height velocity has occurred.

4.2.3 *Monitoring training programs*

Assessment of body composition is an important component of the ongoing monitoring of athletes. Monitoring of skinfolds indicates changes in adipose tissue mass in response to changes in training and energy intake. The Body Mass Index (BMI), or population index of weight status, is not sensitive to changes in body composition (Ross et al. 1988b) and should not be used for monitoring athletes. Girths and corrected girths can be used to monitor changes in muscularity. The skinfold-corrected arm girth is calculated by the following formula (Ward et al. 1989):

$$\text{Skinfold-corrected arm girth (AGRsc)} = \text{AGR} - (3.14 \times \text{TPSK})$$
$$\text{Where AGR} = \text{relaxed arm girth (cm)}$$
$$\text{TPSK} = \text{tricep skinfold (cm)}$$

Usually the skinfold reading will be in millimetres and must therefore be converted to centimetres for the calculation. The skinfold-corrected girths are used in the O-Scale and Oz-scale systems (see Section 4.4.2).

4.2.4 *Determining optimal body composition for weight-category sports*

In weight-category sports, athletes attempt to gain a competitive advantage by making the lowest weight category possible. These sports include the combative sports such as judo, wrestling, boxing, weight-lifting and lightweight rowing. Aesthetic sports such as gymnastics, diving, ballet and figure-skating are in essence weight-category sports, as a low BM is a requirement.

The assessment of body composition, in particular body fat, can be useful in identifying whether the desired weight category is realistic. If an athlete already has low body fat as assessed by the skinfold sum (seven or eight sites), then significant weight loss could only be achieved by loss of lean body mass (LBM). It is important that this issue is discussed with the coach and athlete before weight loss is undertaken as loss of LBM can compromise strength and endurance capacity.

4.3 *METHODOLOGIES FOR ASSESSING BODY COMPOSITION*

Martin and Drinkwater (1991) have suggested three approaches to body composition assessment. The first approach is the direct assessment or Level I method which is based on cadaver analysis. It is important to understand that all body composition methodologies available to assess athletes provide an indirect assessment of body composition. Therefore all other approaches are indirect (Level II methods) or doubly indirect (Level III methods). Level II and III approaches must make certain assumptions to be able to predict the body composition and are therefore termed indirect methods of assessing body composition. For comprehensive reviews on body composition, readers are directed to Martin and Drinkwater (1991), Brodie et al. (1998), and Roche et al. (1996).

4.3.1 *Direct assessment of body composition (Level I)*

The German anatomists reported the earliest data on direct body composition analysis over 100 years ago (Keys & Brozek 1953). Until the 1980s there had been only eight complete adult dissections (Mitchell et al. 1945; Forbes et al. 1953). Clarys et al. (1984) undertook a study to compare surface anthropometry with anatomically dissected cadavers. Twenty-five cadavers sampled from an elderly Belgian population were dissected into the gross tissue masses of skin, adipose tissue, muscle, bone and organs. Comprehensive comparisons were made between the gross tissue weights and the surface anthropometry. This study provided important data, which questioned many of the commonly held assumptions in the techniques for measuring body composition.

4.3.2 *Indirect assessment (Level II)*

Historically, the interest in body composition arose from a desire to measure body fat. The work of Behnke et al. (1942) on naval divers was the first time body density had been used to estimate body fat. In order to predict the percentage of fat from body density it is necessary to assume that the body is composed of two compartments (fat mass (FM) and fat-free mass (FFM)) and that the densities of each are known and are the same for all individuals. Until recently, underwater weighing (UWW) was considered the criterion method or the 'gold standard' for validating other methods of body composition analysis. More recently, however, other techniques have been put forward as possible criterion methods including total body water (TBW), total body potassium (TBK), and dual energy X-ray absorptiometry (DEXA). Multi-component chemical methods which use more than one method have recently been proposed (Heymsfield et al. 1990; Friedl et al. 1992). Considering any method to be the gold standard is misleading because none are absolutely accurate. All methods have assumptions and it is important to be alert to conditions where the assumptions may be violated. In practice, the assessment of body composition must be inexpensive, safe and non-invasive. Therefore, most Level II methods, although safe, are not suitable for everyday use in athletes mainly because they require sophisticated and expensive equipment. Level II methods have a research application and are used to validate Level III methods. The application of UWW and DEXA are outlined below. These methods are covered in more detail, as they are the most commonly used in sports science. The other Level II methods (i.e. TBK, TBW) are outside the scope of this chapter and are limited to research applications. Excellent reviews of their applications are found in Jebb and Elia (1993) and Roche et al. (1996).

4.3.2.1 *Underwater weighing*

Underwater weighing is a technique for the assessment of body density, which is extrapolated to compute the relative fat content of the body. It is based on the principle of buoyancy or relative floatability, a principle first observed by Archimedes (287–212 BC). If the mass and density of an object and the densities of its constituent parts are known, then the mass of each can be calculated.

Using underwater weighing or displacement techniques, with the appropriate corrections for the buoyant force of lung and visceral entrapped air, the density of the body can be determined. One must then assume constant densities of fat (0.90 g/mL) and non-fat (1.10 g/mL) to translate the obtained density value into per cent body fat. The most commonly used equations are the Siri (1961) and Brozek (1960) equations.

Siri: % Fat = $((4.95 / D) - 4.50) \times 100$
Brozek: % Fat = $((4.570 / D) - 4.142) \times 100$
              where D = body density

The review article 'Body fat in adult man' (1953) by Keys and Brozek outlines the rationale for the development of these equations.

To predict body fat from densitometry requires the acceptance of the following assumptions:

- The proportion of all fat-free (FF) tissues (FF muscle, FF bone, FF skin, FF organs) must be fixed.
- The densities of the constituents of the body are constant from person to person.
- An individual differs from a 'standard reference person' only in the amount of adipose tissue.

Anatomical evidence from the Brussels Study (Clarys et al. 1984) does not support these assumptions. In six male and seven female unembalmed cadavers, the dissected muscle mass ranged from 41.9 to 59.4%, bone from 16.3 to 25.7% and the remainder from 24.0 to 32.4%. The most significant variation in the density of the FFM constituents occurs in bone due to differences in bone mineralisation (Jones & Corlet 1980). In the cadaver sample, a range of 1.18 g/mL to 1.33 g/mL for bone density was obtained (Martin 1985).

The negative per cent body fat obtained in a team of Canadian football players gives a strong indication of the errors that can arise by assuming a constant density for the FFM (Adams et al. 1982). Many of the players were black and usually have a higher bone density than Caucasians. In individuals with a lower bone density (for example, amenorrheic athletes, osteoporotics), UWW would overestimate per cent body fat.

In addition to the biological error from the assumptions outlined, there are also measurement errors involved in UWW. The two primary sources of error include the volume of air trapped in the lungs and gastrointestinal tract. To account for gastrointestinal gases a constant of 100 mL has been suggested (Buskirk 1961); however, accurate measurement of the residual volume in the lungs is essential. Residual volume is the volume of air remaining in the lungs after maximal expiration (Jensen et al. 1993). The closed circuit nitrogen/oxygen dilution method of Wilmore (1969) provides an accurate assessment of the residual volume; however, this requires the use of expensive equipment and a high level of technical expertise.

4.3.2.2 *Dual energy X-ray absorptiometry (DEXA) for the assessment of bone mineral density and body composition*

Dual energy densitometers were primarily developed to estimate bone mineral content (BMC (g)) and bone mineral density (BMD (g/cm^2)) of regions of the skeleton and for the whole body. The development of DEXA whole body scan based on a sealed X-ray source with dual-energy photons allowed body composition assessment as well (Mazess et al. 1984). Soft tissue can be distinguished from bone due to the difference in the attenuation co-efficient of the X-ray beam over soft tissue compared to that over bone. The relative attenuation of the photons in soft tissue changes in proportion to the fat content over the soft tissue being scanned (Lohman 1992).

Studies have shown that DEXA is able to estimate body mass of the subject with a high degree of accuracy (Svendsen et al. 1993). This indicates that DEXA is able to predict the soft tissue mass accurately but does not assess how well it can predict the components of the soft tissue, fat and lean body mass (LBM). While several studies have shown close correlation between DEXA and other criterion methods generally, there are systematic differences between the methods. A study in male subjects, which compared underwater weighing (UWW) with DEXA, showed a strong correlation between the methods but DEXA gave lower correlation co-efficients for per cent body fat (Johansson et al. 1993). Studies in females have shown higher values for DEXA compared with UWW (Wang et al. 1989; Van Loan & Mayclin 1992). As all methods are indirect there is no way to determine which method is closest to the true tissue masses.

The ability to account for the bone mineral density for different ages, levels of activity and gender is a major advantage of DEXA over other methods, but there are some limitations of DEXA, as follows. Subjects over 120 kg or more than two metres in stature may not be within the scanning region. However, with the low radiation dose and precision of measurement it seems likely that this method will be adopted as a criterion method in the future. But, before DEXA is considered acceptable as a criterion method, more thorough evaluation needs to be undertaken (Kohrt 1995).

4.3.3 *Doubly indirect (Level III) methods*

Level III methods have been referred to by Martin and Drinkwater (1991) as 'doubly indirect' as they require validation against Level II methods to determine percentage body fat. Therefore the assumptions of the Level II method must also be considered in the interpretation of the result. This is in addition to the assumptions of the Level III method itself. Body fat estimated by these methods, using either whole body conductivity or anthropometry (skinfolds) cannot be supported.

4.3.3.1 *Whole body conductivity*

Two similar techniques based on the differing dielectrical properties of fat and lean tissues of the body (Segal et al. 1985) are known as total body electrical conductivity

(TOBEC) and bioelectrical impedance analysis (BIA). The TOBEC uses uniform current induction to estimate lean body mass (LBM) from the magnitude of the body's electrical conductivity. BIA, however, is a localised method based on differing electrical properties of lean and fat tissue (Harrison 1987). An estimate of fat-free mass (FFM) is then calculated after normalising for stature (Guo et al. 1987). Fat mass (FM) is derived from the total body mass by the subtraction of estimated FFM. Similarly to skinfold equations, BIA equations require validation against a Level II criterion method, and are therefore population specific. Factors that affect the recorded electrical resistance in the BIA technique have been reported. Variations in diet, hydration, ethnicity and diseased states affect the body's electrolyte balance, which in turn influences the FM estimate (Malina 1987; Hutcheson et al. 1988). To date, there is no evidence to justify the use of BIA for the assessment of individual body composition status.

4.3.3.2 *How skinfolds are used to predict body fat*

Skinfold calipers are commonly used in sports science because they are non-invasive, cheap and accessible to most sports scientists and dietitians. A skinfold caliper reading measures the compressed thickness of a double layer of skin and the underlying sub-cutaneous adipose tissue. The sums of skinfold measures have been used to predict FM and per cent body fat.

The observation that skinfolds were correlated with criterion techniques such as UWW has led to a proliferation of regression equations to predict body fat. Since 1950 more than 100 equations to predict body fat from skinfolds have been reported in the literature (Lohman 1981). The problem is that these equations are population specific and should only be used on a similar population to that upon which the specific equation was developed (Johnston 1982).

To predict body fat from skinfold measures requires the acceptance of certain assumptions. A major source of error is the skinfold compressibility, which causes a decrease in the reading after the initial application of the skinfold caliper to the fold (Martin et al. 1985). Skinfold compressibility varies considerably between and within individuals and at different skinfold sites on the same person. The important implication, however, is that two individuals may have identical skinfold values but very large differences in uncompressed adipose tissue thickness.

4.4 ▰ *INDICES OF HEIGHT AND WEIGHT*

Weight–height indices have been used for many years in an attempt to determine the 'ideal weight' for an individual. The best known of these is the Body Mass Index (BMI: weight (kg)/height (m)^2). All indices provide a measure of ponderosity which is not the same as measuring adiposity. For an individual of any given stature, body mass will vary according to the amount and density of LBM as well as the adipose tissue mass. This was identified by Behnke et al. in 1942, who reported that

70% of a sample of American college football players were classified as 'overweight' using weight-for-height indices.

Adolphe Quetelet (1796–1874), the Belgian astronomer and mathematician, was one of the first scientists to collect population statistics, which included height and weight. It was Quetelet's observation that the weight of adults of differing heights is nearly the square of stature (Quetelet 1842). Historically, Quetelet's observation on the dimensional relationship between weight and height is the origin of the BMI. More recently, epidemiologists have used the BMI in the identification of health risk factors (van Itallie & Abraham 1985).

The rationale for the use of the BMI as an indicator of relative fatness lies in the fact that it seems to dissociate height; that is, is maximally correlated with weight and minimally correlated with height. The BMI, however, does not distinguish subcutaneous adiposity from other anthropometric characteristics.

Ross et al. (1988b) examined the relationship between the BMI and anthropometric measures in 19 000 men and women aged 20–70 years. Subjects were grouped according to their BMI table and the sum of five skinfolds. In the combined sample, 26% of those rated with a BMI of less than 20 had a skinfold sum above the 50th percentile and 16% of those with a BMI of greater than 27 had a skinfold sum below the 50th percentile. BMI does not distinguish the body composition or structure of individuals so misclassification is a problem especially in sportspeople with a muscular physique.

4.4.1 *Interpreting anthropometric data*

Anthropometric data has been used in a variety of ways to estimate body composition size and structure. To estimate body fat, a skinfold sum can be determined and compared to normative data for elite athletes (Table 4.1 and Table 4.2) or monitored over time. This approach is preferable to using percentage body equations, which are not reliable for individual predictions (Johnston 1982). As suggested by Johnston (1982), it is better to use anthropometry itself and changes in absolute measures in individuals rather than making predictions of per cent body fat based on questionable assumptions.

When interpreting anthropometric data it is important to recognise the variability in physique between athletes. The physique and level of adiposity which equates to optimal performance in one athlete may not be the same for another athlete. Genetic variability (Bouchard et al. 1988) means that some athletes can maintain a low level of adiposity without having to restrict their energy intake.

4.4.2 *The O-scale and Oz-scale systems*

The O-scale system (Ward et al. 1989) provides a method of comparing individual skinfold results with a normative database categorised by age and gender. The databases were constructed from 1 236 children (Whittingham 1978) and over 19 000 adults from the YMCA Life Project (Bailey et al. 1982). The measures recorded in

Table 4.1 Normative data for international and national level female athletes

Sport	Level	Position/event	Number of subjects	Skinfold sum (mm)* Mean	Range
Athletics[1]	National	SASI Jumps	4	61.1±12.7	41.7 – 72.8
		SASI Throws	9	95.3±49.4	53.0 – 203.7
		SASI Sprint	7	60.3±11.9	45.1 – 83.9
		SASI Middle distance	20	59.2±19.6	37.4 – 110.6
		SASI Long distance	6	51.3±8.8	40.4 – 68.3
Basketball[2]	International	Guard	64	76.6±22.2	36.4 – 143.5
		Forward	65	76.0±20.1	40.9 – 131.7
		Centre	47	88.0±21.1	45.7 – 146.8
Cricket[1]	National		27	90.8±19.7	55.9 – 141.1
Cycling, Road[1]	National		32	61.9±12.0	33.8 – 89.5
Diving[3]	International		39	65.6±17.0	32.1 – 114.3
Gymnastics[1]		SASI Elite	68	37.9±6.1	27.4 – 57.6
		SASI Senior	57	87.4±18.5	48.1 – 140.3
Hockey[1]		SA Senior	33	83.4±17.3	51.5 – 124.0
Netball[1]		SASI Light weight	24	73.4±13.4	55.5 – 105.2
Rowing[1]		SASI Heavy weight	30	87.5±17.8	60.7 – 119.4
Triathlon[4]	International		19	62.8±13.4	40.3 – 98.4
Swimming[3]	International		170	72.6±19.6	37.9 – 147.1
Synchronized swimming[3]	International		137	81.7±22.1	37.5 – 145.8
Volleyball[1]		SASI Senior	29	90.5±25.1	35.8 – 147.1
Waterpolo[3]	International		109	89.8±23.8	39.7 – 151.6

*Sum of 7 skinfolds (unless otherwise indicated) = triceps, subscapular, biceps, supraspinale, abdominal, front thigh, medial calf.

Adapted with permission from the South Australian Sports Institute and published previously by Woolford et al. (1993).

[1] Ackland et al. 1997b.

[2] Note: Sum of 6 skinfolds from Carter and Ackland (1994) = triceps, subscapular, supraspinale, abdominal, front thigh, medial calf.

[3] Note: Sum of 6 skinfolds from Ackland et al. (1998) = triceps, subscapular, supraspinale, abdominal, front thigh, medial calf.

[4] Note: Sum of 8 skinfolds from Ackland et al. (1998) = triceps, subscapular, biceps, iliac crest, supraspinale, abdominal, front thigh, medial calf.

Table 4.2 *Normative data for international and national level male athletes*

Sport	Level	Position/event	Number of subjects	Skinfold sum (mm)* Mean	Range
Athletics[1]	State	SASI Pole	3	46.8±0.3	46.4–47.1
		SASI Sprint	4	56.1±2.2	53.9–58.3
		SASI Middle distance	9	38.6±12.0	25.8–68.2
		SASI Long distance	4	49.8±6.4	41.3–56.4
Australian Rules Football[1]	National	Under 17 years	20	67.2±6.9	44.7–104.1
Boxing[1]	State		13	57.5±17.7	34.2–95.2
Cricket[1]	National		22	77.8±23.0	52.3–135.2
Cycling[1]	State	Road	24	58.1±11.9	42.9–85.0
	National	Track	83	53.9±12.7	26.4–85.3
Diving[2]	International		43	45.9±11.4	28.0–79.7
Gymnastics[1]	State	SASI Elite	41	41.6±7.2	27.5–59.1
Hockey[1]	State	Under 21 squad	22	59.4±17.0	38.7–107.2
Kayaking[1]	State	SASI Senior	64	58.0±14.0	37.4–96.7
Rowing[1]	State	SASI Light weight	27	45.2±6.5	35.8–65.1
	State	SASI Heavy weight	18	66.9±18.0	46.1–111.8
Rugby Union[1]	State	SASI Senior	58	92.2±32.9	50.6–223.2
Triathlon[3]	International		19	48.3±10.2	36.8–85.9
Swimming[2]	International		231	45.8±9.5	26.6–99.9
Volleyball[1]	State	SASI Senior	17	56.8±13.2	36.9–79.6
Weight-lifting[1]	State	SASI Squad	47	74.9±34.4	33.9–190.2
Waterpolo[2]	International		190	62.5±17.7	27.9–112.1

*Sum of 7 skinfolds (unless otherwise indicated) = triceps, subscapular, biceps, supraspinale, abdominal, front thigh, medial calf.

[1]Adapted with permission from the South Australian Sports Institute and published previously by Woolford et al. (1993).

[2]Note: Sum of 6 skinfolds from Carter and Ackland (1994) = triceps, subscapular, supraspinale, abdominal, front thigh, medial calf.

[3]Note: Sum of 8 skinfolds from Ackland et al. (1998) = triceps, subscapular, biceps, iliac crest, supraspinale, abdominal, front thigh, medial calf.

this system were age, gender, height, weight and six skinfolds (triceps, subscapular, supraspinale, abdominal, front thigh and medial calf). From these data, the adiposity (A) and proportional weight (W) ratings can be calculated as shown below.

The A rating is determined from the sum of six skinfolds (Σ6SF) and compared to the appropriate age/sex norm. The Σ6SF is dimensionally scaled to account for individuals of varying size using the equation:

$$p\Sigma FSF = \Sigma 6SF \ (170.18/H)$$
$$\text{where: } p\Sigma FSF = \text{the proportional sum of six skinfolds (mm)}$$
$$H = \text{the subject's height (cm)}$$

The A rating is then determined by reference to normative data shown in Tables 4.3 and 4.4 (Ward et al. 1989).

Table 4.3 / O-Scale system adiposity ratings for female subjects

Age (years)	Stanine threshold values#								
	1	2	3	4	5	6	7	8	9
6		46.8*	56.1	61.7	69.5	77.9	96.7	128.6	144.0
7		44.3	47.4	60.2	68.3	76.1	91.8	113.2	140.0
8		43.7	49.2	63.9	69.8	81.4	94.5	111.7	143.2
9		45.5	53.4	66.1	73.2	87.7	98.6	111.7	143.3
10		49.2	59.6	67.6	78.6	98.3	109.7	143.2	173.5
11		51.9	56.4	66.5	75.6	96.4	108.8	150.0	173.4
12		53.0	59.3	66.5	77.8	98.7	111.4	153.0	175.6
13		46.7	56.9	67.9	77.4	97.7	114.9	153.0	165.5
14		46.7	60.9	69.0	81.9	99.6	113.4	147.4	164.8
15		49.4	62.6	72.4	85.4	99.6	113.2	145.3	162.1
16		53.8	65.0	76.2	90.3	101.1	112.0	142.4	158.1
17		62.1	69.4	78.3	92.8	106.5	117.6	141.4	156.4
18–19		63.4	70.5	78.5	90.2	103.4	118.2	135.9	155.7
20–25		64.0	72.5	81.2	92.0	104.2	118.9	138.0	164.0
25–30		62.2	74.1	82.2	93.0	107.9	122.9	141.0	169.2
30–35		64.1	72.0	81.9	94.6	108.0	126.0	144.3	172.2
35–40		64.5	73.9	85.5	97.9	112.1	131.7	148.0	178.4
40–45		69.5	80.5	90.3	102.4	120.7	140.9	161.1	187.3
45–50		72.5	83.2	97.7	110.5	125.7	141.8	165.1	194.0
50–55		70.0	84.5	96.2	112.5	127.8	144.8	168.3	196.5
55–60		46.9	90.1	102.6	115.7	130.5	152.8	169.9	198.2
60–65		78.3	85.3	96.8	114.6	130.6	146.4	166.0	194.0
65–70		74.3	84.8	97.0	110.4	130.7	140.7	153.4	164.6

Source: Ward et al. 1989

*Proportional sum of six skinfolds (mm).

#Individual adiposity ratings are determined from nine standard intervals (stanines) which provide divisions at the percentile equivalents of P4, 11, 23, 40, 60, 77, 89 and 96.

Table 4.4 *O-Scale system adiposity ratings for male subjects*

Age (years)	Stanine threshold values#								
	1	2	3	4	5	6	7	8	9
6		43.0*	47.4	57.4	63.0	70.0	80.9	92.7	121.0
7		40.2	44.6	51.2	59.0	70.9	83.0	99.5	131.0
8		41.2	45.7	50.7	56.8	65.4	77.6	99.5	137.9
9		43.6	47.1	50.9	55.9	64.2	77.7	105.2	172.4
10		45.1	47.1	53.7	59.1	65.4	83.7	129.1	183.2
11		41.5	45.1	50.8	58.4	68.3	90.9	154.7	193.2
12		37.6	43.1	47.0	53.4	65.7	89.3	126.6	188.9
13		34.8	40.2	44.9	51.7	62.7	86.1	116.4	166.5
14		34.7	37.2	43.4	49.3	57.3	70.9	103.5	146.1
15		33.5	35.7	42.1	47.0	55.9	69.0	100.8	146.1
16		32.3	35.4	40.4	44.6	53.3	63.1	79.4	126.7
17		32.3	35.4	39.5	44.7	53.3	62.4	79.4	107.8
18–19		31.5	34.3	41.7	47.6	57.0	70.3	87.3	109.3
20–25		35.0	40.9	48.1	57.8	71.5	89.0	109.0	130.0
25–30		38.3	45.5	54.5	66.8	81.8	99.5	119.3	144.0
30–35		41.9	49.8	60.3	72.2	87.3	103.9	121.3	145.5
35–40		43.9	53.0	62.3	73.9	88.1	102.5	121.9	143.0
40–45		46.0	53.9	64.2	74.6	87.5	102.5	121.0	142.5
45–50		44.7	55.2	64.8	76.3	90.5	106.8	123.4	147.0
50–55		47.2	56.3	66.3	75.7	87.8	105.0	121.0	140.0
55–60		46.9	56.8	65.8	76.4	87.5	101.1	115.9	136.0
60–65		47.3	53.9	64.8	74.5	87.2	98.3	116.8	134.3
65–70		43.0	53.0	60.5	71.6	84.3	92.9	104.8	121.5

Source: Ward et al. 1989

*Proportional sum of six skinfolds (mm).

#Individual adiposity ratings are determined from nine standard intervals (stanines) which provide divisions at the percentile equivalents of P4, 11, 23, 40, 60, 77, 89 and 96.

The W rating is determined by geometrically scaling the subject's weight to a common height in order to produce a proportional weight (pWT) as follows:

$$pWT = WT (170.18/H)^3$$

where: WT = the subject's weight (kg)
H = the subject's height (cm)

The W rating is then determined by reference to normative data (Ward et al. 1989).

When used in combination, the A and W ratings provide a significant description of the physique and composition of the individual. The A rating indicates 'fatness' with respect to the same age and gender and may be used for intra-individual comparisons over time. The W rating is a ponderosity index and together with the A rating may be used to indicate musculo-skeletal development. A software package is available for personal computers which also includes bone breadths, girths and corrected girths to indicate musculo-skeletal development (Ward et al. 1989). The system was intended to replace prediction of per cent body fat and so does not require the assumption of any biological constraints. A more detailed explanation of the O-Scale system has been reported by Whittingham et al. (1992).

The Oz-scale system is based on the O-scale system but uses Australian normative data and some differences in scaling procedures (Norton et al. 1996). The data required for this system are six skinfolds (triceps, subscapular, biceps, supraspinale, abdominal and calf skinfolds), height, weight, relaxed arm girth, hip girth and waist girth. LifeSize software package (Olds et al. 1994) is available for personal computers and includes calculation of somatotype, percentage body fat and technical error of measurement, in addition to the Oz-scale printout.

4.5 SUMMARY

When evaluating the indirect methodologies available to assess body composition in athletes, a value judgement needs to be made as to the 'best' technique for the particular application. Clearly, indices of height and weight are not appropriate for assessing athletes. In most instances (for those with the required level of skill), anthropometry will provide a useful method of monitoring body composition. These values should not be transformed into estimates of percentage body fat using regression equations since they were based on selected population groups and can only reliably be applied to that group. The individual skinfold values can be summed and compared to normative data or used in the O-scale or Oz-scale computer-based systems. When interpreting any anthropometric or body composition data it is important to be aware of the underlying assumptions and the limitations discussed.

4.6 PRACTICE TIPS

Deborah Kerr and Tim Ackland

ASSESSING PHYSIQUE

- It is essential that the anthropometrist is sensitive to the potential psychological impact of anthropometric assessment on the athlete. Many athletes are preoccupied with their BM and skinfolds. They can be sensitive to comments about their BM from coaches, parents, and especially peers. For this reason, anthropometric assessment should be done in private. Anthropometrists need to be aware of an athlete's response to either the measurement process itself or the results of the total sum of skinfolds. Some athletes are overly concerned about the results, which could be an indication of body image disturbances or a more serious underlying eating disorder. Individual data should be kept confidential and not discussed or displayed publicly. In practice when doing skinfolds on teams, it can be a good idea not to give the athletes their final skinfold sum so that comparisons between individuals can be avoided.

Choice of method to assess physique and body composition

- Dietitians are mostly interested in assessing changes in body composition in athletes in response to training and dietary intervention rather than physique assessment. For individuals, anthropometry measures (including height, BM, skinfolds, girths and often wrist circumferences) are often used. Skinfold measures are used routinely in elite sports programs to provide an estimate of the subcutaneous adipose tissue mass. Usually six skinfold sites (but preferably eight) are taken (tricep, subscapular, supraspinale, abdominal, front thigh and medial calf) using the Oz-scale or O-scale system of measurement (see Section 4.6). Girths and skinfold-corrected girths using the O-scale system software provide an estimate of relative muscularity. These are useful to measure body composition changes in athletes at the beginning and end of a strength training or weight loss program.

Protocol and accreditation in anthropometry

- The recommended measurement protocol is that endorsed by The International Society for the Advancement of Kinanthropometry (ISAK). Definitions of the anthropometric sites have been defined by Ross and Marfell-Jones (1991), Blooomfield et al. (1994) and Norton and Olds (1996). This protocol is taught in the Anthropometry Accreditation Courses and is endorsed within Australia by the Laboratory Standards Assistance Scheme of the Australian Sports Commission. It is recommended that dietitians wishing to take skinfolds on athletes should become accredited in anthropometry. Accreditation courses are run on a regular basis throughout Australia, Canada and New Zealand.

Equipment
Skinfold calipers

- The Harpenden skinfold caliper is the instrument of choice for taking skinfold measurements. The inexpensive Slimguide calipers have the same jaw pressure as the Harpenden caliper and produce almost identical results (Schmidt & Carter 1990).

Anthropometry tapes

- The Lufkin (W606PM) is the preferred tape. This is a flexible metal tape calibrated in centimetres with automatic retraction.

Minimising error in anthropometry

- With training and continual practice, anthropometry can provide accurate and useful data on physique. It is recommended that a minimum of two sets (ideally three) of measurements be taken and the mean of two scores or median (middle) score recorded. Determining the technical error of measurement (TEM) and comparing it to the recommended measurement tolerances, as outlined by Norton et al. (1996), can assess measurement error. Anthropometrists can minimise measurement error by:

  — undertaking accredited training in anthropometry;
  — using a standard protocol;
  — repeating measurements (double or triple measures);
  — using standard equipment; and
  — assessing measurement error (TEM).

ASSESSING AND INTERPRETING ANTHROPOMETRIC DATA

- Once the anthropometric data has been collected on an athlete the next step is interpretation. This requires an understanding of the specific requirements for the sport or team position and the current phase of training. Changes in body composition should always be monitored in relation to performance increments or decrements. It is also important to combine the anthropometric data in relation to the dietary assessment collected by the dietitian. For example, if an athlete has a high skinfold sum and wishes to reduce it then the dietitian needs to assess the current energy intake. Athletes usually have a preferred competition weight or skinfold level. It is unrealistic and unnecessary to attempt to maintain this level throughout the year. Large fluctuations, however, should be avoided. It is also important to assess the athlete's goals for weight and skinfold sum and how realistic these goals are in terms of an individual's physique and genetics. An athlete may already have reduced their energy intake under the guidance of the dietitian but still not achieved the desired reduction in the skinfold sum. If this occurs it may be necessary to adjust the aerobic output. It is essential, however, that this is discussed with the coach and exercise scientist to determine if increasing aerobic output and hence energy expenditure is consistent with the athlete's training goals.

- The skinfold sum may be compared to normative data for elite athletes to provide the athlete with a comparison, but providing such information to a weight-sensitive athlete can be psychologically traumatic and best avoided. Skinfolds in individuals can be tracked over time. The O-Scale computer program or LifeSize (see Section 4.4.2) provides a printout of comparisons with normative data as well as changes in individual data over time.

Targets for skinfolds

- Published values for skinfolds of elite athletes should be used as a guide only and not used to determine a skinfold 'cut-off' for an individual athlete. Such definitive values do not account for individual genetic variability and may not be applicable to recreational athletes. It is also important to explain to the athlete who does not meet elite skinfold values that body composition is only one factor contributing to performance. For some athletes, achieving the 'ideal' skinfold sum may require a severe restriction of their energy intake and may never be achievable.

- The rate of weight loss in relation to reduction in skinfold sum shows individual variation. As a general guide, at higher skinfolds (> 80 mm for sum of seven sites) a one kilogram weight loss will be equivalent to a ten millimetre loss from the total skinfold sum. At lower skinfold sum (< 80 mm for sum of seven sites) a one kilogram weight loss is approximately equivalent to five millimetres of fat loss. This can be used as a guide in determining if a particular weight category is possible. It should be remembered, however, that not all athletes will follow this pattern. Changes in skinfold compressibility may occur with weight loss and athletes may lose body fat from sites not identified with skinfold calipers.

ANTHROPOMETRIC SOFTWARE

O-Scale Physique Assessment System is available from:
Rosscraft
PO Box 2043
Blaine, WA
USA 98231

Tel (604) 531 5049   Fax (604) 538 3362
E-mail: billross@netcom.ca

LifeSize Computer Package is available from Human Kinetics:
Human Kinetics Australia
PO Box 80
Torrens Park
SA 5062
Order: liahka@senet.com.au

Purchasing anthropometric equipment

Anthropometric equipment (Slimguide calipers, small bone caliper, anthropometric tape, full anthropometric kit) can be purchased from Rosscraft at the above address.

REFERENCES

Ackland TR, Blanksby BA, Bloomfield J. Physical growth and motor performance of adolescent males. In: Blanksby BA et al., eds. Athletics, growth and development in children. Chur, Switzerland: Harwood Academic Publishers, 1994:200–15.

Ackland TR, Schreiner AB, Kerr DA. Absolute size and proportionality characteristics of world championship female basketball players. J Sports Sci 1997a;15:485–90.

Ackland TR, Schreiner AB, Kerr DA. Technical note: anthropometric normative data for female international basketball players. Aust J Sci Med Sports 1997b:29:24–6.

Ackland TR, Blanksby BA, Landers G, Smith D. Anthropometric profiles of elite triathletes. J Sci Med Sport 1998;1:51–6.

Adams J, Mottola M, Bagnall KM, McFadden KD. Total fat content in a group of professional football players. Can J Appl Sp Sci 1982;7:36–44.

Bailey DA, Carter JEL, Mirwald RL. Somatotypes of Canadian men and women. Hum Biol 1982;54:813–28.

Behnke AR, Feen BG, Welham WC. The specific gravity of healthy men. JAMA 1942;118:495–8.

Bloomfield J, Ackland TR, Elliott BC. Applied anatomy and biomechanics in sport. Carlton, Victoria: Blackwell Scientific Publications, 1994:65–78.

Bouchard C, Perusse C, Leblanc C, et al. Inheritance of the amount and distribution of human body fat. Int J Obesity 1988;12:205–15.

Brodie D, Moscrip V, Hutcheon R. Body composition measurement: a review of hydrodensitometry, anthropometry, and impedance methods. Nutrition 1998;14:296–310.

Brozek J. The measurement of body composition. In: Montagu MFA, ed. A handbook of anthropometry. Springfield: Charles C Thomas, 1960.

Buskirk ER. Underwater weighing and body density: a review of procedures. In: Brozek J, Henschel A, eds. Techniques for measuring body composition. Washington DC: National Academy of Sciences, 1961:90–105.

Carter JEL, ed. Physical structure of Olympic athletes: Part II, Kinanthropometry of Olympic athletes. Basel, Switzerland: Karger, 1984.

Carter JEL, Ackland TR, eds. Kinanthropometry in Aquatic Sports. Champaign, Illinois: Human Kinetics, 1994.

Carter JEL, Aubrey SP, Sleet DA. Somatotypes of Montreal Olympic Athletes. In: Carter JEL, ed. Physical Structure of Olympic athletes: Part 1, Montreal Olympic Games Anthropological Project. Basel, Switzerland: Karger, 1982:53–80.

Carter JEL, Honeyman Heath B. Somatotyping—development and applications. Cambridge, Great Britain: Cambridge University Press, 1990.

Clarys JP, Martin AD, Drinkwater DT. Gross tissue weights in the human body by cadaver dissection. Hum Biol 1984;56:459–73.

DeRose EH, Crawford SM, Kerr DA, Ward R, Ross WD. Physique characteristics of Pan American Games lightweight rowers. Int J Sports Med 1989;10:292–7.

Faulkner F, Tanner JM. Human Growth, 2nd edn, 3 vols. New York: Plenum Press, 1978.

Forbes RM, Cooper AR, Mitchell HH. The composition of the adult human body as determined by chemical analysis. J Biol Chem 1953;203:359–66.

Friedl KE, DeLuca JP, Marchitelli LJ, Vogel JA. Reliability of body-fat estimations from a four-compartment model by using density, body water, and bone mineral measurements. Am J Clin Nutr 1992;55:764–70.

Guo S, Roche AE, Chumlea WC, Miles DS, Pholman Rl. Body composition predictions from bioelectrical conductivity. Hum Biol 1987;59:221–33.

Harrison GG. The measurement of total body electrical conductivity. Hum Biol 1987;59:311–17.

Heymsfield SB, Lichtman S, Baumgartner RN. Body composition of humans: comparison of two improved four-compartment models that differ in expense, technical complexity, and radiation exposure. Am J Clin Nutr 1990;52:52–8.

Hutcheson L, Latin R, Berg K, Prentice E. Body impedance analysis and body water loss. Res Quart Exerc Sport 1988;59:359–62.

Jebb SA, Elia M. Techniques for the measurement of body composition: a practical guide. Int J Obes 1993;17:611–621.

Jensen MD, Kanaley JA, Roust LR, et al. Assessment of body composition with use of dual-energy X-ray absorptiometry: evaluation and comparison with other methods. Mayo Clinic Proceedings 1993;68:867–73.

Johansson C, Mellstrom D, Rosengren K, Rundgren A. Prevalence of vertebral fractures in 85-year-olds. Acta Orthop Scand 1993;64:25–7.

Johnston FE. Relationships between body composition and anthropometry. Hum Biol 1982;54:221–45.

Jones PRM, Corlett J. Some factors affecting the calculation of human body density: bone mineralisation. In: Ostyn MG, Beunen G, Simons J, eds. Kinanthropometry II. Baltimore, Maryland: University Park Press, 1980.

Keys A, Brozek J. Body fat in adult man. Physiol Rev 1953;33:245–325.

Kohrt WM. Body composition by DXA: tried and true? Med Sci Sports Exerc 1995;27:1349–53.

Lohman TG. Skinfolds and body density and their relationship to body fatness: a review. Hum Biol 1981;53:181–225.

Lohman TG. Advances in body composition assessment. Champaign, Illinois: Human Kinetics Publishers, 1992.

Malina R. Bioelectrical methods for estimating body composition: an overview and discussion. Hum Biol 1987;59:329–35.

Marshall W. Puberty. In: Falkner F, Tanner J, eds. Human growth, Vol 2. London: Bailliere Tindall, 1978:141–78.

Martin AD, Drinkwater DT. Variability in the measures of body fat. Sports Med 1991;1:277–88.

Martin AD, Ross WD, Drinkwater DT, Clarys JP. Prediction of body fat by skinfold caliper: assumptions and cadaver evidence. Int J Obesity 1985;9(S1):31–9.

Mazess RB, Peppler WW, Gibbons M. Total body composition by dual-photon (153Gd) absorptiometry. Am J Clin Nutr 1984;40:834–9.

Mitchell HH, Hamilton TS, Steggerda FR, Bean HW. The chemical composition of the adult human body and its bearing on the biochemistry of growth. J Biol Chem 1945;158:625–37.

Norton K, Whittingham N, Carter L, Kerr D, Gore C, Marfell-Jones M. Measurement techniques in anthropometry. In: Norton K, Olds T, eds. Anthropometrica, Sydney: University of New South Wales Press, 1996:25–75.

Olds TS, Ly SV, Norton KI. LifeSize Computer Software. Sydney: Nolds Sports Scientific, 1994.

Quetelet A. A treatise on man and the development of his faculties. Edinburgh: Chambers, 1842.

Roche AF, Heymsfield SB, Lohman TG, eds. Human body composition. Champaign, Illinois: Human Kinetics, 1996.

Ross WD, Crawford SM, Kerr DA, Ward R, Bailey DA, Mirwald RM. Relationship of the body mass index with skinfolds, girths, and bone breadths in Canadian men and women aged 20–70 years. Am J Phys Anthr 1988b;77:169–73.

Ross WD, De Rose EH, Ward R. Anthropometry applied to sports medicine. In: Dirix A, Knuttgen HG, Tittel K, eds. The Olympic book of sports medicine. London: Blackwell, 1988a.

Ross WD, Marfell-Jones MJ. Kinanthropometry. In: MacDougall JD, Wenger HA, Green HJ, eds. The physiological assessment of high performance athletes. Champaign, Illinois: Human Kinetics, 1991.

Ross WD, Ward R. Proportionality of Olympic athletes. In: Carter JEL, ed. Physical structure of Olympic athletes: Part II, Kinanthropometry of Olympic athletes. Basel, Switzerland: Karger, 1984:110–43.

Ross WD, Wilson NC. A stratagem for proportional growth assessment. Acta Paediatrica Belgica 1974;28(suppl):169–82.

Schmidt PK, Carter JEL. Static and dynamic differences among five types of skinfold calipers. Hum Biol 1990;62:369–88.

Segal K, Gutin B, Presta E, Wang J, Van Itallie T. Estimation of human body composition by electrical impedance methods: a comparative study. J Appl Physiol 1985;58:1565–71.

Siri WE. Body composition from fluid spaces and density: analysis of methods. In: Brozek J, Henshel A, eds. Techniques for measuring body composition. Washington, DC: National Academy of Sciences, 1961:223–44.

Svendsen OL, Haarbo J, Hassager C, Christiansen C. Accuracy of measurements of body composition by dual-energy X-ray absorptiometry in vivo. Am J Clin Nutr 1993;57:605–8.

Tittel K. Tasks and tendencies of sport anthropometry's development. In: Landry F, Orban WA, eds. Biomechanics of sport and kinanthropometry. Miami: Symposia Specialists, 1978:283–96.

van Itallie TB, Abraham S. Some hazards of obesity and its treatment. In: Hirsch J, van Itallie TB, eds. Recent advances in obesity research IV. London: Libbey, 1985.

Van Loan MD, Mayclin PL. Body composition assessment: dual energy X-ray absorptiometry (DEXA) compared to reference methods. Eur J Clin Nutr 1992;46:125–30.

Wang J, Heymsfield SB, Aulet M, Thornton JC, Pierson RN. Body fat from body density: underwater weighing vs. dual-photon absorptiometry. Am J Physiol 1989;256:E829–34.

Ward R, Ross WD, Leyland AJ, Selbie S. The advanced O-scale physique assessment system. Burnaby, Canada: Kinemetrix Inc, 1989.

Whittingham NO. Anthropometric prototypes for boys and girls aged 6 to 18, exemplified by structure analyses of sub-12 year old figure skaters. Unpublished Masters Thesis. Canada: Simon Fraser University, 1978.

Whittingham NO, Ward R, Ross WD. A computer based physique assessment system. Aust J Sci Med Sport 1992;24:39–43.

Wilmore JH. A simplified method for determination of residual lung volumes. J Appl Physiol 1969;27:96–100.

Wilmore JH, Costill DL. Training for sport and activity: the physiological basis of the conditioning process, 3rd edn. Dubuque, Iowa: WC Brown, 1988.

Woolford S, Bourdon P, Craig N, Stanef T. Body composition and its effects on athletic performance. Sports Coach 1993;16:24–30.

CHAPTER 5

Protein and amino acid needs for training and bulking up

Mark Tarnopolsky

5.1 INTRODUCTION

Strength-training athletes have traditionally assumed that a very high protein diet is essential to the promotion of muscle hypertrophy. This concept may be traced to ancient Olympic times where records indicated that athletes consumed inordinate amounts of meat (Harris 1966). In the 18th century, it was felt that muscle contraction was fuelled by protein oxidation (von Liebig 1842). Eventually, the importance of lipid and carbohydrate (CHO) oxidation in muscle metabolism became apparent and the central role of protein oxidation in the supply of energy to muscle waned (Cathcart 1925). During much of the past 50 years there has been debate as to whether physical activity alters the dietary requirement for protein. This chapter shall review the pathways of protein metabolism in skeletal muscle with emphasis on the effect(s) of exercise on pathway regulation. I shall then examine methods to assess the adequacy of dietary protein intakes and review studies that have attempted to determine whether athletes require an increase in dietary protein intake. Throughout the text I shall broadly classify exercise as either 'endurance' or 'resistance' to highlight the two major classifications of exercise that are at the opposite ends of the spectrum with respect to metabolic demand. For example, most persons involved in resistance-type exercise desire strength, power and an increase in muscle mass as outcomes, whereas the endurance athlete seeks metabolic adaptations that enhance long duration power output (i.e. high oxygen consumption and low per cent body fat). Obviously, a given sport may have different proportions of strength and endurance and the athlete and coach must decide how the literature review and recommendations put forth in this chapter are to be applied.

5.2 PROTEIN METABOLISM

Proteins are critical molecules that serve structural and regulatory functions in the human body. Structural proteins include cytoskeletal proteins such as desmin and connective tissue proteins such as collagen, whereas regulatory proteins include enzymes such as lactate dehydrogenase or carbonic anhydrase. Proteins are comprised of amino acids (AA)—compounds containing an amino group ($-NH_2$), a carboxylic acid group ($-COOH$), and a radical group (different for each of the amino acids). There are 20 amino acids that are found bound to proteins or present as free amino acids. Of these amino acids, nine are considered essential (histidine, isoleucine, leucine, lysine, methionine, phenylalanine, threonine, tryptophan, valine) (Pellet 1990). These nine indispensable amino acids must come from the diet and/or from endogenous protein breakdown (for obvious reasons the latter is only a temporising measure). Because proteins serve such a critical role in the survival of the organism, it is not surprising that their metabolism is complex and tightly regulated. The concepts of protein metabolism are extremely intricate and incompletely understood. For this reason, I shall focus on basic and generally accepted concepts that serve to allow for an understanding of protein nutrition under periods of increased metabolic demand (i.e. exercise).

5.2.1 Protein synthesis

Protein synthesis starts with a signal (i.e. nutrient, hormone, mechanical) that induces gene expression. In general, it is considered that each gene ultimately directs the synthesis of one protein. Gene expression begins when a signal is transduced to the nucleus of the cell and binds to regulatory regions on DNA that are in close proximity to the gene. These promoters and enhancers initiate a process called transcription where a messenger RNA (mRNA) is formed from the gene template. Transcription is initiated with a start codon and terminated with a stop codon. The primary transcript is modified by splicing out non-coding regions of the gene called introns and is further processed by capping at the 5' end and polyadenylation at the 3' end. Each amino acid in a given protein is ultimately derived from a 3-DNA base region called a codon. Once in the cytosol, the mRNA is translated into a protein through the process of translation via ribosomes (free in the cytosol or bound to rough endoplasmic reticulum). The process of translation requires a second form of RNA, called transfer RNA (tRNA). The tRNAs are combined with their respective amino acids via specific tRNA syntheses to form amino-tRNA complexes (e.g. leucyl-tRNA, histidinyl-tRNA). Within the ribosome 'scaffolding', the mRNA codons are 'read' by the specific tRNAs to form an amino acid. The process of translation requires three distinct steps termed: initiation, elongation and termination (of the protein). There are a series of simple reviews in the *New England Journal of Medicine* starting with an introduction in the July 7 issue that summarises the aforementioned processes (Rosenthal 1994).

These protein synthetic processes can be broadly divided into four sites of potential regulation: transcriptional (i.e. promoter region binding), post-transcriptional (i.e. mRNA stability, poly-adenylation), translational (i.e. tRNA charging, speed and efficiency of translation), and post-translational (i.e. nascent protein stability, glycosylation, degradation). Exercise is a potent physiological stress that ultimately results in an adaptive response in the cell (i.e. resistance exercise results in an increase in myosin accumulation). Although this is well known by any body builder, the fundamental regulation of these processes is complex and is only just being understood. We have found that protein synthesis is increased in human skeletal muscle within four hours of exercise, with no changes in total RNA (Chesley et al. 1992). We considered that this observation represented post-transcriptional regulation (Chesley et al. 1992). More definitive evidence for translational or post-translational regulation of muscle protein synthesis following resistance exercise came from Welle and colleagues (1999) who recently found increases in muscle protein synthesis with no changes in myosin mRNA content. Others have shown that myosin mRNA increases following a more prolonged training stimulus (Morgan and Loughna 1989), which suggested pre-translational control.

The relationship between exercise and nutrition and these fundamental aspects of protein synthesis remain to be explored more fully. Clearly, there is the potential that a progressive adaptation to an exercise stimulus (training) will alter the relative importance of transcriptional and translational control and this may impact on amino acid requirements. Although exercise-induced training adaptations ultimately result in net protein synthesis, the amino acids for this process may be derived from an increase in dietary intake and/or an increase in the efficiency of amino acid re-utilisation.

5.2.2 *Amino acid oxidation/protein breakdown*

Human skeletal muscle can oxidise at least eight amino acids (alanine, asparagine, aspartate, glutamate, isoleucine, leucine, lysine and valine) (Goldberg & Chang 1978; Wolfe et al. 1984). During exercise, it appears that the branched-chain amino acids (BCAA: isoleucine, leucine, and valine) are preferentially oxidised (Goldberg & Chang 1978; MacLean et al. 1991).

Given the predominance of BCAA oxidation during exercise, it is important to understand the regulation of this pathway. BCAA are transaminated to their keto-acid analogues by branched-chain aminotransferase (BCAAT), and the resultant keto-acid is oxidised by branched-chain oxo-acid dehydrogenase enzyme (BCOAD) (Khatra et al. 1977; Boyer & Odessey 1991). In the cytosol, the amino-N group is usually transaminated with α-ketoglutarate to form glutamate, which is in turn transaminated with pyruvate to form alanine (Wolfe et al. 1984) or aminated via glutamine synthase to form glutamine. Some of the amino-N may end up as free ammonia released from muscle, however, during high-intensity contractions most of the ammonia comes from the myoadenylate deaminase pathway (MacLean et al. 1991; Wagenmakers et al. 1991).

The BCOAD enzyme is rate-limiting in BCAA oxidation (Khatra et al. 1977; Boyer & Odessey 1991). At rest, the per cent of BCOAD that is in the active form is about 5–8% and this increases to 20–25% during exercise (Wagenmakers et al. 1989; McKenzie et al. 2000). This activation is thought to be related to a decrease in the ATP/ADP ratio, an increase in intra-muscular acidity, and a depletion of muscle glycogen (Kasperek 1989; Wagenmakers et al. 1991). The inverse correlation between branched-chain keto-acid dehydrogenase enzyme (BCKAD) per cent activation and muscle glycogen concentration (Wagenmakers et al. 1989, 1991) provides a theoretical basis for CHO loading to attenuate BCKAD-mediated amino acid oxidation during endurance exercise (hence attenuating an increase in protein requirements in athletes). We have recently shown that the provision of glucose drinks (1 g/kg body mass (BM) per hour) during endurance exercise significantly reduced urea output (Partington et al. unpublished observations 1999).

Protein degradation is the process of breaking down the proteins into their constituent amino acids. These amino acids contribute to the intra-cellular free amino acid pool, which may be exported into the plasma, directly oxidised, or re-incorporated back into tissue protein (synthesis). Although most athletes think only of maximising protein synthesis, it is equally logical to try to attenuate degradation. After all, net protein balance is a function of synthesis minus degradation. Therefore, a body builder can achieve net protein retention by decreasing degradation and not changing synthesis.

The three main pathways for protein degradation in human skeletal muscle include the lysosomal and non-lysosomal (ubiquitin and calpain) pathways. The lysosomal pathway degrades endocytosed proteins, some cytosolic proteins, hormones and immune modulators (Mitch & Goldberg 1996). This pathway is not a major contributor to human skeletal muscle protein degradation (Lowell et al. 1986), except when there is significant muscle damage and inflammation (Tidball 1995). The two major non-lysosomal pathways in human skeletal muscle are the ATP-dependent ubiquitin pathway (Mitch & Goldberg 1996), and the calcium-activated neutral protease or calpain pathway (Kameyama & Etlinger 1979; Zeman et al. 1985; Belcastro 1993).

The calpain pathway is felt to play a role in skeletal muscle proteolysis during exercise (Belcastro 1993). The ubiquitin pathway is activated after the targeting of proteins for degradation (i.e. oxidative modification). Following targeting, ubiquitin molecules are linked to lysine residues through a series of pathways catalysed by three enzymes, termed E1, E2, and E3, and are then degraded by the 26S proteosome into peptides (Mitch & Goldberg 1996). This pathway is activated during starvation and muscle atrophy (Medina et al. 1995), and its role in exercise-induced muscle protein breakdown is currently being investigated by several groups, including ourselves.

5.2.3 *Models and measurement of protein turnover*

The amino acids found in the plasma can come from dietary intake (I), protein breakdown (B), and in the case of dispensable amino acids, *de novo* synthesis.

Amino acids can be removed from the plasma, either for protein synthesis (S), oxidation (O), or incorporation into other metabolic pathways after transamination/deamination. For an indispensable amino acid such as leucine, the only sources to enter the body are from I or B. Leucine is also completely oxidised in the human body to CO_2, allowing the measurement of O as well. Therefore, if an amino acid such as leucine is used to study metabolism, the flux (Q) is equal to intake + breakdown, which is in turn equal to synthesis + oxidation (Q = I + B = S + O). This simple model is helpful in the measurement of protein turnover (flux), since amino acid tracers can be used to measure Q and O, and if intake equals zero, then Q = B, and by subtraction, S = Q − O (Tarnopolsky et al. 1992). Isotope studies are used to derive these variables of protein turnover. Isotopes are molecules that share the same atomic number (protons), yet have different numbers of neutrons (atomic mass). Stable isotopes occur naturally and do not emit ionising radiation, whereas radioactive isotopes undergo spontaneous decay. For this reason stable isotopes have become very popular in exercise research (i.e. Tarnopolsky et al. 1991, 1992; Phillips et al. 1993; Tipton et al. 1999; McKenzie et al. 2000). Although useful, this model is very simplistic in that there are multiple pools of amino acids that are turning over at very different rates.

There are many other models of protein turnover at the whole body and tissue level. At the most basic level would be the balance between all protein intake and excretion. This protein balance can be measured using nitrogen balance (NBAL) methods. With the NBAL method the investigator measures all of the nitrogen intake (diet and intravenous) and output (urine, faeces, sweat, and miscellaneous) and calculates a balance. If the balance is positive, the person is in a state of net retention and if it is negative, the person is in a state of net depletion. The measurement of nitrogen is based on the fact that proteins are about 16% nitrogen by weight. Using arteriovenous catheters one can also measure the amino acid balance across a limb, and (with stable isotopic infusions) measure amino acid transport, muscle protein synthesis and breakdown (Biolo et al. 1995; Ferrando et al. 1998; Tipton et al. 1999). Another method to measure protein synthesis is the fractional synthetic rate (FSR). This requires the infusion of an isotope and the measurement of the incremental increase in enrichment into a tissue over time. We, and others, have used muscle biopsies to look at mixed skeletal muscle FSR after exercise with this method (Chesley et al. 1992; Phillips et al. 1997). Myofibrillar and mitochondrial FSR can now be determined using stable isotopic tracer incorporation in combination with a gel separation of the component proteins (Balagopal et al. 1997).

Finally, a major limitation in the understanding of protein turnover has been the lack of a good method to measure muscle protein breakdown. Initially, there was much enthusiasm for the use of 3-methylhistidine (3-MH), which is a post-translational modification of histidine residues in the actin and myosin of skeletal muscle (Young & Munro 1978; Rathmacher et al. 1995). This method requires accurate urinary collections and assumes that most of the 3-MH arises from skeletal myofibrillar proteolysis and that the proportional contribution from other sources relative to muscle remains constant under varying physiological situations (Young & Munro 1978). These limitations are not as much of an issue in crossover studies where the subject is his or her own control, yet the collection is still an issue. A method for the determination of mixed muscle fractional breakdown rate (FBR) using a stable isotopic decay kinetic method has recently been demonstrated in the laboratory of Wolfe and colleagues (Phillips et al. 1997).

It is important to understand the theories and limitations of the model that is used in any study of protein metabolism during exercise. In this way, the reader can understand the validity of the conclusions drawn from the results. A more detailed examination of the limitations of protein and tracer methodology can be found in reviews and texts (Wolfe 1992).

5.3 THE EFFECT OF EXERCISE ON PROTEIN METABOLISM

5.3.1 The effect of acute endurance exercise on amino acid oxidation

The majority of the energy for endurance exercise is derived from the oxidation of lipid and CHO (Table 5.1). As mentioned above, skeletal muscle has the metabolic capacity to oxidise certain amino acids for energy. It is counterproductive to oxidise proteins during exercise since they serve either a structural (i.e. cytoskeletal proteins) or functional (i.e. actin, myosin, succinate dehydrogenase or phosphorylase) role. Amino acid oxidation may be required for exchange reactions in the tricarboxylic acid cycle, and this may increase their net utilisation (Gibala et al. 1997).

Table 5.1 *Energy requirements during a one-hour run at 65–75% of $VO_{2\,max}$*

	Energy (kcal/h)	% fat	% protein	% CHO
Males*	838 (125)	23 (18)	5 (3)	72 (17)
Females	623 (32)	39 (16)	1.5 (1)	59 (17)

Males are different from females in all variables (P < 0.01). Values are mean (SD) from 28 females and 27 males pooled data
(Tarnopolsky et al. 1990; Phillips et al. 1993; Tarnopolsky et al. 1995; and Tarnopolsky et al. 1997)

Initial studies looked at urea excretion as an indicator of protein oxidation (urea is a breakdown product formed in the liver following amino acid oxidation). Several studies found that urinary urea excretion was higher following endurance exercise as compared to rest (Tarnopolsky et al. 1990; Lemon 1998). Studies have also shown that a significant amount of urea is excreted in the sweat during exercise (Lemon & Mullin 1980; Tarnopolsky et al. 1988). Therefore, a person exercising in high ambient temperatures and/or humidity would be expected to have a high urea sweat loss that may contribute to a more negative protein balance. Studies of urea excretion provide only indirect evidence for amino acid oxidation and in some cases do not correlate well with direct measures of amino acid oxidation (Wolfe et al. 1984).

A number of studies have demonstrated that endurance exercise resulted in an increase in leucine oxidation (Rennie et al. 1981; Hagg et al. 1982; Wolfe et al. 1982; Evans et al. 1983; Wolfe et al. 1984; Phillips et al. 1993; McKenzie et al. 2000). Leucine oxidation during endurance exercise shows a positive correlation with exercise intensity (Lemon et al. 1982). Leucine oxidation (Phillips et al. 1993; McKenzie et al. 2000) and plasma urea content (Haralambie & Berg 1976) also increase with exercise duration. Finally, leucine oxidation increases with glycogen depletion, which may partially explain the increase with exercise duration (Wagenmakers et al. 1991). Following endurance exercise, there is a rapid return towards baseline in the elevated leucine oxidation (Phillips et al. 1993). There may be a slight increase in leucine oxidation that persists for up to ten days following eccentric exercise (Fielding et al. 1991). This may partially explain why nitrogen balance is negative at the onset of unaccustomed endurance exercise, yet becomes more positive as the person adapts to the stress (Gontzea et al. 1975).

Clearly, there is an increase in amino acid oxidation during endurance exercise. This may account for 3–6% of the total energy cost of a given exercise bout (Table 5.1). The increase in amino acid oxidation with exercise has been shown with leucine and lysine tracers, yet very few other amino acids have been studied. These results cannot be extrapolated to other amino acids or an intact protein. If only a few of the amino acids are oxidised during endurance exercise, then the predicted effect on protein requirements may be minimal. Conversely, an increase in indispensable amino acid oxidation (i.e. leucine) may affect protein requirements since it can only come from dietary intake and/or protein breakdown.

5.3.2 *The effect of acute resistance exercise on protein synthesis and breakdown*

In contrast to endurance exercise, we have shown that acute, whole-body resistance exercise does not alter leucine oxidation (Tarnopolsky et al. 1991). In this same study we also did not find any effect of acute resistance exercise on whole body protein synthesis, either during exercise or for up to two hours post-exercise (Tarnopolsky et al. 1991). We reasoned that since muscle protein synthesis (MPS) accounted for only 25% of whole body synthesis (Nair et al. 1988), changes in MPS may be either not measurable, or would be negated by a reciprocal change in the synthesis of another protein (i.e. gut).

To measure the acute effect of resistance exercise on muscle protein synthesis, we decided to use the fractional synthetic rate (FSR) tracer incorporation method described above. We demonstrated that mixed muscle FSR was elevated for up to

36 hours following a single bout of resistance exercise (Chesley et al. 1992; Mac-Dougall et al. 1995). Other groups have also shown the increase in muscle protein synthesis after resistance exercise using FSR (Phillips et al. 1997) and arteriovenous balance or tracer (Biolo et al. 1995) methods. Phillips and colleagues (1997) demonstrated that FSR was elevated for up to 48 hours after a single bout of resistance exercise in both males and females. Investigators have also found an increase in post-exercise FSR in the elderly (Yarasheski et al. 1993; Welle et al. 1993). Finally, we have found that resting whole body protein synthesis is greater in well-trained strength athletes as compared to sedentary controls (Tarnopolsky et al. 1992).

Studies have also measured protein breakdown after resistance exercise using the intra-cellular tracer dilution (Phillips et al. 1997) and the arteriovenous balance or tracer (Biolo et al. 1995) methods. Phillips and colleagues (1997) demonstrated that fractional protein breakdown (FBR) was increased after resistance exercise, yet the magnitude of the increase was less than for FSR (i.e. the muscle was in a more positive balance). Furthermore, they showed that FBR returned to baseline values before FSR (Phillips et al. 1997). Biolo and co-workers (1995) found that muscle synthesis and breakdown were increased following an acute bout of resistance exercise. The net balance (synthesis minus degradation) was negative prior to exercise and was more positive (but still net negative) after exercise, for the subjects were in the fasted state.

Taken together, these data indicate that muscle FSR and FBR are increased in the post-exercise period following resistance exercise. In the fasted state, net protein balance is negative, and resistance exercise renders the muscle in a less negative balance. Therefore, the post-exercise time period may be an important time for the delivery of nutrients, as discussed below.

5.3.3 *The effect of exercise training on protein metabolism*

Chronic endurance-exercise training might be expected to achieve adaptations that would attenuate the oxidation of protein for energy. This would be predicted based on the sparing of muscle glycogen that accompanies chronic endurance training (causing lower BCOAD activation). Early work by Gontzea (1975) showed that untrained persons who started endurance training were in a negative nitrogen balance, but as they continued to train the nitrogen balance became less negative. Animal data have yielded conflicting results, with some studies showing that training increased amino acid oxidation (Dohm et al. 1977; Henderson et al. 1985), and another finding showed a reduction in the contribution of leucine to total energy consumption (Hood & Terjung 1987).

To date, human data have not yielded a consistent answer to this issue. Following endurance-exercise training, whole body protein synthesis at rest is increased (Evans et al. 1983; Lamont et al. 1990). There is also a greater proportion of leucine flux at rest diverted towards oxidation in the untrained versus trained athlete (Lamont et al. 1990). However, differences in leucine turnover between trained and untrained subjects disappeared when the data were expressed relative to lean mass (Lamont et al. 1999). These findings are not consistent with the hypothesis that endurance-exercise training attenuates glycogen use and spares protein oxidation. For this reason we designed an experiment to train sedentary individuals for a period of 38 days and to measure their leucine oxidation and BCOAD activation during exercise, before and after the training (McKenzie et al. 2000). We found that leucine oxidation during exercise was lower after training, as was BCOAD activation (McKenzie et al. 2000). These data confirm that chronic endurance training results in a sparing of protein oxidation.

Although there are fewer studies concerning resistance training, it is logical that protein requirements/synthesis would be greater in the early stages of adaptation when the initial hypertrophy is achieved, compared to a long-term maintenance phase. We demonstrated that whole body protein synthesis and degradation were greater in resistance-trained athletes compared to sedentary controls (Tarnopolsky et al. 1992). However, protein requirements were lower for well-trained, strength-trained athletes (Tarnopolsky et al. 1988) compared to those who were starting a training program (Lemon et al. 1992). These observations may seem surprising, however, the efficiency of protein utilisation also needs to be considered. A study of resistance training in the elderly did suggest that protein efficiency was enhanced following a resistance-training program (Campbell et al. 1995). It must be remembered that these studies of resistance training are cross-sectional in design and longitudinal data are needed.

5.3.4 *Diet and protein turnover*

It is obvious that diet has an effect on protein metabolism. For example, in starvation there is a clear net negative protein balance that results in cachexia. Conversely, there is a point at which dietary protein becomes optimal for the growth and maintenance of an organism and above this there is a 'plateau' in synthesis with amino acids being diverted into oxidative (e.g. leucine) or other (e.g. phenylalanine is not oxidised in skeletal muscle) pathways. For years it has been known that both dietary energy and CHO intake have a net positive effect on nitrogen balance (Todd et al. 1984; Lemon & Mullin 1980; Welle et al. 1989; Krempf et al. 1993). The positive effects of CHO on net protein balance are probably due to an insulin-mediated stimulation of protein synthesis and an attenuation of protein breakdown (see Section 5.3.5). A high CHO intake *per se* has positive effects on protein balance (Lemon & Mullin 1980; Welle et al. 1989; Krempf et al. 1993). Carbohydrate loading has been shown to attenuate plasma and sweat urea excretion following endurance exercise (Lemon & Mullin 1980). Furthermore, CHO supplementation increases whole body protein synthesis (Welle et al. 1989) and attenuates proteolysis (Krempf et al. 1993). There are a number of athletes who feel that the human body has an infinite capacity to increase synthesis in response to protein and energy intake and often consume an inordinate amount of each in their diet. If this were the case, everyone could become a world class body builder just by eating a huge amount of energy and protein. Certainly, the supplement companies have marketed products with this premise for years. We have frequently seen body builders consuming daily protein intakes in excess of 4 g/kg BM in their habitual diet; in fact, we have seen a professional American football player consuming a daily intake of 80 egg whites, 4 L of milk and 250 g of protein powder per day! It is not uncommon to see young strength athletes spending over twenty dollars each week on amino acid and protein supplements.

We have shown that the provision of dietary protein at levels above requirement resulted in an exponential increase in amino acid oxidation with no further increase in protein synthesis (Tarnopolsky et al. 1992). In addition, Peter Lemon and I found that the provision of dietary protein at 2.6 g/kg/d during resistance-exercise training in young males did not confer any strength or mass benefits compared to a diet supplying 1.35 g/kg/d (Lemon et al. 1992). During and after endurance exercise, the provision of extra protein (beyond requirement) resulted in an increase in leucine oxidation (Bowtell et al. 1998; Forslund et al. 1998). Taken together these data indicate that protein consumed in excess of need is oxidised as energy and does not have a net anabolic effect *per se*. However, there is a lower limit of protein intake where a further reduction in protein intake will have a negative impact on protein synthesis. It is the determination of these points that ultimately will determine the optimal protein intake for a given type of exercise (see Section 5.5).

There has been an interest in the timing of nutrient delivery and the effects on glycogen synthesis in the recovery from endurance exercise (Ivy et al. 1988; Zawadzki et al. 1992). Studies have demonstrated that glycogen resynthesis is more rapid if the glucose is provided in the immediate post-exercise period versus a two-hour delay (Ivy et al. 1988), and that there may be a synergistic effect from the addition of protein to glucose drinks (Zawadzki et al. 1992). However, in a recent study our group did not find evidence for a synergistic increase in post-endurance exercise glycogen recovery with isoenergetic protein–glucose supplements versus glucose alone (Tarnopolsky et al. 1997). Following resistance exercise, we found that isoenergetic glucose–protein supplements were similar in terms of glycogen resynthesis as compared to glucose supplements (Roy & Tarnopolsky 1998). We also demonstrated that whole body protein synthesis was greater for post-resistance exercise protein–glucose and glucose supplements as compared to placebo (Roy et al. 2000). A series of studies by Burke and colleagues demonstrated that muscle glycogen content 24 hours after endurance exercise was similarly restored whether subjects ate four large meals compared with many small snacks (1996) and whether protein and fat were consumed with the meals (1995).

These results suggest that the timing of post-exercise CHO intake may not be critical if the next performance is not until 24 hours later. However, if a sport requires several workouts or performances per day (e.g. a tournament), then a more rapid glycogen resynthesis may enhance performance. This phenomenon has also been shown for resistance exercise, where a CHO versus placebo supplement given after one bout of exercise resulted in performance enhancement in a subsequent bout four hours later (Haff et al. 1999).

Given the known beneficial effects of CHO intake on protein metabolism (Lemon & Mullin 1980; Welle et al. 1989; Krempf et al. 1993), we became interested in determining whether there were beneficial effects of immediate post-resistance exercise glucose supplements on 24-hour protein balance (Roy et al. 1997). We compared the effect of CHO supplementation (1 g/kg) given immediately and an hour after resistance exercise to the same supplement given with breakfast in eight males (Roy et al. 1997). The post-exercise CHO supplement resulted in a more positive nitrogen balance, and an attenuation of 3-MH excretion (myofibrillar proteolysis) (Roy et al. 1997). It is important to note that this post-exercise strategy had a net positive effect on nitrogen balance over a 24-hour period and not just in the immediate post-exercise period (Roy et al. 1997). It has recently been shown that an insulin infusion decreases protein degradation following resistance exercise (Biolo et al. 1999), which supports the idea that the effects of the post-exercise glucose drink were mediated by insulin. The convenience and relative inexpense of CHO supplementation makes this an attractive strategy to favourably alter net protein balance in resistance sports.

In addition to CHOs, there has been interest in whether amino acids *per se* stimulate net protein balance (i.e. increase synthesis and/or decrease degradation). Certainly, there is good evidence that an intravenous amino acid infusion has a stimulatory effect on muscle protein synthesis (Castellino et al. 1987; Tessari et al. 1987; Garlick & Grant 1988; Svanberg et al. 1996; Biolo et al. 1997) that is independent of the insulin effect (Castellino et al. 1987). Furthermore, the essential and branched-chain amino acids seem to increase the sensitivity of the muscle to the protein stimulatory effects of insulin (Garlick & Grant 1988). On the other side of the equation, amino acids appear to have equivocal effects on protein degradation (Castellino et al. 1987; Tessari et al. 1987; Svanberg et al. 1996). The problem with this body of literature is that it does not directly answer the question about protein requirements, for it is impossible to determine whether the amino acids acted to stimulate protein synthesis during a state of deficiency, as compared to a situation of adequate protein status.

In parallel to the effect of timing of CHO intake on glycogen resynthesis, there also appears to be a potentiation of amino acid transport into muscle after an acute bout of training (Zorzano et al. 1986; Biolo et al. 1997). Following resistance exercise, the stimulatory effects of hyperaminoacidemia (achieved by intravenous amino acids) have been shown to further enhance amino acid transport and muscle protein synthesis (Biolo et al. 1997). The same group (Tipton et al. 1999) has replicated these findings using oral amino acids and found that an indispensable amino acid drink was equivalent to a complete amino acid drink.

Taken together, the aforementioned observations suggest that the immediate post-exercise period is an important time for the resistance athlete to consume protein and CHOs. This may have an impact on protein requirements and permit optimal muscle strength gains with a lower absolute protein intake. For the endurance athlete, the immediate provision of CHOs is not as critical to glycogen resynthesis over the ensuing 24 hours, provided that CHO intake is high (~10 g/kg BM/d). We still need to examine the impact of immediate post-exercise intake of protein and CHO on 24-hour whole body protein retention.

5.3.5 *Hormones and protein turnover*

There are many hormones that directly and indirectly affect protein turnover, including insulin, cortisol, testosterone, growth hormone, and insulin-like growth factor. A complete examination of these effects would require at least a dedicated chapter. Therefore, I will focus briefly on only two of these, namely insulin and testosterone.

I will mention testosterone only because of the significant controversy surrounding its unethical use in sporting events and its potent effects on protein metabolism. For years it was assumed that testosterone had stimulatory effects on net protein synthesis, based on observations of male–female differences in lean mass as well as the increases noted for those who supplemented with pharmacological doses. Only recently have there been proper investigations into the metabolism and efficacy of testosterone administration (Florini 1987; Griggs et al. 1989; Bhasin et al. 1996; Ferrando et al. 1998). Even without resistance exercise testosterone administration can increase lean body mass (Griggs et al. 1989; Bhasin et al. 1996), however, the effects are magnified with a resistance-exercise training program (Bhasin et al. 1996). At the muscle level, testosterone acts by increasing protein synthesis and intra-cellular amino acid re-utilisation and does not affect degradation (Ferrando et al. 1998). It should be kept in mind that acute resistance exercise also increases plasma testosterone concentration (Kraemer et al. 1990; Volek et al. 1997), and no studies have yet compared optimal nutritional intervention to testosterone in a comparative study. Another interesting finding that may serve to reduce the enthusiasm for very high protein intakes was the negative correlation between protein intake and plasma testosterone concentration (P = −0.71) (Volek et al. 1997).

Another key hormone that is important in protein metabolism and is the major factor in the efficacy of CHO–protein nutrition is insulin. Insulin has a net stimulatory effect upon muscle protein synthesis (Biolo et al. 1999). A consistent effect of insulin is a reduction in muscle proteolysis (Castellino et al. 1987; Tessari et al. 1987; Bennett et al. 1989; Moller-Loswick et al. 1994; Newman et al. 1994). The effect of insulin on protein synthesis appears to depend on whether or not there is an abundance of amino acids (Biolo et al. 1999). Several studies have not found a stimulation of insulin on muscle protein synthesis (Castellino et al. 1987; Gelfand & Barrett 1987; Tessari et al. 1987; Melville et al. 1989; McNurlan et al. 1994;

Moller-Loswick et al. 1994), however, it is likely that the hypoaminoacidemia that results from insulin inhibits the stimulatory effect of insulin on protein synthesis (Biolo et al. 1999). When amino acids are provided simultaneously with insulin (to prevent hypoaminoacidemia), there appears to be a stimulation of protein synthesis (Castellino et al. 1987; Tessari et al. 1987; Bennet et al. 1990; Newman et al. 1994; Moller-Loswick et al. 1994). Other studies have found that hyperinsulinemia stimulates both muscle FSR and amino acid transport (Biolo et al. 1995). Finally, the effects of insulin on protein metabolism are different before and after resistance exercise (Biolo et al. 1999). In the resting state, insulin induces a more positive protein balance by increasing synthesis and increasing amino acid transport; after exercise there was no effect on synthesis, yet there was a significant reduction in degradation and a three-fold increase in amino acid transport (Biolo et al. 1999).

These findings provide the theoretical basis for the provision of protein and CHO in the early post-exercise period in athletes performing resistance-type exercise.

5.4 DETERMINING THE ADEQUACY OF PROTEIN INTAKE (DIETARY REQUIREMENTS) DURING EXERCISE

5.4.1 Nitrogen balance

As defined above, nitrogen balance (NBAL) is the method whereby the investigator determines all of the protein that enters a person (diet, intravenous etc.) and all of the nitrogen that is excreted (Elwyn 1990; Pellet 1990). Since the body excretes nitrogenous compounds rather than whole proteins and since proteins are ~16% nitrogen by weight, the technique involves measurement of the total nitrogen intake (N_{IN}), and the total nitrogen excretion (N_{OUT}: urine, faeces, sweat and miscellaneous—i.e. menstrual loss, hair, semen and skin). If the person is in a state of net anabolism, then there is a positive NBAL, whereas if the person is losing protein then there is a negative NBAL. The protein intake requirement for a given physiological state (e.g. exercise, pregnancy and lactation) is determined by feeding the person varying protein intakes and determining the nitrogen balance at each level of intake. From this, one can calculate a regression equation from which a zero NBAL can be interpolated. In order to account for inter-individual variability in the development of general guidelines, two standard deviations are added to the zero estimate. In this way, the 'safe' protein intake level is estimated to cover 97% of the given population. It is important to note that the NBAL experiment must indicate the biological value of the dietary protein used in the study. For example, a protein requirement of 1.0 g/kg/d, based on egg white and milk protein, would have to be higher for a diet based on lower biological value proteins such as grains. Most countries in the world base their dietary protein intake recommendations relative to a biological value estimated to be the mean for the population (Pellett 1990).

In studies of athletes, it is important to recall that CHO and total energy intake can positively affect NBAL (Chiang & Huang 1988; Elwyn 1990; Pellett 1990).

Therefore, athletes with low CHO and energy intakes may require more protein than for those with adequate intakes. These dietary interactions between protein, energy and CHO may have implications for those athletes who habitually consume low energy intakes or fad diets that stress a very low CHO intake.

One of the problems with NBAL is that the protein requirement estimates may under-estimate what is required for 'optimal' functioning. This concern comes from the fact that as protein intake decreases there is an increase in the efficiency of amino acid re-utilisation and a lower overall amino acid flux (Young et al. 1989; Young & Bier 1987; Pellet 1990; Tarnopolsky et al. 1992). Therefore, NBAL may be achieved with a compromise in some physiologically relevant processes. For example, an endurance athlete may slow the induction of aerobic enzyme activity or a resistance athlete may not achieve the same degree of hypertrophy of skeletal muscle over a period of training.

Therefore, the ultimate method to determine the dietary requirements for athletes would be to provide a large group of sedentary individuals with a variety of graded protein intakes over a prolonged period of training and determine which was the optimal intake to achieve maximal improvements in physiological outcome variables (i.e. VO$_2$ max, muscle strength, muscle mass). Furthermore, one would also want to determine that the optimal protein intake resulted in optimal function in other critical areas such as resistance to infections. Unfortunately, this approach would be prohibitively expensive and time-consuming. Such an experiment is not likely to ever be completed.

5.4.2   *Tracer methods*

Because of the limitations in the NBAL method, Young and Bier have been instrumental in devising a conceptual framework from which to determine optimal protein intakes using stable isotopic tracers. They have coined the terms: nutrient deficiency, accommodation, adaptation, and nutrient excess (Young & Bier 1987; Young et al. 1989). In a state of protein deficiency, there would be a maximal reduction in amino acid oxidation and a reduction in protein synthesis to all but the essential organs (e.g. brain), that ultimately would result in muscle wasting (negative NBAL). The state of accommodation would be the state where NBAL would be achieved with a decrease in a physiologically relevant process. The state of adaptation would be the dietary intake that provided for optimal rates of protein synthesis for growth, inter-organ amino acid exchange and immune function. Finally, the state of protein excess would be defined as that intake where amino acids are oxidised for energy or used in fat storage and protein synthesis is not further simulated by a further increase in intake.

The four states above can be determined using amino acid tracers during studies at varied protein intakes. The optimal protein intake would be that where amino acid oxidation starts to increase exponentially and protein synthesis starts to plateau. There have only been a few of these studies performed in athletes.

5.5 ◢ *DIETARY PROTEIN REQUIREMENTS FOR ATHLETES*

5.5.1 *The habitual intakes of athletes—a story of deficiency and excess*

Athletes are a group of individuals who are constantly striving for optimal performance. Because of this, many of them may fall victim to false or unsubstantiated claims concerning diet and nutrient supplements. For example, the protein and amino acid supplement market in the United States is a multi-million-dollar industry sustained by a motive to sell product rather than to encourage optimal nutrition through food. It is common to observe individuals consuming protein and amino acid intakes that would clearly be in gross nutrient excess. Another problem of many supplements is that they replace other components of the diet that may have known factors (e.g. vitamins, minerals, fibre, antioxidants), or as yet unknown factors that are critical for optimal body functioning. There may be a role for limited supplement use, such as when an athlete is travelling to a foreign country and the availability of familiar foods may be limited. In addition, there may be cases where an individual is on a weight-restrictive diet and protein intake may not be adequate to meet the needs of a rigorous training program. For the most part, however, the problem of protein excess is predominantly one affecting strength athletes and not endurance athletes. For the most part, resistance-training athletes, who are not energy restricting, consume protein that is already in excess of their protein requirement (see Table 5.3).

In contrast, some individuals may suffer from protein deficiency where chronically low intakes may lead to a compromise of function and ultimately to loss of body protein (atrophy). This is clearly evident in the extreme case of anorexia nervosa and possibly in sports where weight categories are assigned. In the latter case, athletes may use extreme measures such as sweating and severe fluid and energy restriction to attain the lowest possible weight category (Brownell et al. 1987; Tarnopolsky et al. 1996). This situation is discussed in Chapter 8. There are four groups of athletes who appear to be at highest risk from protein and energy deficiency, including: amenorrheic female runners (Drinkwater et al. 1990; Marcus et al. 1985), male wrestlers (Brownell et al. 1987; Tarnopolsky et al. 1996), male and female gymnasts (Short & Short 1983; Brownell et al. 1987) and female dancers (Short & Short 1983; Brownell et al. 1987). As seen in Table 5.2, most groups of athletes consume adequate amounts of protein and energy. It is important to remember that these nutritional surveys are mean intakes for a group and the range can be wide within a group. For example, in one study, the mean energy and protein intake reported by male gymnasts was 2080 kcal and 1.1 g/kg/d respectively, however some athletes reported intakes as low as 568 kcal and 0.16 g/kg/d (Short & Short 1983). Similarly, in a study of female runners, Deuster and colleagues (1986) found that the mean reported energy and protein intake was 2397 kcal and 1.56 g/kg/d respectively, yet the lowest reported intakes were 1067 kcal and 0.53 g/kg/d.

Table 5.2 *Habitual protein intakes in male and female endurance athletes*

Reference	Subjects	Protein g/kg/d	% E$_{IN}$
Tarnopolsky et al. 1997	N = 8 male	1.9	17
	N = 8 female	1.2	14
Tarnopolsky et al. 1995	N = 7 male	1.8	15
	N = 8 female	1.0	12
Phillips et al. 1993	N = 6 male	1.9	15
	N = 6 female	1.0	13
Schultz et al. 1992	N = 9 female	1.4	13
Tarnopolsky et al. 1990	N = 6 male	1.2	12
	N = 6 female	1.7	13
Saris et al. 1989	N = 5 male	2.2	15
Deuster et al. 1986	N = 51 female	1.6	13
Hellsworth et al. 1985	N = 13 male	2.1	14
Nelson et al. 1986	N = 17 EUM*	1.0	15
	N = 11 AMEN*	0.7	15
Marcus et al. 1985	N = 6 EUM*	1.3	17
	N = 11 AMEN*	1.0	15
Drinkwater et al. 1984	N = 13 EUM*	1.1	13
	N = 14 AMEN*	1.2	16
Approximate mean	male	1.8 (0.4)	14 (2)
	female	1.2 (0.3)	14 (2)

Values are mean (SD)
*EUM = eumenorrheic; AMEN = amenorrheic females
Partially adapted from Tarnopolsky 1999

In summary, the majority of strength and endurance athletes consume adequate protein and energy to meet their needs. Even when one takes into account the modest increases required by certain athletes (see below), most athletes are still above these levels. It appears that the human body homeostatically adapts to exercise by matching protein and energy intakes to cover any increase in demand from the activity in question. In some groups there are extrinsic pressures to restrict intake for weight class or aesthetic reasons. In fact, certain groups may not even be attaining the recommended intake levels for sedentary individuals. Each athlete must be considered as an individual when determining the adequacy of dietary protein and energy intakes. The identification of the 'at risk' groups above may help the nutritionist or coach to be aware of those who may need special nutritional counselling.

Table 5.3 *Habitual protein intakes in resistance athletes*

Reference	Participants	Protein g/kg/d	% E_{IN}
Roy et al. 1998	N = 10 male (trained*)	1.6	18
Tarnopolsky et al. 1992	N = 7 male (footballers)	1.8	16
Lemon et al. 1992	N = 12 male (body builders)	1.4	14
Chesley et al. 1992	N = 12 male (body builders)	1.6	17
Tarnopolsky et al. 1988	N = 6 male (body builders)	2.7	17
Faber et al. 1986	N = 76 male (body builders)	2.4	22
Short and Short 1983	N = 30 male (footballers)	2.5	18
	N = 6 male (body builders)	2.3	20
Burke et al. 1991	N = 18 male (weight lifters)	1.9	18
Burke and Read 1988	N = 56 male (footballers)	1.5	15
Kleiner et al. 1990	N = 8 female (body builders)	2.8	37
	Approximate mean	2.0 (0.5)	18 (2)

Approximate mean = mean (SD)
*trained = weight-trained four times per week for more than two years
Partially adapted from Tarnopolsky 1999

5.5.2 *Protein requirements for endurance sports*

In most countries there are no specific allowances for an effect of physical exercise on protein requirements. It is sometimes stated that these are not required because all athletes consume more energy and subsequently achieve adequate protein intakes. Others have argued that moderate exercise does not increase the requirement for dietary protein (Butterfield & Calloway 1984; Campbell et al. 1995; El-Khoury 1997), and therefore there is no need to provide specific protein requirements for athletes. However, these studies were undertaken using exercise intensities that would be considered recreational by most standards. Clearly, the elite athlete is performing daily exercise at a much higher intensity and for a longer duration than the novice. Therefore, it is critical to qualify the state of training and the daily volume in any study looking at protein requirements in athletes. Although most athletes consume enough protein to cover any potential increase in dietary need, there are individuals who may not even meet minimal requirements and it is for this group that a knowledge of protein requirements is useful. For example, a person who is performing regular strenuous activity while on an energy-restrictive diet may wish to know the minimal protein intake for optimal functional status.

Given that amino acids can be oxidised as energy during exercise, it is theoretically possible that this may impact on the need for extra dietary protein. The determination of dietary protein requirements for endurance athletes is a function of the duration and intensity of exercise, gender, age, training status, and habitual energy and CHO intake. To determine the effect of endurance exercise training on amino acid oxidation, we measured leucine oxidation in six males and six females during endurance exercise at 60% $VO_{2\,peak}$ both before and after a 38-day training program (McKenzie et al. 2000). We found that leucine oxidation and BCOAD activation were significantly attenuated following the training period, yet the total BCOAD maximal activity was increased. This suggests that at the same absolute exercise intensity there is a training induced sparing of protein use, yet the capacity existed to oxidise more protein under the period of energy deficiency, CHO depletion and during high-intensity workouts. This demonstrated the importance of indicating the training status of the group of subjects being studied and also their current training regime.

In a simplistic approach to determining protein requirements it is possible to calculate the estimated need for dietary protein by an athlete, from first principles. For example, if a 70 kg male was running for 1.5 hours at 70% $VO_{2\,peak}$ and protein accounted for 5% of the total energy, he would oxidise about 15 g of protein. If his basal protein requirement was 0.86 g/kg/d (60 g), this would represent an additional 25% increase in his daily protein requirement (1.07 g/kg/d). Most male and female athletes habitually consume more protein than this (Table 5.3). These calculations are only rough estimates and most studies have used NBAL to try to quantify dietary protein requirements for endurance athletes.

Two much-quoted studies from the mid-1970s determined NBAL following the initiation of an endurance-exercise program on a constant protein intake (Gontzea et al. 1975), and while consuming two different protein intakes (Gontzea et al. 1974). In a group of males starting an endurance-exercise program they found that a protein intake of 1.5 g/kg/d was adequate to maintain a positive NBAL, whereas 1.0 g/kg/d was inadequate (Gontzea et al. 1974). In addition, they also found that the subjects on a constant protein intake showed progressive adaptation to the moderate exercise program by improving NBAL over the course of about one week (Gontzea et al. 1975). These latter findings suggested that there were adaptive changes to the stress of exercise (e.g. an increase in amino acid re-utilisation efficiency) and therefore an increased protein intake was needed only at the initiation of an endurance exercise program. This is similar to our findings in men and women following a modest training program (McKenzie et al. 2000).

With moderate-intensity endurance exercise (< 50% $VO_{2\,peak}$), there does not appear to be an increase in protein requirements (Butterfield & Calloway 1984; Todd et al. 1984). At these modest exercise intensities, protein utilisation is enhanced (Butterfield & Calloway 1984) and energy deficits are better tolerated (Todd et al. 1984). In another study of endurance exercise at moderate intensity (46% $VO_{2\,peak}$), El-Khoury and colleagues (1997) used a combined isotopic tracer and nitrogen excretion method and found that a protein intake of 1 g/kg/d was adequate for young males. These results suggest that people performing modest-intensity exercise do not require any increase in dietary protein intake. However, most athletes exercise at intensities of 65–85% of $VO_{2\,peak}$ where there may be a negative impact on protein homeostasis and NBAL.

In contrast, there does appear to be an increase in protein requirements for well-trained endurance athletes (Tarnopolsky et al. 1988; Brouns et al. 1989; Friedman & Lemon 1989; Meredith et al. 1989; Phillips et al. 1993). One study used NBAL to determine the protein requirements in a group of endurance-trained males, who were young (27-years-old; $VO_{2\,peak}$ = 65 mL/kg/min) or middle-aged (52-years-old; $VO_{2\,peak}$ = 55 mL/kg/min) (Meredith et al. 1989). They found that a protein intake of 0.94 g/kg/d was required for NBAL, and whole body protein synthesis (glycine tracer) increased with increasing protein intakes (0.61 → 0.92 → 1.21 g/kg/d). When accounting for inter-individual variability by adding two standard deviations to the zero NBAL intercept, the estimated protein requirement in these males was about 1.28 g/kg/d (Meredith et al. 1989). A study performed in our laboratory found that both male ($VO_{2\,peak}$ = 59 mL/kg/min) and female ($VO_{2\,peak}$ = 55 mL/kg/min) endurance athletes were in negative NBAL while consuming a dietary protein intake that was close to the Canadian, United States, and Australian recommended intake for sedentary individuals (males = 0.94 g/kg/d; females = 0.80 g/kg/d) (Phillips et al. 1993).

There are three studies using NBAL methodology to examine the protein requirements of elite endurance-trained athletes (Tarnopolsky et al. 1988; Brouns et al. 1989; Friedman & Lemon 1989). We performed an NBAL experiment in six elite male endurance athletes ($VO_{2\,peak}$ = 76.2 mL/kg/min) (who were training more than 12 hours per week) to determine what we considered to be close to the upper limit of protein requirements for endurance athletes (Tarnopolsky et al. 1988). We determined the safe protein intake for the elite athletes to be 1.6 g/kg/d, whereas the estimate for a sedentary control group (N = 6) was 0.86 g/kg/d, which was very close to Canadian and United States recommendations (Tarnopolsky et al. 1988). In a simulated Tour de France cycling study, Brouns and colleagues (1989) found that well trained cyclists ($VO_{2\,peak}$ = 65.1 mL/kg/min) required protein intakes of 1.5–1.8 g/kg/min to maintain NBAL. In a final study, Friedman and Lemon (1989) calculated that the protein requirement for five well-trained runners was about 1.49 g/kg/d, using NBAL.

To summarise the available data, it appears that low- and moderate-intensity endurance exercise does not result in an increase in dietary protein requirements. At the initiation of an endurance-exercise program there may be a transient increase in dietary protein need, yet the body rapidly adapts to the increase in need. For the well-trained athlete (training four to five days per week for > 45 min), there appears to be an increase of about 20–25% in dietary protein requirements. In the elite athlete, the increase in dietary protein intake may be as high as 1.6 g/kg/d (or nearly twice the recommended intake for sedentary persons). Given that the Tour de France (Brouns et al. 1989) and the $VO_{2\,peak}$ of the athletes in our study (Tarnopolsky et al. 1988) are respectively among the most demanding and highest reported, I feel that this is probably the highest requirement needed. Clearly, there may be some more demanding events, however, the day-to-day training is not likely to exceed that reported for the athletes in these studies (Tarnopolsky et al. 1988; Brouns et al. 1989). In spite of these elevated requirements, there is no need for supplementation with a mixed diet of adequate energy intake, providing 15% of the energy from protein. For example, with an energy intake of about 3 500 kcal per day (which is still modest), this would amount to about 125 g protein per day (~1.6–1.9 g/kg/d).

One final point about protein requirements for endurance athletes is the possibility of a gender difference. We first found a gender difference in protein metabolism in 1990 (Tarnopolsky et al.) whereby males increased urinary urea excretion on an exercise compared to rest day, whereas females did not. We concluded that this was due to a glycogen-sparing effect seen in the women (Tarnopolsky et al. 1990). In the study where we found that the Canadian recommended intake for protein was inadequate for well-trained endurance athletes, we also found that the females were in a less negative NBAL and their basal leucine oxidation was lower compared to the males (Phillips et al. 1993). In a subsequent study, we also found that females had lower leucine oxidation both at rest and during exercise before and after a 38-day training program compared to males (McKenzie et al. 2000). These findings may indicate that the dietary protein recommendations for endurance athletes (Table 5.4) may be 10–20% lower for females as compared to males.

Table 5.4 *Estimated protein requirements for athletes*

Population	Protein requirement g/kg/d
Sedentary males and females	0.80–1.0
Elite male endurance athletes	1.6
Moderate-intensity endurance athletes*	1.2
Recreational endurance athletes+	0.80–1.0
Football, power sports	1.4–1.7
Resistance athletes (early training)	1.5–1.7
Resistance athletes (steady state)	1.0–1.2
Female athletes	~15% lower than male athletes

Exercising approximately four to five times per week for 45–60 min; + exercising four to five times per week for 30 min at < 55% $VO_{2\ peak}$.
Partially adapted from Tarnopolsky 1999

5.5.3 *Protein requirements for strength sports*

In contrast to endurance exercise, resistance exercise results in muscle hypertrophy (Sale et al. 1987; Lemon et al. 1992) rather than an increase in amino acid oxidation (Tarnopolsky et al. 1991). If there are no changes in efficiency of amino acid retention (see below), there must, at some point, be a protein intake in excess of basal requirements to provide the amino acids required for anabolism. The extent of this increased need is again a function of the basal state of training, the duration and the intensity of the training program.

An early study used NBAL and lean mass measurements to estimate the protein requirements during an isometric exercise training program (Torun et al. 1977). They found that a daily protein intake of 1.0 g/kg (egg white and milk) was required to maintain positive NBAL and lean mass accretion in males performing isometric exercise for 75 min/d (Torun et al. 1977). The equivalent protein intake from a mixed source would be about 1.2 g/kg/d. Similar results were found in young males performing circuit training with both endurance and resistance exercise where even after a 40-day adaptation period, protein requirements were ~1.4 g/kg/d (Consolazio et al. 1975).

Similar to the work with endurance exercise (McKenzie et al. 2000), modest resistance exercise programs can attenuate nitrogen loss at protein intakes close to the United States and Canadian recommended protein intake levels in the elderly (Campbell et al. 1995). This phenomenon has also been observed in young men training with a protein intake of ~0.8 g/kg/d (Hickson et al. 1988). Although there may be the ability to achieve NBAL (through increased nitrogen utilisation efficiency) with modest resistance exercise, this may be indicative of accommodation and not adaptation, because at the lower protein intake (~0.8 g/kg/d) Campbell and colleagues (1995) also found that whole body protein synthesis was lower than for the group who consumed protein intakes of 1.6 g/kg/d. This is another example of the utility of amino acid kinetics to provide more information on the physiological adequacy of a given protein intake.

We performed an NBAL experiment in six well-trained body builders (> two years training experience) and six sedentary individuals and found that the protein requirement for the trained body builders was only 12% greater than that for the sedentary controls (Tarnopolsky et al. 1988). We also found that the body builders in this study were habitually consuming protein intakes of ~2.7 g/kg/d (Tarnopolsky et al. 1988). The error of the NBAL method was demonstrated in this study; if the positive NBAL on the high protein intake was extrapolated to net protein retention (assuming no change in breakdown), there would have been a 200 g/d increase in lean body mass each day! Some lay reports have used these data in support of the high protein intakes consumed by the body builders. However, the magnitude of the positive NBAL cannot be directly extrapolated to an increase in lean mass for two reasons. Firstly, there is an inherent error in the technique, which over-estimates NBAL at high nitrogen intakes (Young 1987), and secondly, protein synthesis and breakdown change in parallel (Phillips et al. 1997).

We embarked on two follow-up studies to more accurately characterise the impact of resistance training on dietary protein needs. In the first study we reasoned that the protein requirements would be highest during the early adaptation period to unaccustomed training, since most of the myofibrillar protein accretion occurs within the first several months of initiating a resistance exercise program.

Therefore, we exposed 12 young males to two months of a supervised resistance exercise program (six days per week, two hours per day, 70–85% 1RM) and measured NBAL, muscle mass, muscle protein and strength before and after a one-month period where they were randomised to receive protein at 1.44 and 2.6 g/kg/d. We calculated the estimated protein requirement during this period to be ~1.65 g/kg/d (Lemon et al. 1992). Strength, muscle protein and lean mass gains following training were not different between the two protein intakes (Lemon et al. 1992). We went on to use the conceptual framework put forth by Young and Bier (1989), and studied the protein kinetic response to graded protein intakes in young males who were performing weight training and high-intensity sprinting/power activities (i.e. football and rugby) (Tarnopolsky et al. 1992). In this study we randomly allocated six sedentary males (S) and seven athletes (SA, as described above) to receive a diet supplying protein at each of three levels (Canadian recommended intake ~0.86 g/kg/d; moderate ~1.4 g/kg/d; and high ~2.4 g/kg/d). We measured NBAL, whole body protein synthesis, leucine oxidation and protein breakdown (Tarnopolsky et al. 1992). We found the estimated safe protein intake to be 0.89 g/kg/d for the sedentary group and 1.76 g/kg/d for the athletes (Tarnopolsky et al. 1992). The whole body protein synthesis was greater for the athletes as compared to the sedentary controls at all protein intakes. Furthermore, whole body protein synthesis was lower at 0.86 g/kg/d as compared to 1.4 and 2.8 g/kg/d, and appeared to plateau at around 1.4 g/kg/d for the athletes (SA). At protein intakes of 2.8 g/kg/d, leucine oxidation increased nearly twofold, which provided evidence that protein intake above the requirement is merely oxidised for energy (Tarnopolsky et al. 1992).

5.6 POTENTIAL SIDE-EFFECTS OF EXCESSIVE PROTEIN INTAKE

In general, there are probably few side-effects arising from daily protein intakes under 2.0 g/kg in healthy people. Perhaps the most definite effect of a very high protein diet would be the cost of protein supplements or protein-rich foods. Even with dietary protein, the ultimate cost to produce a kilogram of beef is more than an isoenergetic amount of wheat. Furthermore, most meat products also contain significant amounts of fat, which if taken at a high enough level may render the diet atherogenic. This is not likely to be a problem with protein intakes below 2.0 g/kg/d.

Although it is likely that many people can safely maintain very high protein intakes for long periods of time, there are several caveats that must be considered. Firstly, a high-protein diet can increase urinary calcium excretion (from the sulphur-containing amino acids), which may be a concern for the female athlete with a low energy intake and amenorrhoea. Secondly, high protein intakes in conjunction with pre-existing renal disease may accelerate the progression of the disease (Brenner 1982). Thirdly, rodents fed very high protein intakes have been found to exhibit morphological changes in the liver mitochondria, which could be pathological (Zaragosa et al. 1987). Finally, some problems may occur if the protein is taken as an amino acid supplement. One possible problem relates to contamination of purified amino acids, as in the case of L-tryptophan supplements that were manufactured in Japan and caused a life-threatening disorder called eosinophilic myalgia syndrome (EMS) (Hertzman et al. 1990; Teman & Hainline 1991). Some sources state that this occurred as a result of an HPLC purified contaminant present from a bacterial processing method (Yamaoka et al. 1994). In addition to the expense involved, large doses of purified amino acids could potentially be carcinogenic and mutagenic. Such warnings are noted on the labels of purified chemical-grade laboratory amino acids, although these problems have not been substantiated in humans. Even if purified amino acids are safe, they are not very palatable, are expensive and the efficacy has not been established in spite of many studies (Slavin et al. 1988; Bucci et al. 1992).

5.7 SUMMARY

Protein is an important component of the diet and is involved in almost every structural and functional component of the human body. In general, endurance exercise may impact on the need for dietary protein by increasing the oxidation of amino acids. Resistance exercise may also have an impact through the need for amino acids to support muscle hypertrophy. At the onset of an endurance exercise program there is a negative effect on NBAL, yet with time the body adapts to the stress and NBAL and leucine oxidation are attenuated. After endurance exercise training, the amount of amino acid oxidised at the same absolute exercise intensity is reduced, yet the capacity of the body to oxidise amino acids is increased. However, only in the elite athlete (who is training very hard every day) is there a significant impact on dietary protein requirements, with a maximal requirement of ~1.6 g/kg/d. For the resistance trained athlete, there also appears to be a homeostatic adaptation to the stress of the exercise, where very well trained athletes require only marginally more protein than sedentary persons and those in the early stages of very intensive resistance exercise may require up to 1.7 g/kg/d. A dietary protein intake that represents 15% of the total energy intake with an energy-sufficient diet should cover the requirements for nearly all endurance athletes. Given the increase in energy intake by most athletes, there is no need to use protein supplements to attain these levels. However, athletes on a low-energy diet and/or a low-CHO diet could have an inadequate protein intake to cover their needs. The timing of nutrient delivery appears to be important for resistance athletes, where an immediate post-exercise intake of CHO and protein will lead to a more positive protein NBAL, probably by reducing protein breakdown. The effect of post-exercise nutritional intake on whole body protein metabolism by endurance athletes is not yet known.

5.8 PRACTICE TIPS

Gary Slater

- Bulking up can be an important component in the development of many athletes but it takes more than a simple desire to 'get bigger'. For most athletes, the intent to bulk up or increase weight is a desire to increase lean body mass and strength. Few athletes intentionally plan to increase fat mass. To ensure gains in lean body mass are prioritised, the combination of a well-designed resistance-training program plus an energy-dense, adequate-protein meal plan is required. Strong rapport and a good working relationship among athletes, coaching staff (including strength and conditioning coaches), and the dietitian will definitely enhance the potential for a positive outcome.

- If gains in lean body mass are a priority, a hypertrophy phase needs to be incorporated into the athlete's yearly training schedule. This period might include consistent allocation of resistance-training sessions each week and a decrease in overall training volume, especially conditioning sessions which will limit the potential for gains in muscle mass. The off-season or early pre-season are ideal times to prioritise lean body mass gains. Too often, athletes identified as too weak or small mid-season are placed on a hypertrophy program that is destined to fail—not because of commitment from the athlete but because of the high energy demands of routine training during that phase of the season.

- Ensure short- and long-term weight gain goals are realistic. An increase in body weight of 0.25–0.5 kg per week may be realistic but will depend on genetics and the resistance-training history of the athlete. Longer training histories inevitably ensure only smaller gains are possible. Significantly greater gains than this are likely to include deposition of fat that may have to be dropped at a later stage. Also ensure overall body composition goals are realistic. Far too many athletes want to increase lean body mass and reduce skinfolds simultaneously. This is not achievable for most athletes as the two goals are mutually exclusive; one aims to increase energy density while the other requires a reduction in energy intake. Priorities must be set and dietary intervention applied accordingly.

- Monitoring body composition during a hypertrophy phase is an important tool for assessing progress. It helps identify if energy intake is adequate to allow gains in muscle mass, and may alleviate fears of body-fat gain for those athletes who are weight focused. Measurement of body weight, skinfolds and girths will generally provide an accurate indication of any changes in body composition. See Chapter 4 for a closer examination of physique assessment.

- Meeting the increased protein needs of resistance-training athletes is essential if gains in muscle mass are to be achieved. Fortunately, the higher food intake of most athletes ensures a generous protein intake; usually well above requirements. As energy intake increases to meet the additional energy demands of training, extra protein requirements can be achieved from a meal plan providing ~15% of total energy as protein. However, be aware of athletes at risk of inadequate protein intake. These include athletes involved in weight restriction or aesthetically judged sports, plus those with disordered or restrictive eating patterns.

- With increased protein requirements, the protein intake of endurance-trained athletes should also be reviewed. While absolute requirements may be lower than those in strength-trained athletes, recommendations relative to body weight are similar. Some ill-informed endurance athletes may be so focused on a high-CHO diet that protein intake becomes compromised. The detrimental effects of a low protein intake should be discussed with the athlete and a meal plan should be developed that meets both macronutrient and micronutrient requirements.

- While most athletes readily ingest 1.5–2.0 g protein per kilogram BM per day, some athletes eat more than 4 g/kg/d believing this will further enhance gains in muscle mass. Such extreme diets are neither necessary nor likely to be beneficial. Excess dietary protein does not have an anabolic effect and will be oxidised for energy production. Routine consumption of high-protein diets does not appear to negatively impact renal function in healthy individuals but may increase fluid requirements, possibly promote urinary calcium loss, displace other important nutrients from the diet and potentially be a major source of saturated fat.

- Food sources of protein are shown in Table 5.5. Meat, poultry and dairy products provide ~50% of the protein intake in a typical western diet, but other sources such as cereals and cereal products like bread, pasta, rice and breakfast cereals also contribute significant amounts (~30% of total intake) of protein.

- Athletes should be guided to choose meal combinations that match protein requirements with other nutrient needs: for example, three or more serves of low-fat dairy foods to provide protein and calcium, one to two serves of lean meat, fish, chicken or vegetarian alternatives daily for protein, iron and zinc.

- Timing of protein intake may also be important. Optimal amino acid levels in the blood are achieved by including a small serve of protein-rich food at each meal and snack. Eating a CHO-rich, moderate-protein snack or meal after training may help to optimise gains in lean body mass by increasing production of anabolic hormones, reducing proteolysis and supplying amino acids for protein synthesis.

Table 5.5 *Common dietary sources of protein*

Food	Typical serve	Protein content (g)
Meat, poultry and seafood:		
Beef/ lamb/ pork, lean	100 g cooked	31
Ham/ salami/ corned beef	1 slice (30 g)	7
Sausage	1 (90 g) cooked	13
Chicken/ turkey, lean	100 g cooked	28
Seafood, flesh only	100 g cooked	23
Dairy food:		
Milk (including soy milk)	250 ml glass	9
Cheese, hard	20 g slice	5
Cheese, cottage	tablespoon (20 g)	3
Yoghurt, flavoured	200 g carton	10
Ice-cream	1 scoop (50 g)	2
Cereals and cereal product:		
Rice	1 cup cooked	5
Pasta	1 cup cooked	7.5
Bread/ fruit loaf/ crumpet	1 slice (30 g)	3
Breakfast cereal	1 cup (30–45 g)	3–5
Miscellaneous:		
Eggs	1 cooked	7
Tofu	100 g	8.5
Baked beans	1 cup (220 g)	10
Nuts	50 g	10
Liquid meal supplement	1 cup (250 ml)	12–30*

Protein content will vary with the supplement. Liquid meal supplements produced by large pharmaceutical/ food companies usually provide smaller amounts of protein with additional amounts of other nutrients while the majority of 'body building formulas' focus primarily on higher amounts of protein per serve.

Source: Commonwealth Department of Health and Community Services (1998)

- Any evaluation of an athlete's protein requirements should also consider the energy content of their diet. For any given protein intake, increasing energy density of the meal plan will enhance nitrogen balance. In fact, the most important dietary component of a weight gain program is an increase in energy density. For some athletes this can be a real challenge. Frequent and/or prolonged training sessions can limit the opportunities for meals and snacks while intense training may suppress an athlete's appetite. Novel strategies like an increased reliance on energy-dense snacks and drinks may be required to overcome such obstacles. Use the following tips when attempting to increase energy density of a meal plan:
    1. Increase meal/snack frequency. Gastrointestinal tract tolerance is generally higher when the frequency of meals is increased rather than the size

of existing meals and snacks. Eating frequently should become a priority, even during busy days. Meal plans with at least 5–6 meals and snacks throughout the day should be encouraged.

2. Make use of energy-dense drinks (e.g. smoothies, milkshakes, powdered liquid meal supplements, fruit juice, cordial, soft drink and sports drinks) and other energy-dense foods (e.g. jams, honey, cereal bars and dried fruit or trail mix). Homemade milk drinks can be fortified with skim-milk powder to add an extra protein and energy boost. These drinks can be particularly useful for athletes unable to tolerate solid food pre- and post-training or those with small appetites.

3. Be moderate with intake of high-satiety and high-fibre options. Look to replace some wholegrain options with white. Low-energy fruit and vegetables, while a great source of nutrients, may also need to be moderated, allowing more room for energy-dense, nutrient-rich options.

4. Athletes may need reminding that the period of increased energy density is not an excuse for gluttony and junk food, rather a period where well-planned, frequent eating occasions are prioritised.

- Many athletes will require advice about lifestyle and time management to allow them to achieve adequate time for eating, sleeping, training and their other daily commitments. Planning the day's intake of food—what and when—may assist some athletes in ensuring suitable foods and drinks are at hand when required. A ready supply of non-perishable snacks in their locker or training bag can be a great idea. This might include tetra packs of UHT flavoured-milk or fruit juice, cereal bars, powdered or prepared liquid meal supplements and sports drinks. The sports dietitian should assess the potential of the athlete's environment for purchasing suitable foods, or for storing snacks brought from home.

- Emotive labelling on products promoted in many gyms, sporting magazines and health food stores ensures dietary supplements are very popular among athletes attempting to increase lean body mass. Athletes can be confronted by a huge array of products from protein powders and amino acid formulas to proclaimed growth enhancers and energy substrates. Some may be of benefit to certain athletes in specific situations but the claims of most supplements do not hold up to the scrutiny of scientific research. It is imperative that the sports dietitian maintains an up-to-date knowledge of existing and newly formulated supplements regarding their claims, scientific support or lack thereof, application, dosage, legality and safety. The goal is to allow an athlete to make an informed decision and see through the emotive claims, identifying those supplements that may assist in enhancing gains in lean body mass. From here a cost-versus-benefit assessment is warranted. Athletes must be reminded that the core of a successful hypertrophy program is a suitably designed training program and well structured meal plan—supplements are not essential! The dietitian should, however, remain unbiased in their opinion of new supplements until research has been undertaken on the supplements' ergogenic potential. Chapter 17 provides a detailed review of the most commonly promoted dietary supplements.

REFERENCES

Allen LH, Oddoye EA, Margen S. Protein-induced hypercalciuria: a longer term study. Am J Clin Nutr 1979;32:741–9.

Balagopal P, Ljungqvist O, Nair KS. Skeletal muscle myosin heavy-chain rate in healthy subjects. Am J Physiol 1997;272:E45–E50.

Beaton GH. Toward harmonization of dietary, biochemical, and clinical assessments: the meanings of nutritional status and requirements. Nutr Rev 1986;44:349–58.

Belcastro AN. Skeletal muscle calcium-activated neutral protease (calpain) with exercise. J Appl Physiol 1993;74:1381–6.

Bennet WM, Connacher AA, Scrimgeour CM, Smith K, Rennie MJ. Increase in anterior tibialis muscle protein synthesis in healthy man during a mixed amino acid infusion: studies of incorporation of $[1^{13}C]$leucine. Clin Sci 1989;76:447–54.

Bhasin S, Storer TW, Berman N, Callegari C, et al. The effect of supraphysiological doses on testosterone on muscle size and strength in normal men. N Eng J Med 1996;335:1–7.

Biolo G, Fleming RYD, Wolfe RR. Physiological hyperinsulinemia stimulates protein synthesis and enhances transport of selected amino acids in human skeletal muscle. J Clin Invest 1996;95:811–19.

Biolo G, Maggi SP, Williams BD, Tipton KD, Wolfe RR. Increased rates of muscle protein turnover and amino acid transport after resistance exercise in humans. Am J Phys 1995;268:E514–E520.

Biolo G, Tipton KD, Klein S, Wolfe RR. An abundant supply of amino acids enhances the metabolic effect of exercise on muscle protein. Am J Phys 1997;273:E122–E129.

Biolo G, Williams BD, Fleming RY, Wolfe RR. Insulin action on muscle protein kinetics and amino acid transport during recovery after resistance exercise. Diabetes 1999;48:949–57.

Bowtell JL, Lesse GP, Smith K, et al. Modulation of whole body protein metabolism, during and after exercise, by variation of dietary protein. J Appl Physiol 1998;85:1744–52.

Boyer B, Odessey R. Kinetic characterization of branched chain ketoacid dehydrogenase. Arch Biochem Biophys 1991;285:1–8.

Brenner BM, Meter TW, Hosteler D. Protein intake and the progressive nature of kidney disease: the role of hemodynamically mediated glomerular sclerosing in aging, renal ablation, and intrinsic renal disease. New Engl J Med 1982;307:652–57.

Brouns F, Stroecken SJ, Thijssen BR, Rehrer NJ, ten Hoor F. Eating, drinking and cycling: a controlled Tour de France simulation study: Part II, Effect of diet manipulation. Int J Sports Med 1989;10:S41–S48.

Brownell KD, Steen SN, Wilmore JH. Weight regulation practices in athletes: analysis of metabolic and health effects. Med Sci Sports Exerc 1987;19:546–56.

Bucci LR, Hichson IF, Wolinsky I, Pivarnik JM. Ornithine supplementation and insulin release in body builders. Int J Sport Nutr 1992;2:287–91.

Burke LM, Collier GR, Beasley SK, et al. Effect of coingestion of fat and protein with carbohydrate feedings on muscle glycogen storage. J Appl Physiol 1995;78:2187–92.

Burke LM, Collier GR, Davis PG, Fricker PA, Sanigorski AJ, Hargreaves M. Muscle glycogen storage after prolonged exercise: effect of the frequency of carbohydrate feedings. Am J Clin Nutr 1996;64:115–19.

Burke LM, Gollan RA, Read RSD. Dietary intakes and food use of groups of elite Australian male athletes. Int J Sport Nutr 1991;2:287–91.

Butterfield GE, Calloway DH. Physical activity improves protein utilisation in young men. Br J Nutr 1984;51:171–84.

Campbell WW, Crim MC, Young VR, Joseph LJ, Evans WJ. Effects of resistance training and dietary protein intake on protein metabolism in older adults. Am J Phys 1995;268:E1143–E1153.

Carraro F, Kimbrough TD, Wolfe RR. Urea kinetics in humans at two levels of exercise intensity. J Appl Physiol 1993;75:1180–5.

Castellino P, Luzi L, Simonson DC, Haymond M, DeFronzo RA. Effect of insulin and plasma amino acid concentrations on leucine metabolism in man. J Clin Invest 1987;80:1784–93.

Cathcart EP. Influence of muscle work on protein metabolism. Physiol Rev 1925;5:225–43.

Chesley A, MacDougall JD, Tarnopolsky MA, Atkinson SA, Smith K. Changes in human muscle protein synthesis after resistance exercise. J Appl Phys 1992;73:1383–8.

Chiang AN, Huang PC. Excess energy and nitrogen balance at protein intakes above the requirement level in young men. Am J Clin Nutr 1988;48:1015–22.

Consolazio CF, Johnson HL, Nelson RA, Dramise JG, Skala JH. Protein metabolism during intensive physical training in the young adult. Am J Clin Nutr 1975;28:29–35.

Department of Health and Welfare. Recommended Nutrient Intakes (Protein), in Nutrition recommendations: The report of the scientific review committee. Ottawa, Canada: Canadian Government Publishing Centre, 1990.

Deuster PA, Kyle SB, Moser PB, Vigersky RA, Singh A, Schoomaker EB. Nutritional survey of highly trained women runners. Am J Clin Nutr 1986;45:954–62.

Dohm GL, Hecker AL, Brown WE, et al. Adaptation of protein metabolism to endurance training. Biochem J 1977;164:705–8.

Drinkwater BL, Bruemmer B, Chesnut III CH. Menstrual history as a determinant of current bone density in young athletes. J Am Med Assoc 1990;263:545–8.

El-Khoury AE, Forslund A, Olsson R, et al. Moderate exercise at energy balance does not affect 24-hour leucine oxidation or nitrogen retention in healthy men. Am J Physiol 1997;273:E394–E407.

Ellsworth NM, Hewitt BF, Haskell WL. Nutrient intake of elite male and female Nordic skiers. Phys Sports Med 1985;13(2):78–2.

Elwyn DH. New concepts in nitrogen balance. Can J Gastroenterol 1990;4(SA):9A–12A.

Evans W, Fisher EC, Hoerr RA, Young VR. Protein metabolism and endurance exercise. Phys Sportsmed 1983;11:63–72.

Faber M, Benade AJS, van Eck M. Dietary intake, anthropometric measurements, and blood lipid values in weight training athletes (body builders). Int J Sports Med 1986;7:342–6.

FAO/WHO/UNU. Energy and protein requirements, in report of a joint FAO/WHO/UNU expert consultation. (Tech. Rep. No.724) Geneva, Switzerland: 1985.

Felder JM, Burke LM, Lowdon BJ, Cameron-Smith D, Collier GR. Nutritional practices of elite female surfers during training and competition. Int J Sport Nutr 1998;8:36–48.

Ferrando AA, Tipton KD, Doyle D, Phillips SM, Cortiella J, Wolfe RR. Testosterone injection stimulates net protein synthesis but not tissue amino acid transport. Am J Physiol 1998;275:E864–E871.

Fielding RA, Meredith CN, O'Reilly KP, Frontera WR, Cannon JG, Evans WJ. Enhanced protein breakdown after eccentric exercise in young and older men. J Appl Physiol 1991;71(2):674–9.

Florini JR. Hormonal control of muscle growth. Muscle and Nerve 1987;10:577–98.

Food and Nutrition Board/Commission on Life Sciences/National Research Council. Recommended daily allowances. Washington, DC: National Academy Press, 1989:(10)52–7.

Forslund AH, Hambraeus L, Olsson RM, El-Khoury AE, Yu YM, Young VR. The 24-hour whole body leucine and urea kinetics at normal and high protein intakes with exercise in healthy adults. Am J Physiol 1998;275:E310–E320.

Friedman JE, Lemon PWR. Effect of chronic endurance exercise on retention of dietary protein. Int J Sports Med 1989;10:118–23.

Furuno K, Goldberg AL. The activation of protein degradation in muscle by Ca^{2+} or muscle injury does not involve a lysosomal mechanism. Biochem J 1986;237:859–64.

Garlick PJ, Grant I. Amino acid infusion increases the sensitivity of muscle protein synthesis in vivo to insulin. Biochem J 1988;254:579–84.

Gibala MJ, MacLean DA, Graham TE, Saltin B. Anaplerotic processes in human skeletal muscle during brief dynamic exercise. J Physiol (Lond) 1997;502:703–13.

Goldberg AL, Chang TW. Regulation and significance of amino acid metabolism in skeletal muscle. Fed Proc 1978;37:2301–7.

Gontzea I, Sutzescu P, Dumitrache S. The influence of muscular activity on nitrogen balance and on the need of man for proteins. Nutr Reports Int 1974;10:35–41.

Gontzea I, Sutzescu P, Dumitrache S. The influence of adaptation to physical effort on nitrogen balance in man. Nutr Reports Int 1975;22:231–6.

Griggs RC, Kingston W, Jozefowicz RF, Herr BE, Forbes G, Halliday D. Effect of testosterone on muscle mass and muscle protein synthesis. J Appl Physiol 1989;66:498–503.

Haff GG, Stone MH, Warren BJ, et al. The effect of carbohydrate supplementation on multiple sessions and bouts of resistance exercise. J Strength Conditioning Res 1999;13:111–17.

Hagg SA, Morse E, Adibi SA. Effect of exercise on rates of oxidation, turnover, and plasma clearance of leucine in human subjects. Am J Physiol 1982;242:E407–E410.

Haralambie G, Berg A. Serum urea and amino nitrogen changes with exercise duration. Eur J Appl Physiol 1976;36:39–48.

Harris HA. Nutrition and physical performance: the diet of Greek athletes. Proc Nutr Soc 1966;25:87–93.

Hasten DL, Morris GS, Ramanadham S, Yarasheski KE. Isolation of human skeletal muscle myosin heavy chain and actin for measurement of fractional synthetic rates. Am J Physiol 1998;275:E1092–E1099.

Henderson SA, Black AL, Brooks GA. Leucine turnover and oxidation in trained rats during exercise. Am J Physiol 1985;249:E137–E144.

Hertzman PA, Blevins WL, Mayer J, Greenfield B, Ting M, Gleich GJ. Association of the eosinophilia-myalgia syndrome with the ingestion of tryptophan. N Engl J Med 1990;322:869–73.

Hickson JF, Hinkelmann K, Bredle DL. Protein intake level and introductory weight training exercise on urinary total nitrogen excretions from untrained men. Nutr Res 1988;8:725–31.

Hood DA, Terjung RL. Effect of endurance training on leucine metabolism in perfused rat skeletal muscle. Am J Physiol 1987;253:E648–E656.

Ivy JL, Katz AL, Cutler CL, Sherman WM, Coyle EF. Muscle glycogen synthesis after exercise: effect of time of carbohydrate ingestion. J Appl Physiol 1988;65:1480–85.

Kameyama T, Etlinger JD. Calcium-dependent regulation of protein synthesis and degradation in muscle. Nature 1979;279:344–6.

Kasperek GJ, Snider RD. Total and myofibrillar protein degradation in isolated soleus muscles after exercise. Am J Physiol 1989;257:E1–E5.

Khatra BS, Chawla RK, Sewell CW, Rudman D. Distribution of branched-chain keto acid dehydrogenases in primate tissues. J Clin Invest 1977;59:558–64.

Kraemer WJ, Marchitelli L, Gordon SE, et al. Hormonal and growth factor responses to heavy resistance exercise protocols. J Appl Physiol 1990;69:1442–50.

Krempf M, Hoerr RA, Pelletier VA, Marks LM, Gleason R, Young VR. An isotopic study of the effect of dietary carbohydrate on the metabolic fate of dietary leucine and phenylalnine. Am J Clin Nutr 1993;57:161–9.

Lamont LS, McCullough AJ, Kalhan SC. Comparison of leucine kinetics in endurance-trained and sedentary humans. J Appl Physiol 1999;86:320–5.

Lamont LS, Patel DG, Kalhan SC. Leucine kinetics in endurance-trained humans. J Appl Physiol 1990;69:1–6.

Lemon PWR. Effects of exercise on dietary protein requirements. Intl J Sport Nutr 1998;8:426–47.

Lemon PWR, Mullin JP. The effect of initial muscle glycogen levels on protein catabolism during exercise. J Appl Physiol 1980;48:624–9.

Lemon P, Tarnopolsky MA, MacDougall JD, Atkinson S. Protein requirements and muscle mass/strength changes in novice body builders. J Appl Physiol 1992;73:767–75.

Lowell BB, Ruderman NB, Goodman MN. Regulation of myofibrillar protein degradation in rat skeletal muscle during brief and prolonged starvation. Metabolism 1986;35:1121–7.

MacDougall JD, Gibala MJ, Tarnopolsky MA, MacDonald JR, Interisano SA, Yarasheski KE. The time course for elevated muscle protein synthesis following heavy resistance exercise. Can J Appl Physiol 1995;20:480–6.

MacLean DA, Spriet LL, Hultman E, Graham TE. Plasma and muscle amino acid and ammonia responses during prolonged exercise in humans. J Appl Physiol 1991;70:2095–103.

Marcus R, Cann C, Madvig P, et al. Menstrual function and bone mass in elite women distance runners: endocrine and metabolic features. Ann Intern Med 1985;102:158–63.

McKenzie S, Phillips S, Carter SL, Lowther S, Gibala MJ, Tarnopolsky MA. Endurance exercise training attenuates leucine oxidation and branched-chain 2-oxo acid dehydrogenase activation during exercise in humans. Am J Physiol 2000;278:E580–E587.

McNurlan MA, Essen P, Thorell A, et al. Response of protein synthesis in human skeletal muscle to insulin: an investigation with L-[^{2}H$_5$] phenylalanine. Am J Physiol 1994;267:E102–E108.

Medina R, Wing SS, Goldberg AL. Increase in levels of polyubiquitin and proteasome mRNA in skeletal muscle during starvation and denervation atrophy. Biochem J 1995 May 1;307(Pt 3):631–7.

Meredith CN, Zackin MJ, Frontera WR, Evans WJ. Dietary protein requirements and body protein metabolism in endurance-trained men. J Appl Physiol 1989;66:2850–6.

Mitch WE, Goldberg AL. Mechanisms of muscle wasting. New Engl J Med 1996;335:1897–905.

Moller-Loswick AC, Zachrisson H, Hyltander A, Korner U, Matthews DS, Lundholm K. Insulin selectively attenuates breakdown of non-myofibrillar proteins in peripheral tissues of normal men. Am J Physiol 1994;266:E645–E652.

Morgan MJ, Loghna PT. Work overload induced changes in fast and slow skeletal muscle myosin heavy chain gene expression. FEBS Lett 1989;255(2):427–30.

Nair KS, Halliday D, Griggs RC. Leucine incorporation into mixed skeletal muscle protein in humans. Am J Physiol 1988;254:E208–E213.

Newman E, Heslin MJ, Wolf RF, Pisters PWT, Brennan MF. The effect of systemic hyperinsulinemia with concomitant amino acid infusion on skeletal muscle protein turnover in the human forearm. Metabolism 1994;43:70–8.

Pellett PL. Protein requirements in humans. Am J Clin Nutr 1990;51:723–37.

Phillips SM, Atkinson SA, Tarnopolsky MA, MacDougall JD. Gender differences in leucine kinetics and nitrogen balance in endurance athletes. J Appl Physiol 1993;75:2134–41.

Phillips SM, Tipton KD, Aarsland A, Wolf SE, Wolfe RR. Mixed muscle protein synthesis and breakdown following resistance exercise in humans. Am J Physiol 1997;273:E99–E107.

Rathmacher JA, Flakoli PJ, Nissen SL. A compartmental model of 3-methylhistidine metabolism in humans. Am J Physiol 1995;269:E193–E198.

Rennie MJ, Edwards RHT, Krywawych S, et al. Effect of exercise on protein turnover in man. Clin Sci 1981;61:627–39.

Rosenthal N. DNA and the genetic code. N Engl J Med 1994;331(1):39–41.

Roy BD, Tarnopolsky MA, MacDougall JK, Fowles J, Yarasheski KE. Effect of glucose supplement timing on protein metabolism after resistance training. J Appl Physiol 1997;82:1811–88.

Roy BD, Fowles JR, Hill R, Tarnopolsky MA. Macronutrient intake and whole body protein metabolism following resistance exercise. Med Sci Sports Exerc, Aug 2000.

Sale DG, MacDougall JD, Alway SE, Sutton JR. Voluntary strength and muscle characteristics in untrained men and women and male bodybuilders. J Appl Physiol 1987 May;62(5):1786–93.

Short SH, Short WR. Four year study of university athletes' dietary intake. J Am Diet Assoc 1983;82:632–45.

Slavin JL, Lanners G, Engstrom MA. Amino acid supplements: beneficial or risky? Phys Sportsmed 1988;16(3):221–4.

Snead DB, Weltman A, Weltman JY, et al. Reproductive hormones and bone mineral density in women runners. J Appl Physiol 1992;72:2149–56.

Steen SN, Brownell KD. Patterns of weight loss and regain in wrestlers: has the tradition changed? Med Sci Sports Exerc 1990;22:762–8.

Svanberg E, Moller-Loswick AC, Matthews DE, Korner U, Andersson M, Lundholm K. Effects of amino acids on synthesis and degradation of skeletal muscle proteins in humans. Am J Physiol 1996;271:E718–E724.

Tarnopolsky MA, Atkinson SA, MacDougall JD, Chesley A, Phillips S, Schwarcz H. Evaluation of protein requirements for trained strength athletes. J Appl Physiol 1992;73:1986–95.

Tarnopolsky MA, Atkinson SA, MacDougall JD, Senor BB, Lemon PWR, Schwarcz HP. Whole body leucine metabolism during and after resistance exercise in fed humans. Med Sci Sports Exerc 1991;23:326–33.

Tarnopolsky MA, Atkinson SA, Phillips SM, MacDougall JD. Carbohydrate loading and metabolism during exercise in men and women. J Appl Physiol 1995;78:1360–8.

Tarnopolsky MA, Bosman M, MacDonald JR, Vandeputte D, Martin J, Roy BD. Post-exercise protein-carbohydrate and carbohydrate supplements increase muscle glycogen in men and women. J Appl Physiol 1997;83:1877–83.

Tarnopolsky MA, Cipriano N, Woodcroft C, et al. Effects of rapid weight loss and wrestling on muscle glycogen concentration. Clin J Sport Med 1996;6:78–84.

Tarnopolsky MA, MacDougall JD, Atkinson SA. Influence of protein intake and training status on nitrogen balance and lean body mass. J Appl Physiol 1988;64:187–93.

Tarnopolsky LJ, MacDougall JD, Atkinson SA, Tarnopolsky MA, Sutton JR. Gender differences in substrate for endurance exercise. J Appl Physiol 1990;68:302–8.

Teman AJ, Hainline B. Eosinophilia-myalgia syndrome. Phys Sportsmed 1991;19(2):81–6.

Tessari P, Inchiostro S, Biolo G, et al. Differential effects of hyperinsulinemia and hyperaminoacidemia on leucine–carbon metabolism in vivo. J Clin Invest 1987;79:1062–9.

Tidball JG. Inflammatory cell response to acute muscle injury. Med Sci Sports Exerc 1995;27:1022.

Tipton KD, Ferrando AA, Phillips SM, Doyle Jr D, Wolfe RR. Post-exercise net protein synthesis in human muscle from orally administered amino acids. Am J Physiol 1999;276:E628–E634.

Tipton KD, Ferrando AA, Williams BD, Wolfe RR. Muscle protein metabolism in female swimmers after a combination of resistance and endurance exercise. J Appl Physiol 1996;81:2034–8.

Todd KS, Butterfield GE, Calloway DH. Nitrogen balance in men with adequate and deficient energy intake at three levels of work. J Nutr 1984;114:2107–18.

Torun B, Scrimshaw NS, Young VR. Effect of isometric exercises on body potassium and dietary protein requirements of young men. Am J Clin Nutr 1977;30:1983–93.

Volek JS, Kraemer WJ, Bush JA, Incledon T, Boetes M. Testosterone and cortisol in relationship to dietary nutrients and resistance exercise. J Appl Physiol 1997;82:49–54.

Von Liebig J. Animal chemistry or organic chemistry in its applications to physiology. G Gregory (Trans) 1842;London:Taylor & Walton.

Wagenmakers AJM, Brooks JH, Coakley JH, Reilly T, Edwards RHT. Exercise-induced activation of the branched-chain 2-oxo acid dehydrogenase in human muscle. Eur J Appl Physiol 1989;59:159–67.

Wagenmakers AJ, Beckers EJ, Brouns F, et al. Carbohydrate supplementation, glycogen depletion, and amino acid metabolism during exercise. Am J Physiol 1991;260:E883–E890.

Welle S, Bhatt K, Thornton CA. Stimulation of myofibrillar synthesis by exercise is mediated by more efficient translation of mRNA. J Appl Physiol 1999;86:1220–5.

Welle S, Matthews DE, Campbell RG, Nair KS. Stimulation of protein turnover by carbohydrate overfeeding in men. Am J Physiol 1989;E413–E417.

Welle S, Thornton C, Jozefowicz R, Statt M. Myofibrillar protein synthesis in young and old men. Am J Physiol 1993;264:E693–E698.

White TP, Brooks GA. [U-14C]glucose,-alanine, and leucine oxidation in rats at rest and two intensities of running. Am J Physiol 1981;241:E155–E165.

Wolfe RR. Radioactive and stable isotope tracers in biomedicine: principles and practice of kinetic analysis. New York: Wiley-Liss, 1992.

Wolfe RR, Goodenough RD, Wolfe MH, Royle GT, Nadel ER. Isotopic analysis of leucine and urea metabolism in exercising humans. J Appl Physiol 1982;52:458–66.

Wolfe RR, Wolfe MH, Nadel ER, Shaw JHF. Isotopic determination of amino acid-urea interactions in exercise in humans. Am J Physiol 1984;56:221–9.

Yamaoka KA, Miyasaka N, Inuo G, et al. 1,1'-Ethylidenebis (tryptophan) (Peak E) induces functional activation of human eosinophils and interleukin 5 production from T lymphocytes: association of eosinophilia-myalgia syndrome with an L-tryptophan contaminant. J Clin Immunol 1994;14:50–60.

Yarasheski KE, Zachwieja JF, Bier DM. Acute effects of resistance exercise on muscle protein synthesis rate in young and elderly men and women. Am J Physiol 1993;265:E210–E214.

Young VR, Bier DM. A kinetic approach to the determination of human amino acid requirements. Nutr Rev 1987;45:289–98.

Young VR, Bier DM, Pellett PL. A theoretical basis for increasing current estimates of amino acid requirements in adult man, with experimental support. Am J Clin Nutr 1989;50:80–92.

Young VR, Munro HN. N-Methylhistidine (3-methylhistidine) and muscle protein turnover: an overview. Fed Proc 1978;37:2291–300.

Zaragosa R, Renau-Piqueras J, Portoles M, Hernandez-Yago J, Jorda A, Grisolia S. Rats fed prolonged high protein diets show an increase in nitrogen metabolism and liver megamitochondria. Arch Biochem Biophys 1987;258:426–35.

Zawadski KM, Yaspelkis III BB, Ivy JL. Carbohydrate–protein complex increases the rate of muscle glycogen storage after exercise. J Appl Physiol 1992;72:1854–9.

Zeman RJ, Kameyama T, Matsumoto K, Bernstein B, Etlinger JD. Regulation of protein degradation in muscle by calcium. J Biol Chem 1985;260(25):13619–24.

Zorzano A, Balon TW, Goodman MN, Ruderman NB. Additive effects of prior exercise and insulin on glucose and AIB uptake by rat muscle. Am J Physiol 1986 Jul;251(1 Pt 1):E21-6.

CHAPTER 6

Energy requirements of the athlete: assessment and evidence of energy efficiency

Melinda Manore and Janice Thompson

6.1 INTRODUCTION

Most individuals, including athletes, maintain a stable body mass (BM) over long periods of time, while paying little attention to the amount of energy consumed or expended each day. However, energy balance is of primary concern to the athlete who wants to alter body mass and/or composition to improve their exercise performance or meet a designated weight requirement for their sport. When energy consumption is insufficient to match that expended, much of the effort of training can be lost, since both fat and muscle will be used for energy. In addition, if energy intake is limited or restricted, the ability to obtain other essential nutrients (e.g. carbohydrate (CHO), protein, fat, vitamins and minerals) necessary for optimal sport performance and good health will also be compromised.

Many athletes, especially female athletes, feel pressured by their coaches, parents, peers and themselves to reduce BM. To maintain a low BM, these athletes restrict energy intake even though their energy expenditure is high. Athletes of any age must consume enough energy to cover the energy costs of daily living, the energy cost of their sport, and the energy costs associated with building and repairing of muscle tissue. Females of reproductive age must also cover the costs of menstruation, while younger athletes must cover the additional costs of growth. What is the consequence of restricting energy intake when energy expenditure is high? It has been hypothesised that this behaviour can increase energy efficiency, thus decreasing the amount of energy actually required to maintain BM.

This chapter will briefly review the concept of energy and macronutrient balance and the factors that contribute to energy balance in an athlete. Manipulating the energy balance equation for either gain or loss of BM for an individual athlete is covered in other sections of this book (see Practice tips in Chapter 5 for BM gain and Chapters 7 and 8 for BM loss). We will then discuss the concept of energy efficiency and the research evidence for and against this phenomenon in the athlete.

6.2 *ENERGY AND MACRONUTRIENT BALANCE*

For BM to be maintained, energy in (total kilojoules or kilocalories consumed and those drawn from body stores) must equal energy expended. Under these conditions an individual is considered to be in energy balance. This concept can be stated using the following equation:

Energy balance occurs when: $E_{in} = E_{out}$
Where E_{in} = Energy in (kJ/d or kcal/d) and E_{out} = Energy expended (kJ/d or kcal/d)

If an athlete is trying to increase BM, then E_{in} must exceed E_{out}. Conversely, if an athlete is trying to reduce BM, E_{out} must exceed E_{in}. Thus, inducing an imbalance in either E_{in} or E_{out} will result in the most dramatic changes in BM. Although a number of popular diets (e.g. high-protein/high-fat diets, low-CHO diets) claim to induce weight loss by just altering diet composition, BM will not be lost unless E_{in} is less than E_{out}. In addition, these types of diets are often detrimental to the serious athlete. Diet composition will only influence long-term changes in BM and body composition when there is an imbalance in E_{in} versus E_{out} (Melby & Hill 1999). In addition to diet composition, maintenance of BM and body composition can also be influenced by a number of other factors, such as genetic make-up, and environmental and lifestyle conditions (Flatt 1993).

We now know that the maintenance of BM and body composition over time requires that $E_{in} = E_{out}$ and that intakes of protein, CHO, fat and alcohol equal their oxidation rates. Therefore, macronutrient balance occurs when:

$Protein_{in} = Protein_{oxidation}$
$CHO_{in} = CHO_{oxidation}$
$Fat_{in} = Fat_{oxidation}$
$Alcohol_{in} = Alcohol_{oxidation}$

where $Protein_{in}$ is the amount of protein intake (g/d) and $Protein_{oxidation}$ is the amount of protein oxidised (g/d). These same notations apply to CHO, fat and alcohol.

The energy and macronutrient balance equations are both dynamic and time dependent, and allow for the effect of changing energy stores on energy expenditure over time. The following example, given by Swinburn and Ravussin (1993), illustrates this point. What would happen if an individual decided to consume an extra 413 kJ (100 kcal) a day for 40 years? The amount of extra energy consumed in this time would equal ~6 million kJ or 1.5 million kcal. If one assumes that there are 31 786 kJ/kg (7 700 kcal/kg) of body fat, the theoretical gain in BM would equal 190 kg over this 40-year period, yet the actual gain would be ~2.7 kg. After a period of positive energy balance, extra energy intake would cause a gain in BM (both fat and lean tissue). The larger body size would cause an increase in energy expenditure that would eventually balance the extra energy consumed. Of course, the actual gain in BM will depend on the amount of extra energy consumed, and to a lesser extent the composition of this energy (i.e. the amount of fat, CHO, protein or alcohol) and overall energy expenditure. Therefore, a gain in BM is the consequence of an initial positive energy balance, but can also be a mechanism whereby energy balance is eventually restored at a higher BM and energy requirement.

6.3 ▮ MACRONUTRIENT BALANCE

As indicated earlier, alterations in either energy intake or expenditure are the primary determinants of BM. However, changes in the type and amount of macronutrients consumed (i.e. protein, fat, CHO, and alcohol) and the oxidation of these macronutrients within the body must be considered when examining long-term weight maintenance. Under normal physiological conditions, CHO, protein and alcohol are not easily converted to body fat (Swinburn & Ravussin 1993; Prentice 1998). Thus, increases in the intake of non-fat nutrients stimulate their oxidation rates proportionally. Conversely, an increase in dietary fat intake does not immediately stimulate fat oxidation, thus increasing the probability that excess dietary fat will be stored as adipose tissue (Abbott et al. 1988; Westerterp 1993; Prentice 1998). In this way, the type of food eaten can play a role in the amount of energy consumed and expended each day (Acheson et al. 1984; Swinburn & Ravussin 1993).

6.3.1 *CHO balance*

Carbohydrate balance is proposed to be precisely regulated such that CHO intake matches CHO oxidation (Acheson et al. 1984; Flatt 1988; Jebb et al. 1996; Prentice 1998). The ingestion of CHO stimulates both glycogen storage and glucose oxidation, and inhibits fat oxidation. Glucose not stored as glycogen is oxidised directly in almost equal balance to that consumed (Flatt et al. 1985). The conversion of excess dietary CHO and protein to triglycerides (de novo lipogenesis) is very limited in normal weight humans except under non-physiological situations (Hellerstein et al. 1991). However, if large amounts of CHO (85% of total energy) are consumed over several consecutive days, and E_{in} exceeds E_{out}, fat in the form of triglyceride is synthesised (Acheson et al. 1988).

6.3.2 *Protein balance*

As with CHO, the body adjusts to a wide range of protein intakes by altering the rate of oxidation of dietary protein. After body protein needs are met, the carbon skeletons of any excess amino acids are diverted into the energy substrate pool and used for energy. The adequacy of total energy intake, and CHO intake in particular, appear to dramatically affect this process. Inadequate intakes of either energy or CHO result in negative protein balance (Krempf et al. 1993). Conversely, excess intake of either energy or CHO will spare protein. This protein is then available to support brief periods of protein accumulation until the protein pool is expanded to a new balance point. At this point, the degradation of endogenous protein matches the available exogenous protein. The excess protein consumed or the protein made available through protein sparing may contribute indirectly to fat storage by diverting dietary fat for storage.

6.3.3 *Fat balance*

Fat balance is not as precisely regulated as CHO balance and protein balance (Prentice 1998). As dietary fat intake increases, the short-term oxidation of fat does not increase proportionately (Astrup et al. 1994; Schrauwen et al. 1997). Over the long term, a positive fat balance, due to excess energy intake from a palatable high-fat diet, will lead to a progressive increase in total body-fat stores as the body attempts to achieve energy balance (Melby & Hill 1999). It has been hypothesised that increases in body-fat stores are due to low rates of fat oxidation relative to fat intake (Flatt 1995). As fat stores expand, they increase the free fatty acid (FFA) concentrations in the blood as a consequence of the constant flux of triglycerides occurring in these stores. This increase in circulation of FFA's may slightly increase fat oxidation; thus the larger adipose tissue mass promotes increased fat oxidation. When the new rate of fat oxidation equals the rate of fat intake, the individual will again achieve fat balance (and hence energy balance) but at a significantly higher body weight.

6.3.4 *Alcohol balance*

Alcohol consumption causes a rapid rise in alcohol oxidation until all the alcohol is cleared from the body. Thus alcohol is used preferentially as an energy source over other substrates and can suppress the oxidation of fat and, to a lesser degree, that of protein and CHO (Shelmet et al. 1988). Alcohol is not converted to triglycerides and stored as adipose tissue, nor can it contribute to the formation of muscle or liver glycogen. It may, however, indirectly divert dietary fat to storage by providing an alternative and preferred energy source for the body (Sonko et al. 1994). Alcohol has an energy density of ~29 kJ/g (7 kcal/g) and, thus, can contribute significantly to total daily energy intake. Individuals who consume alcohol must reduce their consumption of energy from other dietary components in order to maintain energy balance.

6.4 *ENERGY EXPENDITURE*

Determining energy balance requires the direct measurement or estimate of energy in (energy intake from the diet and from stored energy) and energy expended. This section reviews the various components of energy expenditure, how these components are measured, and discusses how physical activity may influence these components. We will also cover methods for predicting energy expenditure based on age, gender and body size.

6.4.1 *Components of energy expenditure*

The components of total daily energy expenditure are generally divided into three main categories (see Figure 6.1):

1. Basal energy expenditure or basal metabolic rate (BMR).
2. The thermic effect of food (TEF).
3. Energy expended in physical activity, or thermic effect of activity (TEA).

BMR is the energy required to maintain the systems of the body and to regulate body temperature at rest. BMR is measured in the morning after an overnight fast, while the individual is resting in a bed. The individual must be comfortable, and free from stress, medications or any other stimulation that would increase metabolic activity. In addition, the room where BMR is measured needs to be quiet, temperature-controlled and free of distractions. Because assessment of BMR requires the individual to stay

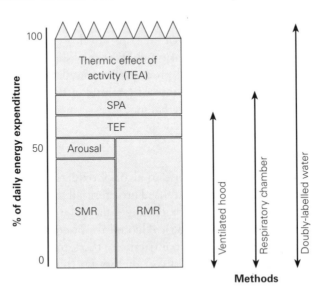

Figure 6.1 *Components of daily energy expenditure in humans (Adapted from: Ravussin E & Swinburn 1993)*

SPA = spontaneous physical activity; TEF = thermic effect of food; SMR = sleep metabolic rate; RMR = resting metabolic rate.

overnight in the laboratory, many researchers measure resting metabolic rate (RMR) instead. Assessment of RMR usually means that the individual slept at home and drove or was driven to the research laboratory, where they rested for a period of time before metabolic rate was assessed. Like BMR, subjects need to have fasted overnight, refrained from strenuous exercise the day before assessment, and be measured in a quiet temperature-controlled room. In general, BMR and RMR usually differ less than 10%. In this chapter, we will use the term RMR (except when a research study specifically reports that BMR was measured), since it is more frequently measured. Dietitians frequently use these terms interchangeably, when in fact they are measured differently.

RMR accounts for approximately 60–80% of total daily energy expenditure in most sedentary healthy adults (Ravussin et al. 1986; Ravussin & Bogardus 1989). However, in an active individual this percentage will vary greatly. Many elite athletes easily expend 4100–8300 kJ/d (1000–2000 kcal/d) in sport-related activities. For example, Thompson et al. (1993) reported that RMR represented only 38–47% of total daily energy expenditure in 24 elite male endurance athletes, while Beidleman et al. (1995) found in ten female endurance runners that RMR represented only 42% of total energy expenditure. During days of repetitive, heavy competition, such as ultramarathons, RMR may represent < 20% of total energy expenditure (Rontoyannis et al. 1989).

The TEF (sometimes called diet-induced thermogenesis (DIT)) is the increase in energy expenditure above RMR that results from the consumption of food throughout the day. The TEF includes the energy cost of food digestion, absorption, transport, metabolism and storage within the body. TEF usually accounts for approximately 6–10% of total daily energy expenditure, with women usually having a lower value (~6–7%) (Poehlman 1989). However, the TEF for an individual will vary depending on the energy content of the meal or the food eaten over the day, the types of foods consumed, composition of the diet, and the degree of obesity (Stock 1999; Westerterp et al. 1999).

Although TEF is frequently used interchangeably with the thermic effect of a meal (TEM), the terms are not synonymous. TEM represents the increase in metabolic rate above RMR after eating a meal. Most researchers measure TEM instead of TEF because of the difficulties in trying to assess the cumulative energy cost of all foods consumed within a day. Thus, most of the research literature examining the energy costs of active individuals reports TEM, unless a metabolic chamber is used to collect data.

TEA is the most variable component of energy expenditure in humans. It includes the energy cost of daily activities above RMR and TEF, such as purposeful activities of daily living (e.g. dressing, shopping, cooking, gardening) or planned exercise events (e.g. running, swimming, or weight lifting). It also includes the energy cost of involuntary muscular activity such as shivering and fidgeting. This type of movement is called spontaneous physical activity (SPA). TEA may be only 10–15% of total daily energy expenditure in sedentary individuals, but may be as high as 50% in active individuals.

There are a number of factors that can increase energy expenditure above normal baseline levels, such as cold, heat, fear, stress, and various medications or drugs (e.g. caffeine, alcohol and smoking) (Manore & Thompson 2000). The thermic effect of these factors is frequently referred to as adaptive thermogenesis (AT). AT represents a temporary increase in thermogenesis that may last for hours or even days, depending on the duration and magnitude of the stimulus. In athletes, a serious physical injury, the stress associated with an upcoming event, going to a higher altitude, or the use of certain medications may all increase RMR above normal levels.

6.4.1.1 *Factors that influence RMR*

A variety of factors can influence RMR for a given individual on any given day; however, some factors appear to have more of an influence than others. It is well documented that RMR is influenced by age, sex and body size, including the size of an individual's fat-free mass (FFM) and fat mass. In fact, these factors are usually included in prediction equations for RMR. Three of these variables (age, sex and FFM) generally explain about 80% of the variability in RMR (Bogardus et al. 1986). Since FFM, especially organ tissue, is very metabolically active, any change in FFM can dramatically influence RMR (Sparti et al. 1997). In general, males have larger RMRs than females because of an increased size and greater FFM; however, there may be other contributing factors to the differences in RMR besides gender. Ferraro et al. (1992) report that females have a lower BMR than males (413 kJ or 100 kcal/d less) even after controlling for differences in FFM, fat mass and age. Age is known to influence BMR, with an estimated decline in BMR of ~1–2% per decade from the second through to the seventh decade of life (Keys et al. 1987). Part of this decrease in RMR is attributed to the decline in quantity and the metabolic activity of FFM that occurs with ageing (Piers et al. 1998), especially if an individual leads a more sedentary lifestyle (Poehlman et al. 1992, 1993).

RMR also has a genetic component, which means that individuals within families may have similar RMRs. For example, Bogardus et al. (1986) found that family membership explained 11% of the variability in RMR (p < 0.0001) when they examined 130 non-diabetic adult south-western native Americans from 54 families. Bouchard and colleagues (1989) at Laval University also found that heritability explained approximately 40% of the variability in RMR in twins, and parent–child pairs after adjusting for age, gender and FFM.

Phases of the menstrual cycle may also influence RMR and total energy balance. Although the current research is equivocal, some studies report that RMR values are lowest during the follicular phase of the cycle (beginning of the cycle) and highest during the luteal phase (end of the cycle) (Solomon et al. 1982; Bisdee et al. 1989). The difference in RMR between these two phases is estimated to be approximately 413–1238 kJ/d (100–300 kcal/d); however, adaptations in energy intake appear to mimic the changes in RMR. A study by Barr et al. (1995) reports that females consume approximately 1238 kJ/d (300 kcal/d) more during the luteal phase of the menstrual cycle as compared with the follicular phase. Thus, the increased energy expenditure, due to a higher RMR during the luteal phase, is compensated for by an increase in energy intake during this period. Additional evidence supporting the impact of menstrual cycle on RMR comes from studies examining the impact of menstrual dysfunction on energy expenditure. Lebenstedt et al. (1999) found that RMR was significantly lower (~460 kJ or 111 kcal/d) in female athletes with menstrual dysfunction (nine periods per year) compared to active controls (12 periods per year), while Myerson et al. (1991) found amenorrheic runners had significantly lower RMRs than eumenorrheic runners and inactive controls. Conversely, Weststrate (1993) and Li et al. (1999) found no effect of menstrual cycle on RMR, and Piers et al. (1995) found no effect of menstrual cycle phase on RMR or energy intake. Thus, until these issues are resolved, menstrual status and the phase of the menstrual cycle should be documented using some type of hormonal data and/or recorded when measuring RMR or energy intake in females, especially active females.

There are a number of ways that exercise might indirectly or directly change RMR. Firstly, exercise may increase RMR indirectly by increasing an individual's FFM, which is a strong determinate of RMR. It is well documented in the research literature that active individuals, especially elite athletes, are leaner (lower per cent body fat) and have greater FFM than their sedentary counterparts. Thus, for a given BM, an athlete with a lower percentage of body fat and higher percentage of FFM will have a higher RMR. Secondly, it has also been hypothesised that exercise training influences RMR; however, data comparing RMR in exercise-trained and sedentary controls have not shown consistent increases in RMR when subjects (athletes and controls) are matched for size and FFM. For example, Poehlman et al. (1990) found a significantly greater (~5%) RMR (expressed as kJ/kg FFM) in active men compared with untrained males of similar size and FFM, while Broeder et al. (1992) found no significant difference in RMR between active and inactive males. Mean RMR was only 3.4% higher in the exercise-trained group. The discrepancies in these results may be due to a number of factors, including level of fitness, type of exercise training program, methods used to measure RMR, and level of energy flux (the amount of energy expended in exercise compared with the amount of energy consumed each day) (Bullough et al. 1995; Manore & Thompson 2000). Thirdly, strenuous exercise may cause muscle tissue damage that requires building and repair after exercise is over, thus indirectly causing an increase in RMR.

An acute bout of strenuous exercise has also been hypothesised to directly influence RMR. It has been observed that RMR is increased for a period of time (minutes or hours) after strenuous exercise; this phenomenon is termed excess post-exercise oxygen consumption (EPOC). How quickly oxygen consumption returns to baseline after exercise is over may depend on a number of factors including level of training, age, environmental conditions, and intensity and duration of the exercise. It appears that to produce a significant increase in EPOC, exercise intensity must be high and/or the duration of exercise must be long. A normal exercise bout of 30–60 minutes of moderate intensity (50–65% $VO_{2\,max}$) does not appear to significantly elevate EPOC for any appreciable amount of time after the exercise is over (Manore & Thompson 2000). After this type of exercise, oxygen levels usually return to normal within one hour. However, if exercise (either aerobic or strength training) is of high intensity and/or of long duration, EPOC appears to be elevated for hours after exercise (Chad & Quigley 1991; Melby et al. 1993; Gillette et al. 1994).

6.4.1.2 *Factors that influence TEF*

A number of factors can influence how our bodies respond metabolically when we consume food. The TEF can last for several hours after a meal and depends on the energy content of the meal consumed, and the composition of the meal (percentage of energy from protein, fat and CHO). In general, the thermic effect of a mixed meal is estimated to be 6–10% of total daily energy intake; however, the total TEF will also depend on the macronutrient composition of the diet. For example, the thermogenic effect of glucose is 5–10%, fat is 3–5% and protein is 20–30% (Flatt 1992). The lower thermic response for fat is due to the lower energy requirement to store fat as triglyceride as compared to the synthesis of proteins from amino acids or glycogen from CHO. The impact of diet composition on TEF has been clearly demonstrated by Westerterp et al. (1999) in women of normal BM. They fed two different diets: high-protein, high-CHO diet (30% energy protein, 60% CHO, 10% fat) and a high-fat diet (10% energy protein, 30% CHO, 60% fat). The diets were isocaloric and isovolumetric, and they were composed of normal foods and matched for taste, smell and appearance. The diets were administered to eight healthy females over two different 24-hour periods in the metabolic chamber. They found a significantly higher TEF (14.6% of total energy intake: 1295 kJ/d or 313 kcal/d) in the high-protein, high-CHO diet compared to the high-fat diet (10.5% of total energy intake: 931 kJ/d or 225 kcal/d).

Acute exercise and chronic training may also influence the TEF. Aerobically-trained males generally have a lower TEF than sedentary males, while studies in trained women do not support a lower TEF (Poehlman 1989). These gender differences might be attributed to the failure to control for the time of the menstrual cycle or menstrual status (e.g. amenorrhoea, oligomenorrhoea or eumenorrhoea) in studies measuring the TEF in active women. For example, Li et al. (1999) found that the thermic effect of feeding sucrose was influenced by the phase of the menstrual cycle, with a significantly higher response in the luteal phase than the follicular phase. The effect of acute exercise on TEF appears to depend on a number of factors, including the level of obesity, the timing of the meal and exercise session, the intensity and duration of the exercise, and the level of fitness. Segal et al. (1992) reported that exercise before a meal had no significant effect on the TEM in lean subjects, but increased the TEM in obese subjects by 40%. However, the absolute increase in total energy was small 40–60 kJ (10–15 kcal) per three hours. Few data are available on the effect of exercise before and after a meal in exercise-trained subjects.

6.4.2 *Measurement of total daily energy expenditure*

Total daily energy expenditure or its components can be measured in the laboratory or estimated using prediction equations. The following section discusses the most commonly used laboratory techniques for measuring the components of energy expenditure. When laboratory facilities are not available, prediction equations can be used to estimate total daily energy expenditure.

6.4.2.1 *Indirect calorimetry*

Energy expenditure in humans is commonly assessed using indirect calorimetry, which measures the rate of oxygen consumption (L/min) and carbon dioxide production (L/min) either at rest or during exercise. The ratio between the volume of carbon dioxide produced (VCO_2) and the volume of oxygen consumed (VO_2) can be calculated (VCO_2/VO_2). This ratio, when considered at the cellular level, is termed the non-protein respiratory quotient (RQ) and represents the ratio between oxidation of CHO and lipid. By knowing the amount of each energy substrate oxidised and the amount of oxygen consumed and carbon dioxide produced, total energy expenditure can be estimated using various published formulae. In general, the consumption of one litre of oxygen results in the expenditure of approximately 19.86 kJ (4.81 kcal) if the fuels oxidised represent a mixture of protein, fat and CHO. Since RQ cannot be directly determined at the cellular level in humans, an indirect measurement is taken by measuring gas exchange at the mouth. The relationship of VCO_2/VO_2 measured by this means is termed the respiratory exchange ratio (RER). RER is considered an accurate reflection of RQ under steady-state conditions. Using the indirect calorimetry method, one can measure total daily energy expenditure in a metabolic chamber, or measure RMR by using a mask, hood, or mouthpiece in which gases are collected and analysed for a specified period of time. Reviews by Schoeller & Racette (1990), Webb (1991), Westerterp (1993) and Montoye et al. (1996) provide additional information on the methods of indirect calorimetry.

RER values depend on the substrate being utilised, ranging from values of 0.7 (oxidation of fat only) to 1.0 (oxidation of pure CHO). Most individuals consuming a mixed diet of protein, fat and CHO will have an RER value of 0.82–0.87 at rest. However, during times of high exercise intensity, RER will increase closer to 1.0, while during times of fasting or low energy intake RER will decrease and be closer to 0.7. Thus, RER depends on the composition of the foods consumed, the energy demands placed on the body, and whether BM is being maintained.

6.4.2.2 *Doubly-labelled water*

Because indirect calorimetry requires that an individual be confined to a laboratory setting or a metabolic chamber, it is difficult to measure an individual's free-living energy expenditure. The development of the doubly-labelled water (DLW) ($^2H_2^{18}O$) method for use in humans has become a valuable tool in determining free-living energy expenditure (Speakman 1998). This method was first developed for use in animals (Lifson et al. 1955) and eventually applied to humans (Schoeller et al. 1986). The DLW method is a form of indirect calorimetry based on the differential elimination of deuterium ($^2H_2$) and ^{18}oxygen (^{18}O) from body water, following a load dose of water labelled with these two stable isotopes. The deuterium is eliminated as water, while the ^{18}O is eliminated as both water and carbon dioxide. The difference between the two elimination rates is a measure of carbon dioxide production (Coward & Cole 1991; Prentice et al. 1991; Speakman 1998). This method differs from traditional indirect calorimetry in that it only measures carbon dioxide production and not oxygen consumption. One advantage to this method is that it can be used to measure energy expenditure in free-living subjects for three days to three weeks, and only requires the periodic collection of urine for measurement of the isotope elimination rates. Another advantage is that it is free of bias, and subjects can engage in normal daily activities and sports without the interruption of writing down activities or wearing a heart-rate monitor. This method has become a valuable tool for the validation of other less expensive field methods of measuring energy expenditure, such as accelerometers (Schoeller & Racette 1990). The major disadvantage of this technique is expense. Another disadvantage is that it has a five-times greater potential for error in estimating energy expenditure because it uses only the energy equivalent of carbon dioxide instead of the energy equivalent of oxygen (Jequier et al. 1987). Finally, the experimental variability of the DLW technique in adult humans appears to be high ($\pm$ 8.5%) (Speakman 1998). This variability is high both when repeating the technique in the same individual and between individuals (Goran et al. 1994).

6.4.2.3 *Predicting total daily energy expenditure*

When laboratory facilities are not available for assessing total energy expenditure, it can be estimated by applying prediction equations to estimate RMR, then multiplying RMR by an appropriate activity factor. A number of prediction equations have been developed to estimate RMR (see Table 6.1). These prediction equations have been developed for different populations that vary in age, gender, level of obesity, and activity level. In general, it is best to use a prediction equation that is the most representative of the population or group of individuals with whom you are working. For example, if you are trying to predict the RMR of young active females, it is best to use an equation that was derived from a study of this population. Table 6.1 summarises some of the commonly used RMR prediction equations and the population from which these equations were derived (Manore & Thompson 2000). It should be noted that most of the prediction equations have been developed using sedentary individuals. In an effort to determine which of these equations works best for active individuals and athletes, Thompson and Manore (1996) compared the actual RMR values measured in the laboratory with predicted RMR values, using equations listed in Table 6.1. They found that for both active males and females the Cunningham (1980) equation best predicted RMR in this population, with the

Harris–Benedict (1919) equation being the next best predictor. Figures 6.2a and 6.2b graphically show how close these equations actually predicted RMR in a group of endurance-trained males and females. Because the Cunningham (1980) equation requires the measurement of lean body mass (LBM) or FFM in kilograms, the Harris–Benedict (1919) equation is easier to use in settings where FFM cannot be directly measured.

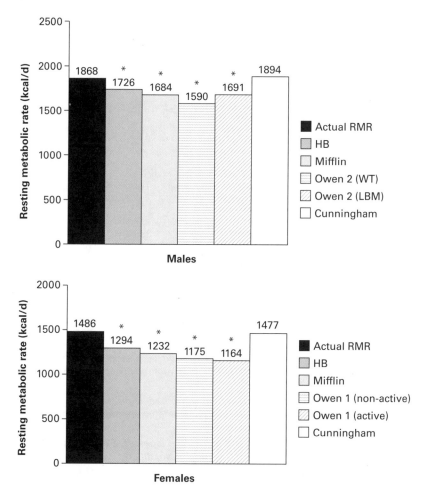

Figure 6.2   *Mean group differences between actual and predicted resting meta-bolic rate (RMR) for 24 male (6.2a) and 13 female (6.2b) highly-trained endurance athletes (Adapted from Thompson & Manore 1996)*

* Indicates values were significantly different from actual measured RMR (P < 0.05)
HB = Harris and Benedict equation (1919); Mifflin = Mifflin et al. equation (1990); Owen 1 = Owen et al. equation (1986) for active and non-active women; Owen 2 = Owen et al. equation (1987) for men using either body weight (WT) or lean body mass (LBM); and Cunningham = Cunningham (1980) equation. Equations are listed in Table 6.1

Table 6.1 *Equations for estimating resting metabolic rate (RMR) in healthy individuals*

Harris–Benedict (1919):[a]
Males: RMR = 66.47 + 13.75 (wt) + 5 (ht) − 6.76 (age)
Females: RMR = 655.1 + 9.56 (wt) + 1.85 (ht) − 4.68 (age)
Owen et al. (1986):[b]
Active females: RMR = 50.4 + 21.1 (wt)
Inactive females: RMR = 795 + 7.18 (wt)
Owen et al. (1987):[c]
Males: RMR = 290 + 22.3 (LBM)
Males: RMR = 879 + 10.2 (wt)
Mifflin et al. (1990):[d]
RMR = 9.99 (wt) + 6.25 (ht) − 4.92 (age) + 166 (sex; male = 1, female = 0) −161
Cunningham (1980):[e]
RMR = 500 + 22 (LBM)
World Health Organization (1985):[f]
Sex and age (yr) range equation to derive RMR in kcal/d

Males				Females		
0–3	(60.9 x wt)	− 54	0–3	(61.0 x wt)	− 51
3–10	(22.7 x wt)	+ 495	3–10	(22.5 x wt)	+ 499
10–18	(17.5 x wt)	+ 651	10–18	(12.2 x wt)	+ 746
18–30	(15.3 x wt)	+ 679	18–30	(14.7 x wt)	+ 496
30–60	(11.6 x wt)	+ 879	30–60	(8.7 x wt)	+ 829
60	(13.5 x wt)	+ 487	> 60	(10.5 x wt)	+ 596

Where wt = weight (kg), ht = height (cm), age = age (yr), and LBM = lean body mass (kg)

a) Harris–Benedict equation was published in 1919, based on 136 men (mean age 27 ± 9 yr; mean wt 64 ± 10 kg) and 103 women (mean age 331 ± 14; 56.5 ± 11.5) (n = 239 subjects). Included trained male athletes. They derived different equations for both men and women. Weight, height and age were variables they included. Research frequently reports that Harris–Benedict equation over-predicts RMR by > 15%. Harris–Benedict equation reports the measurement of basal energy expenditure (BEE), but the methods used were that of RMR (Frankenfield et al. 1998).

b) Owen et al. (1986) equation used 44 lean and obese women; eight women were trained athletes (ages 18–65 yrs; weight range 48–143 kg). No women were menstruating during the study; all were weight stable for at least one month.

c) Owen et al. (1987) equation used 60 lean and obese men (ages: 18–82 yr; weight range 60–171 kg). All were weight stable for at least one month. No athletes were included in this study.

d) Mifflin et al. (1990) equation used 498 healthy lean and obese subjects (247 females and 251 males), aged 18–78 years; weight ranged from 46–120 kg for the women and 58–143 kg for the men. No mention was made of physical activity level.

e) Cunningham (1980) used 223 subjects (120 males and 103 females) from the 1919 Harris and Benedict database. They eliminated 16 males who were identified as trained athletes. In this study, LBM accounted for 70% of the variability of BMR. Age variable did not add much because group age range was narrow. LBM was not calculated in the Harris–Benedict equation so they estimated LBM based on body mass (kg) and age.

f) WHO (1985) derived these equations from BMR data.

Reprinted with permission from: Manore MM, Thompson JL. *Sport nutrition in health and performance.* Champaign, Illinois: Human Kinetics Publishers, 2000

Once RMR has been estimated, total daily energy expenditure can then be estimated by a variety of different factorial methods. These methods vary in how labour intensive they are to use, and the level of subject burden. Manore and Thompson (2000) provide a detailed description of these methods. The easiest method for assessing total energy expenditure multiplies RMR by an appropriate activity factor, with the resulting value representing total daily energy expenditure. This factor may range from as low as 10–20% (0.10–0.20) of RMR for a bed-ridden individual to > 100% (> 1.0) for a very active individual. Although many laboratories establish their own activity factor for their particular research setting, factors of 1.3–1.6 are commonly used with sedentary individuals or individuals doing only light activity. With the activity factor methods, RMR is multiplied by a designated activity factor or factors (see Table 6.2). One activity factor can be applied to the whole day or a weighted activity factor can be determined. This activity factor is then multiplied by the RMR to provide a total daily energy expenditure. For example, if an individual has a RMR of 6 192 kJ/d (1500 kcal/d) and an activity factor of 1.5, then the daily energy expenditure would be 50% above RMR or 9288 kJ/d (2250 kcal/d) (6192 kJ $\times$ 1.5 = 9288 kJ/d). Regardless of the method used to calculate energy expenditure, it should be noted that all values are estimates. How accurate these values are depends on how accurately activity is recorded or reported, how accurate the data base is that is used to generate the energy expended per activity, and how accurately the required calculations are done.

6.5 *ENERGY EFFICIENCY: DOES IT EXIST?*

The potential for energy efficiency among athletes was brought to the attention of researchers through a number of research studies in which active women reported energy intakes that appeared inadequate to meet total daily energy expenditures (Drinkwater et al. 1984; Deuster et al. 1986; Kaiserauer et al. 1989; Dahlstrom et al. 1990; Mulligan & Butterfield 1990; Myerson et al. 1991; Wilmore et al. 1992; Beidleman et al. 1995). In these studies, active women (running 20–60 miles per week; or participating in gymnastics, swimming, triathlons or dancing) were reported to be consuming ≤147 kJ (35 kcal) per kg BM. Despite these low energy intakes and apparent energy deficits, these individuals reported the maintenance of BM over relatively long periods of time.

There are a number of possible explanations for an athlete's ability to maintain BM despite the discrepancy between reported energy intake and energy expenditure. Firstly, this discrepancy may be due to inaccuracies in reported estimates of energy expenditure or energy intakes, particularly due to athletes under-reporting or under-consuming their usual intake during the period of monitoring (Dahlstrom et al. 1990; Wilmore et al. 1992; Schulz 1992). A second explanation is that active individuals become more sedentary during non-exercising portions of the day, thus expending less energy than is estimated (Gorsky & Calloway 1983). Finally, these

Table 6.2 *Approximate energy expenditure, expressed as multiples of RMR, for various activities in relation to resting needs for males and females of average size*

Activity category[a]	Representative values for activity factor per unit of time of activity	Range
Resting Sleeping, reclining	RMR x 1.0	< 1-1
Very light Seated and standing activities, painting trades, driving, laboratory work, typing, sewing, ironing, cooking, playing cards, playing a musical instrument, billiards	RMR x 1.5	1.5–2.5
Light Walking on a level surface at 2.5–3 mph, garage work, electrical trades, carpentry, restaurant trades, house-cleaning, child care, golf, sailing, table tennis, ten-pin bowling, tennis (leisurely pace)	RMR x 2.5	2.0–4.0
Moderate Walking 3.5–4 mph, weeding and hoeing, carrying a load, cycling (slow), skiing, tennis, dancing, cricket, horse-riding, sailing, swimming (slow), stretching, tennis (moderate)	RMR x 4.0	3.0–5.0
Strenuous Jogging/running (7 km/h), tennis (fast pace), ice/roller skating, swimming (moderate pace), gymnastics, aerobic, basketball, football, squash, weight training, walking uphill with a load, soccer	RMR x 7.0	5.0–9.0
Very strenuous Swimming (race pace), rowing (race pace), cycling (race pace), squash (fast pace), running (10–15 km/h)	RMR x 10.0	7.0–13.0

[a]*When reported as multiples of basal needs, the expenditures of males and females are similar.*
Adapted from: National Research Council. *Recommended Dietary Allowances*, 10th edn. Washington DC: National Academy Press, 1989: 27; and Warwick PM. *Predicting food energy requirements from estimates of energy expenditure.* Aust J Nutr Diet 1989;46(suppl):3–29

differences may be due to increased metabolic efficiency (Mulligan & Butterfield 1990; Myerson et al. 1991; Thompson et al. 1993, 1995). If metabolic efficiency is present, then the actual energy requirements of these athletes are lower than those estimated by traditional means and would partially explain their ability to maintain body weight despite a seemingly low energy intake. Thus, they may expend less energy at rest or while performing various daily tasks than those whose energy intake appears adequate.

6.5.1 *Evidence for*

Evidence supporting energy efficiency in 24 male endurance athletes, classified as either low energy intake or adequate energy intake, was reported by Thompson et al. (1993). In this study the low energy balance athletes reported eating 6150 kJ/d (1490 kcal/d) less than the adequate energy balance athletes, while the activity level of both groups was similar. Despite these energy intake differences, both groups had similar FFM and had been weight stable for at least two years. RMR was significantly lower ($p < 0.05$) in the low energy intake group compared with the adequate energy intake groups (~4.9 versus 5.3 kJ/FFM/h or 1.19 versus 1.29 kcal/FFM/h, respectively).

To further examine the above findings, a second study was completed on another group of male endurance athletes classified as having either low or adequate energy intakes (Thompson et al. 1995). This study aimed to determine if there were differences in 24-hour energy expenditure (EE), sleep EE, RMR and spontaneous physical activity (SPA), with these measurements being determined in a respiratory chamber. All subjects were of similar body size and composition. The low energy intake athletes reported a daily energy intake of 6446 ± 2163 kJ (1535 ± 524 kcal) less than estimated EE. The daily 24-hour EE, RMR, sleep EE, and SPA of the low-energy-intake athletes were significantly lower than the adequate energy intake athletes (859 kJ or 208 kcal for 24 h EE, 524 kJ or 127 kcal for RMR and 2890 kJ or 770 kcal for sleep EE, and 43 minutes for SPA). Thus, part of the ability of the low-energy-intake athletes to maintain BM on a seemingly low energy intake appears due to a lower daily sedentary EE.

Myerson et al. (1991) found that amenorrheic runners had a significantly lower RMR than eumenorrheic runners and inactive controls, and the energy intake of these runners was similar to the inactive controls despite higher activity levels. Lebenstedt et al. (1999) studied eumenorrheic and oligomenorrheic active women (runners and triathletes). The menstrual function of the women was determined by assessing salivary progesterone levels, and the women were classified as either having normal menstrual function (12 periods per year) or menstrual disturbances (nine or fewer periods per year). Although the reported energy intake and activity level of these women was not different, the women with menstrual disturbances had a significantly lower RMR and reported significantly higher restrained eating scores. The results of both these studies show that amenorrheic women and women with menstrual disturbances exhibit energy efficiency, which may be either a cause or a consequence of menstrual cycle disturbances.

6.5.2 *Evidence against*

There are a number of studies of female athletes whose results do not support the existence of energy efficiency. Wilmore et al. (1992) and Schulz et al. (1992) found that female athletes reported significantly lower energy intakes than expected for their activity level. After measuring the energy expenditure of these women, it was determined that they under-reported their energy intake, as there was no evidence of energy efficiency. Beidleman et al. (1995) also found large differences between reported energy intake and energy expenditure in female distance runners but could not attribute these differences to metabolic efficiency (i.e. lower RMR and EE during exercise) as compared to untrained controls. However, the data collection period was very brief (three days), and may not have been long enough to detect true differences. Fogelholm et al. (1995) found that gymnasts reported a significantly lower energy balance (energy intake minus energy expenditure) than sedentary controls and soccer players, but the RMR was similar between all groups of athletes.

In most of these studies, metabolic efficiency was examined by comparing the RMR, total daily energy expenditure or energy expenditure during exercise of female athletes to sedentary controls. One criticism of these studies is that they did not attempt to compare the athletes who reported significant energy deficits to the athletes within the group who reported an adequate energy intake. A second criticism is that energy expenditure was not measured during the same time during the menstrual cycle in all studies (Schulz et al. 1992; Wilmore et al. 1992). RMR can change over the menstrual cycle, and is reported to be the lowest in the follicular phase and highest in the luteal phase (Bisdee et al. 1989; Solomon et al. 1982; Barr et al. 1995). Failure to compare women during the same phase of the menstrual cycle or to clearly document and hormonally assess menstrual status could mask any differences in energy expenditure that may exist. Finally, only four studies (Mulligan & Butterfield 1990; Myerson et al. 1991; Beidleman et al. 1995; Lebenstedt et al. 1999) verified ovulation in eumenorrheic athletes, and only Myerson et al. (1991) and Lebenstedt et al. (1999) screened for eating disorders. As demonstrated in the study by Lebenstedt et al. (1999), active females may report regular menstrual bleeding and still have some type of menstrual dysfunction, a condition that may decrease energy expenditure if hormone responses are blunted (Dueck et al. 1996).

6.6 SUMMARY

This chapter has discussed the components that determine energy balance, both those on the energy input side (dietary energy plus the contribution of energy stores within the body) and the energy expenditure side. In addition, we have covered how the various components of energy expenditure can be measured. It appears that some athletes may have an increased energy efficiency, which can impact the energy intake needed to maintain BM. For any one individual the factors that influence energy balance may be numerous, including gender, age, family history, dietary choices, level of daily activity and stress level. If an individual wishes to permanently change body size, then one or more of the components of energy balance need to be altered over an extended time. Methods for doing this are discussed in Chapters 5 and 7.

REFERENCES

Abbott WGH, Howard BV, Christin L, et al. Short-term energy balance: relationship with protein, carbohydrate, and fat balances. Am J Physiol 1988;255:E332–E337.

Acheson KJ, Schutz Y, Bessard T, Anantharaman K, Flatt JP, Jequier E. Glycogen storage capacity and de novo lipogenesis during massive carbohydrate overfeeding in man. Am J Clin Nutr 1988;48:240–7.

Acheson KJ, Schutz Y, Bessard T, Ravussin E, Jequier E, Flatt JP. Nutritional influences on lipogenesis and thermogenesis after a carbohydrate meal. Am J Physiol 1984;246:E62–E70.

Astrup A, Buemann B, Christensen NJ, Toubro S. Failure to increase lipid oxidation in response to increasing dietary fat content in formerly obese women. Am J Physiol 1994;266:592–9.

Barr SI, Janelle KC, Prior JC. Energy intakes are higher during the luteal phase of ovulatory menstrual cycles. Am J Clin Nutr 1995;61:39–43.

Beidleman BA, Puhl JL, De Souza MJ. Energy balance in female distance runners. Am J Clin Nutr 1995;61:303–11.

Bisdee JT, James WPT, Shaw MA. Changes in energy expenditure during the menstrual cycle. Br J Nutr 1989;61:187–99.

Bjorntorp P, Brodoff BN. Obesity. New York: JB Lippincott Co, 1992.

Bogardus C, Lillioja S, Ravussin E, et al. Familial dependence of the resting metabolic rate. New Eng J Med 1986;315:96–100.

Bouchard C, Tremblay A, Nadeau A, et al. Genetic effect in resting and exercise metabolic rates. Metabolism 1989;38:364–70.

Broeder CE, Burrhus KA, Svanevik LS, Wilmore JH. The effect of aerobic fitness on resting metabolic rate. Am J Clin Nutr 1992;55:795–801.

Bullough RC, Gillette CA, Harris MA, Melby CL. Interaction of acute changes in exercise energy expenditure and energy intake on resting metabolic rate. Am J Clin Nutr 1995;61:473–81.

Chad KE, Quigley BM. Exercise intensity: effect on postexercise O_2 uptake in trained and untrained women. J Appl Physiol 1991;70:1713–19.

Coward WA, Cole TJ. The doubly labelled water method for the measurement of energy expenditure in humans: risks and benefits. In: Whitehead RG, Prentice A, eds. New techniques in nutritional research. San Diego, CA: Academic Press, Inc, 1991;139–76.

Cunningham JJ. A reanalysis of the factors influencing basal metabolic rate in normal adults. Am J Clin Nutr 1980;33:2372–4.

Dahlstrom M, Jansson E, Nordevange E, Kaijser L. Discrepancy between estimated energy intake and requirements in female dancers. Clin Physiol 1990;10:11–25.

Deuster PA, Kyle SB, Moser PB, Vigersky RA, Singh A, Schoomaker EB. Nutritional intakes and status of highly trained amenorrheic and eumenorrheic women runners. Fertil Steril 1986;46:636–43.

Drinkwater BL, Nilson K, Chesnut III CH, Bremner WJ, Shainholtz S, Southworth MB. Bone mineral content of amenorrheic and eumenorrheic athletes. N Engl J Med 1984;311:277–81.

Dueck CA, Manore MM, Matt KS. Role of energy balance in athletic menstrual dysfunction. Int J Sport Nutr 1996;6:165–90.

Durnin JVGA. Practical estimates of energy expenditure. J Nutr 1991;121:1907–91.

Ferraro R, Lillioja S, Fontvieille AM, Rising R, Bogardus C, Ravussin E. Lower sedentary metabolic rate in women compared to men. J Clin Invest 1992;90:780–4.

Flatt JP. Importance of nutrient balance in body weight regulation. Diabetes/Metabolism Reviews 1988;4:571–81.

Flatt JP. The biochemistry of energy expenditure. In: Bjorntrop P, Brodoff BN, eds. Obesity. New York: JB Lippincott Co, 1992:100–16.

Flatt JP. Dietary fat, carbohydrate balance, and weight maintenance. Ann NY Acad Sci 1993:683;122–40.

Flatt JP. Use and storage of carbohydrate and fat. Am J Clin Nutr 1995;61(suppl):S952–59.

Flatt JP, Ravussin E, Acheson KJ, Jequier E. Effects of dietary fat on post-prandial substrate oxidation and on carbohydrate and fat balance. J Clin Invest 1985;76:1019–24.

Fogelholm GM, Kukkonen-Harjula TK, Taipale SA, Sievänen HT, Oja P, Vuori IM. Resting metabolic rate and energy intake in female gymnasts, figure-skaters and soccer players. Int J Sport Med 1995;16:551–6.

Frankenfield DC, Murth ER, Rowe WA. The Harris–Benedict studies of human basal metabolism: history and limitations. J Am Diet Assoc 1998;98:439–45.

Gillette CA, Bullough RC, Melby CL. Post-exercise energy expenditure in response to acute aerobic or resistive exercise. Int J Sport Nutr 1994;4:347–60.

Goran MI, Poehlman ET, Danforth E. Experimental reliability of the doubly labelled water technique. Am J Physiol 1994;266:E510–E15.

Goran MI, Poehlman ET, Johnson RK. Energy requirements across the life span: new findings based on measurement of total energy expenditure with doubly labelled water. Nutr Res 1995;15:115–50.

Gorsky RD, Calloway DH. Activity pattern changes with decreases in food energy intake. Hum Biol 1983;55:577–86.

Harris JA, Benedict FG. A biometric study of basal metabolism in man. Carnegie Inst Wash Pub No. 279. Philadelphia: FB Lippincott Co., 1919:227.

Hellerstein MK, Christiansen M, Kaempfer S, et al. Measurement of de novo hepatic lipogenesis in humans using stable isotopes. J Clin Invest 1991;87:1841–52.

Jebb SA, Prentice AM, Goldberg GR, Murgatroyd PR, Black AE, Coward WA. Changes in macronutrient balance during over and under feeding assessed by 12-d continuous whole-body calorimetry. Am J Clin Nutr 1996;64:259–66.

Jequier E, Acheson K, Schutz Y. Assessment of energy expenditure and fuel utilization in man. Ann Rev Nutr 1987;7:187–208.

Kaiserauer S, Snyder AC, Sleeper M, Zierath J. Nutritional, physiological, and menstrual status of distance runners. Med Sci Sports Exerc 1989;21:120–5.

Keys A, Taylor HL, Grande F. Basal metabolism and age of adult man. Metabolism 1987;22:5979–87.

Krempf M, Hoerr RA, Pelletier VA, Marks LM, Gleason R, Young VR. An isotopic study of the effect of dietary carbohydrate on the metabolic fate of dietary leucine and phenylalanine. Am J Clin Nutr 1993;57:161–9.

Lebenstedt M, Platte P, Pirke K-M. Reduced resting metabolic rate in athletes with menstrual disorders. Med Sci Sports Exerc 1999;31:1250–6.

Li ETS, Tsang LBY, Lui SSH. Resting metabolic rate and thermic effects of a sucrose-sweetened soft drink during the menstrual cycle in young Chinese women. Can J Physiol Pharmacol 1999;77:544–50.

Lifson N, Gordon GB, McClintock R. Measurement of total carbon dioxide production by means of doubly labelled water. J Appl Physiol 1955;7:704–10.

Manore MM, Thompson JL. Sport nutrition for health and performance. Champaign, Illinois: Human Kinetics, 2000.

Melby CL, Hill JO. Exercise, macronutrient balance, and body weight regulation. Sports Sci Exchange 1999;112(1):1–6.

Melby C, Scholl C, Edwards G, Bullough R. Effect of acute resistance exercise on post-exercise energy expenditure and resting metabolic rate. J Appl Physiol 1993;75:1847–53.

Mifflin MD, St. Jeor St, Hill LA, Scott BJ, Daugherty SA, Koh YO. A new predictive equation for resting energy expenditure in healthy individuals. Am J Clin Nutr 1990;51:241–7.

Montoye HJ, Kemper HCG, Saris WHM, Washburn RA. Measuring physical activity and energy expenditure. Champaign, Illinois: Human Kinetics Publisher, 1996.

Mulligan K, Butterfield GE. Discrepancies between energy intake and expenditure in physically active women. Br J Nutr 1990;64:23–36.

Myerson M, Gutin B, Warren MP, et al. Resting metabolic rate and energy balance in amenorrheic and eumenorrheic runners. Med Sci Sports Exerc 1991;23:15–22.

National Research Council. Recommended Dietary Allowances, 10th edn. Washington DC: National Academy Press, 1989.

Owen OE, Holup JL, D'Alessio DA, et al. A reappraisal of the caloric requirements of men. Am J Clin Nutr 1987;46:875–85.

Owen OE, Kavle E, Owen RS, et al. A reappraisal of caloric requirements in healthy women. Am J Clin Nutr 1986;44:1–19.

Piers LS, Diggavi SN, Rijskamp J, van Raaij JMA, Shetty PS, Hautvast JGAJ. Resting metabolic rate and thermic effect of a meal in the follicular and luteal phases of the menstrual cycle in well-nourished Indian women. Am J Clin Nutr 1995;61:296–302.

Piers LS, Soares MJ, McCormack LM, O'Deal K. Is there evidence for an age-related reduction in metabolic rate? J Appl Physiol 1998;85:2196–204.

Poehlman ET. A review: exercise and its influence on resting energy metabolism in man. Med Sci Sports Exerc 1989;21:515–25.

Poehlman ET, Berke EM, Joseph JR, Gardner AW, Katzman-Rooks SM, Goran MI. Influence of aerobic capacity, body composition, and thyroid hormones on the age-related decline in resting metabolic rate. Metabolism 1992;41:915–21.

Poehlman ET, Goran MI, Gardner AW, et al. Determinants of decline in resting metabolic rate in aging females. Am J Physiol 1993;264:E450–E5.

Poehlman ET, McAuliffe TL, Van Houten DR, Danforth E. Influence of age and endurance training on metabolic rate and hormones in healthy men. Am J Physiol 1990;259:E66–E72.

Prentice AM. Manipulation of dietary fat and energy density and subsequent effects on substrate flux and food intake. Am J Clin Nutr 1998;67(suppl):S535–S41.

Prentice AM, Diaz EO, Murgatroyd PR, Goldberg GR, Sonko BJ, Black AE, Coward WA. Doubly labelled water measurements and calorimetry in practice. In: Whitehead RG, Prentice A, eds. New techniques in nutritional research. San Diego, CA: Academic Press Inc., 1991:177–207.

Ravussin E, Bogardus C. Relationship of genetics, age and physical fitness to daily energy expenditure and fuel utilization. Am J Clin Nutr 1989;49:968–75.

Ravussin E, Lillioja S, Anderson TE, Christin L, Bogardus C. Determinants of 24-hour energy expenditure in man: methods and results using a respiratory chamber. J Clin Invest 1986;78:1568–78.

Ravussin E, Swinburn BA. Energy Metabolism. In: Stunkard AJ, Wadden TA, eds. Obesity: theory and therapy, 2nd edn. New York: Raven Press Ltd, 1993:98.

Rontoyannis GP, Skoulis T, Pavlou KN. Energy balance in ultramarathon running. Am J Clin Nutr 1989;49:976–9.

Schoeller DA, Racette SB. A review of field techniques for the assessment of energy expenditure. J Nutr 1990;120:1492–5.

Schoeller DA, Ravussine E, Schutz Y, Acheson KJ, Baertschi P, Jequier E. Energy expenditure by doubly labelled water: validation in humans and proposed calculations. Am J Physiol 1986;250:823–30.

Schrauwen P, Lichtenbelt WDV, Saris WHM, Westerterp KR. Changes in fat oxidation in response to a high-fat diet. Am J Clin Nutr 1997;66:276–82.

Schulz LO, Alger S, Harper I, Wilmore JH, Ravussin E. Energy expenditure of elite female runners measured by respiratory chamber and doubly labelled water. J Appl Physiol 1992;72:23–8.

Schutz Y, Tremblay A, Weinsier RL, Nelson KM. Role of fat oxidation in the long-term stabilization of body weight in obese women. Am J Clin Nutr 1992;55:670–4.

Segal KR, Chun A, Coronel P, Valdez V. Effects of exercise mode and intensity on postprandial thermogenesis in lean and obese men. J Appl Physiol 1992;72:1754–63.

Shelmet JJ, Reichard GA, Skutches CL, Hoeldtke RD, Owen OE, Boden G. Ethanol causes acute inhibition of carbohydrate, fat, and protein oxidation and insulin resistance. J Clin Invest 1988;81:1137–45.

Solomon SJ, Kurzer MS, Calloway DH. Menstrual cycle and basal metabolic rate in women. Am J Clin Nutr 1982;36:611–16.

Sonko BJ, Prentice AM, Murgatroyd PR, Goldberg GR, van de Ven MLHM, Coward WA. Effect of alcohol on postmeal fat storage. Am J Clin Nutr 1994;59:619–25.

Sparti A, DeLany JP, de la Bretonne JA, Sanders GE, Bray GA. Relationship between resting metabolic rate and the composition of the fat-free mass. Metabolism 1997;46:1225–30.

Speakman JR. The history and theory of the doubly labelled water technique. Am J Clin Nutr 1998;68(suppl):932S–938S.

Stock MJ. Gluttony and thermogenesis revisited. Int J Obesity 1999;23:1105–17.

Swinburn B, Ravussin E. Energy balance or fat balance? Am J Clin Nutr 1993;57(suppl):S766–S71.

Thompson JL, Manore MM. Predicted and measured resting metabolic rate of male and female endurance athletes. J Am Diet Assoc 1996;96:30–4.

Thompson J, Manore MM, Skinner JS. Resting metabolic rate and thermic effect of a meal in low- and adequate-energy intake in male endurance athletes. Int J Sport Nutr 1993;3:194–206.

Thompson JL, Manore MM, Skinner JS, Ravussin E, Spraul M. Daily energy expenditure in male endurance athletes with differing energy intakes. Med Sci Sports Exerc 1995;27:347–54.

Warwick PM. Predicting food energy requirements from estimates of energy expenditure. Aust J Nutr Diet 1989;46(S):3–29.

Webb P. The measurement of energy expenditure. J Nutr 1991;121:1897–1901.

Westerterp KR. Food quotient, respiratory quotient, and energy balance. Am J Clin Nutr 1993;57(suppl):S759–S65.

Westerterp KR, Wilson SAJ, Rolland V. Diet induced thermogenesis measured over 24h in a respiration chamber: effect of diet composition. Int J Obesity 1999;23:287–92.

Weststrate JA. Resting metabolic rate and diet-induced thermogenesis: a methodological reappraisal. Am J Clin Nutr 1993;58:592–601.

Wilmore JH, Wambsgans KC, Brenner M, et al. Is there energy conservation in amenorrheic compared with eumenorrheic distance runners? J Appl Physiol 1992;72:15–22.

World Health Organization (WHO). Energy and protein requirements. Report of a Joint FAO/WHO/UNU Expert Committee. Technical Report Series 724. World Health Organization, Geneva. 11985:206. (Reprinted in the 1989 RDAs National Research Council.)

Weight loss and the athlete

Helen O'Connor, Terri Sullivan and Ian Caterson

7.1 INTRODUCTION

The stereotype of the lean, toned and strong athlete paints a picture of a population that controls its weight and body composition within tight limits with relative ease. This is not necessarily the case, with many studies providing evidence of athletes experiencing difficulty achieving and controlling desired levels of body weight and fat (Walberg-Rankin 1998). In most cases, the perceived excess weight or fat does not place the athlete at an increased health risk. Usually, the desired level of fatness is less than that which would be considered healthy or normal within the context of public health guidelines (see Chapter 4).

Athletes and coaches are open to just as much misinformation about weight loss and dieting as the rest of the community. In some cases, the methods used to reduce weight, and/or the level of reduction achieved or desired, becomes dangerous, increasing the likelihood of decreased performance, and increasing the risk of detrimental health or psychological effects. This chapter will cover a range of issues related to weight loss in athletes. Specific diets and problems related to 'making weight' for competition will be covered in Chapter 8.

7.2 JUSTIFICATION FOR WEIGHT LOSS IN ATHLETES

Weight or fat reduction in athletes is generally motivated by a desire to either achieve a pre-designated weight in order to compete in a specific weight class or category (e.g. horse racing, light-weight rowing, boxing, weight lifting), or to optimise performance by improving power to weight ratio (e.g. jumping events, distance running, triathlon, road cycling). In aesthetic sports like gymnastics, diving and figure skating, attainment of desired body composition and physical appearance is considered important. Adding to these performance issues are current societal trends which encourage the pursuit of leanness for both men and women (Ballor & Keesey 1991). There is an unrealistic community perception and expectation, of female body size in particular, which is at odds with reality (Cash et al. 1994). Unfortunately, this has become an increasingly important issue in sports where an image of physical attractiveness is created for promotion or advertising. Athletes, or the sport itself, frequently derive significant financial rewards for delivering an image and wearing clothing accentuating physique.

Despite the apparent preoccupation with body weight and fat levels in many sporting groups, there is surprisingly little evidence of the effects of fat reduction on performance, particularly at the elite level. This is partly due to the difficulty in determining the effect of fatness compared with other factors that also impact on performance, such as diet and training. At the elite level, body fatness ranges are often quite narrow, and studies therefore have to be carefully designed using measures sensitive enough that they can accurately attribute any performance effects to an alteration in body fat. However, from a mechanical perspective, excess fat represents an inert load (dead weight), which must be moved, and it has been shown that fatness is negatively correlated with activities which require projection or movement through space (e.g. vertical jumps and running) (Malina 1975; Cureton et al. 1978). From a metabolic perspective, excess fatness is associated with a decreased physical working capacity and increased energy cost of movement (Buskirk & Taylor 1957; Dempsey et al. 1966).

A high level of body fat has been shown to have an adverse effect on performance in a number of sporting activities. Using an experimental approach, Cureton and Sparling (1980) observed a 30% reduction in running performance by loading subjects with additional weight (Cureton and Sparling 1980). Even ignoring the performance change, there was an increase of approximately 0.2 L O_2/kg for each kilometre, costing an additional 4 kJ. Using a mathematical model, Olds et al. (1993) have estimated that an increased fat mass of 2 kg would increase 4 000 m pursuit cycling performance by about 1.5 sec (20 m) and a 40 km time trial by about 15 sec (180 m) (Olds et al. 1993). The energy cost is also altered by the additional body mass increasing the rolling resistance. Although it has been suggested that moderate body fatness may actually enhance swimming performance by improving buoyancy, this has not been shown experimentally (Stager & Cordain 1984), and at the elite level, there is currently a good deal of emphasis placed on maintaining low body-fat levels, especially for competition (Pyne & Lee 2000).

In sports where leanness is desired for aesthetic reasons, the reduction of body fat to extremely low levels may not actually benefit performance *per se*. However, coaches and athletes believe that an appropriate level of leanness is assessed by the 'trained eye' of the judges and that this influences the score for artistic impression. Regardless of the reason, athletes and coaches, even at the recreational level, frequently place great importance on the attainment of desired body weight and fat levels. Yet even in athletes, as in the general population, the distribution and amount of fat is influenced by both genetic and environmental factors as well as the training schedule, the sport, and any attempts at weight control or reduction.

7.3 FACTORS INFLUENCING THE ABILITY TO ACHIEVE OPTIMAL BODY WEIGHT AND COMPOSITION IN ATHLETES

7.3.1 *Genetic factors*

A significant proportion of the inter-individual variance in human fatness is attributable to genetic factors. Over the past 15 years, estimates of the heritability of body fatness and composition from a number of epidemiological studies have been reported. These are quite varied, however a trend in the size of estimates is apparent, with those based on twin studies being the highest (80%) (Bouchard 1993), and those determined from adoption studies, the lowest (10–30%) (Bouchard 1993). Overall it has been suggested that 25–40% of adiposity is due to our genes (Bouchard 1994). Short- and long-term intervention studies examining energy balance in pairs of identical twins suggest that body weight and fat gains in response to over-feeding are under significant genetic control, evidenced by a three-fold higher between-pair (compared to within-pair) variance in weight and fat gain (Bouchard et al. 1990).

Twin studies have also shown a greater similarity in dietary intake and food preference in monozygotic compared with dizygotic twins, suggesting genetic factors contribute to dietary intake (Heller et al. 1988; Perusse et al. 1988). However, it must be remembered that high correlations in dietary variables are observed in individuals sharing the same environment. When expressed as a percentage of total energy intake, carbohydrate (CHO) and fat were characterised by a genetic effect of 20%, while cultural transmission and environmental effects explained 10% and 70% of their intake respectively (Perusse et al. 1988). It appears that food preferences are largely influenced by the environment, but may also be driven by genetic factors. Twin studies may tend to under-estimate the effect of environment on the food choices of athletes. It is likely that athletes are strongly influenced by the culture of the sport in which they participate, and by the focus on the role of nutrition on sports performance or physique.

A number of genes are now known to be associated and/or linked with human obesity. These appear to be 'susceptibility genes', increasing the risk for obesity, but not necessarily its expression. An individual with deficient or unfavourable alleles at a large number of susceptibility genes will be at a higher risk of developing greater levels of body fatness, while a person with a smaller number will be more resistant (Bouchard 1993). Recently a number of single gene mutations producing obesity have been discovered. Other such genes are likely to be discovered in the near future.

The gap between such gene discovery and the application of this knowledge to the problems of obesity in humans, particularly in subgroups such as athletes, is demonstrated by our current knowledge of the protein leptin. In 1973, mouse studies by Coleman demonstrated the presence of a relatively long-lived circulating factor which appeared to be a satiety factor (Coleman 1973). Some animals (*ob/ob* mice) appeared to be deficient in this factor and became obese, others appeared to be insensitive to the factor and also became obese (*db/db* mice). In 1994, Friedman's group reported on a protein, called leptin, which corresponds to this satiety factor (Zhang et al. 1994). Leptin is produced by the adipocyte, and serum levels in both rodents and humans correlate closely with per cent body fat and body mass index (Considine et al. 1996; Rosenbaum et al. 1996). Serum levels appear to act as a signal of adequacy of these energy stores. Leptin binds to receptors in the hypothalamus, influences energy intake, and increases activity in the mouse (Weigle et al. 1995). Despite hopes to the contrary, serum leptin levels are elevated in obese humans and, except in a very few individuals who are lacking this factor (Montague et al. 1997), it is not a cause of obesity. Leptin levels are higher in females than males (Considine et al. 1996), and are elevated by increasing energy and particularly by increasing CHO intake (Jenkins et al. 1997).

In the human it appears that rather than being a satiety factor, leptin acts as a signal of nutritional adequacy and protection against famine. It signals the level of fat stores and is important in the initiation of puberty, and in fertility. Leptin levels are low in anorexia nervosa sufferers (Grinspoon et al. 1996), characterised by amenorrhoea and extreme thinness, and similarly in those sports desirous of low levels of body fatness, it would be expected for leptin to be low. The long-term effect on reproductive potential, or on eating and activity, of such suppressed leptin is not yet known. Human obesity is characterised by resistance to insulin action. Currently a great deal of research is directed at determining whether elevated levels of leptin have any major effect on lipid or CHO metabolism. In athletes, leptin levels appear consistent with reduced body fat, although animal studies suggest there may be an independent effect of exercise in reducing leptin (Kowlalska et al. 1999). After a marathon, leptin levels are further reduced, and it has been suggested that major changes in energy expenditure (as in marathon running) may also alter leptin levels (Leal-Cerro et al. 1998).

Specific metabolic risk factors associated with increased weight gain in certain populations (Ravussin et al. 1988; Ravussin & Swinburn 1993), such as a low resting metabolic rate relative to that predicted for body size, a high 24-hour respiratory quotient which indicates a high rate of CHO relative to fat oxidation (Zurlo et al. 1990), and a lower rate of spontaneous physical activity (Ravussin et al. 1986) almost certainly have a genetic basis. However, the relative contribution of genetic versus environmental factors is unclear. The rapid escalation in the rate of obesity prevalence in western countries highlights the importance of the interaction between genes and the environment in the development of excess body fatness and obesity.

Another factor that needs to be considered when weight loss is attempted or contemplated is the fact that body weight and composition tend to remain stable in most people for significant periods (over years). This suggests to some that it is regulated and has led to the suggestion that there are a series of set points for body weight throughout life. Reductions or increases in weight away from the current baseline, or set point, result in metabolic alterations that resist the maintenance of a new weight and promote weight loss or gain back towards the set point. This may be explained by the difficulty of displacing metabolic equilibria and maintaining this displacement for sufficient time for weight to change and a new equilibrium to be established.

Although most athletes exhibit lower levels of fatness than the general population, genetic factors still influence the relative effort that might be required to attain desired body composition and weight. Athletes often use extreme measures to manipulate body weight and fat to improve performance or appearance. Genetics ultimately influences their ability to successfully and safely achieve and maintain these desired levels.

7.3.2 *Environmental factors*

7.3.2.1 *Energy intake and macronutrient selection*

For many years there was a general consensus that a stable body weight was maintained by a tight control of energy balance, and that each kilojoule had the same value in this balance, independent of whether it came from protein, fat, CHO or alcohol. In this view, excesses of CHO or protein would be converted into lipid and then stored as adipose tissue through the process of *de novo* lipogenesis. Recent evidence suggests, however, that *de novo* lipogenesis does not occur to any great extent in humans on a normal western diet (Acheson et al. 1988). This is in part because lipogenesis is an energetically expensive process and in part because of the diet's composition and energy content. Net *de novo* lipogenesis requires forced overfeeding and does not occur under the conditions of *ad libitum* eating in normal individuals (Astrup & Raben 1992).

The nutrient balance concept, proposed by JP Flatt, suggests that energy and weight balance can only be achieved together with the separate balance of the energy-producing macronutrients (CHO, protein, fat and alcohol) (Flatt 1987). Achievement of macronutrient balance requires that the body's net oxidation of each macronutrient equals the average amounts found in the diet. Weight stability is achieved when the composition of the fuel oxidised by the body (respiratory quotient (RQ)) is equal to the composition of the diet. In Flatt's view, energy balance is achieved when the food oxidised (food quotient (FQ)) is equal to the mean RQ over 24 hours. Positive energy balance occurs when the RQ to FQ ratio is greater than one, indicating the amount of lipid oxidised is less than ingested.

Regulation of CHO balance is strictly controlled as the body has limited CHO stores. Carbohydrates promote their own oxidation by stimulating insulin secretion and cellular glucose uptake (Schutz et al. 1989). Like CHO, protein stores are tightly controlled. Excessive protein in the diet stimulates its own oxidation

(Astrup & Raben 1992). Protein in addition, and perhaps even more so than CHO, regulates appetite by promoting satiety (Blundell & Burley 1990). Alcohol is also an energy-yielding nutrient; however, unlike the other macronutrients, it is preferentially oxidised as there are no body stores. Alcohol, and the other macronutrients eaten in excess of storage requirements, may contribute to fat stores by diverting fat from oxidation to storage while the body is actively metabolising alcohol or the other macronutrients (Suter et al. 1992).

Although it has been assumed that each individual is capable of changing their oxidation of particular nutrients rapidly to match the composition of the diet, the body's ability to increase fat oxidation in response to a diet with a high fat to CHO ratio is limited (Schutz et al. 1989). When a certain ratio of fat to CHO intake is exceeded, some individuals are unable to increase their fat oxidation further, and a positive fat balance ensues. A further increase in fat oxidation can only be achieved by increasing aerobic exercise and/or increasing body-fat stores, the latter facilitating fat oxidation partly through increased circulating non-esterified fatty acids and insulin resistance.

It is important to recognise that macronutrient composition will only impact on body composition when there is also an imbalance in total energy consumption and utilisation. In a 12-day study measuring energy and macronutrient balance in a 24-hour calorimeter after over- and under-feeding, fuel selection was found to be driven by the need to maintain CHO balance (Jebb et al. 1996). During over-feeding, fat oxidation was decreased to ensure CHO oxidation balanced CHO intake. The reduction in fat oxidation increased the risk of body-fat gain. In western countries, avoiding a high-fat, energy-dense diet requires a certain degree of discipline and dedication, even for athletes. Despite efforts to educate athletes about the health and performance benefits of a high-CHO, low-fat diet, dietary surveys frequently show that the proportion of fat reportedly consumed by athletes is similar to that found in the general population (Brotherhood 1984).

Some athletes are protected from weight and fat gain by virtue of adaptations associated with aerobically-based training such as increased oxygen delivery through improved capillarisation (Andersen & Henriksson 1977), greater density of mitochondria (Hoppeler et al. 1973), and elevated concentrations of enzymes required for fat metabolism (Henriksson & Reitman 1976). Others, despite training for many hours each day, may not elevate fat oxidation substantially. Athletes in sports such as gymnastics, diving and figure skating fall into this category as their training is mainly skill based, providing little opportunity to enhance fat oxidation. Despite many hours of training and a low-fat, low-energy intake, some of these athletes face a constant struggle with body weight and fat to achieve the desired physique requirements of their sport. To a degree, the struggle with weight is partially offset at the elite level where there is selective survival of individuals with the genetic propensity to be extremely lean. However, even those more suited to a sport's physique requirements usually need to limit both fat and energy consumption as the desired levels of leanness, at least in females, are below what is biologically natural.

7.3.2.2 *Exercise training and appetite*

Although it is often assumed that additional exercise (particularly aerobic exercise) will result in an energy and fat deficit and hence weight loss, it is entirely possible that individuals partially or even fully compensate for the increased expenditure by consuming more energy. This compensation may be affected by numerous factors, such as the intensity, duration or mode of exercise. The precise nature of the effect of exercise on appetite is yet to be established, but has been investigated more recently by King et al. (1994). Their findings on the acute response to aerobic exercise suggest only a weak, short-term coupling between energy expenditure and energy intake (King et al. 1994). They demonstrated a short-term suppression of hunger and relative energy intake (relative to the energy used during the exercise bout) only after longer duration (60 versus 30 minute) intense exercise (cycling at 70% $VO_{2\ max}$ versus 30% $VO_{2\ max}$). However, in most studies, this short-term, exercise-induced suppression of appetite, possibly related to elevated body temperature (Andersson & Larson 1961), increased levels of lactic acid (Baile et al. 1970) or even higher concentrations of tumour necrosis factor (Grunfield & Feingold 1991), does not appear to impact on energy balance over a longer term (reviewed King et al. 1997).

In a subsequent study, King and Blundell compared treadmill with cycling exercise and failed to observe a difference between running and cycling (King & Blundell 1995). Although there is anecdotal evidence of an increase in appetite after swimming, there are no studies comparing swimming to other modes of exercise directly. There is some evidence that exercise alters macronutrient selection, stimulating the drive for CHO, theoretically to aid replenishment of limited glycogen stores. Tremblay has reported on a relationship between exercise-induced changes in RQ and energy intake, whereby individuals with the greatest reduction in RQ during exercise show the smallest increase in post-exercise energy intake (Tremblay et al. 1985). Taken a step further, feeding a low- versus high-fat diet after exercise has been shown to result in negative energy balance, with a positive balance occurring after the high-fat diet (Tremblay et al. 1985; King & Blundell 1995). This may be due to alterations in appetite associated with the composition of the fuel mix oxidised or, alternatively, due to passive over-consumption as a result of the high palatablity and energy density of the low-CHO diet which is known to have a weak effect on satiation (King & Blundell 1995).

Since appetite is influenced by many factors, it is difficult to tease out the effect of exercise, particularly when there are so many potential combinations of exercise mode, intensity and duration to consider. Most of the work has also been confined to relatively short-term laboratory studies using student or obese populations and the results of these may not reflect free living eating patterns (reviewed by King et al. 1997) or those pertaining to athletes. Clearly, some athletes have difficulty maintaining energy balance when exposed to substantial training loads. In such cases, the chronic exposure to strenuous exercise must fail to drive the consumption of sufficient energy adequately, at least in the shorter term. Anecdotally, this phenomenon is found more commonly in males than females. There is some evidence of gender differences in energy intake in response to exercise training, with females either increasing energy consumption or reducing energy expenditure relative to males (Staten 1991; Westerterp et al. 1992). This has been used to explain differences in the capacity for body-fat losses and may arise from biologically-based evolutionary differences (Tremblay et al. 1984; King et al. 1997).

7.3.2.3 *Physical activity and energy expenditure*

The increasing prevalence of overweight and obesity in the general population has occurred in parallel with a profound change in societal patterns of physical activity (Booth et al. 1997). Cross-sectional studies of active, fit individuals consistently report that they have lower body weight and fat (Barlow et al. 1995). Physical activity affects energy expenditure directly due to the work done, and indirectly through modifications to the type of substrate oxidised and to resting metabolic rate as well as the thermic effect of food (Melby et al. 1998, p. 20). The amount of energy expended during exercise depends on variables attributable to the individual (e.g. body weight and efficiency of performing a particular activity), and on variables related to the activity itself (e.g. frequency, duration and intensity). Greater body mass increases the work required to perform weight-bearing activities, while skills developed in training reduce the energy cost of exercise by improving efficiency. The frequency, intensity and duration of exercise determine the overall energy expended during activity. However, exercise intensity in particular affects the magnitude of the post-exercise elevation in metabolic rate (Bahr & Sejersted 1991). Post-exercise energy expenditure may be significantly elevated in athletes who perform high-intensity, long-duration exercise, even though this component of expenditure is considered to be trivial for most non-athletes (Freedman-Akabas et al. 1985). Genetic predisposition is also important as it ultimately dictates an individual's aerobic capacity and potential to perform sustained, moderate- to high-intensity activity. The interaction of genetic factors with the type, intensity and magnitude of training influence the capacity to oxidise fat and the potential for fat loss through exercise.

Total physical activity includes the athlete's regular training or exercise, plus any incidental activity occurring in non-training hours. Incidental activity can be described as the movement of daily living. It includes walking from place to place, usual work patterns and practices, showering, and other daily care duties. Although incidental activity may be low intensity, it should not be overlooked, as it is a significant contributor to daily energy expenditure and therefore energy balance. An athlete who spends a large amount of their non-exercising time asleep or watching television will be burning less energy than one who performs a full work day. Anecdotally, some elite athletes participating in large volumes of training may experience a decrease in incidental activity, due to the incorporation of daytime rest and limitation of work and leisure activities. Reduction in incidental activity has been observed in the elderly after an increase in organised training (Goran & Poehlman 1992), but not in other groups (Meyer et al. 1991).

Another factor to consider is the seasonal nature of many sports, which may also coincide with Christmas or winter, where there appears to be a significant trend for weight gain (Almeras et al. 1997). Injury or illness will also decrease activity and total energy expenditure and this influences weight control. One of the aims in any off-season or off-training time should be the prevention of excess weight or fat accumulation. Assessment of energy expenditure in athletes therefore requires an understanding of their energy expenditure both during and outside of training.

(i) Effect of physical activity on resting metabolic rate and the thermic effect of food (TEF)

Physical activity has been reported to influence resting metabolic rate (reviewed by Poehlman et al. 1991). It is currently unclear whether there is an independent effect of physical activity on resting metabolic rate (Arciero et al. 1993), or if the increases observed are due to an exercise-related gain in lean body mass (Sharp et al. 1992). Since changes in energy intake and energy balance can affect resting metabolic rate, studies that fail to control for these variables often provide conflicting evidence (Melby et al. 1998, p. 22). Elevation in resting metabolism has been observed in elite athletes with high energy expenditures and intakes (Poehlman et al. 1989). It has been suggested that this increase is an adaptation to a chronic high energy flux. Physical activity of less intensity and duration, such as would be used in a typical prescription for weight loss in the general community, appears less likely to have an impact on resting metabolism (Melby et al. 1998, p. 23).

A number of studies have focussed on the impact of exercise training on TEF (reviewed by Melby et al. 1998, p. 20). This accounts for about 10–15% of daily energy expenditure and is small compared to resting metabolic rate and the potential contribution of physical activity (Reed & Hill 1996). Small deficits in TEF are considered unlikely to contribute significantly to weight gain (Ravussin & Swinburn 1992). Despite a number of studies, in both obese and trained populations, there is no consistent evidence that physical activity has a biologically important effect on TEF (Melby et al. 1998, p. 21).

(ii) Physical activity and substrate utilisation

The intensity of exercise determines which fuel is used to supply energy to the working muscle. Plasma free fatty acids are the predominant fuel during low-intensity exercise ($< 50\%$ $VO_{2\ max}$) (Romijn et al. 1993). As intensity increases there is a greater reliance on muscle glycogen and plasma glucose (Coyle et al. 1986). The amount of CHO utilised during exercise also depends on the training status of the individual. Well-trained athletes oxidise more fat than the untrained due to improved mitochondrial density (Hoppeler et al. 1973) (Davis et al. 1981) and an increased concentration of oxidative enzymes (Oscai et al. 1982; Henriksson

& Reitman 1976). In addition, transport of fatty acids into the mitochondria may be enhanced (Kiens 1977), and at a given sub-maximal workload well-trained athletes have lower levels of circulating catecholamines (Deuster et al. 1989). These adaptations, along with a greater capillary density (Andersen & Henriksson 1977) and an increase in intra-muscular triglyceride (Hurley et al. 1986), enhance the delivery of oxygen and improve the ability to utilise fat, especially during low- to moderate-intensity exercise. Although training also results in adaptations which enhance CHO utilisation, such as an increase in glucose transport and insulin sensitivity, it is the enhanced fat utilisation which mostly aids in weight control. Although endurance exercise rather than high-intensity exercise has been associated with most of the exercise-related adaptations mentioned above, recent research provides evidence that acute glycogen-depleting exercise enhances fat oxidation during recovery. Although relatively few studies have investigated the effect of resistance exercise, there is some evidence that supports greater fat oxidation during recovery from both a single bout (Melby et al. 1993) and a 16-week strength-training program (Treuth et al. 1995). These results provide support for the use of regimens incorporating strength training or shorter duration, high-intensity exercise in the management of excess body fat. Further research is required to confirm these findings and to determine their relative effectiveness against aerobically-based exercise and whether trained or untrained individuals benefit most.

7.3.2.4 *Social and behavioural factors*

Eating behaviours are important in the maintenance of desired body weight (Wing & Jeffery 1979). Although the eating behaviours of athletes have not been studied extensively, there are certain issues specific to athletes that require consideration. These include the sporting environment that may expose athletes to cafeteria or buffet-style eating. This has been associated with over-consumption in other populations (Stunkard & Kaplan 1977), especially when the food is high in fat and palatable. Athletes usually have regimented lifestyles that revolve around training and competition schedules. Food is often the easiest form of recreation or release from the strict daily regimen, as other social or hobby-type activities are necessarily limited. Parental or coach pressure to perform or achieve a particular weight or body fat may result in rebellion against a dietary regimen designed to control body composition. Alternatively, obsession with weight loss may result in disordered eating (Thornton 1990). Lastly, as the typical age group of most athletes is adolescent or young adult, this means that their age-related diet preferences lean toward high-fat fast-foods and take-away foods (Truswell & Darnton-Hill 1981). During this period of life too, alcohol consumption for social reasons and relaxation often begins, and there is potential for over-consumption, particularly in team sports, where alcohol use may be seen as part of a 'team bonding' experience (Burke & Read 1987).

7.3.2.5 *Growth and pubertal changes*

Restriction of dietary energy to control body weight and fat levels may retard and possibly stunt growth in young athletes (Bass et al. 2000). Pubertal development in girls may influence their ability to conform to physique requirements in sports which require extreme leanness, such as gymnastics. The effect of energy restriction and weight loss on growth, maturation, health and performance in young athletes is covered in Chapter 18.

7.3.2.6 *Competition influences*

The training phase immediately prior to competition is an important preparation stage for athletes. During this time, training is usually tapered to facilitate physical recovery and restoration of fuel reserves. In some sports (e.g. swimming), the taper results in a substantial reduction in training which may increase the risk for weight and fat gain if dietary energy is not reduced to accommodate the decrease in energy expenditure. Anecdotally, weight gain during this time is often reported in female swimmers. This problem is sometimes complicated by the need to travel to the competition venue, where dietary intake is more difficult to control. Practical strategies for managing this situation are covered in the Practice tips section at the end of the chapter.

7.4 *APPROACHES TO WEIGHT AND FAT LOSS IN ATHLETES*

7.4.1 *Dietary approaches for weight and fat loss*

7.4.1.1 *Low-fat versus low-energy diets*

There are numerous studies investigating the efficacy of energy-restricted diets versus fat-controlled diets for weight loss, yet there is no definitive conclusion as to which approach is more effective. Although dietary fat intake is significantly correlated with both energy consumption and body weight (Westrate 1995), epidemiological evidence suggests that weight loss is more strongly associated with a reduction in the percentage of energy derived from fat rather than a decrease in total energy intake (Sheppard et al. 1991). The results from numerous clinical trials, however, indicate that the major effect of fat restriction on weight loss comes from a decrease in total energy intake (Powell et al. 1994; Bray & Popkin 1998). Both regimens usually result in a relative reduction of total energy (Schlundt et al. 1993) with energy-restricted diets being typically lower in energy intake than *ad libitum* low-fat eating (Schlundt et al. 1993; Harvey-Berino 1998). Despite the observation of a greater rate of initial weight loss with energy-restricted diets, total weight loss over time appears to be similar (Schlundt et al. 1993; Jeffery et al. 1995; Shah et al. 1996) as does weight regain (Jeffery et al. 1995). Arguments supporting the preferential use of *ad libitum* low-fat eating suggest that these diets are more palatable, are easier to follow, produce greater longer-term compliance, and minimise binge eating, although other studies report no difference between these measures (Schlundt et al.

1993; Shah et al. 1996). An important observation to consider is the increasing prevalence of obesity in western countries despite a reported reduction in fat consumption (Prentice & Jebb 1995). Clearly, fat intake is important, but over time energy intake must be less than expenditure for fat loss to occur.

To our knowledge, a trial of the relative benefits of using a low-fat versus an energy-restricted diet to achieve fat loss in athletes has not been undertaken. In practice, many athletes achieve and maintain an optimal body composition for their sport by following a low-fat eating plan alone. This approach would seem more beneficial as it allows unrestricted consumption of CHO, which assists in optimising glycogen storage. Unfortunately, the popularity of fad dietary regimens supports the view that attainment of a desirable body composition comes at an even higher price for some athletes. This is most probably due to their need to meet a set requirement dictated by the sport (e.g. making weight or conforming to a set range of fatness), or their desire to attain a certain level of weight or fatness for personal or aesthetic reasons. These goals are often below what is biologically normal, therefore, in addition to consuming less dietary fat, these athletes must also achieve a chronic negative energy balance by using energy restriction, additional exercise or a combination of both. Where possible, energy restriction should be minimised to ensure adequate CHO and other nutrients are consumed. This will be possible in most situations where adequate time has been set aside for weight or fat loss. Unfortunately this is often not the case (see Chapter 8). It is interesting to consider that in some situations, the rigour and negative aspects of the diet itself (see Section 7.5) may actually be more detrimental to health and performance than the additional weight or fat itself. Unfortunately, weight and fat loss is one case where athletes and coaches often think in terms of the end justifying the means.

7.4.1.2 *Low-CHO diets*

Low-CHO or CHO-modified diets such as the Doctor Atkins (Atkins 1992), Scarsdale (Tarnower & Baker 1980), and Sugarbusters (Andrews et al. 1998) have enjoyed waves of popularity over the past 25 years. Enthusiasts for this way of eating suggest that dietary CHO is the key factor in the development of excess body fat and obesity, diabetes, heart disease and a number of other medical conditions. However, this assertion is not supported by current scientific evidence. On a normal diet and given normal activity, humans do not synthesise fat, but rather store fat eaten in the diet (see also Section 7.3.2.1). The important factors in body-fat gain are total energy intake and the proportion of fat in the diet. CHO may influence fat gain if it is eaten in excess (increased total energy intake) and with fat (weight gain comes with the increased risk of metabolic disease). Other ways in which CHO may influence disease risk depend on the type of CHO (e.g. starches or sugars), or the glycaemic index. Low-CHO diets do not generally advertise an increase in performance *per se*, but they promise weight and fat loss, which is attractive to many athletes, especially those who have struggled with traditional weight loss approaches.

Most low-CHO diets base their success around a reduction in insulin secretion or a decrease in the insulin to glucagon ratio. As insulin inhibits lipolysis and promotes fat storage, it is plausible that the restriction of CHO facilitates improved lipolysis and weight loss (Lefebvre & Luyckx 1969). In fact, the short-term results of such diets are often outstanding, partly due to the initial loss of water and glycogen (Rosen et al. 1982). Although this is not fat loss, the observation of a reduction in kilograms on the scales can be a powerful motivator. In the medium term, low-CHO diets promote ketosis and nausea (Dwyer 1992, p. 668). In this phase, weight loss continues, partly due to ketosis and low plasma insulin concentration, but also due to a reduction in energy intake (Dwyer 1992, p. 668).

In the long term, low-CHO diets fail to provide adequate nutritional balance and may result in a substantial loss of lean body mass, due to the utilisation of muscle protein to maintain blood glucose concentrations via gluconeogenesis (Dwyer 1992, p. 668). A loss of lean tissue is associated with a reduction in resting energy expenditure; this is detrimental to long-term weight control (Ravussin et al. 1985). Low-CHO diets fail in the long term for a number of reasons. Firstly, they limit CHO intake, which has been shown to drive food consumption in humans (Jebb et al. 1996) (see also Section 7.3.2.2). Severe CHO restriction becomes almost impossible to maintain, as appetite is geared to replenish body CHO stores (Tremblay et al. 1985). This drive would be even greater in athletes because they also deplete CHO stores through exercise on a regular basis. Lack of CHO results in side-effects including ketosis, headaches, fatigue, nausea and bad breath (Van Itallie 1980, p. 15). In the medium to long term, these effects become difficult to tolerate for most individuals. In athletes, these side-effects and the associated reduction in performance make such diets ineffective.

Despite the negative consequences of low-CHO diets, the theme tends to be recycled periodically, with new diets promoting a short-lived revival in popularity. The Zone Diet (see Section 7.4.1.3) is a complicated type of CHO-restricted diet, although the levels of CHO recommended (40% of energy) are less extreme than in the Dr Atkin's (less than 20 g CHO per day) and Scarsdale diets (34.5% CHO or approximately 85 g CHO per day). Newer low-CHO diets are often simultaneously promoted as being high-protein or high-fat, as the proportion of these nutrients is increased to compensate for the reduced CHO content. High-protein diets often promote the virtues of avoidance of fat, as well as the ability of protein to assist in the maintenance of lean body mass. High-protein diets are more satiating and therefore less energy is taken in. Aside from the camouflage provided by the complicated rules and rituals prescribed by these diets, the essential common feature becomes a reduction in total energy intake, via the restriction of CHO (Dwyer 1992, p. 668). This fact however is often not disclosed in the diet's rationale, possibly as followers may be less impressed by the notion that they are really using just another low-energy diet.

Some diets recommend altering the type or glycaemic index, rather than the total amount, of CHO consumed (e.g. Sugarbusters or the GI Factor) (Brand-Miller et al.

1996). Such diets do not promote ketosis and are not associated with most of the negative side-effects mentioned above. Low–glycaemic index diets have been shown to aid weight loss, possibly by enhancing satiety (Holt & Brand-Miller 1994).

7.4.1.3 *The Zone Diet*

In his book *The Zone: A Dietary Road Map* (Sears 1995), Dr Barry Sears targets an athletic market by claiming the diet enhances performance, endurance, fat loss and the maintenance of lean body mass. The diet opposes traditional guidelines for high-CHO eating, recommending that CHO be limited in an effort to reduce insulin secretion and promote favourable changes in the insulin to glucagon ratio. Sears claims that hormonal benefits induced by balancing the insulin to glucagon ratio include increased lipolysis and improved regulation of eicosanoids, in particular the two major types of prostaglandins, series one and two. The series one prostaglandins have an antithrombolytic, vasodilatory action; while series two are vasoconstrictive. The diet claims that increasing the production of series one ('good') prostaglandins and inhibiting series two ('bad') eicosanoids results in less exercise-induced vasoconstriction, thus increasing blood-flow and oxygen delivery to the working muscle. This theoretically improves substrate availability and energy production, and results in enhanced performance. Achieving this state is referred to as 'entering the zone' and is attained by maintaining an energy distribution of 40% CHO, 30% protein and 30% fat (40:30:30), divided into a regimen of three meals and two snacks per day. Meals and snacks are planned by combining prescribed numbers of blocks of fat, protein and CHO foods from lists of food exchanges.

'Eating in the zone' is claimed to increase the intake of precursor fatty acids required for 'good' eicosanoid production. This combined with a decrease in the insulin to glucagon ratio results in competitive inhibition of the 'opposing' series two pathways, facilitating a net balance of more 'good' eicosanoids. Unfortunately, eicosanoid metabolism is complex, with little predictability. Often the theoretical changes expected do not occur in response to dietary manipulation (Stone et al. 1978). Although Sears has based some of his claims on plausible scientific theory, there are many flaws in his arguments and the diet contains opposing and contradictory information. One example of this is the claim that a reduction in CHO intake to 40% of energy, based mainly around low– to moderate–glycaemic index foods will decrease plasma insulin levels. However, a reduction in CHO intake to less than 25% of energy is required before insulin levels are significantly reduced (Coulston et al. 1983). In addition, Sears misclassifies the glycaemic index of a number of foods (e.g. classifying pasta as high glycaemic index) hence basing avoidance on incorrect information.

In practice, 'eating in the zone' is difficult and impractical as most meals and snacks need to be totally redesigned to cater for the 40:30:30 ratio. Interestingly, even the recipes provided in Sear's book do not keep precisely to this macronutrient distribution. Organising snacks that follow the Zone guidelines is also a challenge, however this has been partially solved with the commercial development of specialised snack bars (e.g. PR Bar). The Zone Diet is essentially low in energy, typically providing between 4200–8400 kJ/d (1000–2000 kcal/d). These levels are not easily increased even for individuals in heavy training. It is not surprising that followers lose weight on the program. However, if followed strictly, athletes may experience fatigue and decreased performance due to glycogen depletion. For a comprehensive review of the Zone Diet, see Cheuvront 1999.

7.4.1.4 *Food-combining diets*

Use of the term 'food-combining diet' is almost a misnomer as diets based on this philosophy recommend that certain foods should not be combined. Typically, these diets warn against the combination of protein and CHO foods suggesting that such combinations are difficult to digest and result in a build-up of toxins, which has negative health effects, including excess weight. The 'Fit for life' diet (Diamond & Diamond 1986) is an example of one such diet. In addition to avoiding protein–CHO combinations the 'Fit for life' diet recommends eating fruit only until midday and avoiding eating after 8 pm.

Athletes are often seduced by complex or exotic dietary regimes as they are new, exciting and tend to exaggerate the potential for fast and easy success. Food-combining diets are often supported by reported outstanding early results from a number of devoted followers who adhere strictly to the recommendations. Vigilance to a food-combining diet generally results in an energy and fat intake that is substantially lower than usual and it is this, rather than any special magic derived from the food combinations, that promotes weight loss. The finer details of food-combining diets are often open to variable interpretation, but they generally result in a food intake that is low in fat and energy and relatively low in CHO. They have the potential to be detrimental for athletes as they limit opportunities to consume adequate energy and CHO that may interfere with the athlete's ability to complete training and competition schedules. Inadequate CHO intake may also result in the loss of muscle mass as amino acids may be recycled via the liver to maintain blood glucose levels. Restricting the combination of protein and CHO immediately post-exercise may also be detrimental to recovery (Roy & Tarnopolsky 1998).

7.4.1.5 *Adaptation to high-fat diets*

Adaptation to high-fat diets has been used as a strategy to delay fatigue in endurance exercise by enhancing fat oxidation and sparing CHO stores (Lambert et al. 1994). Although this dietary manipulation is not typically employed to promote weight loss, athletes have been interested in the notion that fat adaptation might result in a permanent up-regulation of fat metabolism and subsequent improvement in body-fat control. The use of this strategy for body-fat management has not been studied specifically, however, several studies have investigated its efficacy for enhancing athletic performance (see Chapter 16). The dietary regimens used vary but typically provide greater than 30% of dietary energy as fat with some as high as 94%.

Overall, the use of high-fat diets is associated with an elevation in the concentration of enzymes used in ß-oxidation and a shift in substrate metabolism to favour lipid utilisation. Despite any suggested benefits to lipid oxidation and body-fat control, fat adaptation regimens have little to offer most athletes, who require adequate CHO stores to maximise higher-intensity phases of training. The use of high-fat diets in the longer term may be associated with an increased risk of cardiovascular disease, although endurance training should attenuate this risk (Sarna & Kaprio 1994). See Chapter 16 for further information.

7.4.1.6 *Very low energy diets (VLEDs)*

Very low energy (VLEDs) or calorie (VLCDs) diets are used therapeutically to facilitate rapid weight loss in the obese. Most provide a daily energy intake of 400–600 kcal (Brodoff & Hendler 1992, p. 683). They generally take the form of a liquid meal made from commercial powder preparations (e.g. Modifast or Optifast). They typically provide less than 100 g CHO/d. As VLEDs are usually prescribed for use exclusively without food, they are supplemented with vitamins and minerals to provide levels approximating the Recommended Dietary Intakes (RDIs). A significant proportion of the energy in VLEDs comes from high biological value protein to assist in the maintenance of lean body mass. Earlier versions of these diets failed to provide adequate protein and this was associated with complications including arrhythmia, heart failure and death (Lantigua et al. 1980).

Very low energy diets initially induce a rapid early weight reduction due to loss of glycogen, water and protein (muscle mass) (Evans & Strang 1929). After glycogen stores are exhausted, stored fat is almost exclusively used to provide energy and this produces substantial ketosis. With only small amounts of CHO provided by the VLED (typically around 100 g/day), blood glucose levels are maintained via gluconeogenesis. Although physical activity is encouraged in the obese to promote additional fat loss, the severe reduction in energy intake below resting metabolic rate ensures substantial weight loss, even without physical activity (Kreitzman 1989). Potential side-effects of VLEDs include: nausea, halitosis (bad breath), hunger (which may decrease after the initiation of ketosis), headaches, hypotension, light-headedness and precipitation of gout (Brodoff & Hendler 1992, p. 688).

Although weight loss induced by VLEDs is large and rapid (1.5–2 kg per week) (Donnelly 1991), it is often not sustained (Perri 1995). These diets are therefore a short-term weight loss tool for the very obese. Serious negative side-effects, including glycogen depletion, loss of lean body mass, dehydration, electrolyte imbalance and hypotension, make VLEDs unsuitable and dangerous for athletes. Apart from insufficient energy and macronutrient intake, the levels of vitamins and minerals may not be adequate for athletes. They would most certainly result in fatigue, decreased concentration and a fall in exercise performance. It is unlikely that most athletes would be able to complete their usual training program while using VLEDs.

7.4.1.7 *Weight loss groups and centres*

These groups or centres (e.g. Weight Watchers, Jenny Craig) are designed for the general public, to provide support for weight loss. Many of these now have professional input from dietitians, psychologists and medical practitioners to aid in keeping their programs safe, effective and relevant for clients. The programs are not designed specifically for athletes, however, some have the facility to provide additional energy and CHO in their meal plans or diet meals. Athletes seeking to use this method of weight loss need to choose an accredited program that has professional input and the capacity to cater for their special needs.

7.4.2 *Exercise prescriptions for weight and fat loss*

Exercise complements dietary approaches to weight loss by increasing energy expenditure and inducing negative energy balance. Although the effectiveness of exercise for weight or fat loss in obese populations has been questioned (Garrow 1995), problems encountered with the obese, such as low levels of motivation, poor compliance and ability to complete a useful amount of exercise, are less likely to be present in athletic individuals. Athletes may, however, have difficulty finding time to add extra training purely for weight or fat loss; alternatively there may be issues with over-use, injury risk (especially with running programs) or fatigue. Exercise prescriptions for weight or fat loss in athletes need to be developed with these factors in mind. This may result in a program that is less than optimal from a fat loss perspective but one which compliments their athletic pursuits and offers the best chance of safe and effective weight management.

7.4.2.1 *High- versus low-intensity exercise for fat loss*

Most prescriptions for fat loss in overweight populations revolve around the incorporation of low-intensity (approximately 50% $VO_{2\ max}$), medium-duration (approximately 60 minutes) aerobic activity. This prescription is reported to be most effective in promoting weight and fat loss, and is the type of exercise that overweight individuals are most likely to be able to do (Déspres et al. 1991). In addition, this type of exercise has been associated with an improvement in insulin sensitivity, lipoprotein profile and blood glucose control, important for many overweight individuals, who frequently experience these metabolic abnormalities (Déspres et al. 1991). Although it would seem logical for athletes to try to increase the volume of low-moderate intensity activity to maximise lipid oxidation, such low-intensity activity may not be the most efficient prescription for fat loss in fit individuals. While the proportion of fat utilised is greater at low to moderate intensities, well-trained athletes still oxidise substantial proportions of fat at higher intensities, providing this is less than their anaerobic threshold. The effectiveness of high- versus low-intensity training on body fatness and skeletal muscle metabolism was investigated by Tremblay et al. (1994). In this study, young adults (eight men and nine women) were randomised to either high- or low-intensity, intermittent or endurance training for 15 or 20 weeks respectively. The mean cost of the high-intensity program (57.9 MJ) was significantly lower than the endurance training (120.4 MJ). However, despite its lower energy cost, the high-intensity exercise program produced a nine-fold greater reduction in skinfold measurements of subcutaneous fat. In addition, the high-intensity program resulted in a greater increase in 3-hydroxyacyl coenzyme A dehydrogenase (HAD), a marker of β-oxidation.

Although a lower proportion of fat is utilised in the fuel mix oxidised at higher exercise intensities, a greater energy deficit occurs in less time and this results in a higher total fat utilisation (Romijn et al. 1993). Fat oxidation may also be greater in the post-exercise recovery period and there are potentially other benefits including an increase in resting metabolic rate and the thermic effect of food (see Section 7.3.2.3). The efficiency of high-intensity exercise may also be attractive to many athletes who have little time to incorporate extra training that expends 200–500 kcal just for fat loss.

7.4.2.2 *Mode of exercise and fat loss*

Weight-bearing exercise, in particular running, is often used to promote weight and fat loss in athletes. Apart from it being practical, runners tend to be leaner and lighter than other highly trained athletes in aerobically-based sports such as swimming or cycling. Flynn et al. (1990) demonstrated that swimming utilised similar energy to running, but proposed that the higher proportion of body fat in swimmers may be due to differences in post-exercise energy expenditure or appetite. It is also possible that control of thermoregulation and the recovery from the impact of running contribute to higher post-exercise energy expenditure. Although there is as yet no explanation for the superior weight control benefits of running, it is frequently used for this purpose. The choice of other modes of exercise is often due to factors such as avoidance of the high impact and injury risk associated with running, because use of different muscle groups is required and/or because running is not preferred by the athlete.

7.5 ▰▰ NEGATIVE ASPECTS OF WEIGHT CONTROL IN ATHLETES

7.5.1 *Menstrual and endocrine disturbance*

Loss of body weight and fat may produce menstrual disturbance in female athletes (Brownell et al. 1987). Although it was once believed that a critical level of body fat was required to initiate (17% body fat) and then sustain (22% body fat) the menstrual cycle (Frisch & McArthur 1974), more recent evidence suggests that the threshold for regular menstrual function is individual, with no particular critical level of body fatness identified (Sanborn et al. 1987). It may be the level of leptin that is the signal of adequacy of fat stores. Dieting or energy restriction itself is often associated with cycle interruption (Kaiserauer 1989). This may be related to the magnitude or rate of loss of body fat (Brownell et al. 1987) or be a response to an inadequate energy or protein intake (Loucks & Horvath 1985). Dietary factors such as a low-fat (Deuster et al. 1986), high-fibre (Lloyd et al. 1987) intake, or vegetarianism (Carlberg et al. 1983) have also been associated with lower levels of circulating oestrogen, and this rather than the specific energy or protein level may require consideration. Although strenuous training programs have been associated with cycle interruption, there appears to be a consensus that it is a combination of factors that place female athletes most at risk (Keizer & Rogol 1990). Loss of the menstrual cycle, with consequent lower levels of oestrogen, increases the risk of osteopaenia. This in the short term, combined with other risk factors, may increase the potential for stress fractures (Lloyd et al. 1986). Bone demineralisation after prolonged periods of menstrual disruption may not be completely reversible. In the long term, low bone density in female athletes may predispose them to premature osteoporosis (for further information see Chapter 10).

Weight loss in males is also associated with endocrine changes, in particular, reductions in testosterone and prolactin (Strauss et al. 1993). This is especially the case when body-fat levels are severely decreased. These reductions in testosterone concentration may make it difficult to optimise lean body mass and performance.

7.5.2 *Reduced lean body mass and resting metabolic rate*

Resting metabolic rate is primarily determined by lean body mass. Even modest energy restriction is associated with a reduction in lean body mass. Substantial decreases in resting metabolic rate (15% decrease) have been observed in obese individuals on very low energy diets (Leibel et al. 1995). Although the decrease in resting energy expenditure is closely related to the loss of lean body mass, the changes in resting metabolism are not totally explained by lean mass changes. It is possible that some may be due to alterations in thyroid hormones (Strauss et al. 1993).

Weight loss brought about by dieting usually results in a reduction in metabolic rate, making weight loss more difficult (Jeffery et al. 1984; Leibel et al. 1995). As exercise promotes the increase, or at least maintenance, of lean body mass, there is interest in whether athletes experience reductions in resting metabolic rate with dieting as the obese do. Although there is limited evidence, athletes appear to lose lean body mass with dieting, even with heavy resistance-training as in body building (Heyward et al. 1989). Greater reductions are observed in the athletes who consume the least energy. There appears to be the potential to reduce losses by maintaining an adequate protein intake (Walberg-Rankin et al. 1994) and allowing the body to adapt to energy restriction as losses in lean body mass appear to decline over time.

Repeated cycles of weight loss and gain theoretically decrease lean mass and increase fat mass over time. This is because with each weight loss cycle, lean mass, and hence resting metabolic rate, is reduced, facilitating a gain in body fat when energy restriction ceases. Although there is some evidence to support this theory from cross-sectional studies, longitudinal studies do not support this view. In fact, there is good evidence that metabolic rate returns to a level appropriate for a person's lean body mass after the acute effects of dieting have been lifted, even though this may take some months. In a prospective study designed specifically to test the effects of repeated weight loss–weight regain cycles in an obese population using very low energy diets, basal metabolic rate was not suppressed significantly after three weight loss cycles (Jebb et al. 1991). In an extensive review of both animal and human research, including large-scale population studies, Wing et al. concluded that there was little evidence to support a permanent fall in metabolic rate with cycles of dieting (Wing 1992) if overall weight loss has not been achieved.

Controlled studies in athletic populations have been mainly performed in wrestlers. While a cross-sectional study suggested resting metabolic rate was lower than non-cycling counterparts (Steen et al. 1988), these results were not verified in a longitudinal study (Melby et al. 1990). The available data do not support the contention that weight cycling reduces metabolic rate. However, the research thus far has been mainly in wrestling and this may not reflect what occurs in other sports (for further information see Chapter 9).

7.5.3 *Illness and immunity*

There is a popular perception that dieting increases the risk for illness in athletes. This is partly due to the potential inadequacy in energy, protein or vitamin and mineral intake while energy is restricted. Inadequate micronutrient intake in athletes on restricted diets has been reported in a number of studies, especially in female gymnasts, ballet dancers, and runners (Barr 1987). Unfortunately, most of this information comes from food diaries, which are notoriously inaccurate. In addition, the collection period used to assess the intake of certain micronutrients may not be of adequate duration. Groups of athletes who appear to be most at risk include those in sports where leanness is prized or where there is the need to make weight (Barr 1987).

Recently, the importance of adequate CHO and n-3 fatty acids for the maintenance of immunity has been highlighted (reviewed by Pedersen et al. 1999). Adequate CHO appears to attenuate the cortisol and growth hormone response to exercise, resulting in fewer perturbations in blood immune cell counts (Nieman et al. 1997). There also appears to be a role for fat intake, as shifting the ratio of n-6 to n-3 fatty acids towards a higher proportion of n-3s has been shown in animal research to counteract the production of a prostaglandin hormone (PGE_2) and subsequent suppression of the cellular immune system (Johnson et al. 1993 cited in Pedersen et al. 1999). It is possible that dieting may result in an inadequate CHO and fat intake and that this impacts on immunity. As most diets recommend higher intakes of fruit and vegetables, it is likely that the intake of antioxidants remains reasonable with dieting. Antioxidants are thought to have a protective effect on the immune system (Peters et al. 1993).

7.5.4 *Psychological effects and disordered eating*

Energy restriction itself may induce a dysphoric mood and increase the risk of disordered eating. Mood disturbance has frequently been reported in the overweight during dieting (Leon & Chamberlain 1973). However, more recently this negative aspect of restrictive eating has also been reported in athletes (Horswill et al. 1990).

A higher prevalence of disordered eating has been reported in sports where leanness is prized (Davis & Cowles 1989). Dieting is one of the known triggers for disordered eating, and this together with other factors such as performance pressure and age-related body image issues may significantly increase the risk of eating problems (for further information see Chapter 9).

7.5.5 *Performance*

Studies investigating the effects of dieting on performance have mainly concentrated on acute weight loss where athletes need to make weight. These effects are discussed in Chapter 8.

7.6 *ADJUNCTIVE AGENTS FOR WEIGHT AND FAT LOSS*

7.6.1 *Dietary supplements*

A number of dietary supplements have been touted as assisting with weight control; these include L-carnitine, chromium picolinate, hydroxy-methyl-butarate (HMB) and pyruvate. The basis of these claims and an assessment of their efficacy related to weight loss are covered in Chapter 17. The efficacy of other over-the-counter supplements touted to assist weight loss, including Cellasene, Chitosan, St Johns Wort, Brindleberry, capsaicin, and grape seed extract, have recently been reviewed elsewhere (Egger et al. 1999).

7.6.2 *Pharmacological agents*

Pharmacological agents may be used to regulate or alter weight in both the short and medium-to-long term. It needs to be stated at the outset that many of these agents are not permitted by sports drug agencies and they should be used only in the appropriate situation and under appropriate medical care.

7.6.2.1 *Drugs for short-term weight loss or weight control*

Diuretics are the drugs used for this purpose. No diuretics are permitted for use by athletes as they can be 'masking agents' for other proscribed drugs. Diuretics, as the name implies, cause a diuresis of extra fluid and some electrolytes by the kidneys. They produce short-term weight loss, but weight (fluid) is rapidly regained once they have ceased being taken. Their effect lasts hours to a day. Side-effects include hypokalaemia (which may affect muscle functioning and produce weakness), hyponatraemia, hypotension and dehydration. These agents should not be taken in hot environments without adequate fluid and electrolyte replacement being at hand.

7.6.2.2 *Drugs which produce weight loss in the medium term*

These drugs can act either locally (on the gastrointestinal tract) or centrally (on appetite or thermogenic mechanisms).

(i) Drugs acting on the gastrointestinal tract

Drugs used previously were generally bulking agents, providing a sense of fullness and therefore satiety. Methylcellulose is the only such agent that has been shown to be effective in a controlled trial (Enzi et al. 1980). Acarbose, a glucosidase inhibitor, which prevents the breakdown of sucrose, and therefore the absorption of sugar, has helped obese patients maintain lower body weight, when it was given in high doses (Caterson 1990). There are many other agents in this category, with no evidence of effectiveness, that are still used. A recent article (Egger et al. 1999) discusses bulking agents and other popular therapies and shows that most are not effective at producing weight loss.

Orlistat is a new drug which produces weight loss. It is a pancreatic lipase inhibitor which prevents fat breakdown in the gut and therefore its absorption. Some 30% of ingested fat is malabsorbed and passed through the bowel when on a course of Orlistat. This loss of energy from fat results in weight loss. Orlistat is given at a dosage of 120 mg three times a day, one tablet with each meal. Because of the fat loss in the stool, a low-fat diet must be prescribed (and adhered to) with Orlistat, otherwise diarrhoea and fat or oil loss by anus may result. Over a six- to 12-month period, some 10 kg is lost with Orlistat treatment compared to 6 kg on placebo (Sjostrom et al. 1998). The side-effects of treatment with Orlistat are abdominal discomfort, diarrhoea, anal leakage and the potential to have loss of fat-soluble vitamins (to date this has not been demonstrated, though levels decline over a two-year course of treatment). As well as weight loss, Orlistat has other beneficial effects. These include a lowering of serum cholesterol, reduction in blood pressure, and better control of diabetes.

There is no data available on the use of Orlistat in athletes. It has the potential benefit of reducing fat absorption while allowing normal CHO absorption, and so should not interfere with CHO loading and/or the accumulation of muscle glycogen. As athletes are not at a health risk through excess weight, it becomes an ethical question as to whether drugs like Orlistat should be used, even though their use does not contravene the International Olympic Committee policy on drug use in sport.

(ii) Drugs acting centrally or on thermogenesis to produce weight loss

Fenfluramine and its isomer, dexfenfluramine, are effective weight loss agents (O'Connor et al. 1995). They act by altering serotonin concentrations in the hypothalamus and are appetite suppressants. However they have been withdrawn world-wide because of the occurrence of cardiac valve lesions (Connolly et al. 1997). This valvulopathy occurred particularly when these drugs were used in combination with phentermine (see below) and for more than three months, possibly due to high circulating serotonin concentrations. Although effective, they are no longer available.

Ephedrine and caffeine have been and are used for weight reduction in obese patients. This combination has been used particularly in Denmark. Ephedrine is a sympathomimetic drug and acts on the catecholamine receptors. In addition to its other properties and actions, such as bronchodilation, it can suppress appetite and increase thermogenesis (Astrup & Raben 1992). Ephedrine at a dose of 150 mg daily can produce weight loss (Astrup et al. 1992), but best results are produced with the ephedrine–caffeine combination. The doses used were 20 mg ephedrine and 200 mg caffeine daily, and these were effective when combined with a reduced energy diet (Astrup et al. 1992, 1996; Astrup & Toubro 1993). Caffeine, though used for weight loss, does not seem to be effective alone. It must be said that this method of weight reduction, with ephedrine and caffeine combinations, is not much utilised worldwide. The side-effects of ephedrine are tremor and nervousness, elevated blood pressure, increased heart rate and arrhythmias. While useful for those with asthma, ephedrine should not be used by those with diabetes, hypertension or hyperthyroidism. While ephedrine alone, or the combination of ephedrine–caffeine, is effective in producing weight loss (1.7 kg and 3.8 kg more than placebo over 24 weeks respectively), ephedrine is not approved by sports drug agencies, and caffeine ingestion needs to be limited to prevent urinary levels exceeding the legal level. These drugs have been shown to be effective in obese patients—a total weight loss of some 16 kg in 24 weeks when used with a reduced energy intake (Astrup & Raben 1992)—but there is little if any data on their effectiveness or use in athletes. In lean subjects, ephedrine and caffeine (together with theophylline) have been shown to increase thermogenesis and energy expenditure.

Nicotine too may suppress appetite and increase resting energy expenditure. Smokers have higher resting energy expenditure at night and for a short while post-smoking (Audrain et al. 1995). Smokers tend to be thinner and certainly there is weight gain on the cessation of smoking (Flegal et al. 1995; Rasky et al. 1996). This being said, the health consequences of smoking (particularly vascular disease and cancer), and the effect of smoking on athletic performance make this an inappropriate way for athletes to attempt to lose weight.

There are older appetite suppressant agents still available. These drugs include phentermine, benzphetamine, phendimetrazine, mazindol and diethylpropion. They are effective in producing weight loss over a period of months when used with a lifestyle program including diet and exercise (Atkinson & Hubbard 1994). Again, most of the experience is in obese subjects, and there is little experience of the use of these drugs in athletes for weight control. They are amphetamine derivatives and tend to have stimulatory side-effects on the central nervous and cardiovascular systems. Another older drug, phenylpropanolamine, is available in some countries in over-the-counter preparations for weight loss. It is related to both noradrenalin and the amphetamine derivatives. It can be effective, but has the potential to stimulate cardiovascular and central nervous systems. They are effective in the short term, but are stimulatory and are not permitted by sports regulatory agencies.

Fluoxetine is a member of a newer class of antidepressants, the selective serotonin reuptake inhibitors (SSRIs). It acts by increasing serotonin levels locally in the central nervous system. In depressed patients, it can produce weight loss and may be useful, at higher than normal doses, in producing weight loss in non-depressed individuals. However, a derivative of this class of agent, sibutramine, is an effective weight loss agent. It has both serotonergic (appetite suppressant) and noradrenergic (thermogenic) effects. At a dose of 10–15 mg/d, combined with an appropriate lifestyle program of diet and exercise, it produces significant weight loss (some 10 kg compared to 6 kg on placebo) which can be maintained for a year (Stock 1997; McNeely & Goa 1998). This drug does increase the pulse rate marginally (by two to three beats per minute), and with treatment and weight loss, blood pressure may not fall as much as it does on placebo. There are no reports of its use for weight control in athletes.

There are effective pharmacologic measures available for reducing weight, but there is little if any information about the use of such agents in athletes. The use of such drugs by athletes must be considered carefully and raises an ethical question. These drugs were designed to assist those at health risk, not young fit individuals. It is better if they not be used except where there is a risk to health of weight.

7.7 GUIDELINES FOR FAT LOSS

Recommendations for safe weight loss in non-athletes are generally in the vicinity of 0.5–1 kg per week. These guidelines also seem reasonable for many athletes. Loss of this weight equates to an approximate energy deficit of 2 100–4 200 kJ (500–1 000 kcal). This deficit can be initiated via changes in diet, training or a combination of both. The main aim of dietary change is to promote a moderate total energy restriction without compromising CHO intake or other nutritional and performance goals (e.g. protein status and micronutrient needs). Energy restriction is best achieved by the implementation of a low-fat diet (15–25% of energy) and a moderate-high CHO intake (6–8 g/kg body weight per day). Protein intake should be approximately 1.5–2 g/kg body weight per day. The upper level of protein intake is recommended if energy restriction is substantial, as this may assist the maintenance of lean body mass and help promote satiety. The incorporation of foods high in fibre and/or of low glycaemic index may assist with appetite control in some athletes.

Exercise complements dietary approaches to weight loss by increasing energy expenditure and inducing negative energy balance. Although lower-intensity, aerobically-based exercise has been recommended extensively as 'best' for fat loss, this prescription may not be the most efficient in athletes. Higher-intensity exercise that can be maintained for a reasonable duration (30–60 min/d) in addition to an athlete's standard training may be a useful and perhaps even better approach to weight loss (see Section 7.4.2.1). Consideration should be given to issues such as the risk of fatigue and injury when additional exercise is prescribed. This will also influence the choice of exercise mode. As with dietary intervention, exercise prescriptions should be tailored to an athlete's individual needs.

7.8 SUMMARY

Athletes may need or desire to lose weight for many reasons. Although most will not need to lose weight for health reasons, they may wish to improve power to weight ratio or attain a desired body composition in a sport that has an aesthetic ideal. Some athletes need to make a pre-designated weight in order to compete. It is these groups that may consider losing or controlling weight.

It needs to be remembered that body weight and composition is determined by many factors, both biological and environmental. Genes have a significant influence on the susceptibility for weight or fat gain and indeed the potential to attain a particular physique. Genes may act through food preferences and appetite, energy expenditure or through metabolic factors such as substrate partitioning (i.e. selecting which fuel is oxidised).

Currently alteration in environmental or lifestyle factors is the only way to manipulate body weight and composition. The two major factors influencing energy balance are energy intake and expenditure. Approaches that manipulate dietary intake to facilitate weight or fat loss range from modest reductions in dietary fat and energy intake through to severe reductions in total energy and CHO consumption. There is evidence demonstrating that approaches utilising reductions in fat intake, and not total energy, produce better compliance and results. Such dietary approaches are also less likely to result in glycogen depletion. Some athletes however will also need to restrict total energy to achieve their desired goals. There is little to no scientific evidence supporting the effectiveness of particular food combinations, or low-CHO diets, for anything more than an acute, short-term weight loss.

Physical activity affects energy expenditure directly due to the work done, and indirectly through potential alterations in resting metabolic rate and TEF. However, the effect on these latter components is small in most individuals and unlikely to make a significant contribution to energy balance, except perhaps in those athletes with high energy flux (high energy intakes and expenditures). Although it is often assumed that additional exercise will result in an energy and fat deficit and thus produce weight loss, it is possible that an individual may compensate, partially or even fully, for increased energy expenditure by consuming more. This may occur through changes in appetite, but the precise nature of the effect of exercise is yet to be established over the medium to long term. There appears to be an acute, post-exercise suppression of appetite, and in some studies, an increase in the preference for CHO. Despite this, athletes, like the general community, are susceptible to weight gain when physical activity ceases or decreases, especially during the off-season or through periods of illness or injury. Careful planning of food intake and the maintenance of some physical activity is important to help prevent weight or fat gain at this time.

Exercise prescriptions for weight loss in athletes are similar to those designed for the overweight, incorporating low-intensity (50% $VO_{2\,max}$), medium-duration (60 min) aerobic activity. This prescription may not be the most efficient for fat loss in fit individuals. Exercise regimens using shorter duration, medium- to high-intensity exercise and possibly strength training components may also be an effective way to reduce excess body fat. This latter approach may be attractive to many athletes because of the limited time available to incorporate extra training for the specific purpose of weight or fat reduction.

Athletes and coaches are open to just as much misinformation about weight loss and dieting as the rest of the community. Unfortunately this often results in the use of unbalanced dietary regimens, nutrition supplements, and drugs which lack scientific support or which are not permitted by sports drug agencies. Such approaches may result in decreased performance and have negative health consequences. The promotion of safe and effective weight loss strategies is an important role of the sports medicine team.

7.9   *PRACTICE TIPS*

These tips are designed to assist practitioners with assessment and management of the athlete presenting for weight or fat loss.

Assessment of the need to lose weight or fat

- The initial assessment for weight or fat loss in an athlete should include measurement of weight, height, adiposity and muscularity, ideally using a standardised measurement protocol. Surface anthropometry is frequently used as it is portable, inexpensive and non-invasive. Anthropometric measures should be performed in duplicate by a trained operator. Other methods of assessing body composition and their relative benefits and pitfalls are discussed in Chapter 4.

- The error associated with the measurement of anthropometry should be explained to the athlete, coach or trainer and (where appropriate) the parent or guardian (see Chapter 18 for specific management of children and adolescents where growth also needs to be assessed). An understanding of the error of any body composition method used is critical to the interpretation of the measurements collected. This is especially important for determining whether a true change in body composition has occurred when serial measurements are performed.

- Body composition assessment should be complemented with a history of personal and family weight patterns. If previous difficulties have been encountered, information about the methods of weight management that have been used and their efficacy both in the short and medium-to-long term need to be determined.

- As with any paramedically-based assessment, information should be gathered regarding past and current medical history, including injuries. An informal assessment of the potential for disordered eating should also be incorporated into the history taking. In females, information about menarche and the regularity of the menstrual cycle should be obtained. Recent biochemical, haematological and bone density results should be considered.

- In athletes with no contraindications to weight or fat loss (e.g. problems with health, or disordered eating) their goals and those of their coach or trainer need to be considered within the context of information which has been gathered in the history (especially personal weight history, previous success with weight control and the methods used). This needs to be weighed up against current weight and body composition results and the optimal ranges of athletes within the sport.

- Goals for weight and fat loss need to be realistic, ideally not greater than 0.5 kg per week or for body fat a maximum of 5 mm per week. The goal of weight or fat loss should not compromise health or performance.

Dietary assessment

- The dietary assessment should gather information about current eating patterns. Generally a dietary history with a food frequency checklist is ideal for this purpose. However, food diaries can be useful to complement this information.

- Dietary histories of athletes presenting for weight or fat loss also need to include questions related to eating away from home, strategies used when travelling to competition, cooking skills, comfort or stress eating, and use of alcohol.

- A measurement or estimate of resting metabolic rate is useful to assess the accuracy of reported food intake. Resting metabolic rate can be measured directly using a total body calorimeter, however resting gas measurements are more often available (see Chapter 6, Section 6.4.2.1). Alternatively, resting metabolic rate can be estimated using a number of regression equations derived for this purpose (see Section 6.4.2.3). In practice the Harris–Benedict or Cunningham equations appear to be best for athletic populations (see Chapter 6, Table 6.1 and Section 6.4.2.3). When reported energy intake is less than 1.3 times resting metabolic rate, under-reporting of food intake should be suspected (Goldberg et al. 1991). Ratios less than this have been considered unrealistic, if not impossible, even for sedentary individuals. In fact, for most athletes, an energy expenditure (which should equate to the reported energy intake if the athlete is in energy balance) to resting metabolic rate ratio should be greater than 1.5. If under-reporting is suspected there may be issues of body image or parental or coach pressure, which need to be explored. The assistance of a clinical or sport psychologist may be warranted. In most cases, confronting the athlete in an understanding manner with the unrealistic nature of their reported food intake can help to reveal practical or psychological issues which are impeding weight or fat loss.

- It appears that some athletes may be fuel efficient (see Section 6.5)—requiring less energy to perform daily tasks and training than might be expected. Apart from incorporating additional training and ensuring an appropriate energy and macronutrient intake which maintains health and vitality and optimises lean body mass, there is little else that can be done to improve the energy balance situation. These athletes may eventually need to reassess their capacity to obtain certain body-weight and body-fat goals, and it may be preferable for them to direct their energies into sports where the physique requirements are less extreme.

Training, exercise and physical activity assessment

- Assessment needs to be made of the total energy expenditure of the athlete. This includes training, occupational expenditure and incidental activity. An estimate of this can be obtained by multiplying resting metabolic rate (see above) by an activity factor appropriate to the athlete's level of training (see Table 6.2). Although these factors were designed to calculate energy expenditure in general recreational and occupational settings, they can provide very approximate estimates of daily energy expenditure in athletes. Food intake can also do this, although it is notoriously inaccurate (see above).

- Ideally a complete training program for the period of weight or fat loss is required, and it is desirable that a 12-month plan be available to assist planning for peaking, tapering and off-season phases.

- Athletes need to be aware that any program needs to be adaptable to cater for changes in training, especially those that may be forced by illness or injury.

Assessment checklist

- A clear indication of goals and how realistic they may be for the athlete.

- Stature, weight and body composition assessment (ideally measuring adiposity and muscularity or lean body mass). Error of the method needs to be acknowledged and considered in planning and follow-up.

- Dietary assessment (see above) with consideration of potential for eating disorders and under-reporting of food intake.

- Physical activity assessment and the potential for adding activity to increase daily expenditure and enhance fat oxidation.

- Any medical or physical therapy assessments need cross-referral to the appropriate professional. These are important if illness or injury is present or suspected.

Dietary approach

- In most cases it is preferable to start the athlete on a low-fat diet which is only moderately restricted in energy. This should produce a gradual weight loss of 0.5–1 kg per week in the majority of individuals.

- In sports where extreme leanness is crucial to competition, energy intake may need to be restricted more substantially. However, care should be taken to ensure that the diet is nutritionally balanced and provides adequate protein, CHO and micronutrients. Diets providing less than 6300 kJ (1500 kcal) should be carefully considered.

- To assist with satiety, a protein choice at each main meal and perhaps at snacks should be considered. Ensuring the diet is high in dietary fibre may also help to satisfy the appetite of a hungry athlete. Regular meals and snacks also prevent the build up of hunger over the day. Organisation is an important factor in successful weight loss, as impulse eating is often a problem, especially for the busy athlete.

- The dietary consultation should also assess the ability of the athlete (or their parents/guardian) to shop and cook for themselves in an appropriate way. Shopping trips and cooking classes provide a practical and enjoyable means of delivering this sort of education. A list of suitable cookbooks and resources is also helpful.

Training, exercise and physical activity

- Additional training or physical activity is a means of increasing energy expenditure and promoting weight or fat loss. Although additional exercise alone may produce satisfactory results, some athletes may increase their food intake sufficiently to compensate for the additional expenditure, negating the benefit. It is preferable for additional exercise to be combined with a sensible eating plan to offset this problem.

- Medium- to longer-term duration (60 minutes), low-intensity (50–60% $VO_{2\ max}$) exercise has been promoted specifically for its benefit in producing weight or fat loss. This prescription, however, may not be the most efficient means of promoting weight or fat loss in athletes. Medium-duration (30–60 minutes), higher-intensity activity (65–70% $VO_{2\ max}$ or below anaerobic threshold) utilises more energy and subsequently more fat, even though the proportion of fat oxidised may be less than for lower-intensity exercise. Higher-intensity programs can therefore be an efficient means of enhancing daily energy expenditure.

- Although resistance training would seem less beneficial for promoting weight and fat loss, there is evidence that this type of training can also enhance fat oxidation, in addition to improving lean body mass, which may improve resting energy expenditure. These benefits should be considered within the context of the program devised.

- The best mode of exercise is generally determined by considering issues of access, time, injury risk and propensity for over-use of certain muscle groups. While running or weight-bearing activity appears (at least anecdotally) to produce superior weight loss results, other forms of aerobic exercise, such as swimming or cycling, may be selected as they result in less impact on the skeleton.

Psychological aspects and behaviour modification

- Approaches used in the management of the overweight or obese client can also be useful with athletes. These include the use of food diaries and visual analogue scales to measure hunger and food cravings. These strategies often help to identify triggers to inappropriate eating. A host of behaviour modification techniques can then be used to manage, control or avoid problem eating behaviours.

- Referral to a clinical or sport psychologist is often integral to the success of weight loss programs as the mental approach is a major factor in the client's confidence and subsequent compliance to a sound approach to the problem.

Travelling and special athlete considerations

- Travelling can often disrupt weight loss plans, as the appropriate food is not always available and the daily routine is interrupted. There are several strategies which may assist. These include: organisation of special low-fat, low-energy or athlete meals on airline flights, development of a travelling meal plan and shopping list if meals are to be self-prepared, or an organised menu plan for the caterers who attend to the meals while the athlete is away. Providing the athlete with a list of appropriate low-fat options from restaurants or take-away outlets is also useful. Avoidance of high-fat snacks on long road trips is easier if low-fat, nutritious alternatives have been packed beforehand.

- Prior to competition, athletes often have a tapered training program. This may require that they consume less, rather than more, food. If weight gain is a problem during the competition phase then a special meal plan devised to maintain energy balance at this time is required.

- As with competition, there are other times when training is reduced or interrupted, such as when the athlete is injured or ill or, during the 'off season'. These are times when athletes prone to weight gain need to adjust their food intake to accommodate the reduction in energy expenditure.

- Athletes are often exposed to buffet-style eating, especially in athlete villages during competition, in dining halls at training camps, or at residential training facilities. Buffets tend to encourage over-consumption and the inclusion of foods that might not be typically consumed as part of the athletes' usual training or competition diet. In this situation it is important that athletes consume similar amounts of food to their usual plan, not use the opportunity to eat as much as they can. The inclusion of high-fat treats should be kept to an occasional addition. Where a stay is to be extended, weight gain and boredom can be offset by advising the athlete to avoid obligatory sampling of each dish on the buffet. Rather, they should select a protein, CHO and several vegetable options as would be typical of a home-prepared meal. After a short time, this means of selection will result in the athlete sampling all options on the menu cycle in a way that keeps the options new and fresh, preventing complaints as to the sameness of and boredom with the buffet options.

- Fad or unscientific dietary regimens often appeal to athletes because they promise quick, effective weight loss. Most of these are unbalanced, providing insufficient energy and CHO for training. Their use while promoting short-term weight loss may also result in fatigue and decreased performance. Athletes need to be advised on sound diet and training approaches to facilitate weight loss, and these need to be supported by their coach or trainer and (where possible) their parent, guardian or partner. The use of the sports medicine team, including a sports dietitian, is essential.

- Like fad diets, the use of supplements and/or drugs to assist weight loss is a major temptation for athletes. Despite claims, dietary supplements promoted for weight loss lack scientific support. Although a number of drugs have proven efficacy for weight loss, these are either deemed illegal by sports drug agencies, or their use would seem unethical in athletes who are not at a medical risk of excess weight.

REFERENCES

Acheson KJ, Schutz Y, Bessard T, et al. Glycogen storage capacity and de novo lipogenesis during massive carbohydrate overfeeding in man. Am J Clin Nutr 1988;48:240–7.

Almeras N, Lemieux S, Bouchard C, Tremblay A. Fat gain in female swimmers. Physiolog Behav 1997;61:811–17.

Andersen P, Henriksson J. Capillary supply of the quadriceps femoris muscle of man: adaptive response to exercise. J Physiol 1977;270:677–90.

Andersson B, Larson B. Influence of local temperature changes in the preoptic area and rostral hypothalamus in the regulation of food and water intake. Acta Physiol Scand 1961;52:75–89.

Andrews S, Balart LA, Bethea MC, Steward HL. Sugarbusters. London: Vermillion, 1998.

Arciero P, Goran MI, Poehlman ET. Resting metabolic rate is lower in women than in men. J Appl Physiol 1993;75:2514–20.

Astrup A, Breum L, Toubro S, Hein P, Quaade F. The effect and safety of an ephedrine–caffeine compound compared to ephedrine, caffeine and placebo in obese subjects on an energy restricted diet: a double blind trial. Int J Obes 1992;16:269–77.

Astrup A, Raben A. Obesity: an inherited metabolic deficiency in the control of macronutrient balance? Eur J Clin Nutr 1992;46:611–20.

Astrup A, Toubro S. Thermogenic, metabolic and cardiovascular responses to ephedrine and caffeine in man. Int J Obes 1993;17(suppl)1:S41–S3.

Astrup AD, Hansen DL, Toubro S. Ephedrine and caffeine in the treatment of obesity. Int J Obes 1996;20:1–3.

Atkins RC. Doctor Atkins' new diet revolution. New York: Avon Books, 1992.

Atkinson RL, Hubbard VS. Report on the NIH workshop on pharmacological treatment of obesity. Am J Clin Nutr 1994;60:153–6.

Audrain JE, Klesges RC, Klesges LM. Relationship between obesity and the metabolic effect of smoking in women. Health Psychol 1995;14:116–32.

Bahr R, Sejersted OM. Effect of intensity of exercise on excess postexercise oxygen consumption. Metabolism 1991;40:836–41.

Baile CA, Zinn WN, Mayer J. Effects of lactate and other metabolites on food intake of monkeys. Am J Physiol 1970;219:1606–13.

Ballor DL, Keesey RE. A meta-analysis of factors affecting exercise-induced changes in body mass, fat mass and fat-free mass in males and females. Int J Obes 1991;15:717–26.

Barlow CE, Kohl HWI, Gibbons LW, Blair SW. Physical fitness, mortality and obesity. Int J Obes 1995;19(suppl)4:S41–S4.

Barr S. Women, nutrition and exercise: a review of athletes' food intakes and a discussion of energy balance in active women. Prog Food Nutr Sci 1987;11:307–61.

Bass S, Bradley M, Pearce G, et al. Short stature and delayed puberty in gymnasts: influence of selection bias on leg length and the duration of training on trunk length. J Paed 2000: In press.

Blundell JE, Burley VJ. Evaluation of the satiating power of dietary fat in man. In: Aihaud G, Guy-Grand B, Lafontan M, Ricquier D, eds. Obesity in Europe 90. London: John Libbey, 1990.

Booth ML, Bauman A, Owen N, Gore CJ. Physical activity preferences, preferred sources of assistance and perceived barriers to increased activity among physically active Australians. Prev Med 1997;26:131–7.

Bouchard C. Recent advances in the molecular and genetic basis of human obesity. In: Aihaud G, Guy-Grand B, Lafontan M, Ricquier D, eds. Obesity in Europe 93. London: John Libbey, 1993:1–8.

Bouchard C. Genetics of obesity: overview and research directions. In: Bouchard C, ed. The genetics of obesity. Boca Raton: CRC Press, 1994:223–33.

Bouchard C, Tremblay A, Déspres J-P, et al. The response to long-term overfeeding in identical twins. N Engl J Med 1990;322:1477–82.

Brand-Miller J, Foster-Powell K, Colagruri S. The GI factor. Sydney: Hodder Headline, 1996.

Bray GA, Popkin BM. Dietary fat does not affect obesity! Am J Clin Nutr 1998;68(6):1157–73.

Brodoff BN, Hendler R, eds. Very low calorie diets in obesity. Philadelphia, USA: Lippincott JB, 1992.

Brotherhood JR. Nutrition and sports performance. Sports Med 1984;1:350–89.

Brownell KD, Steen SN, Wilmore JH. Weight regulation practices in athletes: analysis of metabolic and health effects. Med Sci Sports Exerc 1987;19:546–56.

Burke LM, Read RSD. Alcohol use by elite Australian Rules football players (abst). Proc Nutr Soc Aust 1987;12:127.

Buskirk ER, Taylor HL. Maximum oxygen intake and its relation to body composition with special reference to chronic physical activity and obesity. J Appl Physiol 1957;22:72.

Carlberg KA, Buckman MT, Peake GT, Riedesel ML. A survey of menstrual function in athletes. Eur J Appl Physiol 1983;51:211–22.

Cash TF, Novy PL, Grant JR. Why do women exercise? Factor analysis and further validation of the reasons for exercise inventory. Perc Motor Skills 1994;78:539–44.

Caterson ID. Management strategies for weight control: eating, exercise and behaviour modification. Drugs 1990;30(suppl)3:20–32.

Cheuvront SN. The Zone Diet and athletic performance. Sports Med 1999;27:213–28.

Coleman DL. Effects of parabiosis of obese mice with diabetes and normal mice. Diabetologia 1973;9:294–8.

Connolly HM, Crary JL, McGoon MD, et al. Valvular heart disease associated with fenfluramine-phentermine. N Engl J Med 1997;337:581–8.

Considine RV, Sinha MK, Heiman MK, et al. Serum immunoreactive-leptin concentrations in normal-weight and obese humans. N Engl J Med 1996;334:292–5.

Coulston AM, Liu GC, Reaven GM. Plasma glucose, insulin and lipid responses to high-carbohydrate, low-fat diets in normal humans. Metabolism 1983;32:52–6.

Coyle EF, Coggan AR, Hemmett MK, Ivy JL. Muscle glycogen utilization during prolonged strenuous activity when fed carbohydrate. J Appl Physiol 1986;61:165–72.

Cureton KJ, Sparling PB. Distance running performance and metabolic responses to running in men and women with excess weight experimentally equated. Med Sci Sports Exerc 1980;2:288–94.

Cureton KJ, Sparling PB, Evans BW, et al. Effect of experimental alterations in excess weight on aerobic capacity and distance running performance. Med Sci Sports 1978;10:194–9.

Davis C, Cowles M. A comparison of weight and diet concerns and personality factors among female athletes and non-athletes. J Pschosoma Res 1989;33:527–36.

Davis KJ, Packer L, Brooks GA. Biochemical adaptation of mitochondria, muscle and whole-animal respiration to endurance training. Arch Biochem Biophys 1981;209:539–54.

Dempsey JA, Reddan W, Baike B, Walberg-Rankin J. Work capacity determinants and physiologic cost of weight-supported work in obesity. J Appl Physiol 1966;22:181–5.

Déspres J-P, Prud'Homme D, Tremblay A, Bouchard C. Contribution of low intensity exercise training to treatment of abdominal obesity: importance of metabolic fitness. In: Aihaud G, Guy-Grand B, Lafontan M, Ricquier D, eds. Obesity in Europe 91. London: John Libbey & Co, 1991:177–81.

Deuster PA, Chrousos GP, Luger A, et al. Hormonal and metabolic responses of untrained, moderately trained and highly trained men to three exercise intensities. Metabolism 1989;38:141–8.

Deuster PA, Kyle SB, Moser PB, Vigersky RA, Schoomaker EB. Nutritional intakes and status of highly trained amenorrhoeic and eumenorrheic women runners. Fertil Steril 1986;46:636–43.

Diamond H, Diamond M. Fit for life. Sydney: Angus and Robertson, 1986.

Donnelly JE, Jakicic J, Gunderson S. Diet and body composition: effect of very low calorie diets and exercise. Sports Med 1991;12:237–49.

Dwyer JT. Treatment of obesity: conventional programs and fad diets in obesity. In: Björntorp P, Brodoff BN, eds. Obesity. Philadelphia, USA: Lippincott JB, 1992:662–82.

Egger G, Cameron-Smith D, Stanton R. The effectiveness of popular, non-prescription weight loss supplements. Med J Aust 1999;171:604–8.

Enzi G, Inelman EM, Crepaldi G. Effect of hydrophilic mucilage in the treatment of obese patients. Pharmatherapeutica 1980;2:421–8.

Erickson JC, Hollopeter G, Palmiter RD. Attenuation of the obesity syndrome of obob mice by loss of neuropeptide Y. Science 1996;274:1704–7.

Evans FA, Strang JM. A departure from the usual methods of treating obesity. Am J Med Sci 1929;147:339–42.

Flatt JP. The difference in the storage capacity for carbohydrate and for fat, and its implications in the regulation of body weight. Ann NY Acad Sci 1987;499:104–23.

Flegal KM, Troiano RP, Pamuk ER, Kuczmarski RJ, Campbell SM. The influence of smoking cessation on the prevalence of overweight in the United States. N Engl J Med 1995;333:1165–70.

Fleury C, Neverova S, Collins S, et al. Uncoupling protein 2: a novel gene linked to obesity and hyperinsulinaemia. Nature Genetics 1997;15:269–72.

Flynn MG, Costill DL, Kirwan JP, et al. Fat storage in athletes: metabolic and hormonal responses to swimming and running. Sports Med 1990;11:433–40.

Freedman-Akabas S, Colt E, Kissileff HR, Pi Sunyer FX. Lack of sustained increase in VO_2. Am J Clin Nutr 1985;41:545–9.

Frisch RE, McArthur JW. Menstrual cycles: fatness as a determinant of minimum weight for height necessary for their maintenance or onset. Science 1974;185:949–51.

Fumeron F, Durack-Brown I, Betoulle D, et al. Polymorphisms of uncopuling protein (UCP) and ß3 adrenoreceptor genes in obese people submitted to a low calorie diet. Int J Obes 1996;20:1051–4.

Garrow JS. Exercise in the treatment of obesity: a marginal contribution. Int J Obes 1995;19:S126–S9.

Goldberg GR, Black AE, Jebb SA, et al. Critical evaluation of energy intake data using fundamental principles of energy physiology: 1. Derivation of cut-off limits to identify under-recording. Eur J Clin Nutr 1991;45(12):569–81.

Goran MI, Poehlman ET. Endurance training does not enhance energy expenditure in healthy elderly persons. Am J Physiol 1992;263:E950–E7.

Grinspoon S, Gulick T, Askari H, et al. Serum leptin levels in women with anorexia nervosa. J Clin Endocrinol Metab 1996;81:3861–3.

Grunfield C, Feingold KR. The metabolic effects of tumour necrosis factor and other cytokines. Biotherap 1991;3:143–58.

Harvey-Berino J. The efficacy of dietary fat versus total energy restriction for weight loss. Obes Res 1998;6(3):202–7.

Heller RF, O'Connell DL, Roberts DCK, et al. Lifestyle factors in monozygotic and dizygotic twins. Genet Epidemiol 1988;5(5):311–21.

Henriksson J, Reitman JS. Quantative measures of enzyme activities in type I and type II muscle fibres of man after training. Acts Physiol Scand 1976;97:392–7.

Heyward VH, Sandoval WM, Colville BC. Anthropometric, body composition, and nutritional profiles of body builders during training. J Appl Sports Sci Res 1989;3:22–9.

Holt S, Brand-Miller J. Particle size and the glycaemic response. Eur J Clin Nutr 1994;48:496–502.

Hoppeler H, Luthi P, Claasen H, Weibel ER, Howald H. The ultrastructure of the normal human skeletal muscle: a morphometric analysis on untrained men, women and well-trained orienteers. Plfugers Arch 1973;344:217–32.

Horswill CC, Hickner RC, Scott JR, Costill DL, Gould D. Weight loss, dietary carbohydrate modifications, and high intensity physical performance. Med Sci Sports Exerc 1990;22:470–7.

Hurley BF, Nemeth PM, Martin WH, et al. Muscle triglyceride utilization during exercise: training effect. J Appl Physiol 1986;60:562–7.

Jackson RS, Creemers JW, Ohagi S, et al. Obesity and impaired prohormone processing associated with mutations in the human prohormone convertase 1 gene. Nature Genetics 1997;16:303–6.

Jebb SA, Goldberg GR, Coward WA, Murgatroyd PR, Prentice AM. Effects of weight cycling caused by intermittent dieting on metabolic rate and body composition in obese women. Int J Obes 1991;15(5):367–74.

Jebb SA, Prentice AM, Goldberg G, et al. Changes in macronutrient balance during over and underfeeding assessed by 12-d continuous whole body calorimetry. Am J Clin Nutr 1996;64:259–66.

Jeffery RW, Björnson WM, Rosenthal BS, et al. Correlates of weight loss and its maintenance over two years of follow-up among middle-aged men. Prev Med 1984;13(2):155–68.

Jeffery RW, Hellerstedt WL, French SA, Baxter JE. A randomised trial of counselling for fat restriction versus calorie restriction in the treatment of obesity. Int J Obes 1995;19:132–7.

Jenkins AB, Markovic TP, Fleury A, Campbell LV. Carbohydrate intake and short-term regulation of leptin in humans. Diabetologia 1997;40:348–51.

Kaiserauer S, Snyder AC, Sleeper M, Zierath J. Nutritional, physiological and menstrual status of distance runners. Med Sci Sports Exerc 1989; 21:120–5.

Kalra SP, Dube MG, Piu S. Interacting appetite-regulating pathways in the hypothalamic regulation of body weight. Endocr Rev 1999;20:68–100.

Keizer HA, Rogol AD. Physical exercise and menstrual cycle alterations. What are the mechanisms? Sports Med 1990;10:218–35.

Kiens B. Effect of endurance training on fatty acid metabolism: local adaptations. Med Sci Sports Exerc 1977;29:640–5.

King NA, Blundell JE. High-fat foods overcome energy expenditure due to exercise after cycling and running. Eur J Clin Nutr 1995;49:114–23.

King NA, Burley VJ, Blundell JE. Exercise-induced suppression of appetite: effects on food intake and implications for energy balance. Eur J Clin Nutr 1994;48:715–24.

King NA, Tremblay A, Blundell JE. Effects of exercise on appetite control: implications for energy balance. Med Sci Sports Exerc 1997;29:1076–89.

Kowlalska J, Straczkowski M, Gorski J, Kinalska I. The effect of fasting and physical exercise on plasma leptin concentrations in high-fat fed rats. J Physiol Pharmacol 1999;50:309–20.

Kreitzman SN. Lean body mass, exercise and VLCDs. Int J Obes 1989;13(suppl)2:17.

Lambert EV, Speechly DP, Dennis SC, Noakes TD. Enhanced endurance in trained cyclists during moderate intensity exercise following two weeks adaptation to a high fat diet. Eur J Appl Physiol 1994;69:287–93.

Lantigua RA, Amatruda JM, Biddle TL. Cardiac arrhythmias associated with a liquid protein diet for the treatment of obesity. N Engl J Med 1980;303:735–8.

Leal-Cerro A, Garcia-Luna PP, Astorga R, et al. Serum leptin levels in male marathon athletes before and after the marathon run. J Clin Endocrinol Metab 1998;83:2376–9.

Lefebvre P, Luyckx A. Effect of insulin on glucagon enhanced lipolysis in vitro. Diabetologia 1969;5:195–7.

Leibel RL, Rosenbaum M, Hirsch J. Changes in energy expenditure resulting from altered body weight. N Engl J Med 1995;332(10):621–8.

Leon GR, Chamberlain K. Comparison of daily eating habits and emotional states of overweight persons successful or unsuccessful in maintaining weight loss. J Consult Clin Psychol 1973;41(1):108–15.

Lloyd T, Buchanen JR, Bitzer S. Interrelationship of diet, athletic activity, menstrual status, and bone density in collegiate women. Am J Clin Nutr 1987;46:681–4.

Lloyd T, Triantafyllou SJ, Baker ER. Women athletes with menstrual irregularity have increased musculoskeletal injuries. Med Sci Sports Exerc 1986;18:374–9.

Loucks AB, Horvath SM. Athletic amenorrhoea: a review. Med Sci Sports Exerc 1985;17:56–72.

Malina RM. Anthropometric correlates of strength and motor performance. Exercise Sports Sci Rev 1975;3:249.

McNeely W, Goa KL. Sibutramine: a review of its contribution to management. Drugs 1998;56:1093–124.

Melby CL, Commerford SR, Hill JO. Exercise, macronutrient balance and weight control. In: Lamb D, Murray R, eds. Perspectives in exercise science and sports medicine: exercise, nutrition and weight control. Carmel USA: Cooper Publishing Group, 1998:1–60.

Melby CL, Schmidt WD, Corrigan D. Resting metabolic rate in weight-cycling collegiate wrestlers compared with physically active, noncycling control subjects. Am J Clin Nutr 1990;52:409–14.

Melby CL, Scholl C, Edwards G, Bullough R. Effect of acute resistance exercise on postexercise energy expenditure and resting metabolic rate. J Appl Physiol 1993;75:1847–53.

Meyer GAL, Janssen GME, Westerterp KR, et al. The effect of a month endurance training programme on physical activity: evidence for a sex-difference in the metabolic response to exercise. Eur J Appl Physiol 1991;62:11–17.

Montague CT, Farooqi IS, Whitehead JP, et al. Congenital leptin deficiency is associated with severe early-onset obesity in humans. Nature 1997;387:903–8.

Nieman DC, Henson DA, Garner EB, et al. Carbohydrate affects natural killer cell redistribution but not activity after running. Med Sci Sports Exerc 1997;29:1318–24.

O'Connor HT, Richman RM, Steinbeck KS, Caterson ID. Dexfenfluramine treatment of obesity: a double blind trial with post trial follow-up. Int J Obes 1995;19:181–9.

Olds TS, Norton KI, Craig NP. Mathematical model of cycling performance. J Appl Physiol 1993;75:730–7.

Oscai LB, Caruso RA, Wergeles AC. Lipoprotein lipase hydrolyzes endogenous triacylglycerols in muscle of exercised rats. J Appl Physiol 1982;52:1059–63.

Pedersen BK, Bruunsgaard H, Jensen M, et al. Exercise and the immune system—influence of nutrition and ageing. J Sci Med Sport 1999;2(3):234–52.

Perusse L, Tremblay A, Leblanc C, et al. Familial resemblance in energy intake: contribution of genetic and environmental factors. Am J Clin Nutr 1988;47(4):629–35.

Peters EM, Goetzsche JM, Grobbelaar B, Noakes TD. Vitamin C supplementation reduces the incidence of post-race symptoms of upper-respiratory-tract infection in ultramarathon runners. Am J Clin Nutr 1993;57:170–4.

Poehlman ET, Melby CL, Badylak SF, Calles J. Aerobic fitness and resting energy expenditure in young adult males. Metabolism 1989;38:85–90.

Poehlman ET, Melby CL, Goran MI. The impact of exercise and diet restriction on daily energy expenditure. Sports Med 1991;11:78–101.

Powell JJ, Tucker L, Fisher AG, Wilcox K. The effects of different percentages of dietary fat, exercise, and calorie restriction on body composition and body weight in obese females. Am J Health Promot 1994;8(6):442–8.

Prentice AM, Jebb SA. Obesity in Britain: gluttony or sloth? BMJ 1995;311:437–9.

Pyne D, Lee H. Physiological testing of elite Australian swimmers. In: Proceedings of the XIIIth FINA Sports Medicine Congress, 2000: In press.

Rasky E, Stronegger WJ, Freidl W. The relationship between body weight and patterns of smoking in women and men. Int J Epidemiol 1996;25:1208–12.

Rau H, Reaves BJ, O'Rahilly S, Whitehead JP. Truncated human leptin (delta133) associated with extreme obesity undergoes proteasomal degradation after defective intracellular transport. Endocrinology 1999;140:1718–23.

Ravussin E, Brunand B, Schutz Y. Energy expenditure before and during energy restriction in obese patients. Am J Clin Nutr 1985;41:753.

Ravussin E, Lillioja S, Anderson TE, Christin L, Bogardus C. Determinants of 24 hour energy expenditure in man: methods and results using a respiratory chamber. J Clin Invest 1986;78(6):1568–78.

Ravussin E, Lillioja S, Knowler WC, et al. Reduced rate of energy expenditure as a risk factor for body-weight gain. N Engl J Med 1988;318(8):467–72.

Ravussin E, Swinburn BA. Pathophysiology of obesity. Lancet 1992;340(8816):404–8.

Ravussin E, Swinburn BA. Metabolic predictors of body weight gain: cross-sectional versus longitudinal data. Int J Obes 1993;17:528–31.

Reed GW, Hill JO. Measuring the thermic effect of food. Am J Clin Nutr 1996;63(2):164–9.

Rohner-Jeanrenaud F, Gusin I, Sainsbury A, Kakrzewska KE, Jeanrenaud B. The loop system between neuropeptide Y and leptin in normal and obese rodents. Horm Metab Res 1996;28:642–8.

Romijn JA, Coyle EF, Sidossis L. Regulation of endogenous fat and carbohydrate metabolism in relation to exercise intensity. Am J Physiol 1993;265:E380–E91.

Rosen JC, Hunt DA, Sims EA, et al. Comparison of carbohydrate containing and carbohydrate restricted hypocaloric diets in the treatment of obesity: effects on appetite and mood. Am J Clin Nutr 1982;36:464–72.

Rosenbaum M, Nicholson M, Hirsch M, et al. Effects of gender, body composition and menopause on plasma concentrations of leptin. J Clin Endocronol Metab 1996;81:3424–7.

Roy BD, Tarnopolsky MD. Influence of differing macronutrient intakes on muscle glycogen resynthesis after resistance exercise. J Appl Physiol 1998;84:890–6.

Sanborn CF, Albrecht BH, Wagner WW. Athletic amenorrhoea: lack of association with body fat. Med Sci Sports Exerc 1987;19:202–12.

Sarna S, Kaprio J. Life expectancy of former athletes. Sports Med 1994;17:149–51.

Schlundt DG, Hill JO, Pope-Cordle J, et al. Randomized evaluation of a low fat ad libitum carbohydrate diet for weight reduction. Int J Obes 1993;17:623–9.

Schutz Y, Flatt JP, Jéquier E. Failure of dietary fat intake to promote fat oxidation: a factor favouring the development of obesity. Am J Clin Nutr 1989;50(2):307–14.

Schwartz MW, Seeley RJ. Neuroendocrine responses to starvation and weight loss. New Engl J Med 1997;336:1802–11.

Sears B. The Zone: a dietary road map. New York: Harper Collins, 1995.

Shah M, Baxter JE, McGovern PG, Garg A. Nutrient and food intake of obese women on a low-fat or low-calorie diet. Am J Health Promot 1996;10(3):179–82.

Sharp TA, Reed GW, Sun M, Abumrad NN, Hill JO. Relationship between aerobic fitness level and daily energy expenditure in weight stable humans. Am J Physiol 1992;263:E121–E8.

Sheppard LO, Kristal AR, Kushi LH. Weight loss in women participating in a randomized trial of low-fat diets. Am J Clin Nutr 1991;54(5):821–8.

Sjostrom L, Rissanaen A, Andersen T, et al. Randomised placebo-controlled trial of Orlistat for weight loss and prevention of weight regain in obese patients. Lancet 1998;352:167–72.

Stager JM, Cordain L. Relationship of body composition to swimming performance in female swimmers. J Swim Res 1984;1:21–4.

Staten M. The effect of exercise on food intake in men and women. Am J Clin Nutr 1991;53:27–31.

Steen SN, Opplinger RA, Brownell KD. Metabolic effects of repeated weight loss and regain in adolescent wrestlers. J Am Med Assoc 1988;260:47–50.

Stock MJ. Sibutramine: a review of the pharmacology of a novel anti-obesity agent. Int J Obes 1997;21:S25–S9.

Stone KJ, Willis AL, Hart M, et al. The metabolism of dinomo-gamma-linolenic acid in man. Lipids 1978;14:174–80.

Strauss RH, Lanese RR, Malarkey WB. Decreased testosterone and libido with severe weight loss. Phys Sports Med 1993;21(2):64–71.

Stunkard AJ, Kaplan D. Eating in public places: a review of reports of the direct observation of eating behaviour. Int J Obes 1977;1(1):89–101.

Suter PM, Schutz Y, Jéquier E. The effect of ethanol on fat storage in healthy subjects. N Engl J Med 1992;326(15):983–7.

Tarnower H, Baker SS. The complete Scarsdale medical diet. New York: Bantam Books, 1980.

Thornton J. Feast or famine: eating disorders in athletes. Phys Sports Med 1990;18(4):116–23.

Tremblay A, Déspres J-P, Bouchard C. The effects of exercise-training on energy balance and adipose tissue morphology and metabolism. Sports Med 1985;2:223–33.

Tremblay A, Déspres J-P, Leblanc C, Bouchard C. Sex dimorphism in fat loss in response to exercise training. J Obesity Weight Reg 1984;3:193–203.

Tremblay A, Simoneau JA, Bouchard C. Impact of exercise intensity on body fatness and skeletal muscle metabolism. Metabolism 1994;43(7):814–8.

Treuth MS, Hunter GR, Weinsier RL, Kell SH. Energy expenditure and substrate utilization in older women after strength training: 24-hr calorimeter results. J Appl Physiol 1995;78:2140–6.

Truswell AS, Darnton-Hill I. Food habits in adolescence. Nutr Rev 1981;39(2):73–88.

United States Department of Health and Human Services. Cardiac calvulopathy associated with exposure to fenfluramine or dexfenfluramine: United States Department of Health and Human Services interim public health recommendations. Morbidity and mortality weekly report centre for disease control and prevention 1997;Nov:1061–6

Van Itallie TB. Weight reduction: mechanisms of action and physiological effects. London: John Libbey, 1980.

Walberg-Rankin J, ed. Changing body weight and composition in athletes. Carmel, IN: Cooper Publishing Group, 1998.

Walberg-Rankin J, Hawkins CE, Fild DS, Sebolt DR. Effect of weight loss and refeeding diet composition on anaerobic performance in wrestlers. Med Sci Sports Exerc 1994;28:1292–9.

Weigle DS, Bukowski TR, Foster DC, et al. Recombinant ob protein reduces feeding and body weight in the ob/ob mouse. J Clin Invest 1995;96:2065–70.

Westerterp KR, Meijer GAL, Janssen GME, Saris WHM, Ten Hoor F. Long-term physical activity on energy balance and body composition. B J Nutr 1992;68:21–30.

Westrate JA. Fat and obesity. Int J Obes 1995;19(suppl)5:S38–S43.

Wing RR. Weight cycling in humans: a review of the literature. Ann Behav Med 1992;14:113–9.

Wing RR, Jeffery RW. Outpatient treatments of obesity: a comparison of the methodology and clinical results. Int J Obesity 1979;3(3):261–79.

Yeo GS, Farooqi IS, Aminian S, et al. A frameshift mutation in MCR4 associated with dominantly inherited human obesity (letter). Nature Genetics 1998;20:111–12.

Zhang Y, Proenca R, Maffei M, et al. Positional cloning of the mouse obese gene and its human homologue. Nature 1994;372(6505):425–32.

Zurlo F, Lillioja S, Esposito-Del Puente A, et al. Low rate of fat to carbohydrate oxidation as a predictor of weight gain: study of 24h RQ. Am J Physiol 1990;259(5 pt 1):E650–E7.

CHAPTER 8

Making weight in sports

Janet Walberg-Rankin

8.1 INTRODUCTION

Lose three kilograms in two days? This is not a rate of weight loss recommended by nutritionists as safe and nor is it likely to result in long-term weight change, but it is a common scenario for athletes who compete in a variety of sports that involve weight divisions or restrictions. For example, wrestlers must be weighed in the presence of an official prior to their match to compete in their designated weight category. If body mass is even slightly higher than the category allows, the athlete will be disqualified from competing in that match. This provides a powerful motivation to achieve the required weight, and officials have reported a variety of desperate efforts by wrestlers to lose those last few grams, including drastic dehydration, spitting, and forced nose bleeds. The most dramatic and unfortunate result of effort to lose weight in wrestling was the death of three collegiate wrestlers in 1997 (American Medical Association 1998). All died while they were trying to 'make weight' for a competition weigh-in.

In order for nutritionists and medical personnel to assist athletes to make weight safely, it is important to be familiar with the rules and specific constraints of the sport regarding weight divisions/restrictions, as well as the typical practices of the athletes to reduce body mass. This chapter will review these issues as well as the research concerning the potential health and performance hazards of rapid loss of body mass. Although body mass (BM) is the correct term, this chapter will use the terms 'weight' or 'body weight' interchangeably with this, since these are the common terms used by those involved in weight division sports. Finally, suggestions will be made for safe and effective means of making weight and recovering afterwards, based on the available research.

8.2 SPORTS WITH WEIGHT DIVISIONS OR RESTRICTIONS

A variety of sports involve weight divisions or restrictions for competition purposes, and each has its own procedures for prescribing and monitoring competition weights for its participants. As mentioned above, wrestlers compete in a number of designated weight categories; for example, collegiate wrestling involves ten weight classes. Light-weight rowers must meet restrictions placed on individual competitors as well as the total boat crew: male rowers can weigh no more than 72.5 kg with a crew average of 70.0 kg; while female competitors must be 59.0 kg or less, with a crew average of 56.7 kg. Light-weight football is played at a minority of institutions in the United States but allows participation of individuals who are too light to be competitive on most football teams. Players are required to be less than 71.8 kg (158 lb) two days prior to the game. In horse racing the body weight of jockeys may be controlled to provide a 'handicap' to the competing horse. The target weight (including the saddle) for flat-race jockeys may be as light as 47.7 kg (105 lbs) and for jump jockeys 60.4 kg (133 lb) (King & Mezey 1987).

The intention of weight categories is to even the playing field for sports where the larger individual will have a clear advantage. It would be expected that an athlete who has greater muscle mass and reach can generate more power in strength events, or be more competitive in combative sports than a smaller and lighter opponent. Thus matching individuals of similar body weight should theoretically make these sports safer and fairer. The reality is that athletes will dehydrate or otherwise achieve rapid weight loss to make a lower weight division, hoping to recover between the weigh-in and the competition, and compete with an advantage over a smaller opponent. Of course, since most of the athletes go through a similar procedure, there is typically little advantage achieved. However, the atypical athlete who does not lose weight acutely for the weigh-in may worry that they will be at a disadvantage.

Most wrestlers believe that weight loss is a critical part of the culture of wrestling. For example, 70% of the high-school wrestlers interviewed from nine rural teams claimed that losing weight during the season was 'very important' for winning, and 23% thought it was 'important' (Marquart & Sobal 1994). Most of the wrestlers thought making weight was hard; 31% worked 'very hard' while 47% 'somewhat hard'. So, losing weight clearly adds to the stresses and complexities of competing in sports. As discussed later in this chapter, it also increases the risks of the sport.

8.3 METHODS USED TO MAKE WEIGHT

8.3.1 Wrestlers

Some of the earliest studies of weight loss methods of wrestlers were undertaken with high-school wrestlers in Iowa in the late 1960s. Eighty-three per cent of the 528 wrestlers surveyed claimed they used food restriction to lose weight; 77% used fluid restriction, and 83% increased exercise to lose weight (Tipton & Tcheng 1970). More recent surveys of high-school wrestlers have uncovered other clearly inappropriate methods used for weight loss, including fasting (60%), sauna (45%), rubber suits (26%), laxatives (13%) and vomiting (13%) (Steen & Brownell 1990).

Most high-school wrestlers reported that they began losing weight an average of four days prior to the match and lost an average of 1.8 kg (4 lb) (Marquart & Sobal 1994). Our laboratory has seen similar values in wrestlers; the mean and highest weight losses before a match were reported to be 1.9 kg and 4.3 kg for high-school wrestlers and 3.7 kg and 5.4 kg for college wrestlers, respectively (Pesce et al. 1996). This suggests that greater weight losses are undertaken as the athletes become more elite. Several studies have provided an estimate of weight lost for weigh-in by measuring the weight gain between weigh-in and the match. The average gain was about 5% both for collegiate wrestlers followed over four matches in the season and for 668 wrestlers studied at the National Collegiate Athletic Association (NCAA) championships.

8.3.2 *Light-weight rowers*

Many rowers lose a similar magnitude of weight as wrestlers in order to meet the requirements of light-weight competition. Morris and Payne (1996) followed 18 light-weight rowers over their rowing season and found that the women dropped an average of 5.9% of their body weight while men dropped 7.8% of their body weight during the competitive season compared to pre-season. They achieved this most often via additional exercise (73.3%), food restriction (71.4%), and fluid restriction (62.9%).

8.3.3 *Jockeys*

Fourteen jockeys in England responded to a survey distributed to 48 stables (King & Mezey 1987). They were an average of 13% below the population weight for their height, with the lightest being 21% below average. Jockeys reported that weight control was a priority over most other aspects of their lives during the racing season. They used a variety of methods to reduce their already low body weight—food avoidance, sauna, laxatives, diuretics and appetite suppressants. The use of saunas was especially popular with jockeys spending up to four hours in the sauna in a single session. A fast of up to six days was reported by one of the jockeys.

8.3.4 *Light-weight American football*

The five United States colleges with a light-weight football program were invited to participate in a study of the weight loss practices and attitudes of their players (Depalma et al. 1993). A total of 131 players from the four schools that agreed to participate described their weight loss practices in a survey. Sixty-six per cent of the sample admitted to fasting during the previous month. Even more surprisingly, 26% fasted once per week and almost 20% fasted more than once per week. Seventeen per cent used vomiting, 4% used laxatives, and 2.5% used diet pills, diuretics or enemas for weight loss. Not surprisingly, these dramatic efforts to lose weight were perceived as interfering with thoughts and extracurricular activities 'often' or 'always'.

8.4 ▌ WEIGHT LOSS AND COMPETITIVE SUCCESS

Most athletes in weight-division sports think weight loss behaviours are important to their success in the sport. Does research verify this? This question has been examined in wrestlers by determining whether the acute weight gain after weigh-in (assumed to reflect weight lost) is predictive of success during the wrestling match. There was no evidence that magnitude of weight gain affected the outcome of the match for 11 collegiate wrestlers over four matches in their season (Utter & Kang 1998) or for 668 wrestlers at a National Collegiate Athletic Association (NCAA) tournament in the United States (Horswill et al. 1994; Scott et al. 1994). However, virtually all the wrestlers were losing weight for the weigh-in and there was only a small range in the weight losses undertaken at competition. Thus, these studies were not able to test whether athletes who did not lose weight for weigh-in would be at a disadvantage upon competition. Ninety-five per cent of the wrestlers at the NCAA tournament gained at least 1.4 kg over the 20 hours between weigh-in and match, with the overall average gain of 4.9% of body mass.

8.5 ▌ POTENTIAL NEGATIVE CONSEQUENCES TO WEIGHT LOSS

Most weight-category sports are based on anaerobic energy utilisation, with an emphasis on muscle power (e.g. wrestling, boxing, judo, power lifting, and light-weight football). Rapid weight loss by athletes in these sports is typically achieved with drastic dietary or body fluid changes. The goal of all these athletes is to reduce body mass through loss of body fat or fluid, rather than lean tissue, and to recover any water loss prior to the competition. In addition, they intend to maintain physical performance and health while making weight, or at least are able to recover their performance to pre-weight-loss levels after the weigh-in. There is evidence that at least some athletes do not achieve these goals and, in fact, experience impairment of performance or health. The following section provides information that should be used to educate athletes concerning possible negative outcomes of inappropriate weight loss.

8.5.1 *Plasma volume loss and susceptibility to heat illness*

The three collegiate wrestlers who died all used dehydration as part of their weight loss strategy (American Medical Association 1997). Before their deaths, all had exercised in vapour-impermeable suits and hot environments; one of these individuals had a body temperature of 108°F upon death. There is no doubt the acute dehydration coupled with the use of heat and excessive exercise contributed to their deaths. Dehydration reduces the ability of the body to produce sweat and therefore increases the risk of heat injury. A large drop in plasma volume may be expected as a result of dehydration strategies. In one study where wrestlers used a sauna to lose 3.8% of body weight, plasma volume fell 7.5% in these athletes (Greiwe et al. 1998). Another study sought to determine whether the rate of weight loss influenced the change in plasma volume. Collegiate wrestlers were asked to lose about 6% of their weight within a five-day period using their own methods and pattern. Some lost the weight gradually, others moderately, or rapidly (Yankanich et al. 1998). The drop in plasma volume (11%) was independent of the pattern of weight loss. Thus, use of dehydration can have dramatic effects on plasma volume and this change does not appear to be dampened by gradual, as compared to rapid, weight loss.

8.5.2 *Lean tissue maintenance or growth*

It is difficult to maintain lean tissue mass with dramatic weight loss. Although most of the energy deficit is made up from a reduction in body-fat stores, some body protein may be used for gluconeogenesis. Thus, dietary protein needs are higher during periods of low energy consumption. We found that resistance-trained athletes who lost weight over a week while consuming a formula diet of 75 kJ/kg (18 kcal/kg) lost body protein if they were given the Recommended Dietary Allowance (RDA) (0.8 g/kg) for protein, but were in nitrogen balance (no net body protein loss) if the diet contained twice the RDA for protein (Walberg et al. 1988).

Several studies have verified that wrestlers and rowers have less lean tissue than age-matched controls over the competitive season. For example, one study reported a reduction in the fat-free mass of female rowers during their season compared to pre-season measurements (McCargar et al. 1993). Wrestlers had lower increases in arm and thigh muscle cross-sectional areas over the wrestling season compared to non-wrestling classmates (Roemmich & Sinning 1997). Fortunately, they found no effect on linear growth and during the off-season the wrestlers showed a rebound in muscle growth to bring them up to the average for controls. Concurrent with the drop in lean tissue was a depression of growth-inducing hormones. Like the muscle cross-sectional area, these hormonal disruptions were normalised during the post-season (Roemmich & Sinning 1997).

Although these changes appeared to be temporary in these older athletes, there is question whether a chronic negative energy balance could affect linear growth in younger athletes. Theintz et al. (1993) examined the estimated bone age and predicted height in a cross-sectional study of young elite gymnasts and swimmers for over two years. Over the period studied they reported stunting of leg length growth, and thus predicted height, in the gymnasts but not in the swimmers. They concluded that early, heavy training can alter growth rate, particularly in a sport known to have high emphasis on low body-fat levels and energy restriction. It is important to point out that there were no dietary measures performed in this study. However, the information is provocative and suggests that severe emphasis on body weight in young athletes may have long-term effects on growth.

In summary, athletes practising repeated weight loss over a season are likely to inhibit lean tissue growth. At least in older athletes, there appears to be catch-up of lean growth during the off-season. Although all individuals should be encouraged to have a well-balanced diet, involving moderate energy restriction for long-term weight loss, this is particularly important for young athletes.

8.5.3 *Metabolic rate and weight loss*

Early research noted that wrestlers who reported repeated weight loss and gain (termed weight cyclers) had a lower metabolic rate than those who were not cyclers (Steen et al. 1988). This suggested the possibility that weight cycling caused the metabolic rate to drop. However, later studies which used longitudinal measures of metabolic rate in wrestlers over a season and in post-season did not verify a permanent effect of weight loss on metabolic rate (Melby et al. 1990). The almost 18% decrease in resting metabolic rate during season disappeared in post-season (Melby et al. 1990). However, a drop in metabolic rate during the season will make weight loss more difficult since more restriction in energy intake will be required to cause a negative energy balance. In summary, it appears from the literature that resting metabolic rate is likely to drop significantly during the wrestling season and will alter the energy intake prescription for weight loss. However, the evidence that these metabolic changes continue after the season is not strong.

8.5.4 *Cognitive function*

Not surprisingly, most people do not feel mentally sharp and at their peak while dieting. This has been shown in chronic dieters; eight body builders who were dieting over 12 weeks showed significant increases in fatigue, tension, depression, and confusion (Newton et al. 1993). Even short-term weight loss can have adverse effects on mood and cognitive abilities. Horswill et al. (1990a) showed that rate of perceived exertion during a performance test designed to simulate wrestling was 7% higher when the athletes had lost weight over four days. So, wrestling workouts as well as matches will feel more difficult for those trying to lose weight. Another set of 14 collegiate wrestlers were tested for mood and cognitive ability before and after loss of an average of 6.2% of their body weight, and again after a 72-hour recovery period of food and fluid consumption (Choma et al. 1998). Four of the five sub-scales of the profile of mood test (tension, depression, anger, fatigue, confusion) revealed a higher score, indicating more negative mood following the weight loss. In addition, the wrestlers had poorer short-term memory ability after weight loss. All these changes returned to baseline after 72 hours. The researchers suggest that some of the cognitive and mood disturbances could be mediated by the significantly lower blood glucose noted in the wrestlers after weight loss (Choma et al. 1998).

In summary, athletes are not likely to feel or perform mental tasks as well during periods of weight loss. There is no research at this point to determine whether particular dieting strategies may dampen these mental disturbances.

8.5.5 *Nutritional status*

It is unlikely that a period of brief dieting or weight loss by itself will have a negative effect on nutritional status. Our bodies can typically handle brief periods of low nutrient intake. One study confirmed that the dietary intakes reported by wrestlers while making weight were very low for many nutrients; e.g. 30% and 48% of them had diet records with less than 67% of the RDA for vitamin C and vitamin A, respectively (Steen & McKinney 1986). Although self-reported dietary records showed low intakes of almost all nutrients during rapid weight loss in wrestlers (and judo athletes in another study), none of the blood biochemical indicators showed abnormal nutrient status (Folgelholm et al. 1993).

Problems with nutritional status may arise in those athletes who are repeatedly restricting their diet for weight loss or are dieting over a prolonged period. Biochemical evidence of nutritional deficiency was observed in athletes who lost weight over a three-week period but not for those dieting over just a few days (Fogelholm et al. 1993). Horswill et al. (1990b) found that the repeated dieting of wrestlers was associated with a significant reduction in pre-albumin and retinol-binding protein, which are plasma indicators of protein status. Similarly, another study found low serum pre-albumin levels in adolescent wrestlers during their season (Roemmich & Sinning 1997). Protein intake, as assessed with food records, showed that average reported intake of protein was 0.9 g/kg above the RDA. However, as stated earlier, a negative energy balance may increase protein requirements.

In summary, the diets of most athletes attempting rapid weight loss are likely to be low in many nutrients. A single weight-loss effort is unlikely to cause problems in nutrient status but repeated weight loss over a season is more likely to cause a deterioration of nutritional status. More research is required to determine the specific changes expected. Counselling an athlete to choose a higher nutrient density diet with sufficient micronutrients and protein will lessen the likelihood of nutritional deficiencies.

8.5.6 *Bone*

Four days of fasting has been reported to cause a 40–50% reduction in markers of bone synthesis and resorption in healthy females (Grinspoon et al. 1995). This lower bone-turnover may result in lower bone-mass over time. A recent study in light-weight male rowers has confirmed a negative effect of a briefer period of reduced energy intake on bone metabolism (Talbott & Shapses 1998). A 24-hour fast that caused a 1.7 kg reduction in body weight influenced markers of bone formation and breakdown. Serum osteocalcin, a marker of bone synthesis, was reduced by 20%. Urinary pyridinoline and deoxypyridinoline cross-links, indicative of bone resorption, decreased 27% and 22% respectively (Talbott & Shapses 1998). In summary, athletes, particularly females who have menstrual disturbances and there-fore have an elevated risk of reduced bone mass, should be educated on the potential effect on bone of repeated weight loss.

8.5.7 *Performance*

The effect of rapid weight loss on performance appears to depend on the method of weight loss, the magnitude of weight loss, and the type of exercise performance test utilised (Fogelholm 1994; Walberg-Rankin 1998). The detrimental effect of weight loss on aerobic performance via dehydration is well documented, but the effect on muscle power or strength is less clear. One study (Viitasalo et al. 1987) found a 7.8% reduction in isometric muscle strength in athletes who lost 3.4% of their body weight via dehydration in a sauna. Another study showed that a 3.8% loss of body weight using sauna exposure had no effect on muscle isometric strength and endurance (Greiwe et al. 1998).

Adding energy restriction to dehydration, or dieting alone, appear to be more con-sistent in causing impairments of muscle performance. Athletes who followed a very low calorie diet (600 kJ/d) for 60 hours, followed by a diuretic to dehydrate, showed a decline in muscle isometric strength (Viitasalo et al. 1987). A series of studies in our laboratory has looked at the effect on anaerobic performance of short-term weight loss through energy restriction without dehydration. Resistance-training athletes who lost 3.8 kg over seven days (50% carbohydrate (CHO) formula diet) had a significant reduction in quadriceps isometric endurance (Walberg et al. 1988). Muscle dynamic strength of the quadriceps and biceps brachii was reduced by about 8% in athletes who lost 3.3 kg over a ten-day period of dieting (Walberg-Rankin et al. 1994). In sum-mary, there is evidence for a reduction in muscle strength and endurance in a number of studies examining acute weight loss in athletes. Addition of energy restriction to dehydration appears to be more likely to cause impairments than dehydration alone.

Tests using intermittent bouts of high-intensity work have been developed to attempt to mimic the pattern of muscle use in sports, including wrestling. Weight loss using a formula diet (102.8 kJ/kg) over three days significantly reduced the amount of work accomplished during a six-minute intermittent test (Hickner et al. 1991). Similarly, Horswill et al. (1990a) and Walberg-Rankin et al. (1996) showed reduction in performance of 6.3% and 7.6% in similar intermittent upper-body sprint tests when wrestlers lost weight over four and three days respectively. Thus, there is ample evidence that weight loss in the range of 5% of body weight using energy restriction alone or with dehydration can depress high-intensity intermittent-exercise performance.

It is interesting that many wrestlers perceive their performance to be impaired by their weight-loss efforts. Sixty-three per cent of high-school wrestlers surveyed perceived a depression of muscle strength, 56% speed, 42% agility, and 42% concentration as a result of weight loss (Marquart & Sobal 1994). Studies looking at muscle performance of wrestlers over their season have confirmed a depression in muscle strength for adolescent wrestlers compared to their non-wrestling classmates (Roemmich & Sinning 1997). This performance decrement was correlated with the lower muscle cross-sectional area in the wrestlers during their season.

In summary, acute weight loss in the range of 5% of body weight has been shown in some studies to reduce performance in athletes, particularly in repeated high-intensity sprint tests. It is valuable to point out that the weight loss used in many of these studies is very close to the typical weight loss observed in wrestlers under competitive situations. A reduction in physical performance over a season of repeated weight loss may be secondary to limited growth of lean tissue. Many of the athletes already believe that weight loss hurts their performance.

8.6 STRATEGIES FOR WEIGHT LOSS

8.6.1 *Dehydration*

Since dehydration is banned by the NCAA for wrestlers and some high-school wrestling associations (see later discussion), it is not ethical to recommend any degree of dehydration as a means of making weight. Athletes involved in sports that do not ban dehydration and who intend to use dehydration for weight loss are cautioned to not lose more than 2% of BM with this method, as performance and tolerance to heat is probably impaired with greater degrees of dehydration. In addition, as shown in later sections, short recovery periods do not allow full rehydration of individuals with body-weight losses due to dehydration in the 5% range.

8.6.2 *Diet*

A few researchers have compared the effects of rapid compared to gradual weight loss in athletes. Fogelholm et al. (1993) had judo and wrestler athletes lose weight rapidly with energy restriction and dehydration over 2.4 days (6% of body weight) or reduce weight more gradually (5% of body weight) with more modest energy restriction alone over three weeks. Neither strategy was shown to be superior with regard to changes in performance.

Another study compared the effects of losing similar amounts of weight over either two or four months in national calibre light-weight rowers (Koutedakis et al. 1994). Six rowers were studied over two years; the rapid weight-loss strategy (3.8 kg over two months) was implemented in the first, and the gradual approach (4.7 kg over four months) was used in the following year. Neither method was able to exclusively cause fat loss; about 50% of the weight lost with both strategies was a reduction in fat-free mass. However, the more rapid weight loss was associated with a decline in lactate threshold and leg strength, while these measures, as well as $VO_{2\,max}$ and anaerobic power, were actually increased during the slower weight-loss period. This study suggests that a more gradual weight loss is superior for maintenance or increases in performance but does not affect body composition change.

One study has examined the effect of altering frequency of eating on weight loss in athletes. Boxers ate 5020 kJ (1200 kcal) per day for two weeks as either two meals per day or six meals per day (Iwao et al. 1996). The same weight loss was noted but more reduction in lean body-mass occurred for the two meals per day pattern.

Several studies have demonstrated the value of CHO in a weight-loss diet. Wrestlers could maintain high power performance on a high-CHO diet (66–70% of energy respectively) but not when they consumed a modest CHO (41–55%) diet for weight loss (Horswill et al. 1990a; McMurray et al. 1991). A practical suggestion, based on these studies, is to maximise CHO intake within other dietary goals in an energy-restricted diet (e.g. to include at least 60–70% of energy as CHO in a weight-loss diet).

The high CHO intake recommended above should not be at the expense of dietary protein since it has been shown that protein requirements are increased during weight loss using energy restriction (see Section 8.5.3). This research suggests that dietary protein should be at least 1.2 g/kg during weight loss. Since this might contribute up to 20% of energy, this leaves a suitable dietary fat content of weight-loss diets at $\leq 20\%$.

8.7 RECOVERY STRATEGIES

8.7.1 Fluids and electrolytes

Recovery of fluids lost through dehydration may take 24–48 hours, longer than is commonly appreciated by athletes (Costill et al. 1973). A loss of 5% of BM, accompanied by a 12.5% reduction in plasma volume was not eliminated by a two-hour rehydration period with 1.5 L of water (Burge et al. 1993). Performance of a rowing test was depressed following the rehydration period as compared to prior to weight loss. The cause of performance decrement may have been the continued depression of plasma volume (still 6% lower than baseline) but also could have been related to the reduced muscle glycogen observed in the rowers after weight loss plus rehydration. Nevertheless, this study shows that consumption of a large volume of water over two hours following an acute weight loss typical of wrestlers and rowers was not sufficient to totally rehydrate the athletes and bring their performance to optimal levels.

It is important to note that water was not provided *ad libitum* in this study, thus it is possible that athletes would have spontaneously ingested more water. Although the traditional recommendation has been to ingest about one litre of fluid for each kilogram lost due to dehydration, more recent research suggests that increasing this recommendation to consume 150% of volume fluid lost due to dehydration is more effective (Shirreffs et al. 1996). Consuming fluid in volumes greater than that lost is preferable due to the loss of some of the fluid ingested via urine production (see Chapter 15, Section 15.4.2).

In the dehydration study with rowers, rehydration was attempted using tap water containing no electrolytes nor other nutrients in the water consumed (Burge et al.

1993). Research shows that rehydration will occur more rapidly if electrolytes are included in the fluid consumed (Shirreffs et al. 1996). The benefit of sodium in a rehydration fluid appears to be related to the stimulatory effect of sodium on water absorption in the gut as well as the maintenance of thirst drive. Ingestion of water will reduce the osmolality of the blood and reduce the desire to drink, which is counterproductive to rehydration (see Section 15.4.2).

Provision of CHO in the recovery fluid may also be important in accelerating rehydration. Research suggests that a modest CHO concentration in the beverage will enhance total water absorption in the gut, but excessive CHO content will counteract this effect; Shi et al. (1995) showed that an 8% CHO solution allowed less water absorption than a 6% CHO beverage. Thus, it is not surprising that juices and soft drink beverages (CHO content typically greater than 10%) have been shown to be less effective than a sports drink in increasing plasma volume following dehydration from exercise (Gonzalez-Alonso et al. 1992). Chapter 15 provides a detailed discussion on optimal rehydration strategies.

8.7.2 *CHO*

Weight loss in athletes has been associated with reduced muscle CHO storage. Wrestlers losing 5% of their weight with food and fluid restriction had a 54% decline in muscle glycogen (Tarnopolsky et al. 1996). A similar weight loss in rowers over just 24 hours was accompanied by a 30% drop in muscle glycogen content (Burge et al. 1993). Sub-optimal muscle glycogen levels can be overcome with time and adequate CHO intake (see Chapter 15, Section 15.2), but this may not be realistically achieved between the weigh-in and the start of competition. Wrestlers who lost about 5% of their weight with energy restriction and were re-fed a 50% CHO diet over five hours did not recover their performance to baseline levels while those fed a higher CHO diet (70%) had a performance similar to baseline after the recovery (Walberg Rankin et al. 1996). Although we did not measure muscle glycogen, we would expect that it was reduced by weight loss and increased more with the higher CHO re-feeding diet. We found that most collegiate wrestlers did consume a high-CHO diet (66%) between weigh-in and the match, but the range in reported energy intake from CHO during re-feeding was 28–87% (Pesce et al. 1996). Thus, since energy restriction to produce weight loss is likely to cause a drop in muscle and liver glycogen, which may contribute to impairment of performance if recovery time is short, athletes should be counselled to eat a high-CHO diet during recovery from energy restriction to make weight.

No studies have studied the role of different types of CHO on recovery rate of glycogen following weight-making strategies. However, it is likely that this situation would be similar to that of recovery of muscle glycogen after prolonged endurance exercise (Burke et al. 1993); an enhanced rate of glycogen resynthesis would be likely if CHO-rich foods with a high glycaemic index are consumed. Strategies to enhance recovery of muscle glycogen are summarised in greater detail in Chapter 15.

8.8 NEW MEASURES TO REDUCE DANGEROUS WEIGHT-LOSS PRACTICES

8.8.1 Introduction

It is obvious from descriptive studies that athletes who compete in weight-class sports are highly motivated to use weight-making strategies, as they perceive moving into a lower weight division to be an important determinant of their success. Eighty per cent of high-school wrestlers surveyed listed winning as the biggest influence on their decision to lose weight (Marquart & Sobol 1994). Coaches were identified by 64% of the wrestlers as a major influence on their intention to lose weight. Thus, the wrestlers are self-motivated in addition to receiving some external pressure to lose weight.

Many athletes could use assistance to develop a plan for weight loss. When a group of high-school wrestlers were asked who helped them plan their weight-loss efforts, 'nobody' was the second highest answer (42%) after coaches (44%) (Marquart & Sobol 1994). Most coaches are not trained in nutrition and thus may not be able to appropriately advise athletes on safe weight loss. Sossin et al. (1997) demonstrated a poor knowledge of issues of making weight in a group of high-school wrestling coaches: correct answers on a nutrition knowledge survey were 64% for weight loss, 59% for training diets, 57% for dehydration, and 52% for body composition. Although this could be improved through coach education, the best approach is to use health professionals for counselling in this area. A minority of the wrestlers used trainers (11%), doctors (7%), or dietitians (3%) (Marquart & Sobal 1994). Although it is likely that collegiate and especially Olympic-level athletes have greater access to medical and nutrition professionals, there are no data on the sources of information used by more elite athletes. However, there may be resistance by some coaches and athletes to use nutritionists for fear they will discourage weight loss. It is important for nutritionists to understand the stresses placed on the athletes and attempt to help them in a way that will be least likely to cause health problems.

8.8.2 High-school wrestlers

New rules made by some governing bodies in sport promote greater use of health professionals in educating athletes about weight issues. These changes are best illustrated by recent programs in wrestling. The Wisconsin Interscholastic Athletic Association set up a pilot program in 1989 with a goal to reduce unsafe weight loss in high-school wrestlers (Oppliger et al. 1995). This program included new rules for determining weight class based on body composition and maximum weight losses that can occur per week. Body composition testers were trained and certified to do skinfold analysis of high-school wrestlers throughout the state. Minimum competitive weights were based on BM calculated to be no lower than 7% body fat for that individual. In addition, wrestlers were not to lose more than 1.4 kg (3 lb) per week during the season. These rules were paired with development of nutrition education materials to educate the athletes on appropriate weight-loss methods (developed with the help of state nutrition organisations such as Wisconsin Dietetic Association). Following the pilot year, 1990 was a voluntary year for use of the program, with mandatory implementation of the new rules in 1991. The scope of this program can be realised when one knows that more than 9 000 body-fat tests were required each year. Body-fat assessments must be done prior to the start of the season with data being sent to the state wrestling association. An appeal process was in place such that athletes could opt for hydrostatic weighing to verify skinfold measurement. Only 1% of athletes appealed in 1993. Change was difficult for athletes and coaches. Originally 60% of coaches opposed the project but by 1993, 95% felt positive about the changes. Some were pleased to be free of the responsibility for choosing weight class for each athlete.

There is published evidence that this program has significantly reduced inappropriate weight-loss practices. Oppliger et al. (1998) examined weight loss in wrestlers a year before and after implementation of this program. The maximum amount of weight loss fell from an average of 3.2 to 2.6 kg; average weight loss to certify: 2.8–2.4 kg; weekly weight cycled: 1.9 to 1.6 kg; longest fast: 20.5–16.5 h; and frequency of weight cutting 6.2 to 4.7 times per season. Use of fluid restriction and rubber suits also declined. Thus, these rule changes reduced but did not totally eliminate inappropriate weight-loss methods.

The success of this program was instrumental in the development of similar recommendations in the American College of Sports Medicine position stand concerning weight loss in wrestlers published in 1996 (American College of Sports Medicine 1996).

8.8.3 *Collegiate wrestlers*

Although collegiate wrestling governing bodies were slower to implement new rules, the deaths of the collegiate wrestlers in 1997 accelerated the development of programs for safer weight-management practices. Recently, the NCAA added new rules to wrestling that reflected those begun in Wisconsin in high-school wrestlers. Their stated goal was to 'emphasize the competitive element of wrestling and minimize the emphasis on making weight' (National Collegiate Athletic Association News, March 2 1998). The rule changes recommended by the NCAA wrestling committee include the following features (National Collegiate Athletic Association Press Release, January 13 1998 and April 13 1998):

- Prohibition of dehydration. Guidelines to discourage dehydration were included in the NCAA Sports Medicine Handbook since 1985. These guidelines were expanded and changed to rules. Hot rooms (defined as rooms hotter than 79°F), use of vapour-impermeable suits, excessive food or fluid restriction, laxatives and vomiting are now prohibited.
- An increase in weight allowance of seven pounds (3.2 kg) to each weight class.

- Limitations for wrestlers to compete only in the weight classes that were achieved at the beginning of the season.
- Rescheduling of weigh-ins to be closer to the event to discourage the potential for recovery after severe weight-making strategies: weigh-ins shall be held no more than two hours before the first match in a regular meet. The weigh-in for a multiple-day tournament will occur two hours before competition on the first day and one hour before competition on subsequent days.
- Prohibition of artificial rehydration techniques (e.g. intravenous hydration).

Since these recommendations are recent, it is not known how smoothly they will be implemented and enforced. It is possible that these new rules will be modified as experience is gained. Thus, health professionals are encouraged to keep up with new developments on rule changes regarding body weight in specific sports.

8.9 SUMMARY

Athletes competing in sports with weight categories are highly motivated to acutely lose weight prior to weigh-in. Many will use drastic dietary restriction or dehydration to achieve a temporary weight loss. Quick losses of 5% of body weight, typical in many of these sports, have been shown to result in reductions in physical performance, abnormalities of bone metabolism, impairments in cognitive function and increased susceptibility to heat illness. Prolonged or repeated weight-loss attempts are likely to cause nutritional deficiencies and limit lean tissue growth.

Weight-loss goals and strategies should be determined with the assistance of health-care professionals (e.g. team physicians, nutritionists) to ensure appropriate and safe weight loss. Regular monitoring of health and performance of the athlete will help in making decisions to adjust the weight-loss plan.

More research is needed to compare different dietary strategies for weight loss to determine the method most likely to cause weight loss while maintaining performance and health. The limited research available suggests that modest energy restriction using a high-CHO, moderate-protein and low-fat diet is recommended. Risk of nutrient deficiencies can be reduced by consumption of nutrient-rich foods. Due to the potentially fatal consequences of dehydration, this method should be used modestly or not at all.

8.10 PRACTICE TIPS

Greg Cox

- There is no specific set of nutrition guidelines to address weight-management issues for all weight-making sports. When counselling athletes on weight-making strategies it is essential to consider the physiological requirements specific to their sport, the rules governing weigh-in procedures and the traditions within the sport. The practice tips outlined below reflect current research findings and personal experience gained from dealing with athletes competing in weight-making sports. Counselling such athletes often involves compromising your professional opinion in order to facilitate a working relationship. In many instances, successful counselling is as simple as attempting to minimise the negative impact of the athlete's current weight-making strategies.

- Before any nutrition intervention is commenced, present dietary habits and weight-making strategies of the athlete should be assessed. Many elite athletes in weight-making sports have established strategies to reduce body weight prior to competition. These strategies are often based on personal experience and practices of other athletes in the sport. Be prepared to hear stories of drastic weight-loss techniques such as food and fluid restriction, excessive exercise, and use of saunas, laxatives and diuretics.

- It is useful to develop a yearly weight management plan with the athlete. This should consider the length of the competition season, the number of times they are expected to compete throughout the year, the type of training they perform and the weigh-in procedures of the sport. Make allowances for their weight to fluctuate between the off-season and competition season, as it is difficult for most athletes to maintain their competition weight year-round.

- It is important to understand the rules that govern weigh-in procedures in the various weight-making sports. Be careful to clarify rules governing weigh-in procedures, since these differ between sports and sometimes differ within the same sport (for example: weigh-in procedures for professional boxing differ from amateur boxing; and NCAA wrestling weigh-in procedures differ from those of international wrestling). Weight categories, the time between weighing-in and competition, the length of the tournament and the number of occasions athletes are required to weigh-in vary between sports. These factors ultimately determine the nutrition advice provided to these athletes for making weight and should be investigated prior to the interview or during the interview process. Table 8.1 outlines weight categories and issues relevant to making weight in numerous sports.

- Allowances for growth should be considered for adolescent athletes competing in weight-making sports. Many athletes competing in lighter divisions in boxing, wrestling and judo are still in adolescence. It is common for younger athletes competing in open competition to move across weight categories as they mature.

- Many athletes use extreme short-term measures to make weight in the week immediately preceding competition, rather than implementing long-term

Table 8.1 Summary of specific issues in making weight for weight division sports

Sport	Competition	Weight categories (kg)		Weigh-in procedures
		Male	Female	
Wrestling—Senior International Includes Greco-Roman and Freestyle wrestling	1 bout = 2 × 3 min rounds for international competition and may require an additional 3 min round if match is tied or inadequate points are scored Competition sessions last no longer than 3 h Individual weight categories are contested over a maximum of 2 days 4 or fewer bouts each day of competition	48–54 <58 <63 <69 <76 <85 <97 97–125	41–46 <51 <56 <62 <68 68–75	Weigh-in in the evening before competition, 6–8 pm Weigh-in period lasts 30 min Expected to weigh-in only once at start of competition
Boxing—Amateur	Each bout is 4 × 2 min rounds Competitors box every second day and may be expected to box 4–5 times during the tournament	Male <48 48–51 51–54 54–57 57–60 60–63.5 63.5–67 67–71 71–75 75–81 81–91 91 >	Light fly weight Fly weight Bantam weight Feather weight Light weight Light welter weight Welter weight Light middle weight Middle weight Light heavy weight Heavy weight Super heavy	All competitors weigh-in on the first day of competition at an hour appointed between 8–10 am On following days only those who are drawn to box shall appear to weigh-in between 8–10 am Boxing shall not commence earlier than 3 h after the time appointed for the close of weigh-in

Boxing—Professional	Australian National and the various World Association	Weight divisions vary from amateur boxing, and may vary slightly between countries and boxing associations	In Australia, competitors weigh-in 8–10 h before a title fight, but may weigh-in anywhere up to half an hour before a fight.
	Title fights are fought over 12 × 3 min rounds	Below are the weight divisions of the Australian National Boxing Federation	Competitors weigh-in 24 h prior to a fight when contesting a fight under one of the world boxing organisations
	Fights may vary between 4–12 × 3 min rounds	< 47.63 Straw weight	
	Competitors usually fight 3–4 times per year	47.63–49.89 Junior fly weight	
		49.89–50.80 Fly weight	
		50.80–52.16 Junior bantam weight	
		52.16–53.52 Bantam weight	
		53.52–55.34 Junior feather weight	
		55.34–57.15 Feather weight	
		57.15–58.97 Junior light weight	
		58.97–61.23 Light weight	
		61.23–63.50 Junior welter weight	
		63.50–66.68 Welter weight	
		66.68–69.85 Junior middle weight	
		69.85–72.57 Middle weight	
		72.57–76.20 Super middle weight	
		76.20–79.38 Light heavy weight	
		79.38–86.18 Cruiser weight	
		> 86.18 Heavy weight	

(continues)

(continued)

Sport	Competition	Weight categories (kg)		Weigh-in procedures
Horse racing—Jockeys	Races are conducted over various distances, usually 1 000–2 000 m (lasting 1–2 min), however may be as long as 3 200 m (i.e. the Melbourne Cup) Jockeys may have up to 6–8 rides during one racing session which lasts roughly 5–6 h	Minimum weight for any race in Australia as sanctioned by the Australian Rules is 43.5 kg including saddle and accessories Minimum weight varies between states and within states (country versus city) for local races Minimum weight also varies between countries Horses are weight-handicapped according to ability or age		All jockeys weigh-in roughly 30 min before racing for each race they compete in Jockeys on horses that earn prize money (plus the next best finisher) have to weigh-in directly after the race
Olympic weight lifting	Competitors have 3 lifts in each discipline: Clean-and-jerk and snatch Competition for any one competitor is conducted over 1 day	Male <56 <62 <69 <77 <85 <94 <105 105+	Female <48 <53 <58 <63 <69 <75 75+	Weigh-in is 2 h before the start of competition and lasts for 1 h Lifters are required to weigh-in once during the course of competition
Karate	Have team and individual events—no weight categories in team events 3 min bout for males and a 2 min bout for females	Male <60 60.01–65.00 65.01–70.00 70.01–75.00	Female <53 53.01–60.00 60.01 >	At international level, weigh-in is usually conducted the day before competition starts, however is up to the discretion of the tournament organising

	Competitors may be expected to fight 6–8 times, depending on the number of competitors in the tournament Competition for a weight category is completed over 1 day	75.01–80.00 80.01 >	committee
Light-weight rowing	Race over 2 000 m course Competition is over 7 days Expected to compete every second day	Male Average weight of crew shall not exceed 70 kg No individual shall weigh more than 72.5 kg A single sculler shall not weigh more than 72.5 kg Female Average weight of crew shall not exceed 57 kg No individual shall weigh more than 59 kg A single sculler shall not weigh more than 59 kg Coxswain Minimum weight of a coxswain is 55 kg for men and 50 kg for women and mixed crews To make this weight a coxswain may carry up to 10 kg of dead weight	Weigh-in is not less than 1 h and not more than 2 h before race start Competitors are expected to weigh-in each day and for each event they are competing in

(continues)

(continued)

Sport	Competition	Weight categories (kg)			Weigh-in procedures
Judo	Each bout is 4 min for females and 5 min for males. Competition is 1 day only. Can be expected to contest 4–5 bouts during the competition. Minimum of 10 min between bouts	Male	Female		Have a trial 1 h weigh-in period followed by an official 1 h weigh-in period. Minimum time between weigh-in and start of competition is 2 h
		< 60	< 48		
		66	52		
		73	57		
		81	63		
		90	70		
		100	78		
		100 >	78 >		
Taekwondo	Each bout involves 3 × 3 min rounds with 1 min between rounds. Competition is 1 day only. Can be expected to contest 5–8 bouts during the competition	At Olympic Games there are 4 weight divisions whereas at World Championships there are 8			Weigh-in period is 1 h on the morning of competition. Usually 1–2 h between weigh-in and start of competition
		Male	Female	Division	
		< 58	< 49	Fly weight	
		58–68	49–57	Feather weight	
		68–80	57–67	Welter weight	
		80 >	67 >	Heavy weight	

strategies to reduce body fat and body weight to reach the competition target. The first strategy of these athletes should be to reduce body-fat levels in order to maximise their power to weight ratio and make a given weight category safely. Chapter 7 outlines dietary strategies to promote decreases in body-fat levels.

- In most situations, qualification tournaments are scheduled months in advance of major international tournaments such as World Championships and Olympic Games. When discussing an ideal weight category for an athlete, account for the practicality of maintaining a weight category between these tournaments, particularly in light of potential growth sports in adolescent athletes. Athletes are only eligible to compete in the weight category for which they originally qualified.

- The motivation of athletes to compete in a given weight category is determined primarily by their current weight. However, they may also be influenced by their likelihood of winning or qualifying in a given weight category or the expectations of coaches, parents, or trainers. In some situations, the added pressures may lead to unrealistic weight category goals for these athletes. Objective anthropometric data such as height, weight and body-fat levels should remain important in determining the chosen weight category.

- For some athletes in weight division sports, the primary purpose for seeking nutritional advice may be to gain weight. Lean athletes with low body-fat levels may recognise the difficulties associated with reducing weight to meet a lower division. However, they may also find themselves at a disadvantage being at the lower end of the next weight category, and competing against heavier and stronger opponents. Gaining muscle mass and strength may help them to become competitive in this new division. Chapter 5 outlines strategies to increase lean body mass and strength in athletes.

- The harsh reality of weight-division sports is that athletes will always endeavour to compete in a weight category below their usual weight. Many athletes practise dehydration techniques such as restricting fluids, exercising in sweat-promoting suits, and using saunas in order to make weight. Sometimes these practices start seven days before competition starts, impairing exercise performance for the entire week leading up to competition. Against these practices, 24 hours of moderate dehydration (< 2% body weight), mild food restriction and a low residue diet in the day immediately prior to competition, combined with appropriate refuelling and rehydrating strategies between weigh-in and competition, might be less deleterious to health and competition performance. In sports where athletes weigh-in the evening before competition (international amateur wrestling) or several hours before competition starts (international amateur boxing) this technique may be warranted.

- Low-residue diets can be achieved over the 12–24 hours before weigh-in by using low-residue, low-fibre food and fluids combined with commercially available meal supplements and replacements. Replacement of normal dietary intake with a low-residue diet may allow for a 'weight' loss of 300–400 g by reducing usual gastrointestinal contents.

- Many athletes increase their exercise load immediately prior to competition in order to facilitate sweat losses and promote weight loss. Athletes involved in weight-making sports that involve significant aerobic training such as boxing are more likely to cope with increased exercise loads immediately prior to competition. Some athletes who do not routinely include aerobic conditioning in their training may struggle to recover from increased exercise loads implemented to facilitate weight loss immediately prior to competition.

- Implementing appropriate nutritional strategies following weigh-in will facilitate recovery for athletes making weight. Use of sports drinks, liquid meal replacements and high-carbohydrate, low-fat foods may all enhance recovery following weigh-in. For athletes who weigh-in on consecutive days of a tournament, careful planning is imperative to maximise recovery and minimise the likelihood of body-weight fluctuations.

- As with any competition nutrition strategy, weight-making tactics should be practised prior to competition. This is best achieved by making a weight allowance and having athletes weigh-in under similar circumstances to those of competition. For instance, amateur boxers should practise weighing-in every second day with a weight allowance of one kilogram, combined with a series of sparring to mimic competition exercise demands.

REFERENCES

American College of Sports Medicine. Position stand on weight loss in wrestlers. Med Sci Sports Exerc 1996;28:ix–xii.

American Medical Association. Hyperthermia and dehydration-related deaths associated with intentional rapid weight loss in three collegiate wrestlers–North Carolina, Wisconsin, and Michigan, November–December 1997. JAMA 1998;279:824–5.

Burge CM, Carey MF, Payne WR. Rowing performance, fluid balance, and metabolic function following dehydration and rehydration. Med Sci Sports Exerc 1993;25:1358–64.

Burke LM, Collier GR, Hargreaves M. Muscle glycogen storage following prolonged exercise: effect of the glycemic index of carbohydrate feedings. J Appl Physiol 1993;75:1019–23.

Choma CW, Sforzo GA, Keller BA. Impact of rapid weight loss on cognitive function in collegiate wrestlers. Med Sci Sports Exerc 1998;30:746–9.

Costill DL, Sparks KE. Fluid replacement following thermal dehydration. J Appl Physiol 1973;34:299–303.

Depalma MT, Koszewski WM, Case JG, Barile RJ, Depalma BF, Oliaro SM. Weight control practices of light weight football players. Med Sci Sports Exerc 1993;25:694–701.

Fogelholm GM. Effects of bodyweight reduction on sports performance. Sports Med 1994;18:249–67.

Fogelholm GM, Koskinen R, Laakso J, Rankinen T, Ruokonen I. Gradual and rapid weight loss: effects on nutrition and performance in male athletes. Med Sci Sports Exerc 1993;25:371–7.

Gonzalez-Alonso JC, Heaps I, Coyle EF. Rehydration after exercise with common beverages and water. Int J Sports Med 1992;13:399–406.

Greiwe JS, Staffey KS, Melrose DR, Narve MD, Knowlton RG. Effects of dehydration on isometric muscular strength and endurance. Med Sci Sports Exerc 1998;30:284–8.

Grinspoon S, Baum H, Kim V, Coggins C, Klibanski A. Decreased bone formation and increased mineral dissolution during acute fasting in young women. Clin Endocrinol Metabol 1995;80:3628–33.

Hickner RC, Horswill CA, Welker JM, Scott J, Roemmich JN, Costill DL. Test development for the study of physical performance in wrestlers following weight loss. Int J Sports Med 1991;12:557–62.

Horswill CA, Hickner RC, Scott JR, Costill DL, Gould D. Weight loss, dietary carbohydrate modifications, and high intensity physical performance. Med Sci Sports Exerc 1990a;22:470–7.

Horswill CA, Park SH, Roemmich JN. Changes in protein nutritional status of adolescent wrestlers. Med Sci Sports Exerc 1990b;22:599–604.

Horswill CA, Scott JR, Dick RW, Hayes J. Influence of rapid weight gain after the weigh-in on success in collegiate wrestlers. Med Sci Sports Exerc 1994;26:1290–4.

Houston, ME, Marrin DA, Green HJ, Thompson JA. The effect of rapid weight loss on physiological functions in wrestlers. Phys Sportsmed 1981;9(11):73–8.

Iwao S, Mori K, Sato Y. Effects of meal frequency on body composition during weight control in boxers. Scand J Med Sci Sports 1996;6:265–72.

King MB, Mezey G. Eating behaviour of male racing jockeys. Psychol Med 1987;17:249–53.

Koutedakis Y, Pacy PJ, Quevedo RM, et al. The effects of two different periods of weight-reduction on selected performance parameters in elite light weight oarswomen. Int J Sports Med 1994;15:472–7.

Marquart L, Sobal J. Weight loss beliefs, practices and support systems for high school wrestlers. J Adol Health 1994;15:410–15.

McCargar LJ, Crawford SM. Anthropometric changes with weight cycling in wrestlers. Med Sci Sports Exerc 1992;24:1270–5.

McCargar LJ, Simmons D, Craton N, Taunton JE, Brimingham CL. Physiological effects of weight cycling in female light weight rowers. Can J Appl Physiol 1993;18:291–303.

McMurray RG, Proctor CR, Wilson WL. Effect of caloric deficit and dietary manipulation on aerobic and anaerobic exercise. Int J Sports Med 1991;12:167–72.

Melby CL, Schmidt WD, Corrigan D. Resting metabolic rate in weight-cycling collegiate wrestlers compared with physically active, non-cycling control subject. Am J Clin Nutr 1990;52:409–14.

Morris FL, Payne WR. Seasonal variations in the body composition of light weight rowers. Br J Sports Med 1996;30:301–4.

National Collegiate Athletics Association. USA: NCAA News, March 2 1998.

National Collegiate Athletics Association. USA: NCAA press release, January 13 1998 and April 13 1998.

Oppliger RA, Harms RD, Herrmann DE, Streich CM, Clark RR. The Wisconsin wrestling minimum weight project: a model for weight control among high school wrestlers. Med Sci Sports Exerc 1995;27:1220–4.

Oppliger RA, Landry GL, Foster WW, Lambrecht AC. Wisconsin minimum weight program reduces weight-cutting practices of high school wrestlers. Clin J Sport Med 1998;8:26–31.

Pesce T, Walberg Rankin J, Thomas E, Sebolt D, Wojcik J. Nutritional intake and status of high school and college wrestlers prior to and after competition. Med Sci Sports Exerc 1996;28:S91.

Roemmich JN, Sinning WE. Weight loss and wrestling training: effects on nutrition, growth, maturation, body composition, and strength. J Appl Physiol 1997;82:1751–9.

Scott JR, Horswill CA, Dick RW. Acute weight gain in collegiate wrestlers following a tournament weigh-in. Med Sci Sports Exerc 1994;26:1181–5.

Shi X, Summers RW, Schedl HP, Flanagan SW, Chang R, Gisolfi CV. Effects of carbohydrate type and concentration of solution osmolality on water absorption. Med Sci Sports Exerc 1995;27:1607–15.

Shirreffs SM, Taylor AJ, Leiper KB, Maughan RJ. Post-exercise rehydration in man: effects of volume consumed and drink sodium content. Med Sci Sports Exerc 1996 28:1260–71.

Sossin K, Gizis F, Marquart LF, Sobal J. Nutrition beliefs, attitudes, and resource use of high school wrestling coaches. Int J Sport Nutr 1997;7:219–28.

Steen SN, Brownell KD. Patterns of weight loss and regain in wrestlers: has the tradition changed? Med Sci Sports Exerc 1990;22:762–8.

Steen SN, McKinney S. Nutrition assessment of college wrestlers. Phys Sportsmed 1986;14(11):100–16.

Steen SN, Oppliger RA, Brownell KD. Metabolic effects of repeated weight loss and regain in adolescent wrestlers. J Am Med Assoc 1988;260:47–50.

Talbott SM, Shapses SA. Fasting and energy intake influence bone turnover in light weight male rowers. Int J Sport Nutr 1998;8:377–87.

Tarnopolsky MA, Cipriano N, Woodcroft C, Pulkkinen WJ, Robinson DC, Henderson JM, et al. Effects of rapid weight loss and wrestling on muscle glycogen concentration. Clin J Sport Med 1996;6:78–84.

Theintz GE, Howald H, Weiss U, Sizonenko PC. Evidence for a reduction of growth potential in adolescent female. J Pediatr 1993;122:306–33.

Tipton CM, Tcheng TK. Iowa wrestling study: weight loss in high school students. JAMA 1970;214:1269–74.

Utter A, Kang J. Acute weight gain and performance in college wrestlers. J Strength Cond Res 1998;12:157–60.

Viitasalo JT, Kyrolainen H, Bosco C, Alen M. Effects of rapid weight reduction on force production and vertical jumping height. Int J Sports Med 1987;8:281–5.

Walberg JL, Leidy MK, Sturgill DJ, Hinkle DE, Ritchey SJ, Sebolt D. Macronutrient content of a hypoenergy diet affects nitrogen retention and muscle function in weight lifters. Int J Sports Med 1988;9:261–6.

Walberg-Rankin J. Changing body weight and composition in athletes. In: Lamb D, Murray R, eds. Perspectives in exercise and sports medicine. Vol 11: Exercise, nutrition, and control of body weight. Carmel: Cooper Publishing Company, 1998:199–242.

Walberg-Rankin J, Hawkins CE, Fild DS, Sebolt DR. The effect of oral arginine during energy restriction in male weight trainers. J Strength Cond Res 1994;8:170–7.

Walberg-Rankin J, Ocel JV, Craft LL. Effect of weight loss and refeeding diet composition on anaerobic performance in wrestlers. Med Sci Sports Exerc 1996;28:1292–9.

Yankanich J, Kenney WL, Fleck SJ, Kraemer WJ. Precompetition weight loss and changes in vascular fluid volume in NCAA Division I college wrestlers. J Strength Cond Res 1998;12:138–45.

CHAPTER 9

Eating disorders and disordered eating in athletes

Linda Houtkooper

9.1 INTRODUCTION

'For women, eating disorders are like steroids for men. You'll get results, but you'll pay for it' (Noden 1994). Such are the feelings of a successful female cross-country runner, recovering from anorexia, on the pressure and rewards related to thinness in her sport. Of course, this must be seen against the backdrop of contemporary culture in which the archetype of physical perfection for women is a thin, lean body (Rodin & Larson 1992; Rodin 1993). In the 1960s, the model Twiggy became a symbol of an ideal body type for young women, with a reported height of 166 cm, body mass (BM) of 41 kg and bust, waist, and hip measurements of 79, 56, 79 cm, respectively (Woscyna 1991). The extreme model represented by Twiggy served as a turning point in the ever-increasing cultural idolisation of slimness. Thinness has become equated with beauty, acceptance, competence, control, power, and goodness for young women (Root 1991; Mortenson et al. 1993). Adolescent girls and women are placed under increasing pressure to restrict food intake to achieve thin physiques (Beals & Manore 1994).

Female athletes face considerable pressures to conform to specific aesthetic requirements of their sports, which often also prize leanness, and performing well in these sports (Wilmore 1991). In some sports, a certain physique or a low BM is considered to be essential for optimal performance, leading to the credo of 'get thin and win' (Thornton 1990). Participation in these sports is associated with a higher risk of eating disorders. These sports are categorised into three groups: 1) 'aesthetic sports' such as diving, figure skating, gymnastics, and synchronised swimming; 2) sports in which low BM and body-fat levels are considered a physical or biomechanical advantage, such as distance running, road cycling and triathlon; and

3) sports that require weight categories for competition, such as light-weight rowing, weight lifting, and wrestling (Benardot et al. 1994).

Research has clearly demonstrated that biological factors significantly influence body shape and BM (Bouchard 1992). This means that some individuals will be prevented from achieving substantial changes to their body shape. Indeed many females are pressured to achieve 'ideal physiques' that are excessively lean, arbitrarily chosen and essentially unrealistic to attain (Leon 1991; Manore 1996). Striving to achieve such an unrealistic goal can lead to disordered thoughts about food, and to pathogenic weight-control practices. These disordered eating and weight-control behaviours occur in a spectrum ranging from mild pathological eating practices to severe clinical eating disorders such as anorexia nervosa and bulimia nervosa. Anorexia nervosa and bulimia nervosa are psychological disorders with dysfunctional implications for eating and exercise-related practices (Wilmore 1991; Sundgot-Borgen 1993b; American Psychiatric Association 1994; Beals & Manore 1994; Brownell 1995). Current estimates indicate that more than 90% of the clinical eating disorders of anorexia and bulimia nervosa occur in females, however, the prevalence of these disorders in males and in athletes (in comparison to the general population) is unclear (American Psychiatric Association 1994; Anderson 1995; Brownell 1995). This chapter will investigate the prevalence and suggested causes of the range of disordered eating and dysfunctional body-image problems in athletes, extending the discussion begun in Chapters 7 and 8 about the challenges of achieving ideal BM and physique in sport.

9.2 ◼ TOOLS FOR ASSESSING DISORDERS OF EATING AND BODY IMAGE

Since disordered eating and weight-control behaviours occur in a spectrum it is important to consider the methods by which these problems can be assessed or diagnosed. Eating disorders as defined by the DSM-IV criteria of the American Psychiatric Association (American Psychiatric Association 1994) are difficult to detect and diagnose, even for professionals, because of the complex and secretive nature of these disorders. Typically, the diagnosis of eating disorders includes self-reports of eating-related behaviours. Several questionnaires and other diagnostic tools have been developed by investigators especially for use in the study of populations or groups. These standardised instruments include the Eating Attitudes Test (EAT) (Garner & Garfinkel 1979) and the Eating Disorder Inventory (EDI) (Garner et al. 1984).

The EAT is the questionnaire most commonly used in the assessment of eating disorders (Brownell & Rodin 1992; Beals & Manore 1994). While the original version of the EAT contained 40 items (EAT-40), a more recent version has been developed containing 26 items (EAT-26) (Gamer et al. 1982). The EAT questionnaire asks individuals to report how well various statements apply to them by using a six-point rating scale ranging from 'rarely' to 'always'. Examples of statements include 'I like eating with other people', 'I am terrified about being overweight', 'I feel like food controls my life', 'I wake up early in the morning', and 'I enjoy trying rich new foods'. Patients diagnosed with clinical anorexia nervosa typically rank scores of 30 or higher on the EAT-40 and 20 or higher on the EAT-26.

The EDI, which has also been used to assess the occurrence of eating disorders, has 64 items that focus on eight sub-scales (Garner et al. 1984). The first three sub-scales (body dissatisfaction, bulimia and drive for thinness) assess behaviours and attitudes regarding body image, eating and dieting, whereas the remaining sub-scales (interpersonal distrust, perfectionism, introspective awareness, maturity fears and ineffectiveness) assess psychopathology related to individuals with clinical anorexia nervosa. A newer version, the EDI-2 (Garner 1991), contains 91 items and three additional sub-scales that assess asceticism, impulse regulation, and social insecurity. The EDI has been used for diagnostic screening in both clinical and non-clinical settings (Brownell & Rodin 1992). However, according to Garner (1991) the total EDI score should not be used to measure disordered eating pathology because each sub-scale of this instrument is intended to measure a conceptually independent trait. Instead, it is recommended that each sub-scale score be compared to a standardised patient score.

It is important to recognise that neither the EAT or the EDI were originally designed to make clinical diagnoses of eating disorders. Rather, they were developed for use in non-clinical settings as screening devices to assess attitudes and behaviours exhibited by individuals who met the clinical diagnoses of anorexia nervosa or bulimia nervosa (Garner & Garfinkel 1979; Garner et al. 1982; Leon 1991). In essence these instruments assess attitudes and behaviours that coexist with those exhibited by people with eating disorders; these instruments are not able to distinguish factors that are causative of, or exclusive to, the problems. Although high reliability and validity have been reported for both instruments when used in non-athletic populations (Garner & Garfinkel 1979; Garner et al. 1982; Garner 1991), they have not been well validated in athletic populations.

Reports from validation studies of the EDI in athletes have yielded conflicting results. In one study, Sundgot-Borgen (1993b) reported that 48% of the athletes who met the EDI classification for being at risk of having an eating disorder actually met the criteria of anorexia nervosa or bulimia nervosa when they completed in-depth clinical interviews. However, another study failed to find any relationship between results of the EDI and subsequent diagnosis of clinical eating disorders in the athletes (Wilmore 1991). The discrepancies in these findings have been attributed to the different methodologies used in the two studies, including different criteria for classifying the athletes as at risk of eating disorders and different numbers of athletes in each study (Sundgot-Borgen 1994b).

Other methodologies used in studies to determine the occurrence of eating disorders in a group of athletes include asking participants to self-diagnose these problems based on descriptions of anorexia and bulimia provided to them. This approach was used by a recent study of 30 aerobic dance instructors, and found that 40% of subjects reported having these eating disorders (Olson et al. 1996). Other studies have used questionnaires that assessed dieting practices, preoccupation with weight, and attitudes about eating without reporting the reliability and validity of these questionnaires (Brownell & Rodin 1992). An exception is a questionnaire developed by Steen and Brownell (1990) designed to assess eating, dieting and weight-control practices in athletes competing in weight-controlled sports such as wrestling and rowing. Currently this is the only questionnaire that has been developed for use with athletes that has assessed criteria for validity and reliability.

In summary, caution must be exercised when drawing conclusions about the presence of eating disorders on the basis of scores on tools like the EAT or EDI, or from non-standardised instruments. Many EAT or EDI scores in the elevated ranges associated with patients with eating disorders have been shown to be false positives when they are compared with information obtained from in-depth clinical interviews (Szmukler & Russell 1985; Sundgot-Borgen 1993b). The validity of these tools may be questionable when used with athletes (Brownell & Rodin 1992; O'Connor et al. 1995), particularly when there is some concern that individuals can be identified from their responses. Athletes may not truthfully respond to the items in the instruments if they believe that being identified as having an eating disorder would jeopardise their status or retention on a team. On these occasions, the instruments may under-estimate the true prevalence of eating disorder symptoms among athletes. All such instruments are best used as initial screening devices (Leon 1991). A check list assessing each of the DSM-IV diagnostic criteria for eating disorders, combined with a psychiatric clinical interview and measures that more specifically assess the presence of diagnostic criteria, provide the most effective means of determining the presence of clinical eating disorders (Leon 1991; Sundgot-Borgen 1993b; American Psychiatric Association 1994).

9.3 CLASSIFICATIONS OF CLINICAL EATING DISORDERS

The key functional requirements for behaviour to be clinically defined as an eating disorder are that the behaviour must no longer be under personal control and/or must cause significant adverse changes in psychological, social or physical functioning (Anderson 1990b). The most severe clinical eating disorders are anorexia nervosa and bulimia nervosa, both of which can lead to serious physical damage and even death (American Psychiatric Association 1994). In recognition that many individuals exhibit behaviours and attitudes to eating and their body image that are disordered without fully meeting the criteria set for anorexia or bulimia, the American Psychiatric Association has also established a separate category for 'Eating disorder not otherwise specified'.

9.3.1 *Anorexia nervosa*

Although anorexia nervosa is often portrayed as a disorder of the twentieth century, it was first described in 1689 in a textbook of medicine by Richard Morton, a fellow of the College of Physicians (Silverman 1995). Morton described a condition that he referred to as 'nervous consumption' caused by sadness and anxious cares. The descriptions were based on his clinical observations and included both a female and male case. However, it wasn't until the 1960s that work by Doctor Hilde Bruch lead to a revolution in the understanding of the psychopathology of anorexia nervosa (Silverman 1995).

The diagnostic criteria for anorexia nervosa, defined in the fourth edition of the *Diagnostic and statistical manual of mental disorders* (DSM-IV) of the American Psychiatric Association (1994), include issues of behaviour, psychopathology and biological outcomes. As summarised in Table 9.1, the criteria involve the *behaviour* of self-induced starvation leading to BM below a minimal level considered normal for age and height; the *psychopathological* intense fear of becoming fat or gaining weight; a significant disturbance in the perception of body shape and size that is out of proportion to reality; and, in post-menarchal females, a *biological* abnormality of reproductive hormone functioning leading to amenorrhoea (American Psychiatric Association 1994).

Table 9.1 *Diagnostic criteria for anorexia nervosa*

A.	Refusal to maintain BM over a minimal normal weight for age and height, e.g. weight loss leading to maintenance of BM 15% below that expected; or failure to make expected weight gain during period of growth, leading to BM 15% below that expected.
B.	Intense fear of gaining weight or becoming fat, even though underweight.
C.	Disturbance in the way in which one's BM, size, or shape is experienced, undue influence of body weight or shape on self-evaluation, or denial of the seriousness of the current low body weight.
D.	In post-menarchal females: amenorrhoea, i.e. the absence of at least three consecutive menstrual cycles. (A woman is considered to have amenorrhoea if her periods occur only following hormone administration.)

Type of anorexia nervosa	
Restricting type	During the current episode of anorexia nervosa, the person *has not* regularly engaged in binge-eating or purging behaviour (i.e. self-induced vomiting or the misuse of laxatives, diuretics or enemas)
Binge-eating/purging type	During the current episode of anorexia nervosa, the person *has* regularly engaged in binge-eating or purging behavior (i.e. self-induced vomiting or the misuse of laxatives, diuretics or enemas)

Adapted from the *Diagnostic and statistical manual of mental disorders IV*, Washington DC: American Psychiatric Association 1994

Criterion A for the diagnosis of anorexia specifies that a BM lower than 85% of what is considered normal for a person's age and height is the cut-off for a minimal BM. This value for minimal BM can be calculated from the Metropolitan Life Insurance table values for adults, or from growth charts used for children and youths up to 18 years of age. An alternative measure of minimal BM is a BM index (mass (kg)/height (m)^2) of 17.5 (American Psychiatric Association 1994). Restriction of food intake is the primary means of weight loss for the restricting type of anorexia nervosa. Individuals may start dieting by excluding foods perceived to be high in kilojoules and/or fat, but most eventually follow a very restricted diet that is often limited to only a few foods (American Psychiatric Association 1994). The binge-eating/purging type of anorexia nervosa is distinguished by regular use of binge-eating and purging behaviours such as self-induced vomiting to achieve weight loss (American Psychiatric Association 1994).

Criterion B specifies that the individual with this eating disorder exhibits intense fear of gaining weight or becoming fat, and this fear is not alleviated by weight loss. In fact, distress about weight gain will often increase as BM continues to decrease (American Psychiatric Association 1994). The experience and significance of BM and shape are distorted in individuals with this disorder (Criterion C). While some individuals feel overweight in all parts of their physique, others realise that they are thin but are still concerned that parts of their body are too fat. The self-esteem of individuals with anorexia is highly dependent on their BM and shape, and they are obsessive about weighing themselves and measuring body parts. Weight loss is viewed as a sign of an impressive achievement of self-control, whereas weight gain is perceived as an unacceptable failure of self-control. Although some individuals with this disorder may acknowledge being thin, they typically deny the serious health implications of their condition.

Criterion D stipulates that amenorrhoea is present in post-menarchal females, and menarche is delayed in pre-pubertal females (American Psychiatric Association 1994). In post-menarchal females with this disorder, amenorrhoea is related to abnormally low levels of oestrogen secretion, which is the result of a decreased secretion of follicle-stimulating hormone and luteinising hormone (see Chapter 10).

9.3.2 *Bulimia nervosa*

The term 'bulimia' is derived from the Greek words for 'ox' and for 'hunger.' Although the definition of the syndrome bulimia nervosa was only recently proposed (Russell 1979), the term 'bulimia' has been traced in Western European sources for more than two centuries, with remarkable consistency of meaning. Bulimia has been defined as a state of pathological voraciousness that leads to ingesting excessive quantities of food (Parry-Jones & Parry-Jones 1995). Bulimia nervosa is characterised by a history of rapidly ingesting large amounts of food in a discreet time period against a person's initial resistance, and is usually followed by purging (American Psychiatric Association 1994). During these binge-eating episodes the individual has feelings of being unable to stop eating or to control what or how much is eaten. The binge-eating episodes are associated with feelings of being out of control as well as of depression and/or guilt. Bulimic behaviours occur in a continuum between the extremes of the anorexic with mild bulimia, who feels she has binged when she has eaten a salad against her will, and the other extreme of a normal-weight bulimic who may ingest large amounts of food containing up to 2–2.5 MJ (8000–10 000 kcal) in a brief time and then purge (Anderson 1990b; American Psychiatric Association 1994). Typical purging methods include self-induced vomiting; misuse of laxatives, diuretics or enemas; fasting; and excessive exercise. The diagnostic criteria for bulimia nervosa, defined by the American Psychiatric Association (DSM-IV), are summarised in Table 9.2.

Table 9.2 *Diagnostic criteria for bulimia nervosa*

A.	Recurrent episodes of binge eating. An episode of binge eating is characterised by both of the following: (1) eating, in a discrete period of time (e.g. within any two-hour period), an amount of food that is definitely larger than most people would eat during a similar period of time and under similar circumstances (2) a sense of lack of control over eating during the episode (e.g. a feeling that one cannot stop eating or control what or how much one is eating).
B.	Recurrent, inappropriate, compensatory behaviour in order to prevent weight gain, such as self-induced vomiting; misuse of laxatives, diuretics, enemas or other medications; fasting; or excessive exercise.
C.	The binge eating and inappropriate compensatory behaviours both occur, on average, at least twice a week for three months.
D.	Self-evaluation is unduly influenced by body shape and mass.
E.	The disturbance does not occur exclusively during episodes of anorexia nervosa.

Type of bulimia nervosa	
Purging type	During the current episode of bulimia nervosa, the person has regularly engaged in self-induced vomiting or the misuse of laxatives, diuretics, or enemas
Non-purging	During the current episode of bulimia nervosa, the person has used other inappropriate compensatory behaviours, such as fasting or excessive exercise, but has not regularly engaged in self-induced vomiting or the misuse of laxatives, diuretics or enemas

Adapted from the *Diagnostic and statistical manual of mental disorders IV*, Washington DC: American Psychiatric Association 1994

9.3.3 *Eating disorder not otherwise specified*

The American Psychiatric Association has recently added another category to the DSM-IV criteria to include disorders of eating that do not meet the criteria for any specific eating disorder (American Psychiatric Association 1994). Examples are summarised in Table 9.3.

Table 9.3 *Diagnostic criteria for eating disorder not otherwise specified*

This category is for disorders of eating that do not meet the criteria for any specific eating disorder. Examples include:
A. For females, all of the criteria for anorexia nervosa are met except that the individual has regular menses.
B. All of the criteria for anorexia nervosa are met except that despite significant weight loss the individual's current BM is in the normal range.
C. All of the criteria for bulimia nervosa are met except that the binge eating and inappropriate compensatory mechanisms occur at a frequency of less than twice a week or for less than three months.
D. The regular use of inappropriate compensatory behaviour by an individual of normal BM after eating small amounts of food (e.g. self-induced vomiting after the consumption of two cookies).
E. Repeatedly chewing and spitting out, but not swallowing, large amounts of food.
F. Binge-eating disorder: recurrent episodes of binge eating in the absence of the regular use of inappropriate compensatory behaviours characteristic of bulimia nervosa.

Adapted from the *Diagnostic and Statistical Manual of Mental Disorders IV*, Washington DC: American Psychiatric Association 1994

9.3.4 *Diagnostic criteria in males*

The diagnostic criteria for anorexia in males are similar to those for females (Anderson 1995). These criteria include self-induced starvation, a morbid fear of fatness, and relentless pursuit of thinness, but they differ in the reproductive hormone abnormalities. Males with anorexia nervosa are characterised by lower testosterone levels, causing decreased sexual drive and performance (Anderson 1995). The diagnostic criteria for bulimia are gender independent (Anderson 1995). Studies of anorexia nervosa indicate that the psychosocial and clinical characteristics are essentially indistinguishable between females and males (Hsu 1980; Crisp & Burns 1983). Nevertheless, males who develop eating disorders are more likely than are females to have experienced medically defined, pre-morbid obesity (Anderson 1995).

9.4 *SUB-CLINICAL EATING DISORDERS*

A substantial number of individuals show signs of disordered eating and distorted concerns regarding BM, fatness or shape, but fail to meet the strict DSM-IV criteria for eating disorders. Such people may be considered to exhibit sub-clinical eating disorders (American Psychiatric Association 1994; Beals & Manore 1994). The concept of sub-clinical anorexia was first identified in female college students (Button & Whitehouse 1981) and later in adolescents who had growth failure or delayed puberty due to malnutrition resulting from self-imposed calorie restriction based on a fear of becoming obese (Pugliese et al. 1983). Whereas individuals diagnosed with anorexia nervosa and bulimia nervosa exhibit severe emotional distress and/or specific psychopathologies that go beyond concerns about BM and use of weight-reduction methods (Leon 1991; American Psychiatric Association 1994). These psychopathological profiles are generally not present in individuals with subclinical eating disorders (Leon 1991; Sundgot-Borgen 1993b; Wichmann & Martin 1993).

9.4.1 *Athletes and sub-clinical eating disorders*

Athletes with sub-clinical eating disorders may exhibit some of the psychological traits associated with clinical eating disorders, such as high achievement orientation, obsessive-compulsive tendencies, and perfectionism. Because these traits are also generally associated with success in athletic performance, this has led to the belief that sub-clinical eating disorders are more common among athletes than among the general population (Leon 1991). Anecdotal reports and research with methodological limitations have provided indirect evidence suggesting that the prevalence of sub-clinical eating disorders is quite high in female athletes, particularly among athletes participating in sports that require a low BM and/or level of body fatness (Gadpaille et al. 1987; Davis & Cowles 1989; Leon 1991; Brownell & Rodin 1992; Stoutjesdyk & Jevne 1993; Beals & Manore 1994).

The term 'anorexia athletica' has been used to describe a sub-clinical eating disorder syndrome characterised by disordered eating and compulsive exercising (Pugliese et al. 1983; Sundgot-Borgen 1993b). The essential feature of anorexia athletica is an intense fear of gaining weight or becoming fat, even though the individual weighs at least 5% less than the expected normal weight for age and height. Weight loss is achieved by restriction of food intake, extensive compulsive exercise, or both (Sundgot-Borgen 1993b). Frequently the athlete also reports bingeing, selfinduced vomiting, or the use of laxatives or diuretics. The criteria for sub-clinical eating disorders have not been well defined. Thus, better-designed research is needed to define and determine the prevalence, incidence, and consequences of sub-clinical eating disorders in athletes.

It is important to recognise differences between primary and secondary occurrences of eating disorders related to people who exercise (Leon 1991). The clinical features of both anorexia nervosa and bulimia nervosa often include a strong exercise component expressed by intensive and highly ritualised daily activities, such as performing a specific number of sit-ups or aerobic exercises. For individuals with a primary eating disorder, exercise is a pathway for expression of the disorder, but little is known about the prevalence of compulsive exercise in these patients. It is possible that these individuals gravitate to organised sporting activities as an outlet or camouflage for their exercise behaviours and interest in nutrition.

By contrast, a secondary eating disorder may develop in an athlete as a result of participating in a sport in which low BM or low body-fatness is stressed as ideal for optimal performance (Leon 1991). As an occupational hazard of their involvement in sport, some athletes become excessively concerned about their BM or fatness and use pathological weight-control practices, such as the use of diuretics, laxatives or self-induced vomiting. These concerns and behaviours often resolve after the athletic season or when the athlete's career is over (Leon 1991). However, a sub-set of these athletes may be psychologically vulnerable to the development of an eating disorder. Even after the season is over they may continue to have intense concerns regarding BM and shape, and persist in engaging in disordered eating and weight-control practices, until they have developed a clinically diagnosable eating disorder.

9.5 ▌ *DEVELOPMENT AND PREVALENCE OF EATING DISORDERS*

According to Anderson (1990b), eating disorders usually begin as a voluntary restriction of food intake but progress by stages in predisposed individuals into a syndrome in which personal control of behaviour is lost. There is a continuum of eating behaviour, which ranges between 'normal' and 'abnormal', with no clear break points to indicate when a problem occurs. Many people can skip a meal or over-indulge in food within the context of a change in their lifestyle or timetables without causing significant damage. However, repeated unwillingness to eat adequate amounts of food that leads directly to a state of starvation or indirectly to binge eating (and is not a consequence of involuntary deprivation or the result of a primary medical or psychiatric illness) defines the behaviour as psychiatrically abnormal (Anderson 1990b). At the extremes of clinical anorexia nervosa and bulimia nervosa, it is usually clear when an eating behaviour is abnormal.

9.5.1 *Prevalence of anorexia nervosa and bulimia nervosa among non-athletes*

Anorexia and bulimia nervosa appear to be more prevalent in industrialised countries, in which there is an abundance of food and in which being considered attractive is linked to being thin (American Psychiatric Association 1994). Little systematic work has been done to examine the prevalence in other cultures (American Psychiatric Association 1994). Studies examining the prevalence of clinical eating disorders among females in late adolescence and early adulthood have reported rates of 0.5–1.0% for cases that meet full criteria for anorexia nervosa and 1–3% for bulimia nervosa (American Psychiatric Association 1994). In clinical studies in the United States, individuals presenting with bulimia nervosa are primarily white, but the disorder has also been reported among other ethnic and racial groups (American Psychiatric Association 1994; French et al. 1995). There are limited data concerning the prevalence of eating disorders in males, but some evidence indicates that occurrence may be greater than previously believed (Anderson 1990a; 1995). Typically, the rate of reporting of disorders in males is approximately one-tenth of that in females.

Eating disorders usually begin in late adolescence or early adult life. Individuals make transitions in both directions between having anorexia nervosa and bulimia nervosa. The most common transition is changing from a food-restricting sub-type of anorexia nervosa to the bulimia nervosa sub-type or to bulimia nervosa, while maintaining a normal weight (Anderson 1990b). The course of bulimia may be chronic or intermittent, with periods of remission alternating with recurrences of binge eating and purging.

9.5.2 *Prevalence of clinical eating disorders in athletes*

Because of heightened body awareness and pressures in some sports to have a low BM and body fatness, there has been speculation that an increased risk of eating disorders may occur. Importantly, many athletes share psychological qualities similar to those of non-athletes with eating disorders, such as perfectionism, and drive and ability to achieve a narrow focus. There is some evidence that supports the assumption that eating disorders are more common among athletes, and that the prevalence of eating disorders is greatest in sports in which low body weight is related to improved performance in the sport (Brownell & Rodin 1992; Sundgot-Borgen 1994b).

The prevalence of eating disorders reported in groups or populations of athletes ranges from as low as 1% to as high as 39% (Dick 1991; Brownell & Rodin 1992; Beals & Manore 1994; Sundgot-Borgen 1994a). The disparity in these estimates is attributed to the differences in methodology used to assess the occurrence of eating disorders. As indicated in Section 9.2, some studies use criteria derived from the strict diagnostic definitions of eating disorders established by the American Psychiatric Association, whereas other surveys estimate prevalence using questionnaires or standardised instruments that assess behaviours and attitudes exhibited by people with clinical eating disorders. These instruments have not been adequately validated in athletic populations. In addition to problems caused by the type of diagnostic tools chosen, most studies are limited by including participants in only a single sport, failing to include an appropriate control group or undertaking inappropriate statistical analyses (Brownell & Rodin 1992; Sundgot-Borgen 1993b; Brownell 1995). These limitations must be considered when interpreting results of studies regarding prevalence of eating disorders.

9.5.2.1 *Comparisons between athletes and non-athletes*

Studies investigating the prevalence of eating disorders among athletes (using standardised assessment instruments such as the EAT and EDI) have shown findings to be inconsistent. The studies reviewed below have variously reported a lower prevalence in athletes than in non-athletes, no difference between the two groups, and a higher prevalence in athletes than in non-athletes. These discrepancies may be due to inconsistencies in the definition of eating disorders among studies, differences in non-athletic control groups, and lack of appropriate statistical analyses (Brownell & Rodin 1992; Sundgot-Borgen 1994a; Brownell 1995). For example, one study determined that university athletes have a lower prevalence of eating disorders than students who were not athletes. The 126 athletes in the study had lower EDI scores than did 590 non-athletic student controls in five comparison groups, but no statistical comparisons among the groups were made (Kurtzman et al. 1989).

A recent study indicated that there were no differences in EDI-2 sub-scale scores between collegiate female athletes and non-athletes who had high academic achievement (Ashley et al. 1996). The study included 145 female intercollegiate athletes and, as a control group, 14 non-athletes who had a high grade-point average in an advanced collegiate program of study. The percentage of respondents scoring above the norms for anorexia nervosa on any EDI-2 sub-scale did not differ between the groups. Furthermore, the athletes did not have significantly higher scores on any of the EDI-2 sub-scales, compared to non-athletes, and there were no significant differences among the 'lean' athletic group, 'other' athletic group or the control group on any of the EDI-2 sub-scales. The African-American athletes did have significantly lower scores on the body dissatisfaction sub-scale than did the white athletes, indicating they were more satisfied with their bodies. Similarly, another investigation found no significant differences between 25 collegiate female gymnasts and 25 non-athletic controls matched for age, height and BM with respect to mean EDI-2 sub-scale scores (O'Connor et al. 1995). Finally, in a study comparing EDI-2 scores of 68 male body builders to a control group of 50 male college students, Anderson et al. (1996) found that average scores did not indicate the presence of eating disorder tendencies in either group. The student control group scores were higher than those of body builders on the 'body dissatisfaction' sub-scale.

By contrast, in the most comprehensive study to date, Sundgot-Borgen found that eating disorders were more prevalent among female athletes than among non-athletic controls (Sundgot-Borgen 1993b). This investigation included 522 elite Norwegian female athletes representing 35 different sports, and 448 non-athletic control subjects, and compared data obtained using the EDI to results of in-depth clinical interviews. On the basis of EDI scores (greater than or equal to 40), 22% of the athletes and 26% of the control subjects were classified as being at risk of developing eating disorders. However, when subsequent clinical evaluations and personal interviews were undertaken with at-risk subjects using the model described by Johnson (1986), 18% of the athletes and 5% of the non-athletic controls were found to meet the criteria for anorexia nervosa, bulimia nervosa, and anorexia athletica. If the diagnosis of anorexia athletica was excluded, only 9% of the at-risk athletes met the criteria for the clinical eating disorders of anorexia nervosa and bulimia nervosa. The athletes who had eating disorders participated in sports in which leanness or maintaining a specific weight was considered important. The study also found that these elite athletes under-reported the use of purging practices such as vomiting and use of diuretics and laxatives and over-reported the use of binge eating. In addition, the athletes who reported having an eating disorder indicated that they had anorexia nervosa; however, most of the athletes actually met the criteria for bulimia nervosa or sub-clinical eating disorders. Other studies have also shown that athletes have a higher prevalence of eating disorders than do non-athletes, but all of these studies have methodological limitations (Davis & Cowles 1989; Benson et al. 1990; Loosli & Benson 1990; Sundgot-Borgen 1993b).

9.5.2.2 *Comparisons of eating disorders among sports*

Many studies have reported that disordered eating practices are prevalent among athletes irrespective of what practices might occur in a non-athletic comparison group (Rosen et al. 1986; Dummer et al. 1987; Rosen & Hough 1988; Sundgot-Borgen 1993b). For instance, a study with 42 collegiate gymnasts showed that all of these athletes were dieting and that 62% had used at least one pathogenic weight-control method (Rosen & Hough 1988). In a comparison study of athletes in 'thin-build' sports with athletes in 'normal-build' sports, Davis and Cowles (1989) reported that there were no overall differences in EAT scores. However, the thin-build athletes (n = 64; gymnasts, synchronised swimmers, divers, figure skaters, long distance runners, and ballet dancers) had lower body weights, greater weight concerns, more body dissatisfaction, and more assiduous dieting than did athletes participating in sports that do not stress a thin physique (n = 62; basketball, field hockey, sprinting, downhill skiing, and volleyball).

Interest in pathogenic eating behaviours of male athletes has focused mainly on the effects of rapid weight loss by body builders (Hickerson et al. 1990; Kleiner 1990), wrestlers (Tipton & Oppliger 1984; Brownell et al. 1987; Webster et al. 1990) and light-weight college football players (DePalma et al. 1993). All studies noted unhealthy practices used for weight control, such as dehydration, severe energy restriction, and laxative or diuretic abuse. The issues related to weight-making sports have been reviewed in Chapter 8. In the survey of light-weight football players, discriminant factor analysis yielded several variables that in 70–85% of the cases correctly identified individuals in the sample who were at risk of pathogenic eating behaviours. The risk index model developed in this study needs to be cross-validated in other groups of athletes to determine its usefulness for identifying athletes at risk of developing eating disorders.

9.5.2.3 *Comparisons of female and male athletes within a sport*

Few studies have compared the prevalence of eating disorders between females and males in a sport, but the available data show a higher prevalence in females than in males. An investigation of competitive ice skaters (23 females, 17 males) indicated that the mean score on the EAT was 29 for the females and 10 for the males

(Rucinski 1989). Forty-eight per cent of the females had EAT scores greater than 30, which is the cut-off point for a screening assessment of anorexia nervosa. Another study compared female and male athletes in rowing, a sport with a weight-limited division and a heavy-weight category for both females and males (Sykora et al. 1993). The study included 82 heavy-weight rowers (56 females, 26 males; no weight limitations) and 80 weight-limited light-weight rowers (17 females and 63 males). The similar athletic training of the two groups allowed the heavy-weight rowers to serve as a comparison group for the light-weights. A questionnaire developed by the investigators, and the EAT-26 tool, were used to examine eating, weight control, and dieting practices among the four groups. Results indicated that average scores for females and males were greater than 30, the cut-off point related to anorexia nervosa, and that the females had higher average EAT scores than did the males. Contrary to expectations, there were no significant differences between the average EAT scores of the light-weights and heavy-weights or between the female and male average scores within the light-weight and heavy-weight groups. Likewise, light-weights and heavy-weights, and males and females did not differ significantly in the reported frequency of binge eating. However, a greater percentage of females (20%) than of males (12%) reported bingeing more than two times per week for at least three months, which is one diagnostic criterion for bulimia nervosa. The investigators concluded that rowing joins the growing list of sports where eating disorders occur and that male athletes may be more vulnerable to these problems than previously recognised (Sykora et al. 1993).

9.6 *RISK FACTORS FOR THE DEVELOPMENT OF DISORDERED EATING*

Several factors contribute to the development of disordered eating practices and sub-clinical or clinical eating disorders, although the specific factors that precipitate the development of these problems are unique for each person. An inherited tendency appears to exist: there is an increased risk of anorexia nervosa and bulimia nervosa among first-degree biological relatives or individuals with these disorders (American Psychiatric Association 1994). Furthermore, studies of anorexia nervosa in twins have reported concordance rates for identical twins to be significantly higher than those for fraternal twins (Holland et al. 1988). However, what distinguishes the people who voluntarily start dieting or exercising to control their weight, body composition or body shape but then go on to develop either anorexia or bulimia nervosa is of great theoretical interest and practical concern.

9.6.1 *Psychological factors*

A number of psychological characteristics are associated with people with eating disorders. These include perfectionism (Davis & Cowles 1989; Warren et al. 1990;

Yates 1989, 1992; Brownell & Rodin 1992), a feeling of personal ineffectiveness, guilt, and distrust (Klemchuk et al. 1990), obsessive personality traits (Davis & Cowles 1989; Yates 1989), and high achievement expectations (Yates 1989, 1992; King 1989; Warren et al. 1990). Characteristics associated with people who develop bulimia instead of anorexia include impulsiveness, intolerance to hunger or other continued psychological distress, and narcissism, whereas anorexic individuals tend to be in the sensitive, obsessional, perfectionist, and avoidant group (Piran et al. 1988; Anderson 1990b).

Low self-esteem is another trait associated with eating disorders (Silverstone 1992; Thompson & Sherman 1993) and could be a precipitating factor in the development of these problems (Lindeman 1994). Studies investigating the association between exercise and self-esteem indicate that in general, exercise participation enhances self-esteem (Lindeman 1994), however, little is known about whether athletes have greater self-esteem than do non-athletes.

9.6.2 *Exercise participation*

The role of exercise participation as a risk factor for developing eating disorders merits examination. Wolf and Akamatsu (1994) investigated the relationship between exercise and disordered eating attitudes and behaviours in Caucasian male (n = 120) and female (n = 168) college undergraduate students. Results showed that females in general, and female exercisers in particular, scored higher on the various measures of disordered eating attitudes and behaviours than did the males and non-exercisers. In the study, 'exercisers' were defined as individuals who participated in an organised sport or regular exercise at least three times per week and included activities such as dance, gymnastics, basketball, football, running, swimming, and cross-training. Non-exercisers were defined as individuals who did not participate in any organised sport or regular exercise and participated in informal exercise less than three times per week. The participants completed demographic questionnaires and the EDI-64 and EAT-40, where a cut-off of 30 on the EAT and a criterion of 15 on the EDI Drive for Thinness Scales are indicative of disordered eating concerns and behaviours. The researchers reported that 22% of the female exercisers exceeded the EAT cut-off, compared with 10% of female non-exercisers, suggesting a higher rate of disordered eating concerns and behaviours among female exercisers. Twenty per cent of female exercisers exceeded the cut-off on the EDI 'drive for thinness' scale, compared with 8% of the female non-exercisers.

Separate discriminant function analysis, using the EDI sub-scale scores as predictor variables, was undertaken to determine if female exercisers and non-exercisers with EAT scores higher than 30 could be distinguished from each other and from the other females with lower scores. Results indicated that two discriminant functions were significant. Overall, the authors concluded that although female exercisers and non-exercisers with disordered eating concerns were similar in the pursuit of thinness, they differed in regard to personality dimensions characteristic of eating disorders. The exercisers had some characteristics of females with eating disorders (anorexic/bulimic eating attitudes and greater drive for thinness), but they did not have the full behavioural and psychological syndrome common to clinical eating disorders.

9.6.3 *Sport-related factors*

The most comprehensive study of disordered eating in athletes has helped to identify a number of factors related to sport that may increase the risk or precipitate an eating disorder. In this study, 603 elite female athletes in Norway completed EDI questionnaires to identify individuals at risk of eating disorders (Sundgot-Borgen 1994b). Athletes defined as at risk (n = 103) completed structured clinical interviews, and 92 of these athletes met the criteria for anorexia nervosa, bulimia nervosa or anorexia athletica. Members of a control group of 30 athletes chosen at random from a pool of not-at-risk athletes matched for age, community of residence, and sport were also interviewed. Compared with controls, athletes with eating disorders began sport-specific training and dieting earlier and felt that puberty occurred too early for optimal performance. The athletes with eating disorders reported several key trigger factors that they associated with their development of eating disorders. These factors are listed in Table 9.4. Additional studies are needed to determine if these trigger factors are also identified by female and male athletes in other ethnic or racial groups.

Table 9.4 *Trigger factors associated with onset of eating disorders in athletes*

- Prolonged periods of dieting or weight fluctuations.
- Traumatic events such as:
  - illness or injury to self or family member
  - new coach
  - leaving home
  - failure at school or work
  - family problems
  - problems with relationships
  - death of significant other
  - sexual abuse
  - work transition.
- Large increase in training volume and significant weight loss associated with this.
- Belief that menarche has been reached too early.
- Early start of sport-specific training.
- Large discrepancy between self-defined ideal BM and actual BM.
- Recommendation to lose weight without guidance.

Sundgot-Borgen 1994b

9.7 CONSEQUENCES OF EATING DISORDERS ON PERFORMANCE AND HEALTH

Disordered eating of any degree leads to adverse health consequences, with risk of morbidity, impaired athletic performance, and even death; increasing as the severity of disordered eating increases. The weight loss, food restriction, and purging practices associated with eating disorders have powerful physiological and psychological effects. These effects can include a decrease in exercise capacity, increased risk of injury, and medical complications. These complications include depression, nutrient deficiencies, fluid and electrolyte imbalances, and adverse changes in the cardiovascular, digestive, endocrine, skeletal and thermoregulatory systems, some of which can be fatal. Specific issues related to chronic inadequate energy and nutrient intake, or the practices associated with making weight, have been summarised in Chapters 7 and 8. This chapter will consider briefly the special problems that have come to be identified as the female athlete triad. Further details on some aspects of this syndrome can be found in Chapter 10.

9.7.1 Female athlete triad

Attaining and maintaining unrealistically low body weight through disordered eating and exercise practices can put young women at risk of developing two associated disorders: amenorrhoea and osteoporosis (Brooks-Gunn et al. 1987; Nattiv et al. 1994; Yeager et al. 1993; Putukian 1994). The female athlete triad refers to the interrelations among disordered eating, amenorrhoea and osteoporosis. Alone, each disorder is of medical concern, but when all three components of the triad are present, there is the potential for more serious impacts on health, and risk of death (De Souza & Metzger 1991; Yeager et al. 1993; Nattiv et al. 1994; Putukian 1994; American College of Sports Medicine 1997).

Primary amenorrhoea, or delayed menarche, is present when menses has not begun by 16 years of age, whereas secondary amenorrhoea is defined as the absence of at least three to six consecutive menstrual cycles (Nattiv et al. 1994). The reported prevalence of these problems appears higher in athletes than in the general population (Keizer & Rogol 1990; Yeager et al. 1993). Menstrual dysfunction associated with athletics is related to many factors, including a history of weight fluctuations; rigorous training schedules, and inadequate energy intake causing an 'energy drain'; social pressures associated with competition; and nutrient deficiencies (Loucks 1990; Otis 1992; Wilmore et al. 1992; Dueck et al. 1996b). Disordered eating and eating disorders have also been identified as a key risk factor. These issues are discussed in greater depth in Chapter 10.

It is a common misconception among some athletes, coaches, and trainers that amenorrhoea is a benign consequence of strenuous exercise, and an indicator that body-fat levels and training are at an optimal level for a sport (Dueck et al. 1996b). In fact, the altered hormonal environment is a risk factor for the development of impaired bone health and osteoporosis. Osteoporosis in the young female athlete refers to inadequate bone formation and premature bone loss, resulting in low bone mineral density and increased risk of fracture (Van de Loo & Johnson 1995). Studies conducted with female athletes have shown that premature osteoporosis may occur as a result of menstrual dysfunction and may be partially irreversible, despite resumption of menses, oestrogen replacement, or calcium supplementation (Cann et al. 1984; Drinkwater et al. 1986, 1990; Rencken et al. 1996). An increase in the risk of stress fractures has been reported in athletes with amenorrhoea, and this appears to be related to low bone mineral density (Van de Loo & Johnson 1995). This issue is discussed in greater detail in Chapter 10.

9.8 PRACTICAL ISSUES IN THE PREVENTION AND TREATMENT OF EATING DISORDERS

The course and outcome for individuals with eating disorders are highly variable. Some people fully recover after a single bout with anorexia nervosa, others exhibit a fluctuating pattern of weight gain followed by a relapse, and others experience a chronically deteriorating course of the illness over many years. In some cases, hospitalisation is required to help restore weight and to manage fluid and electrolyte imbalances. The long-term consequences of intractable anorexia nervosa can be fatal. In the treated, non-athletic population, anorexia nervosa has a 10–18% mortality rate (Ratnasuriya et al. 1991), with death most commonly resulting from starvation, suicide, or electrolyte imbalance. The long-term outcome of bulimia nervosa is unknown (American Psychiatric Association 1994).

Clinical eating disorders rarely occur before puberty, but there are indications that when they do, the severity of associated mental disturbances may be greater and prognosis for recovery is poorer than when they begin in early adolescence, between ages 13 and 18 years (American Psychiatric Association 1994). Recovery from eating disorders also varies with the stage of development of the disorder, duration of the disorder, and previous history of counselling intervention, but early intervention tends to improve the chances for a better outcome (Szmukler & Russell 1986). With specific regard to sport, one study has shown that symptoms of eating disorders abate after retirement from the sport (O'Connor et al. 1996).

There are limited opportunities for primary prevention of eating disorders by professionals because they have little control of the many factors that contribute to the development of eating disorders (Thompson & Sherman 1993). Instead, professionals should focus on secondary interventions, by providing education about reducing risk factors for the development of disordered eating, and the value of early identification and treatment aimed at minimising the severity and duration of eating disorders.

The early identification of eating disorders plays an important role in improved treatment. An awareness of risk factors for eating disorders, as well as signs and symptoms of disordered eating patterns and their health and sport performance consequences, may help detect problems early and initiate prompt treatments (Grooms 1996). Education should be targeted to a range of levels (athletes, parents, coaches, training staff, physicians and athletic administrators) and provide information on methods to screen for eating disorders; the importance of and guidelines for healthy eating and exercise practices; appropriate expectations concerning body weight and body composition; and available local resources for prevention and treatment of eating disorders. In addition, coaches, trainers and parents need to be educated on how they may influence the development of eating disorders in their athletes.

9.8.1 *Warning signs for the development of eating disorders*

Since disordered eating practices are typically well-kept secrets, it is important for those working with athletes to be aware of subtle warning signs that can be related to the presence of disordered eating or exercise practices. Table 9.5 summarises typical warning signs for anorexia nervosa and bulimia nervosa, as provided in education material distributed to coaches, athletes and athletic officials by the National Collegiate Athletic Association in the United States (Brownell & Rodin 1992).

Table 9.5 *Warning signs for eating disorders*

Warning signs of anorexia nervosa
- Dramatic weight loss
- A preoccupation with food, calories and BM
- Wearing baggy or layered clothing
- Relentless, excessive exercise
- Mood swings
- Avoiding food-related social activities

Warning signs of bulimia nervosa
- A noticeable BM loss or gain
- Excessive concern about BM
- Bathroom visits after meals
- Depressive moods
- Strict dieting followed by eating binges
- Increased criticism of one's body

9.8.2 *Approaches to the treatment of eating disorders*

A planned approach to the prevention of, intervention in and treatment of eating disorders, involving the team of people who work with the athlete, improves the probability that those who develop problems will get support and treatment. The plan should include identification of the risk factors and triggering events that precipitate the development of eating disorders, and the implementation of a screening program to identify athletes who fit these profiles. Team members should be able to recognise warning signs and symptoms, know what treatment options are available in the community, and have guidelines for what steps to take if a problem is suspected or identified (Grandjean 1991; Leon 1991; American Dietetic Association 1994; Johnson 1994; Nattiv & Lynch 1994; Van de Loo & Johnson 1995; Grooms 1996).

A pre-participation physical examination, educational meetings, or workshops can be used to conduct screenings for signs and symptoms of disordered eating and other triad disorders. Screening instruments that address both the behavioural and psychological characteristics of eating disorders should be used. If athletes are assessed using several of the standardised questionnaires, it is important to be aware that they are likely to produce spuriously high 'eating-disordered' scores in relation to questions about rigorous exercise patterns (Wolf & Akamatsu 1994). Athletes who are identified by a screening program to have disordered eating attitudes or practices should be approached carefully to initiate appropriate interventions. Guidelines on how to approach these athletes and refer them to appropriate treatment have been published (Thompson & Sherman 1993; Clark 1994, 1996).

The preservation of the athlete's health and mental well-being are the first goal of treatment (Nattiv & Lynch 1994). A multidisciplinary team involving people experienced in the management of eating disorders provides the ideal treatment approach (Johnson 1994). Each team member should have a specific role.

- A physician should monitor medical status, rule on athletic participation, and often co-ordinate the care provided by the team.
- A dietitian or nutritionist should provide appropriate nutritional guidance.
- A psychologist, psychiatrist or counsellor should address issues of mental well-being.
- Trainers, coaches and exercise physiologists should assist with and support a training program or performance monitoring as appropriate.
- In the case of young athletes who live at home, family involvement in treatment is often necessary.

Individuals who exhibit the full range of symptoms and signs of sub-clinical and clinical eating disorders require comprehensive treatment plans. However those with only a limited array of disordered eating concerns and practices may benefit from an appropriate preventive, educational or dietary intervention within their sporting program. Well-designed preventive educational programs, including seminars, workshops, and individual consultations, can all help increase awareness of warning signs and symptoms as well as provide guidance for how to obtain appropriate prevention and treatment assistance for eating disorders. There is extensive literature related to specific guidelines for screening for and treating people with eating disorders and other disorders of the female athlete triad (Grandjean 1991; Woscyna 1991; Clark 1993, 1994; Sandri 1993; Thompson & Sherman 1993; Wichmann & Martin 1993; Johnson 1994; Lindeman 1994; Nattiv & Lynch 1994; Nattiv et al. 1995; Dueck et al. 1996b; Manore 1996).

Private organisations, sport governing bodies, and sports medicine organisations have developed educational resources for use in eating disorder prevention programs.

9.9 DIRECTIONS FOR FUTURE RESEARCH

The presence of the spectrum of eating disorders has been determined in most studies by the use of self-report questionnaires that typically include various forms of the EAT and EDI questionnaires. These instruments need to be validated in athletes, and conditions need to be identified under which truthful responses are likely to be given. Because of their limitations, a diagnosis of clinical eating disorders cannot be based solely on responses obtained with these instruments. In future studies, the use of psychiatric interviews or other clinical measures that more specifically assess the presence of diagnostic criteria for eating disorders will help determine the actual prevalence of clinical and sub-clinical eating disorders (Leon 1991; Sundgot-Borgen 1993b; American Psychiatric Association 1994).

Research is particularly needed, via well-designed longitudinal studies, to determine if the prevalence and incidence of eating disorders are higher in athletes than in non-athletes and among athletes in specific sports. The key question that needs to be addressed by these studies is whether or not participation in some sports causes the disturbances or if individuals with eating problems or with psychosocial problems that increase the risk of eating disorders are drawn to certain sports (Brownell 1995). Currently, with the exception of anorexia athletica, classifications for cases of sub-clinical eating disorders are not based on unique diagnostic criteria (Sundgot-Borgen 1993b; Beals & Manore 1994). The features of anorexia athletica as described by Sundgot-Borgen (1993b) need to be refined (Beals & Manore 1994). Therefore, research is needed to further define and describe the unique characteristics of sub-clinical eating disorders such as anorexia athletica, and to determine the prevalence of these disorders in the athletic population. Recommendations on how to proceed in conducting this research have been proposed (Beals & Manore 1994).

There are many theories that might be examined in relation to the development of eating disorders. For example, it is interesting to consider why many of the young athletes who are concerned about their body weight and shape do not develop eating disorders. It has been hypothesised that psychological traits associated with eating disorders, such as depression, stress reactivity, sexual and maturity concerns, autonomy, and control needs, are less likely to occur in young athletes (French et al. 1994). As a result, sports participation could represent a protective factor for the development of eating disorders by increasing self-esteem and feelings of autonomy, control, and social support, while decreasing feelings of depression and stress (French et al. 1994). Prospective research is needed to evaluate these provocative hypotheses as well as to determine the role of genetics and environment in the development of eating disorders.

In addition to the need for further research in all the areas related to determining the development, prevalence, risk factors, consequences and treatment of eating disorders, there is also a critical need to evaluate the effectiveness of approaches to the prevention and treatment of disordered eating and exercise practices. Additional research is needed to develop models that can accurately identify athletes who are at risk of eating disorders. Development of more effective ways for athletes, coaches, trainers, parents and physicians to treat eating disorders and to prevent the development of eating disorders is essential to good health and success in sports.

9.10 SUMMARY

Defined according to diagnostic criteria specified by psychology experts, clinical eating disorders include anorexia nervosa, bulimia nervosa, and eating disorders not otherwise specified. These represent the extreme end of a spectrum of disordered eating and exercise patterns that can result in significant morbidity and even death. Disturbances in the perception of body shape and weight are essential characteristics of both of these eating disorders. Anorexia nervosa is further distinguished by refusal to maintain the minimal healthy BM and by the presence of amenorrhoea in post-menarchal females. Bulimia nervosa is characterised by repeated episodes of binge eating, fear of inability to stop eating, and use of purging behaviours to avoid weight gain. Individuals with bulimia nervosa are able to maintain body weight at or above the minimal healthy BM.

Studies show that recreational exercisers and competitive athletes can suffer from pathological eating and weight-control practices and the psychological aspects of eating disorders, such as preoccupation with body shape and mass. Methodological limitations of studies estimating the prevalence of eating-related problems in these groups prevent definitive information on the prevalence of eating disorders related to exercise, and among athletes, from being available. Disordered eating appears to be more prevalent in females than in males, and in sports where low BM or low body-fatness is considered important to performance (e.g. distance running, cycling, or weight-division sports), or in aesthetic sports (e.g. body building, diving, gymnastics, and figure skating).

Various factors, including sociocultural, biological, psychological, exercise, and sport participation may predispose athletes to the development of disordered eating and exercise practices and subsequent adverse health and performance consequences. The term 'female athlete triad' is used to describe the interrelationships of disordered eating, menstrual dysfunction, and osteoporosis in physically active females, and represents a serious challenge to the health and performance of the athlete. Recovery from eating disorders varies according to age of onset, duration of the disorder, extent of disturbed relationships, and previous history of counselling, but early intervention tends to improve the chances for a better outcome. Prevention and early detection of disordered eating and exercise practices is essential to enabling athletes to participate and succeed in their sports in the healthiest and safest way.

In societies that place a great deal of emphasis on thinness and specific ideal body images, some people will use extreme means to try to reshape their bodies. Athletes who are pressured to meet a rigid definition of physique or lose weight because they think it will improve performance are at risk of developing dysfunctional eating and exercise practices. Until society in general and sport leaders in particular eliminate the pressures that encourage these behaviours, there will be a need to recognise, treat and prevent disordered eating and exercise practices.

9.11 PRACTICE TIPS

Belinda Dalton

Practical tips for identifying athletes with eating disorders

- Many athletes are at risk of disordered eating developing into clinical eating disorders. Dietitians need to screen all athletes for their present dietary practices and beliefs to assess those at risk. Some athletes will talk freely about their problems while many deny any issues with weight or food.

- The DSM-IV criteria are useful when assessing for clinical eating disorders, however, the awareness of warning signs may allow the dietitian (or coach, or parent) to identify problems at an earlier stage, and this often results in better outcomes with treatment (see Table 9.5).

- Many athletes with disordered eating practices gradually reduce the variety of 'allowed/safe' foods in their diets; omitting fatty foods first, then sugary foods and other foods like meat, dairy, breads and cereals until only a handful of different foods remain safe. Deciding to become a vegetarian is also common in athletes with disordered eating. For most, this is not vegetarianism for religious or environmental reasons. Nor does it usually involve eating a variety of legumes, grains, seeds, nuts and other vegetarian foods. Most simply avoid meat, usually claiming it makes them feel 'heavy' or 'is too hard to digest'. Detailed examination of the rationale for dietary restriction (including beliefs about various foods), and of the adequacy of the variety and quantity of the food intake, may disclose disordered eating practices and inaccurate nutrition knowledge.

- Athletes with eating disorders are often obsessed with quantities of foods and can report exact amounts eaten (measured with cups and spoons, or weighed), energy and fat content of foods and their dietary intakes of these. They also often have rigid timing of food patterns and avoid eating out or in public. When taking a diet history, it is useful to ask the athlete questions that establish if these obsessive behaviours are present.

- It is also useful to question training practices as these may reveal excessive exercise patterns, obsessive pursuit of training even when fatigued or injured, and an obsessive knowledge of the kilojoule expenditure of training sessions.

- Being present when athletes are eating (such as when travelling with teams or conducting cooking classes) provides an ideal opportunity to observe athletes' eating practices.

Managing athletes with eating disorders

- The most difficult situations are when:
  — the athlete does not admit to an eating disorder;
  — the athlete's coach (or parent) insists on very low BM or body-fat levels;
  — BM has dropped to a level that is inconsistent with heavy training and evidence of side-effects may be present (e.g. amenorrhoea, stress fractures, anaemia).

- Treatment of eating disorders requires a multidisciplinary approach with a specialist psychologist/counsellor, medical practitioner and dietitian all being involved. Dietitians need to refer the athlete for specialist treatment if they lack experience in dealing with this complex area.

- A client often presents for treatment unwillingly or is ambivalent about it. It is necessary to establish rapport and trust with them and show an interest in understanding their condition. Dietary intake should be increased very gradually (small nutritious snacks six times a day), commencing with the perceived 'safe' foods and progressing to foods and eating situations that create more anxiety for the client. Force-feeding large quantities to someone with an eating disorder is inappropriate and physiologically dangerous. It is safer and easier on the mind and body of the client to encourage slow, safe weight gain and/or reduce the feeling of fullness that often increases the urge to exercise or purge. Weight gain should not be the focus of treatment unless the client is medically compromised. Regular medical assessment (blood tests, blood pressure (postural drop), heart rate and body temperature) is essential throughout treatment, with hospitalisation required for the most severe cases.

- In sports where low BM or low body-fat levels are desirable, some athletes or coaches are sometimes unrealistic in setting goals of BM and composition. A discussion with the athlete or coach can sometimes be effective in resetting BM and body-fat levels to a more realistic and healthy level.

Objective information for athletes with eating disorders and disordered eating

- It may be useful to provide athletes, coaches and parents with objective information about the disadvantages of inadequate eating patterns and inappropriate BM/body-fat goals. These are summarised in Table 9.6.

- The dietitian may need to justify the nutritional benefit of every food recommended for the athlete to consume, since irrational phobias about some foods may exist.

- A frank explanation of the medical complications of eating disorders is essential.

Table 9.6 *Disadvantages of inappropriate BM/body-fat goals*

- Much of the weight loss is due to loss of muscle tissue.
- Training is ineffective and cannot be sustained with low levels of lean body tissue.
- Adequate carbohydrate intake is essential for muscle glycogen stores; inadequate intake will also limit the effectiveness of training.
- Low kilojoule intake and low muscle mass depress resting metabolic rate.
- Eating disorders may precipitate amenorrhoea and increase the risk of bone mass loss and stress fractures.
- Dehydration from the use of laxatives, diuretics, and fluid restriction will significantly impair performance.
- Restricted intake of a variety of foods may lead to nutrient inadequacies, affecting health as well as performance.
- The medical complications of severe eating disorders can be fatal.

Distinguishing between eating disorders and dietary extremism

- The DSM-IV criteria can be useful to distinguish between fad dieting, disordered eating, and eating disorders. However, disordered eating is not without risk to the health and mental well-being of the athlete and should be treated. It is also important to remember that all eating disorder sufferers have dieted at one time, and often the dieting progresses to the more extreme behaviours displayed with eating disorders.

Final comments

- It is useful to present case examples of successful athletes who do not follow fad diets and those who have a healthy and happy relationship with their physique and food. It is also helpful to point out that some athletes are successful in spite of, not because of, dietary extremism.

- Personal example is always the best teacher, so it is important that dietitians practise the guidelines of normal, healthy eating, without extremism. This is especially important where dietitians are attached to a team and may be in regular contact with a group of athletes.

- Among athletes, many diets, supplements and fads concerning foods are popular. It is important for a dietitian working with athletes to be familiar with these. Information on dietary supplements and ergogenic aids used by athletes is provided in Chapter 17, and popular fad diets are discussed in Chapter 7.

REFERENCES

American College of Sports Medicine. Position Stand: The female athlete triad. Med Sci Sport Exerc 1997;29:1–9.

American Dietetic Association. Position of the American Dietetic Association: Nutrition intervention in the treatment of anorexia nervosa, bulimia nervosa, and binge eating. J Am Diet Assoc 1994;94:902–7.

American Psychiatric Association. Diagnostic and statistical manual of mental disorders IV (4th edn). Washington DC: American Psychiatric Association, 1994;539–50.

Anderson AE. Diagnosis and treatment of males with eating disorders. In: Anderson AE, ed. Males with eating disorders. New York: Brunners/Mazel Publishers, 1990a:133–62.

Anderson AE. A proposed mechanism underlying eating disorders and other disorders of motivated behavior. In: Anderson AE, ed. Males with eating disorders. New York: Brunners/Mazel Publishers, 1990b:221–54.

Anderson AE. Eating disorders in males. In: Brownell KD, Fairburn CG, eds. Eating disorders and obesity. New York: The Guilford Press, 1995:177–82.

Anderson SL, Zager K, Hetzler RK, Nahikian-Nelms M, Syler G. Comparison of eating disorder inventory (EDI-2) scores of male body builders to the male college student subgroup. Int J Sport Nutr 1996;3:255–62.

Ashley CD, Smith JF, Robinson JB, Richardson MT. Disordered eating in female collegiate athletes and collegiate females in an advanced program of study: a preliminary investigation. Int J Sport Nutr 1996;6:391–401.

Beals KA, Manore MM. The prevalence and consequences of subclinical eating disorders in female athletes. Int J Sport Nutr 1994;4:175–95.

Benson JE, Allemann GE, Theintz GE, Howard H. Eating problems and calorie intake levels in Swiss adolescent athletes. Int J Sports Med 1990;11:249–52.

Bernardot D, Engelbert-Fenton K, Freeman K, Hartsough C, Nelson Steen S. Eating disorders in athletes: the dietitian's perspective. Sports Sci Exchange Roundtable 1994;5:1–8.

Bouchard C. Genetic aspects of human obesity. In: Bjorntorpp P, Brodoff BN, eds. Obesity. Philadelphia: Lippincott, 1992:343–51.

Brooks-Gunn J, Warren MP, Hamilton LH. The relation of eating problems and amenorrhoea in ballet dancers. Med Sci Sport Exerc 1987;19:41–4.

Brownell KD, Nelson Steen S, Wilmore JH. Weight regulation practices in athletes: analysis of metabolic and health effects. Med Sci Sport Exerc 1987;19:546–55.

Brownell KD, Rodin J. Prevalence of eating disorders in athletes. In: Brownell KD, Rodin J, Wilmore JH, eds. Eating, body weight and performance in athletes: disorders of modern society. Philadelphia: Lea & Febiger, 1992:128–45.

Brownell KD. Eating disorders in athletes. In: Brownell KD, Fairburn CG, eds. Eating disorders and obesity. New York: The Guilford Press, 1995:191–6.

Button EJ, Whitehouse A. Subclinical anorexia nervosa. Psychol Med 1981;11:509–16.

Cann EE, Martin MC, Genant HK, Jaffe RB. Decreased spinal mineral content in amenorrheic women. JAMA 1984;251:626–9.

Clark N. How to help the athlete with bulimia: practical tips and a case study. Int J Sport Nutr 1993;3:450–60.

Clark N. Counseling the athlete with an eating disorder: a case study. J Am Diet Assoc 1994;94:656–8.

Clark N. How to handle eating disorders among athletes. Gatorade Sports Sci Institute Coaches Corner, 1996.

Crago M, Shisslak CM, Estes LS. Eating disturbances among American minority groups: a review. Int J Eat Disord 1996;19:239–48.

Crisp A, Burns T. The clinical presentation of anorexia nervosa in males. Int J Eat Disord 1983;2:5–10.

Davis C, Cowles M. A comparison of weight and diet concerns and personality factors among female athletes and non-athletes. J Psychosom Res 1989;33:527–36.

DePalma MT, Koszewski WM, Case JG, Barile RJ, DePalma BF, Oliaro SM. Weight control practices of lightweight football players. Med Sci Sport Exerc 1993;25:694–701.

De Souza MJ, Metzger DA. Reproductive dysfunction in amenorrheic athletes and anorexic patients: a review. Med Sci Sport Exerc 1991;23:995–1007.

Dick RW. Eating disorders in NCAA athletic programs. Athletic Training JNATA 1991;26:136–40.

Drinkwater BL, Bruemmer J, Chestnut CH. Menstrual history as a determinant of current bone density in young athletes. JAMA 1990;263:545–8.

Drinkwater BL, Nilson K, Ott S, Chestnut CH. Bone mineral density after resumption of menses in amenorrheic athletes. JAMA 1986;256:380–2.

Dueck CA, Manore MM, Matt KS. Role of energy balance in athletic menstrual dysfunction. Int J Sport Nutr 1996b;6:165–90.

Dueck CA, Matt KS, Manore MM, Skinner JS. Treatment of athletic amenorrhoea with a diet and training intervention program. Int J Sport Nutr 1996a;6:24–40.

Dummer GM, Rosen LW, Heusner WW, Roberts PJ, Counsilman JE. Pathogenic weight-control behaviours of young competitive swimmers. Phys Sportsmed 1987;15(5):75–84.

Eichner ER. General health issues of low body weight and undereating in athletes. In: Brownell KD, Rodin J, Wilmore JH, eds. Eating, body weight and performance in athletes: disorders of modern society. Philadelphia: Lea & Febiger, 1992:191–201.

Emmons L. Predisposing factors differentiating adolescent dieters and nondieters. J Am Diet Assoc 1994;84:725–8, 731.

Evers CL. Dietary intake and symptoms of anorexia nervosa in female university dancers. J Am Diet Assoc 1987;87:66–8.

French SA, Perry CL, Leon CR, Fulkerson JA. Food preferences, eating patterns, and physical activity among adolescents: correlates of eating disorders symptoms. J Adolesc Health 1994;15:286–94.

French SA, Story M, Downes B, Resnick MC, Harris LJ, Blum R. Frequent dieting among adolescents: psychosocial and health behavior correlates. Am J Public Health 1995;85:695–701.

Friday KE, Drinkwater BL, Bruemmer B, Chestnut C, Chait A. Elevated plasma, low-density lipoprotein and high-density lipoprotein cholesterol levels in amenorrheic athletes: effects of endogenous hormone status and nutrient intake. J Clin Endocrin Metab 1993;77:1605–9.

Frusztajer NT, Dhuper S, Warren MP, Brooks-Gunn J, Fox RP. Nutrition and the incidence of stress fractures in ballet dancers. Am J Clin Nutr 1990;51:779–83.

Gadpaille WJ, Sanborn CF, Wagner WW. Athletic amenorrhoea, major affective disorders and eating disorders. Am J Psychiatry 1991;144:939–42.

Garner DM. Eating disorder inventory-2: professional manual. Odessa, Florida: Psychological Assessment Resources, 1991.

Garner DM, Garfinkel PE. The eating attitudes test: an index of the symptoms of anorexia nervosa. Psychol Med 1979;9:273–9.

Garner DM, Olmstead MP, Bohr Y, Garfinkel PE. The eating attitudes test: psychometric features and clinical correlates. Psychol Med 1982;12:871–8.

Garner DM, Olmsted MP, Polivy J. Manual of eating disorder inventory (EDI). Odessa, Florida: Psychological Assessment Resources, 1984.

Grandjean AC. Eating disorders—the role of the athletic trainer. Athletic Training JNATA 1991;26:105–12.

Grooms AM. The female athlete triad. J Florida MA 1996;83:479–81.

Hamilton LH, Brooks-Gunn J, Warren MP, Hamilton WG. The role of selectivity in the pathogenesis of eating problems in ballet dancers. Med Sci Sport Exerc 1988;20:560–5.

Hetland MD, Haarbo J, Christiansen C. Running induces menstrual disturbances but bone mass is unaffected, except in amenorrheic women. Am J Med 1993;95:53–60.

Hickerson JF, Johnson TE, Lee W, Sidor RJ. Nutrition and the precontest preparations of a male body builder. J Am Diet Assoc 1990;90:264–7.

Holland AJ, Sicotte N, Treasure J. Anorexia nervosa: evidence for a genetic basis. J Psychosom Res 1988;32:561–71.

Hsu LKG. Outcome of anorexia nervosa: a review of the literature (1954 to 1978). Arch Gen Psych 1980;37:1041–6.

Ibrahim H, Morrison N. Self-actualization and self-concept among athletes. Res Q 1976;47:68–79.

Johnson C. Initial consultation for patients with bulimia and anorexia nervosa. In: Garner DM, Garfinkel PE, eds. Handbook of psychotherapy of anorexia nervosa and bulimia. New York: Guilford Press, 1986:19–33.

Johnson MD. Disordered eating in active and athletic women. Clin Sports Med 1994;13:355–69.

Joy E, Clark N, Ireland ML, Martire J, Nattiv A, Varechok S. Team management of the female athlete triad, part 1: what to look for, what to ask. Phys Sportsmed 1997b;25:94–6, 101–2, 104, 107–8, 110.

Joy E, Clark N, Ireland ML, Martire J, Nattiv A, Varechok S. Team management of the female athlete triad, part 2: optimal treatment and prevention tactics. Phys Sportsmed 1997b;25:55–7, 60–1, 65–9.

Joyce JM, Warren DL, Humphries LL, Smith AJ, Coon JS. Osteoporosis in women with eating disorders: comparison of physical parameters, exercise and menstrual status with SPA and DPA evaluation. J Nucl Med 1990;31:325–31.

Kaiserauer SK, Snyder AC, Sleeper M, Zierath J. Nutritional, physiological and menstrual status of distance runners. Med Sci Sport Exerc 1989;21:120–5.

Kezer HA, Rogol AD. Physical exercise and menstrual cycle alterations: what are the mechanisms? Sports Med 1990;10:218–35.

King M. Eating disorders in a general practice population: prevalence, characteristics and follow-up at 12 to 18 months. Psychol Med 1989;14:S3–S11.

Kirchner EM, Lewis RD, O'Connor PJ. Bone mineral density and dietary intake of female college gymnasts. Med Sci Sport Exerc 1995;27:543–9.

Kirchner EM, Lewis RD, O'Connor PJ. Effect of past gymnastics participation on adult bone mass. J Appl Physiol 1996;80:226–32.

Kleiner SM, Bazzarre TL, Litchford MD. Metabolic profiles, diet, and health practices of championship male and female body builders. J Am Diet Assoc 1990;90:962–7.

Klemchuk HP, Hutchinson CB, Frank RI. Body dissatisfaction and eating-related problems on the college campus: usefulness of the Eating Disorder Inventory with a nonclinical population. J Counsel Psychol 1990;37:297–305.

Kurtzman FD, Yager J, Landsverk J, Wiesmeier E, Bourka DC. Eating disorders among selected female student populations at UCLA. J Am Diet Assoc 1989;89:45–53.

Leon GR. Eating disorders in female athletes. Sports Med 1991;12:219–27.

Lindeman AK. Self-esteem: its application to eating disorders and athletes. Int J Sport Nutr 1994;4:237–52.

Loosli AR, Benson J. Nutritional intake in adolescent athletes. Pediatr Clin North Am 1990;37:1143–52.

Loucks AB. Effects of exercise training on the menstrual cycle: existence and mechanisms. Med Sci Sport Exerc 1990;22:275–80.

Loucks AB, Vaitukaitis J, Cameron JL, et al. The reproductive system and exercise in women. Med Sci Sport Exerc 1992;24:S288–S93.

Manore MM. Chronic dieting in active women: what are the consequences? Women's Health Issues 1996;6:332–41.

Mortenson GM, Hoerr SL, Garner DM. Predictors of body satisfaction in college women. J Am Diet Assoc 1993;93:1037–9.

Nattiv A, Agostini R, Drinkwater B, Yeager K. The female athlete triad. Clin Sports Med 1994;13:405–18.

Nattiv A, Lynch L. The female athlete triad: managing an acute risk to long-term health. Phys Sportsmed 1994;22:60–8.

Noden M. Special report: dying to win. Sports Illustrated 1994;81:52–60.

O'Connor PJ, Lewis RD, Kirchner EM. Eating disorder symptoms in female college gymnasts. Med Sci Sport Exerc 1995;27:550–5.

O'Connor PJ, Lewis RD, Kirchner EM, Cook DB. Eating disorder symptoms in former female college gymnasts: relations with body composition. Am J Clin Nutr 1996;64:840–3.

Olson MS, Williford HN, Richards LA, Brown JA, Pugh S. Self-reports on the eating disorder inventory by female aerobic instructors. Percep & Motor Skills 1996;82:1051–8.

Otis C. Exercise-associated amenorrhoea. Clin Sports Med 1992;11:351–62.

Parry-Jones B, Parry-Jones WL. History of bulimia and bulimia nervosa. In: Brownell KD, Fairburn CG, eds. Eating Disord Obesity. New York: The Guilford Press, 1995:145–50.

Piran N, Lerner P, Garfinkel PE, Kennedy SH, Brouilette C. Personality disorders in anorexic patients. Int J Eat Disord 1988;7:589–99.

Pugliese MT, Lifshitz F, Grad G, Fort P, Marks-Katz M. Fear of obesity: a cause of short stature and delayed puberty. New Engl J Med 1983;309:513–18.

Putukian M. The female triad. Med Clin North Am 1994;78:345–56.

Ratnasuriya RH, Eisler I, Szmukler GI, Russell GF. Anorexia nervosa: outcome and prognostic factors after 20 years. Brit J Psychol 1991;158:495–502.

Rencken ML, Chesnut CH, Drinkwater BL. Bone density at multiple skeletal sites in amenorrheic athletes. JAMA 1996;276:238–40.

Robinson TL, Snow-Harter C, Taaffe DR, Gillis D, Shaw J, Marcus R. Gymnasts exhibit higher bone mass than runners despite similar prevalence of amenorrhoea and oligomenorrhoea. Bone Min Res 1995;10:26–35.

Rodin J. Cultural and psychosocial determinants of weight concerns. Ann Intern Med 1993;119:643–5.

Rodin J, Larson L. Societal factors and the ideal body shape. In: Brownell KD, Rodin J, Wilmore JH, eds. Eating, body weight and performance in athletes: disorders of modern society. Philadelphia: Lea & Febiger, 1992:146–58.

Root MP. Persistent, disordered eating as a gender-specific, post traumatic stress response to sexual assault. Psychotherapy 1991;28:96–102.

Rosen LW, Hough DO. Pathogenic weight-control behaviours of female college gymnasts. Phys Sportsmed 1988;16:141–4.

Rosen LW, McKeag DB, Hough DO, Curley V. Pathogenic weight-control behavior in female athletes. Phys Sportsmed 1986;14:79–86.

Rucinski A. Relationship of body image and dietary intake of competitive ice skaters. J Am Diet Assoc 1989;89:98–100.

Russell G. Bulimia nervosa: an ominous variant of anorexia nervosa. Psych Med 1979;9:429–48.

Sandri SC. On dancers and diet. Int J Sport Nutr 1993;3:334–42.

Silverman JA. History of anorexia nervosa. In: Brownell KD, Fairburn CG, eds. Eating disorders and obesity. New York: The Guilford Press, 1995:141–4.

Silverstone PH. Is chronic low self-esteem the cause of eating disorders? Med Hypotheses 1992;39:311–15.

Slemenda CW, Johnson CC. High intensity activities in young women: site specific bone mass effects among female figure skaters. Bone Miner 1993;20:125–32.

Snow-Harter CM. Bone health and prevention of osteoporosis in active and athletic women. Clin Sports Med 1994;13:389–404.

Steen SN, Wilmore JH. Weight regulation practices in athletes: analysis of metabolic and health effects. Med Sci Sport Exerc 1987;19:546–56.

Steen SN, Brownell KD. Patterns of weight loss and regain in wrestlers: has the tradition changed? Med Sci Sport Exerc 1990;22:762–8.

Stephenson JN. Medical consequences and complications of anorexia nervosa and bulimia nervosa in female athletes. Athlete Training JNATA 1991;26:130–5.

Stoutjesdyk D, Jevne R. Eating disorders among high performance athletes. J Youth Adolesc 1993;22:271–82.

Sundgot-Borgen J. Prevalence of eating disorders in female athletes. Int J Sport Nutr 1993a;3:29–40.

Sundgot-Borgen J. Nutrient intake of female elite athletes suffering from eating disorders. Int J Sport Nutr 1993b;17:176–88.

Sundgot-Borgen J. Eating disorders in female athletes. Sports Med 1994a;17:176–88.

Sundgot-Borgen J. Risk and trigger factors for the development of eating disorders in female elite athletes. Med Sci Sport Exerc 1994b;26:414–19.

Sykora C, Grilo CM, Wilfley DE, Brownell KD. Eating, weight, and dieting disturbances in male and female lightweight and heavyweight rowers. Int J Eat Disorder 1993;14:203–11.

Szmukler G, Russell G. Outcome and prognosis of anorexia nervosa. In: Brownell KD, Rodin J, Wilmore JH, eds. Handbook of eating disorders: physiology, psychology and treatment of obesity, anorexia, and bulimia. New York: Basic Books, 1985:283–300.

Thompson RA, Sherman RT. Helping athletes with eating disorders. Champaign, Illinois: Human Kinetics, 1993:97–170.

Thornton JS. Feast or famine: eating disorders in athletes. Phys Sportsmed 1990;18:116–22.

Tipton CM, Oppliger RA. The Iowa wrestling study: lessons for physicians. Iowa Med 1984;74:381–5.

Van de Loo DA, Johnson MD. The young female athlete. Clin Sports Med 1995;14:687–707.

Walberg JL, Johnston CS. Menstrual function and eating behaviour in female recreational weight lifters and competitive body builders. Med Sci Sport Exerc 1991;23:30–6.

Warren BJ, Stanton AL, Blessing DL. Disordered eating patterns in competitive female athletes. Int J Eat Disorders 1990;9:565–9.

Webster S, Rutt R, Weltman A. Physiological effects of a weight loss regimen practiced by college wrestlers. Med Sci Sport Exerc 1990;22:229–34.

Wichmann S, Martin DR. Eating disorders in athletes. Phys Sportsmed 1993;21:126–217.

Wilmore JH. Eating and weight disorders in the female athlete. Int J Sport Nutr 1991;1:104–17.

Wilmore JH, Wambsgans KC, Brenner M, et al. Is there energy conservation in amenorrheic compared with eumenorrheic distance runners? J Appl Physiol 1992;72:15–22.

Wolf EM, Akamatsu TJ. Exercise involvement and eating-disordered characteristics in college students. Eating Disorders: J Treat Prev 1994;2:308–18.

Woscyna G. Nutritional aspects of eating disorders: nutrition education and counseling as a component of treatment. Athletic Training JNATA 1991;26:141–7.

Yates A. Current perspectives on the eating disorders: I. History, psychological and biological aspects. J Am Acad Child Adolesc 1989;6:813–28.

Yates A. Biologic consideration in the etiology of eating disorders. Pediatr Ann 1992;21:739–44.

Yeager KK, Agostini R, Nattiv A, Drinkwater B. The female athlete triad: disordered eating, amenorrhoea, osteoporosis. Med Sci Sport Exerc 1993;25:775–7.

CHAPTER 10

Bone, exercise, nutrition and menstrual disturbances

Deborah Kerr, Karim Khan and Kim Bennell

10.1 INTRODUCTION

Bone is a tissue that has gained increasing attention in the past two decades because of the media attention afforded stress fractures and the increasing rate of osteoporotic fractures. Furthermore, the advances in imaging bone have allowed researchers to better understand this dynamic tissue. Thus, the sports dietitian must become familiar with the new concepts of bone physiology, the evidence regarding the optimal types of exercise for bone health, and the influence of calcium and nutrition on bone. Also, athletes and clients expect the sports dietitian to be a resource regarding the clinical aspects of menstrual disturbance and bone health, and stress fractures.

We begin by summarising the fundamental concepts of bone physiology that sports dietitians will come across in their reading, their interaction with fellow health-care providers, and with clients who read widely and search the Internet. We explain the vital concepts of bone remodelling and the site-specific nature of bone's response to exercise; we explain how bone is measured, and we define osteoporosis and sports osteopenia. We then summarise the growing body of evidence regarding the effect of exercise on bone. The reader may be surprised to find that genetics plays a huge role, and that the effect of exercise, although important, is not massive, even with quite intense exercise. The subject of calcium and bone is clearly central to the sports dietitian, but the answer to the question 'Does calcium promote bone health' is not as straightforward as was once presumed. We summarise the many studies that the sports dietitian must be familiar with.

The final sections of the chapter relate to abnormalities of physiology, and the role of nutrition in prevention and treatment. We discuss the influence of menstrual disturbance on bone health, as this is a large and apparently increasing problem among female athletes. The sports dietitian must know how to advise these athletes. Also, we discuss the risk factors for stress fracture and focus on the role that nutrition might play in preventing this injury. Finally, we provide practice tips for sports dietitians.

10.2 THE FUNDAMENTALS OF BONE PHYSIOLOGY

Bone is a dynamic tissue, which reflects the biological principle of adaptation of structure to function and the metabolic role of mineral homeostasis. The skeleton is made up of two types of bone. The outer bone is known as cortical and the inner softer core is known as trabecular (the more metabolically active bone). The skeleton is designed to provide strength needed to withstand the mechanical forces of daily weight-bearing. Structurally, the long bones of the skeleton are often referred to as appendicular bones, and the bones of the trunk, as the axial skeleton.

Exercise generates loading within the skeleton, which effects the structure at the skeletal site at which the strain is developed. Physical activity is protective of bone, and studies of athletes show a higher bone mass than those who are inactive. In amenorrhoea, however, bone loss occurs due to the absence of oestrogen. But there is some evidence that if the mechanical load is sufficient it may be protective of bone mass at the site of loading (Young et al. 1994; Robinson et al. 1995).

Bone is continually being broken down and rebuilt in a process known as remodelling, under the regulation of systemic hormones and local growth factors. The remodelling cycle consists of five successive events: quiescence, activation, resorption, reversal and formation (Parfitt 1984). Following resorption of a packet of bone by the osteoclast, new bone is laid down by the osteoblast. When bone resorption exceeds formation, bone loss occurs, which if prolonged can lead to osteoporosis and increased risk of fracture. The hormonal status interacts with the mechanical environment to influence bone remodelling. In conditions of low oestrogen, such as amenorrhoea or after menopause, bone loss occurs, even if physical activity is high. Compared with the general female population, female athletes have a higher prevalence of menstrual alterations, including delayed menarche, anovulation, abnormal luteal phase, oligomenorrhoea and amenorrhoea (Malina et al. 1978; Kaiserauer et al. 1989; Bennell et al. 1997).

The bone remodelling cycle takes between four to six months to complete in adults (Epstein 1988). This is an important concept when evaluating the bone density literature. Ideally intervention studies are the best way to study exercise effects on bone, and these studies should be of at least 12 months duration.

10.2.1 Mechanical loading principles

Loading of the skeleton occurs from the force induced by the contracting muscle (muscle pull) and the gravitational-induced strain. In response to the mechanical loading of bone, strain-related potentials are produced. Frost (1990) proposed that there was a minimum effective strain (MESm) for bone modelling and remodelling and that only when bone strain exceeds the MESm will there be a net gain in bone. If the strain is greater than is optimum for the area of bone under strain an osteogenic response is induced so that the bone can withstand the new loading situation. By rearranging the internal structure the strain is reduced to optimum levels. This is thought to be mediated by increased osteoblast activity, but the mechanism by which the mechanical strain is transduced into a chemical signal at the cellular level is unknown.

There may be a variety of load thresholds for different bones (Martin & McCulloch 1987). Weight-bearing bones, such as the calcaneus, may require a much greater load to induce a change in bone mass than non-weight-bearing bones (Harber et al. 1991). Weight-bearing bones are acted on by both gravitational forces and muscular pull, whereas the forces on non-weight-bearing bones are mostly muscle pull.

Several studies have examined the effect of weight-supported exercise on bone density. In exercises such as swimming and cycling, muscle pull, but not gravitational force, is in operation. Orwoll et al. (1989) found in female masters swimmers there was no significant difference in bone density compared to non-exercisers. However, in the male swimmers, the forearm and lumbar spine bone density was significantly greater compared with non-exercisers. It was unclear why the results were different between the sexes, as both males and females had been swimming for a similar number of years and trained for a similar amount of time. It was suggested that the muscle pull may have been greater in the males compared with the females. A more recent study in eumenorrheic elite female athletes compared the effects of swimming and gymnastics on bone density (Taaffe et al. 1995). The gymnasts had a higher bone density at the femoral neck than the swimmers. At the lumbar spine and whole body sites, when adjusted for body weight, the spine bone mineral density (BMD) was higher in the gymnasts compared with the swimmers and controls. The femoral neck BMD in the swimmers was less than the controls, even though the swimmers participated in some resistance training. The authors suggested that the amount of time spent in a weight-supported environment may negate the effects of resistance training. However, an intervention study is needed to confirm these findings.

These studies indicate the importance of both gravitational forces and muscle pull in maintaining bone density. Also that the action of exercise is specific to the site of loading and that response will be determined by the location within the skeleton. Weight-bearing bones require both muscle pull and gravitational forces and therefore a much greater load threshold compared with non-weight-bearing bones which may only require muscle pull.

10.2.2 *The measurement of bone mineral density*

Bone densitometry measures the average bone mineral within the region scanned, known as the bone mineral density (BMD). The sites measured are the hip, forearm and lumbar spine, which are the most common fracture sites. The whole body scan can estimate the total bone density and body composition. The BMD can be measured by single and dual energy absorptiometry (DXA) and quantitative computerised tomography. The most common method is DXA, but ultrasound is being used increasingly. Low bone mass is defined in terms of how far the measurement falls below the reference range for the young healthy female. A 'fracture threshold' or a cut-off point is used to define osteoporosis and is based on the range of BMD measurements in the population with vertebral or hip fractures.

10.2.3 *Definition of sports osteopenia and osteoporosis*

Osteoporosis is a condition of low bone mass associated with greater bone fragility and increased risk of fractures (World Health Organisation 1994). Clinically, osteoporosis is defined in terms of the BMD that is below the age-adjusted reference range. An individual is considered osteoporotic if their BMD is 2.5 standard deviation (SD) or more below the young adult mean for bone density. Osteopenia is a condition of low bone mass in which the BMD is more than one SD below the young adult mean, but less that 2.5 SD below this value. Sports osteopenia refers to low bone mass, seen most commonly in female athletes.

The risk of developing osteoporosis and subsequent fractures is largely determined by the peak bone mass, achieved in adolescence and early adulthood. Up to 60–80% of the variability in bone density has been attributed to genetic factors (Pocock et al. 1987; Krall et al. 1993). BMD is strongly linked to bone strength, and resistance to fracture.

10.3 *EXERCISE EFFECT ON BONE IN ATHLETES AND HEALTHY PEOPLE*

Exercise is critical for maintaining both the architecture and mass of the skeleton. Throughout the skeleton there appears to be different strain thresholds for particular bones, which are genetically coded. Weight-bearing bones appear to require both muscle pull and gravitational forces, whereas bones in the upper limbs, not subject to the forces of weight bearing, may require only muscle pull for the maintenance of bone mass. In amenorrhoea, weight-bearing bones may be partially protected by mechanical loading, whereas non-weight-bearing bones may not (Young et al. 1994).

10.3.1 *Cross-sectional studies of exercise and bone mass*

Early evidence for the positive effect of exercise on bone mass has come from cross-sectional studies which have shown a higher bone density in both male and female athletes than more sedentary controls (Nilsson et al. 1971; Dalen et al. 1974; Huddleston et al. 1980; Lane et al. 1986). Higher bone densities observed in male athletes, however, may have been confounded by their use of anabolic steroids (Nilsson et al. 1971; Colletti et al. 1989; Karlsson et al. 1993). However, studies in women participating in weight-bearing activities show higher bone densities (Ballard et al.

1990; Risser et al. 1990), as do those of women involved in weight-training programs (Davee et al. 1990; Heinrich et al. 1990).

There is evidence for the site-specific effects of muscle pull from studies in tennis players. In a group of professional tennis players the cortical thickness of the playing arm was greater by 34.9% in the men and 28.4% in the women, compared with the control side (Jones et al. 1977). In the study by Huddleston and colleagues (1980), a group of 35 elderly male tennis players who had been playing for at least 20 years had a greater bone mineral content in the radius of the playing arm compared with the non-playing arm.

When comparing athletes with non-athletic controls or different athletic groups, there are often differences in body size. In the study by Heinrich et al. (1990) the body builders were significantly heavier than the other athletes, and had the highest bone density. A large study of young women aged 18 to 35 years found the best predictors of BMD were weight, age, family history and physical activity (Rubin et al. 1999). Body weight explained over half of the variability in BMD at the hip and spine.

These results stress the importance of controlling for body weight in studies of bone mass and exercise. Another problem with cross-sectional studies of athletes is that a pre-selection bias may exist. Athletes may already have a higher bone density before commencing an exercise program or may be able to continue exercising without injury because of a high bone mass (Marcus & Carter 1988).

10.3.2 *Randomised interventions for endurance*

Studies of exercise intervention on bone density have shown variable results, but generally suggest that weight-bearing exercise (e.g. jogging, walking, running and gymnastics) has a positive effect on bone mass. Results of some of these studies have been criticised for several reasons. In early studies of bone density, the selection of the site for measuring bone density was not specific to the exercise regimen due to the inability to measure bone density at all sites (Smith et al. 1981; Sandler et al. 1987; Prince et al. 1991). Also, a number of studies have had small sample sizes or the subjects had not been truly randomised (thus biasing interpretation) (Aloia et al. 1978; Krolner et al. 1983; Simkin et al. 1987; Cavanaugh et al. 1988; Nielsen et al. 1992; Bloomfield et al. 1993).

Intervention studies in younger women have examined the effect of high-impact aerobic exercise on the skeleton. Bassey and Ramsdale (1994) used a combination of a home- and gym-based program, with one group randomised to a low-impact group and the other to a high-impact group. Bone density was assessed by DXA at the lumbar spine and neck of femur. At six months the low-impact group was crossed over to join the high-impact group. The number of subjects recruited at baseline was not recorded but there were 27 subjects at six months and 19 subjects who completed the study. Improvements in leg strength were only recorded for the first six months and were unimpressive (10% for the low-impact group; 12% for the high-impact group). However, a 3.4% increase in trochanteric BMD was seen in the high-impact group at six months.

10.3.3 *Randomised interventions for strength*

Although animal studies would suggest that strength training may have a beneficial effect on bone mass, few prospective studies have been undertaken in pre-menopausal and postmenopausal women. In several studies the number of subjects has also been too small to provide definitive conclusions about the effect of strength training on bone density (Rockwell et al. 1990; Notelovitz et al. 1991; Snow-Harter et al. 1992; Vuori et al. 1994). Some studies have allowed subjects to choose which group they would like to be in rather than randomly allocating subjects into groups (Gleeson et al. 1990; Rockwell et al. 1990; Peterson et al. 1991). Other studies have not used a resistance-training program that would ensure high skeletal loading (Chow et al. 1987; Gleeson et al. 1990).

In younger premenopausal women, strength training has shown a positive effect at the lumbar spine in several studies (Snow-Harter et al. 1992; Friedlander et al. 1995; Lohman et al. 1995). In an 18-month strength-training program in pre-menopausal women, Lohman et al. (1995) showed a significant increase in bone mass in women in the exercise intervention group at the lumbar spine and femur trochanter compared with the control group.

A randomised intervention study over eight months in young women found a significant exercise effect at the lumbar spine from running and resistance training (Snow-Harter et al. 1992). The progressive resistance-exercise program consisted of three sets of eight to 12 repetitions, performed three times a week, while the running group progressively increased their running so that they were running about ten miles by the end of the study. There was a significant increase at the lumbar spine for both the running group (1.3 ± 1.6%) and the resistance-trained group (1.2 ± 1.8%) compared with the control group, but no change at the neck of femur site. The number of repetitions from running may have been sufficient to stimulate bone formation equivalent to resistance training. This suggests that in young women, running may be equally as effective as resistance training in increasing bone mass.

Two randomised studies using strength-training intervention have been conducted on postmenopausal women (Nelson et al. 1994; Kerr et al. 1996). Nelson et al. (1994), in a randomised controlled trial of one year of strength training in post-menopausal women, found a significant effect at the femoral neck and lumbar spine. In a unilateral exercise study, Kerr et al. (1996) compared two strength-training regimes that differed only in the number of repetitions of the weight lifted. The strength program significantly increased bone density at the hip and forearm sites whereas the endurance program had no significant effect (Figure 10.1). This study indicates that strength training was specific to the site of loading, and dependent on the weight lifted.

10.1a Trochanter hip site

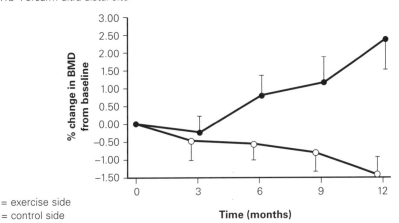

10.1b Forearm ultra-distal site

● = exercise side
○ = control side

Figure 10.1 *The effects of a one-year unilateral strength-training intervention percentage change (SEM) in bone mineral density, comparing the exercise with control side at (a) the trochanter hip site (p < 0.01); (b) forearm ultra-distal site (p < 0.01) from the control side (Reproduced from J Bone Miner Res 1996;11:218–25 with permission of the American Society for Bone and Mineral Research)*

From studies in both premenopausal and postmenopausal women, strength training appears to be effective in either slowing or preventing bone loss. Women of all ages should be encouraged to regularly participate in either weight-bearing activity or strength training.

10.4 CALCIUM INTAKE AND BONE MINERAL AT VARIOUS LIFE STAGES

The human skeleton retains the rather primitive function of serving as both a depot for the storage of excess calcium and as a reservoir, available to replenish calcium during times of deprivation. This portable supply of calcium, however, is a double-edged sword. When the calcium reserve, our skeleton, is called upon to meet dietary insufficiencies, bone strength is compromised.

Calcium balance is determined by the balance between the dietary intake of calcium, the amount of calcium absorbed from the intestine, and the amount excreted in the urine. The plasma calcium levels are tightly regulated by hormonal control. Hence, when negative balance occurs due to low oestrogen levels, demineralisation from the skeleton will follow. The dietary calcium requirement is based on the amount of dietary calcium, which will maintain calcium balance and optimal bone accretion rates.

Balance studies suggest there may be a threshold effect for calcium intake. This means that calcium retention will increase up to a threshold, beyond which further calcium does not result in increased calcium retention. Calcium absorption from the small intestine occurs by active absorption at low levels, but by passive absorption at higher levels of calcium intake. Calcium requirements are determined from balance studies by the intake at which calcium intake and losses are equal. This is not the same as the Recommended Dietary Intake (RDI) or Recommended Dietary Allowance (RDA) which are set to meet the calcium requirements of 95% of the population. The Australian RDIs are currently under review. The National Health & Medical Research Council (1991) in Australia recommended that the dietary intake of calcium be increased from 800 mg/d in premenopausal women to 1000 mg/d in postmenopausal women. This increase accounts for the accelerated loss of calcium from the skeleton after menopause.

10.4.1 *Effect of calcium intake during childhood and adolescence on bone mineral*

To help make sense of the various studies that we are about to summarise, it is useful to review one aspect of gastrointestinal physiology. There is a complex homeostatic control between the amount of calcium ingested, the amount retained after obligatory losses from the various sites (digestive tract, skin, nails, hair, sweat and urine) and the amount that is finally incorporated into the skeleton. The amount of calcium that is retained in bone is called calcium retention.

A recent longitudinal study in growing children documented calcium retention efficiencies of 33% for boys and 29% for girls (Bailey et. al. 2000). Higher calcium efficiencies appear to compensate for low dietary intakes of calcium. In another study, when calcium intakes dropped to 400 mg/d, absorption efficiency rose to 50% (Abrams et al. 1997). This is striking when compared with the calcium retention of 4–8% in the adult with skeletal deficiency. It is, therefore, only in severe cases of dietary restriction that bone mineral accrual is compromised. Such cases are seldom observed in western cultures. In severe cases bone growth may proceed at a slower rate and bones are usually of normal shape and size but have lower than normal bone mineral mass. Bone growth relates directly to the genetic and mechanical (and not the dietary) control of linear growth and periosteal and endosteal expansion.

Against this background of physiology, all the calcium consumed is not directly transferred into the bone reservoir. Randomised, double-blind, placebo-controlled studies of children found that calcium supplementation given during the growing years increased bone mineral by about 1–3%, independently of energy intake or other nutritional factors (Johnston et al. 1992; Lloyd et al. 1993; Lee et al. 1994, 1995; Nowson et al. 1995, 1997). In most follow-up studies, however, after withdrawal of supplementation, the benefit achieved by the formerly supplemented group decreased or disappeared (Slemenda et al. 1993, 1997; Nowson et al. 1995; Lee et al. 1996). In one of these calcium supplementation studies, serum osteocalcin (a marker of bone formation) was 15% lower in the supplemented than in the placebo group, but after the intervention ceased, this difference disappeared (Johnston et al. 1992).

One study in pre-pubertal girls demonstrated a positive effect on BMD when calcium as milk extract was added to food products (Bonjour et al. 1997). One year after supplementation was withdrawn, girls with habitually low dietary calcium intakes, who had previously been supplemented, still had greater increments in BMC and BMD in the femoral shaft than the previously unsupplemented children.

Results of calcium intervention studies in adolescent girls are similar to those performed in younger children. Teenage girls (mean age 14, range 10–17) supplemented with 1000 mg of calcium for 18 months had a 1.5% increase in BMD at both the spine and total hip. The greatest effect occurred during the first six months of supplementation (Nowson et al. 1997).

Exposure to high calcium intakes, even for three years prior to puberty, appears then to have no long-term effect on bone mineral. Although seemingly surprising, this finding is consistent with the hypothesis that bone changes following supplementation with dietary calcium are due to reversible changes in bone remodelling (Kanis 1994). As an extension of this argument, Kanis contends that the calcium RDA for young healthy individuals is unknown and that 'there is no good evidence to suggest that variations in dietary intake of calcium are prejudicial for skeletal health in young individuals who take a reasonably balanced diet' (Kanis 1994).

These findings are consistent with recent findings from the *University of Saskatchewan pediatric bone mineral accrual study* (Bailey 1997). Children appear to have the ability to absorb and retain calcium at levels that at least partially compensate for low levels of dietary calcium (Martin et al. 1997). Thus, although children have enormous skeletal demand for calcium during the years of peak bone mineral accrual, they may be able to meet these demands by a combination of increased calcium absorption efficiency, which may rise to as high as 80% (Kanis & Passmore 1989; Martin et al. 1997), and by borrowing calcium from the cortical shell (Bailey et al. 1989; Parfitt 1994).

Once peak bone mass is achieved, it is primarily the mechanical forces acting on the skeleton that stimulate bone formation. We are not only 'what we eat' as the adage suggests, we are also 'what we do'.

10.4.2 *Effect of calcium intake on BMD during the premenopausal years*

During the premenopausal years, when most women are oestrogen replete, calcium retention and absorption operate at peak adult efficiency. This results in lower dietary calcium requirements than at any other time during life. A prospective study of young women suggested that bone mineral mass may even be augmented after the cessation of linear growth—perhaps into the third decade (Recker et al. 1992).

There have been very few calcium intervention studies in adult premenopausal women. Smith et al. (1989) found no effect of four years of calcium supplementation on wrist BMC. Baran and colleagues found that increasing calcium intake from 960 to 1600 mg/d prevented bone loss over a three-year period. However, this study has been criticised for its small numbers (Mazess & Barden 1991). In large longitudinal studies with a large sample size there has been no effect (on BMD or rates of bone loss) in subjects with high or low levels of calcium intake (Riggs et al. 1987; Mazess & Barden 1991).

As studies comparing BMD in adult communities that have different intakes of calcium do not reveal differences in bone mass, the effect of genetic and other environmental factors on bone mass may be greater than that of dietary calcium (Kanis 1994). Even the strongest proponents of calcium for bone health concede that 'the evidence for a relation between bone density, bone loss, and estimated calcium intake in individuals is somewhat inconclusive' (Nordin & Heaney 1990). The difficulties in measuring current and retrospective intakes in free-living people in combination with other nutrients (phosphorus, protein and sodium), and individual differences in obligatory calcium losses, contribute to this uncertainty (Avioli & Heaney 1991).

10.4.3 *Effect of calcium intake on BMD during the early postmenopausal years*

It appears that the biological response to calcium differs between women of early postmenopausal years and late postmenopausal years. Thus, we summarise the data for women in each of these life stages separately. We use the term 'perimenopause' to describe the years on both sides of the final menstrual period, when the hormonal milieu is in flux. We distinguish studies in women who were less than five years postmenopausal from those in women who were more than five years postmenopausal.

Evidence for the benefits of calcium during the perimenopausal and early postmenopausal years is either conflicting or non-existent. It is accepted that decreased bone mass at the menopause is related to diminished hormone levels, which is akin to raising the bone bending 'set point'. Decreases in bone mass in perimenopausal women, therefore, are not related to nutrient deficiency but to oestrogen withdrawal, and are not even substantially influenced by high doses of calcium. There may be a one-time, rapid downward adjustment of bone mass of as much as 15% of premenopausal levels (Heaney 1990).

There are several key studies of calcium and bone in this age group. A daily calcium supplement of 500 mg did not retard early postmenopausal lumbar spine bone loss in either Danish women who had a mean dietary calcium intake of 1 000 mg/d (Nilas et al. 1984) or in American women who had mean dietary calcium intakes of around 700 mg/d (Ettinger et al. 1987; Dawson-Hughes et al. 1990). Although calcium supplementation to 2 000 mg/d slowed forearm and total body cortical bone loss compared with placebo, it did not slow trabecular bone loss at the spine or ultra-distal radius (Nilas et al. 1984).

Cumming (1990) performed a meta-analysis of six calcium intervention studies (Horsman et al. 1977; Recker et al. 1977; Ettinger et al. 1987; Polley et al. 1987; Riis et al. 1987; Smith et al. 1989) conducted in 'healthy' women with a mean age around 50 years and found a positive effect of calcium on BMD that ranged from 0–1.7% with a mean increase of 0.8% per year. Based on these studies 'a calcium supplement of around 1 000 mg/d in early postmenopausal women can prevent loss of just under 1% of bone mass per year at all bone sites except at the vertebrae' (Cumming 1990). This effect size is intermediate between hormone replacement therapy and no treatment. Studies published since Cumming's meta-analysis support his conclusions (Dawson-Hughes et al. 1990; Elders et al. 1994).

10.4.4 *Effect of calcium intake during the later postmenopausal years on BMD*

Postmenopausal osteoporosis is associated with accelerated remodelling and accelerated bone loss (Heaney et al. 1978; Stepan et al. 1987). Notably, calcium supplementation in later postmenopausal women is associated with the maintenance, and not gain, of skeletal mass (Albanese et al. 1975; Smith et al. 1975; Horsman et al. 1977; Recker et al. 1977; Lamke et al. 1978; Smith et al. 1981; Recker & Heaney 1985; Dawson-Hughes 1991; Heaney 1993; Prince et al. 1995). For example, in healthy women who were more than five years postmenopausal and had dietary calcium intake of less than 400 mg/d, supplementation to 800 mg/d significantly reduced bone loss (Dawson-Hughes et al. 1990). However, no benefit was observed at even moderate intakes of calcium. This supports the argument that calcium is a 'threshold nutrient'.

Reid (1993) and others (Horsman et al. 1977; Recker et al. 1977; Smith et al. 1989; Prince et al. 1991) found that appendicular bone loss slows with calcium supplementation. These authors also found a positive effect of calcium supplementation on axial bone loss in women who had been postmenopausal an average of 10 years. This is consistent with findings that such supplementation was ineffective in women who had just reached menopause (Ettinger et al. 1985; Riis et al. 1987). Reid demonstrated a positive effect of calcium on BMD at the proximal femur (Reid et al. 1993).

Studies that have found calcium supplementation to be effective (Baran et al. 1989; Dawson-Hughes et al. 1990; Elders et al. 1991; Prince et al. 1991) used soluble calcium salts or dairy products as the supplement; whereas calcium carbonate has not been found to be an effective supplement (Ettinger et al. 1985; Riis et al. 1987; Dawson-Hughes et al. 1990). There are differences in the short-term bioavailability of different calcium preparations (Reid et al. 1986) that might contribute to their effect on bone loss. Long-term (four-year) studies have followed calcium-supplemented women (aged 10–15 years postmenopausal) and shown a protective effect of calcium supplementation on bone density (Prince et al. 1995; Reid et al. 1995).

The mechanism whereby calcium attenuates bone loss in postmenopausal women is most likely via decreased activation of new remodelling sites, and continuation of early bone formation at the previously existing bone remodelling sites (Kanis 1994). This phenomenon is known as the 'bone remodelling transient' (Heaney 1994). Because there is still a deficit between the calcium lost in resorption and the calcium replaced in formation, bone continues to be lost, albeit at a slower rate, despite calcium supplementation.

10.5 MENSTRUAL DISTURBANCE IN ATHLETES

With increased participation in vigorous exercise by women, menstrual disturbances have become more common. The term 'athletic amenorrhoea' has been used to describe the menstrual disturbance which occurs in female athletes. Amenorrhoea refers to the absence of menstrual bleeding. Primary amenorrhoea is defined as where no menstrual bleeding has occurred by 16 years of age; whereas secondary amenorrhoea refers to the absence of menstrual cycles in women who have had established periods. The definition for the diagnosis of amenorrhoea varies, but is usually the absence of menstrual period for three to six months (American College of Sports Medicine 1992). Oligomenorrhoea refers to an irregular menstrual cycle. In athletic women the diagnosis of 'athletic amenorrhoea' should only be made after a thorough examination and exclusion of other possible causes (Highet 1989). As eating disorders are not uncommon in sports where low body weight is desirable, this should be considered a possible cause of 'athletic amenorrhoea'.

10.5.1 Mechanisms of menstrual disturbances in athletes

Various mechanisms have been proposed to explain menstrual disturbances in athletes, including body composition, training intensity and diet. To date it appears that no single factor is solely implicated, and a variety of factors may be involved. The main factors implicated will be discussed briefly. Excellent reviews of athletic amenorrhoea are found in Highet (1989) and Chen and Brzyski (1999).

10.5.1.1 *Body composition*

Body composition and body weight are commonly linked with menstrual disturbances and amenorrhoea. This notion has been popular since Frisch and McArthur (1974) put forward the 'critical fat' hypothesis, in which it was proposed that a minimum level of 17% body fat was required for menarche to occur and 22% body fat for menstrual cycles to be maintained. This hypothesis has been strongly criticised (Scott & Johnston 1985), because the formula used to calculate percentage body fat used only weight and height and has since been shown to be grossly inaccurate (Loucks et al. 1984). The difficulty in linking body composition with amenorrhoea depends entirely on the accuracy of the prediction of body fat. Authors who have examined this issue have not used consistent methodologies (Calberg et al. 1983; Sinning et al. 1984; Sanborn et al. 1987; Kaiserauer et al. 1989), therefore it is difficult to draw conclusions. However, a role for body composition or changes in body composition in menstrual dysfunction cannot be entirely eliminated at this time.

10.5.1.2 *Training intensity*

The intensity of training appears to be linked to menstrual disturbances in athletes. Highet (1989) suggested that researchers should examine the percentage of maximal aerobic capacity at which athletes train. Ballet dancers, who train at high intensity but short duration, resume menses after a reduction in training intensity (Abraham et al. 1982). Other studies in runners have also found menstrual irregularities increase with training intensity (Sanborn et al. 1987; Cokkinades et al. 1990).

The rate at which the intensity of training is increased may also be important in the onset of athletic amenorrhoea. Bullen and colleagues (1985) were able to induce menstrual disturbance in a group of female recreational athletes during an eight-week intensive training program, particularly if accompanied by weight loss.

Details of training volume, frequency and duration of training have not always been reported, making interpretation difficult (Keizer & Rogol 1990). To determine the effect of training on amenorrhoea, there is a need for carefully designed studies where these factors are documented.

10.5.1.3 *Diet*

Linking diet with menstrual disturbances relies on the accuracy of being able to measure the dietary intake. This is inherently difficult due to the problems of underreporting when subjects are asked to keep dietary records. Studies have demonstrated that amenorrheic athletes have lower energy intakes than eumenorrheic athletes (Marcus et al. 1985; Nelson et al. 1986; Kaiserauer et al. 1989). Amenorrheic athletes are, therefore, expending the same amount of energy despite a lower reported energy intake. This has led authors (Nelson et al. 1986; Kaiserauer et al. 1989) to suggest that energy imbalance or nutritional inadequacy may contribute to athletic amenorrhoea. Lower fat intakes (Deuster et al. 1986; Kaiserauer et al. 1989) and vegetarianism (Brooks et al. 1984; Kaiserauer et al. 1989) are also more common in amenorrheic athletes. Fibre intake was the only factor found to be significantly higher when oligomenorrheic and amenorrheic runners were compared to regularly menstruating runners (Micklesfield et al. 1995). Other studies have not found any differences between amenorrheic and eumenorrheic athletes (Drinkwater et al. 1984; Moen et al. 1998).

The conflicting results observed may be explained by the lack of power in these studies due to small sample sizes and the difficulty of obtaining accurate dietary intakes in athletes.

Most studies that have examined the role of diet in amenorrhoea have not reported whether athletes with eating disorders have been excluded (Drinkwater et al. 1984; Marcus et al. 1985; Nelson et al. 1986; Kaiserauer et al. 1989; Micklesfield et al. 1995). The reported lower energy intakes and increased frequency of vegetarianism observed in amenorrheic athletes would indicate that eating disorders may be more common in this group and confound the results. A number of studies have reported eating disturbances are more common in amenorrheic athletes (Gadpaille et al. 1987; Walberg & Johnston 1991). Carefully planned studies are clearly needed before conclusions can be made between diet and amenorrhoea.

10.5.2 *Prevalence of menstrual disturbances in athletes*

Reports of the prevalence of menstrual disturbances in female athletes vary considerably depending on the definition of menstrual disturbance and on the population surveyed in terms of sport, age, activity level, parity and nutritional status. The prevalence in athletes (1–44%) is, however, greater than in the general population (2–5%) (Loucks & Horvath 1985). Younger, leaner athletes who train intensely appear to be particularly at risk. In a questionnaire survey of 226 elite athletes, the prevalence of menstrual disturbances was higher in ballet (52%), gymnastics (100%), light-weight rowing (67%) and distance running (65%) than in swimming (31%) or team sports (17%) (Wolman et al. 1989). Menstrual disturbances therefore represent a significant problem in the female athletic community. The effects of prolonged amenorrhoea on bone health are reviewed in the following section.

10.5.3 *Effects of amenorrhoea on bone mass*

The effects of prolonged amenorrhoea on bone health are reviewed in this section. The effects of athletic amenorrhoea on bone mass were first identified in the 1980s by several authors (Cann et al. 1984; Drinkwater et al. 1984; Linnell et al. 1984; Marcus et al. 1985). These studies and others indicate that amenorrheic athletes have lower bone mass than eumenorrheic athletes (Table 10.1).

Interpreting the results of studies on the effects of amenorrhoea on bone mass is difficult, as the sample sizes have been small and the majority of studies have been cross-sectional, which increases the risk of type II errors. There is considerable evidence to show that body mass (BM) is a significant predictor of bone mass.

Table 10.1 Studies of the effects of amenorrhoea on bone mass in athletic women

Reference	Sample size[a]	Population (wt in kg)	Scan sites	Results	Comments
Drinkwater et al. 1984	AM = 14 EU = 14	Runners & rowers (AM = 54.4, EU = 57.9)	DPA—lumbar spine SPA—radius	AM significantly lower BMD than EU at lumbar spine.	NS difference in weight, height or exercise between subjects.
Linnell et al. 1984	AM = 10 EU = 12 C = 15	Runners (AM = 51.4, EU = 54.5, C = 60.3)	DPA—radius	NS difference in BMD at the radius between the groups.	Controls significantly heavier than runners.
Marcus et al. 1985	AM = 11 EU = 6	Distance runners (AM = 49.7, EU = 53.8)	SPA—radius CT—lumbar spine	AM significantly lower BMD than EU at lumbar spine. NS difference at radius.	Groups matched. AM lower BMD due to low oestrogen.
Wolman et al. 1990	LW = 19 R = 18 D = 9 AM = 25 EU = 21	Runners, dancers & rowers (AM = 52.6, EU = 56.0, LW = 59.8, R+D = 51.3)	CT—lumbar spine	BMD at lumbar spine sign. < for AM compared with EU. LW > BMD than R & D.	LW significantly taller & heavier than R & D.
Harber et al. 1991	C = 14 EU = 17 AM = 11	Athletes (C = 63.1, EU = 60.6, AM = 54.3)	Comptom scatter— calcaneus	NS difference between groups at calcaneus.	Weight significantly lower for AM group compared with EU & C.

(continues)

(continued)

Reference	Sample size[a]	Population (wt in kg)	Scan sites	Results	Comments
Snead et al. 1992	AM = 11 EU = 24 OL = 8	Runners (AM = 59.6, OL = 57.6, EU = 58.7, C = 61.0)	DXA—lumbar spine & femur	AM & OL significantly lower at lumbar spine. NS difference at femoral bone sites between groups.	Results suggest gonadal steroids affect lumbar spine BMD but little affect on femoral BMD.
Hetland et al. 1993	R = 28 RR = 89 C = 88	Runners (R = 57.3, RR = 62.1, C = 62.3)	DXA—lumbar spine, proximal femur, whole body, SPA forearm	AM 10% lower spinal BMD than EU (adjusted for age and BMI).	Sex hormone disturbances significantly related to distance run.
Rutherford et al. 1993	EU = 16 AM = 15	Triathletes & distance runners (EU = 60.2, AM = 55.3)	DXA—lumbar spine & whole body	AM significantly lower lumbar spine, arm, trunk BMD.	No control group. Menstrual status explained 32% variation BMD.
Young et al. 1994	AM B = 44 AN = 18 C = 23	Ballet dancers (B = 49.6, AN = 43.3, C = 58.5)	DXA—whole body & regional	Lumbar spine similar among AM B & AN. Weight-bearing sites similar among AM B & C. No significant difference in whole body BMD between groups.	Non-weight-bearing sites for AM B similar to AN.
Micklesfield et al. 1995	EU = 15 10 = OL/AM	Ultra-marathon runners (EU = 58.3, AM = 57.2)	DXA—lumbar spine, femur	Lumbar spine significantly lower in OL/AM group.	OL/AM—included 4 with history of OL/AM. Small sample size.

Study	N	Population	Method/site	Findings	Comments
Robinson et al. 1995	R = 20 G = 18 C = 19	Young athletes (R = 52.8, G = 55.0, C = 60.2)	DXA–lumbar spine, proximal femur, whole body	G higher femoral neck BMD than R & C, R lower lumbar spine BMD than G & C.	G & R had a similar prevalence of amenorrhoea, oligomenorrhoea & eumenorrhoea.
Rencken et al. 1996	AM = 29 EU = 20	Runners (AM = 55.3, EU = 56.1)	DXA–lumbar spine, proximal femur, tibia, fibula	AM significantly lower BMD at lumbar spine, femoral neck, trochanater, intertrochanteric region, femoral shaft, tibia. NS difference at fibula.	Suggests amenorrhoea may result in low BMD at multiple skeletal sites.
Moen et al. 1998	AM = 10 EU = 10 C = 10	Runners (AM = 51.8, EU = 50.7, C = 57.5)	DXA–lumbar spine	No significant differences.	Small sample size.
Pettersson et al. 1999	AM = 10 EU = 10 S = 16	Distance runners (AM = 52.4, EU = 59.0, S = 64.6)	DXA–whole body	AM significantly lower compared with EU for whole body, humerus, lumbar spine, pelvis, head of femur.	Suggests AM affects trabecular & corticol bone. Size differences not accounted for.

AM = amenorrheic athletes, B = ballet, BMD = bone mineral density, C = regularly menstruating non-athletic controls, CT = computer tomography, D = dancers, DPA = dual photon absorptiometry, DXA = dual energy X-ray absorptiometry, EU = eumenorrheic athletes, G = gymnasts, LW = light-weight rowers, NS = no significant, OL = oligomenorrheic athletes, R = runners, RR = recreational runners, S = soccer, SPA = single photon absorptiometry.

Therefore, it is important to account for size differences, as amenorrheic athletes often weigh less than eumenorrheic athletes (Linnell et al. 1984; Marcus et al. 1985; Wolman et al. 1990; Harber et al. 1991; Young et al. 1994). Differences in bone mass may be partly explained by differences in BM, but when BM has been controlled for, the results are not consistent. In a study of ballet dancers (Young et al. 1994) at non-weight-bearing sites, bone density was similar between dancers and girls with anorexia nervosa, after controlling for BM. The importance of BM was seen in a study of ballet dancers (Warren et al. 1991). Significant effects of amenorrhoea on BMD were demonstrated at the spine, wrist and metatarsal. All effects of amenorrhoea were eliminated by controlling for weight.

In a study of 97 young athletes (Drinkwater et al. 1990), there was a significant linear relationship between the current vertebral BMD and the athletes' past and present menstrual patterns. Women who had always had regular menses had the highest vertebral bone mass. BM was a significant predictor of both vertebral and femur BMD. Once BMD was adjusted for BM, only the vertebral BMD remained significantly lower by menstrual status.

An early study by Drinkwater et al. (1984) showed amenorrheic athletes had a significantly lower vertebral BMD than eumenorrheic athletes. This finding has been confirmed by other researchers (Marcus et al. 1985; Wolman et al. 1990).

There is some evidence that amenorrhoea may affect non-weight-bearing bones to a greater extent than weight-bearing bones (Marcus et al. 1985; Young et al. 1994). This may be because exercise may offer some protection at weight-bearing sites. A study which examined the bone mass of gymnasts and runners with a similar prevalence of menstrual disturbances found gymnasts had a higher femoral neck BMD than the runners or controls (Robinson et al. 1995). Higher-impact forces from the gymnastics training were thought to account for the differences.

Bone mass in amenorrheic athletes is, however, well below age-matched normal controls at weight-bearing sites (Cann et al. 1984; Drinkwater et al. 1984; Lindberg et al. 1984; Warren et al. 1986). The lumbar spine BMD is significantly less in amenorrheic athletes compared to eumenorrheic athletes (Drinkwater et al. 1984; Lindberg et al. 1984).

10.5.4 *Effects of resumption of menses on bone mass*

The reversibility of bone loss observed with amenorrhoea has been a concern due to the long-term consequences on bone mass. Drinkwater et al. (1986) followed up athletes with amenorrhoea 15.5 months after they regained menses and compared them to eumenorrheic controls. There was a 6% increase in the vertebral BMD in the amenorrheic athletes who had regained menses. The resumption of menses was also associated with an increase in BM and a reduction in exercise level. It was noted at the time that it was premature to assume that the bone mass would return to the same level for their age group.

It was later reported (Drinkwater et al. 1990) that the gain ceased after two years, suggesting that the bone mass may never fully recover. When the amenorrheic athletes were followed up after eight years (Keen & Drinkwater 1997), despite several years of normal menses or use of oral contraceptives, the vertebral BMD remained lower than the athletes who had always had regular menses. Micklesfield et al. (1998) also showed that despite resumption of menses, previously irregularly menstruating runners still had reduced vertebral bone mass compared with regularly menstruating runners. History of menstrual irregularity is detrimental to the attainment of peak bone mass and early intervention is recommended, in order to minimise the long-term risks of osteoporosis (Keen & Drinkwater 1997).

10.5.5 *Mechanisms of low bone mass in amenorrhoea*

Low levels of endogenous oestrogen are thought to be responsible for the continued bone loss (Cann et al. 1984; Drinkwater et al. 1984; Marcus et al. 1985). Snead et al. (1992) found lower oestradiol and progesterone levels in combination with lower lumbar spine BMD in oligomenorrheic and amenorrheic runners, compared with eumenorrheic runners and controls. The view that amenorrhoea is related to oestrogen deficiency is consistent with the model ovarian failure and menopause. Recently, however, it has been suggested that oestrogen deficiency may not be the primary cause of bone loss in amenorrheic athletes (Zanker 1999). Evidence for this is related to the fact that amenorrheic athletes appear to be less responsive to oestrogen therapy (Hergenroeder 1995) in studies of bone turnover (Zanker & Swaine 1998).

The mechanism by which the low oestrogen levels reduce bone mass is by decreasing the rate of bone turnover (Zanker & Swaine 1998). Amenorrheic runners were found to have bone formation markers below the normal reference range (Zanker & Swaine 1998). The authors suggested under-nutrition as the mechanism which reduced bone formation. Bone formation markers were lowest in the amenorrheic runners who had a body mass index less than 17.5.

A study which compared anorexia nervosa subjects with amenorrheic controls showed a greater incidence of osteopenia in the anorexia nervosa subjects (Grinspoon et al. 1999). This data suggests that nutritional factors, independent of oestrogen, are important in determining bone mass.

10.5.6 *Role of calcium and nutritional factors in amenorrhoea*

Calcium is required for the normal maintenance and development of the skeleton and teeth, therefore requirements are increased during periods of rapid growth, such as during childhood, adolescence, pregnancy and lactation, and in later life.

To date there have been no randomised control trials in amenorrheic athletes to examine the effects of calcium supplementation on slowing bone loss. It is still thought, however, that calcium, if given in sufficient amounts, may modulate the effects of hypogonadism in female athletes. Since calcium deficiency is a stimulus for bone resorption, the effect of calcium deficiency and hypogonadism may be additive (Dalsky 1990). This was supported by the findings of Wolman et al. (1992) who reported a linear relationship between calcium intake and trabecular bone density at the lumbar spine in both amenorrheic and eumenorrheic athletes. However, at all levels of calcium intake, bone density was significantly lower in amenorrheic athletes. Therefore, even though amenorrheic athletes with higher calcium intakes can achieve better bone mass than amenorrheic athletes with lower calcium intakes, this still cannot compensate for the effects of amenorrhoea on the skeleton.

Although intervention trials are lacking in athletic populations, it is generally agreed that 1500 mg/d is recommended for athletes with amenorrhoea (Nativ & Armsey 1997). This is also consistent with the United States National Institute of Health (NIH 1994) consensus guidelines for postmenopausal women not taking oestrogen. The Australian RDIs for calcium are currently under review. Other nutritional factors, such as sodium and protein, can increase urinary calcium losses. Adding 100 mmol of sodium (2.3 g) to the daily diet will result in a calcium loss of 1 mmol (40 mg) (Nordin et al. 1993). The effects of sodium and protein on calcium excretion are most affected when the person is in negative calcium balance (Nordin 1997). High calcium intake with meals can inhibit iron absorption (see Chapter 11, Section 11.5.2.2). Therefore, in athletes with high iron requirements, calcium supplements should be taken at bedtime (Halberg 1998).

10.6 STRESS FRACTURES IN ATHLETES WITH MENSTRUAL DISTURBANCES

A stress fracture is a partial or complete fracture of bone, which results from the bone's inability to withstand non-violent stress that is applied in a repeated, subthreshold manner (McBryde 1985). It arises from accumulation of bone micro-damage which cannot be adequately repaired by the remodelling process. Any factor which increases the applied load, decreases bone strength or interferes with the repair process has the potential to increase the risk of stress fracture (Bennell et al. 1996). The diagnosis of stress fracture is based on the clinical findings of a history of exercise-related bone pain with local bony tenderness on examination.

10.6.1 Role of menstrual factors in stress fractures

Menstrual factors may have an effect on stress fracture aetiology through the influence of reduced levels of reproductive hormones on bone remodelling and bone density (Heaney et al. 1978; Slemenda et al. 1987). Studies have reported that stress fractures are more common in athletes with current or past menstrual disturbances with a relative risk for stress fracture that is between two to four times greater than their eumenorrheic counterparts (Lindberg et al. 1984; Marcus et al. 1985; Lloyd et al. 1986; Warren et al. 1986; Nelson et al. 1987; Barrow & Saha 1988; Frusztajer et al. 1990;

Myburgh et al. 1990; Cameron et al. 1992; Kadel et al. 1992; Bennell et al. 1996) (see Figure 10.2). However, most studies have been cross-sectional designs where women are specifically recruited according to certain criteria, either stress fracture history or menstrual status. In these studies, cohorts are often small, categorisation of menstrual status is based on number of menses per year, rather than on analysis of hormonal levels, and definitions vary. Where hormonal assessment is included, most are single measurements, often non-standardised with respect to menstrual cycle phase.

The relationship between age of menarche and risk of stress fracture is uncertain. Some authors have found that athletes with stress fractures have a later age of menarche (Warren et al. 1986; Carbon et al. 1990; Warren et al. 1991) while others have found no difference (Frusztajer et al. 1990; Myburgh et al. 1990; Kadel et al. 1992). In a prospective study by Bennell et al. (1996), the age of menarche was an independent risk factor for stress fracture, with the risk increasing by a factor of 4.1 for every additional year of age at menarche.

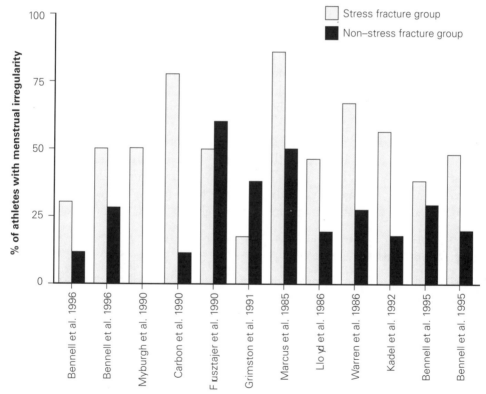

Figure 10.2 *Studies where the percentage of athletes/recruits with menstrual irregularity could be compared in groups with and without stress fracture (From Brukner P, Bennell K, Matheson G. Stress fractures. Blackwell Science, Asia: 1999: 65–66.)*

Some authors have claimed that the oral contraceptive pill (OCP) may protect against stress fracture development. Barrow and Saha (1988) found that runners using the OCP for at least one year had significantly fewer stress fractures (12%) than non-users (29%). This was supported by the findings of Myburgh et al. (1990) but not by others (Kadel et al. 1992). Since these studies are retrospective in nature, it is not known whether the athletes were taking the OCP prior to, or following, the stress fracture episode. In addition, athletes may or may not take the OCP for reasons which in themselves could influence stress fracture risk. It is not known whether the risk of stress fracture is reduced in athletes with menstrual disturbances who subsequently take the OCP after incurring a fracture.

Theoretically, low bone density could contribute to the development of a stress fracture by decreasing the fatigue resistance of bone to loading and increasing the accumulation of micro-damage (Carter et al. 1981). A limited number of cross-sectional studies have compared regional bone density in small groups of female athletes with and without stress fracture but results have been conflicting. The discrepancy may reflect differences in population, type of sport, measurement techniques and bone regions. However, the findings of the only prospective study to date indicate that lower bone density, assessed by DXA, is a risk factor for stress fractures in female track and field athletes (Bennell et al. 1996). Nevertheless, the athletes who developed stress fractures still had bone density levels that were similar to or greater than less-active subjects. This implies that the level of bone density required by athletes for short-term bone health is greater than that required by the general population.

In summary, it would appear that there is a higher prevalence of current and past menstrual disturbances in female athletes with stress fractures than in those without stress fractures. A later age of menarche and lower bone density may also contribute to an increased risk of this over-use bone injury. Use of the OCP may afford protection against stress fractures, although this is yet to be fully elucidated.

10.7 SUMMARY

The skeleton represents a complex interaction between the hormonal environment and the stresses and strains placed upon it. Weight-bearing exercise or strength training have been shown to be effective in slowing or preventing bone loss in both premenopausal and postmenopausal women. In amenorrheic athletes, however, the evidence is not as clear, partly due to the lack of well-designed intervention studies. Nevertheless, amenorrhoea is clearly detrimental to bone health and early intervention is recommended. Calcium has been shown to be effective in decreasing bone loss, and the intake should be increased after menopause or in amenorrhoea. The prevalence of stress fractures is also higher among athletes with menstrual disturbances. Athletes need to be aware of the consequences of menstrual disturbances on bone health.

10.8 PRACTICE TIPS

Deborah Kerr, Karim Khan and Kim Bennell

- It is important that female athletes and their coaches are aware of the long-term consequences of amenorrhoea, particularly on bone health. The sports dietitian can play an important role in the education of athletes and coaches on this issue. In dietary counselling, female athletes should be questioned about their menstrual history, and athletes who have been amenorrheic for more than six months should be referred to a sports physician for assessment.

- The sports dietitian needs to be alert to the possible presence of eating disorders, which can cause serious and irreversible bone loss. Dietary practices that may increase urinary calcium losses should also be assessed. These include excessive intakes of sodium, protein, caffeine and alcohol. These are of greater significance if the dietary calcium intake is low. Therefore focus on increasing the calcium intake first, as at higher calcium intakes (at least > 800 mg/d) excessive sodium, protein and caffeine are of less importance. Cigarette smoking can also have deleterious effects on bone health.

- There are currently no recommended dietary allowances for amenorrheic athletes. However, 1500 mg/d has been proposed. This is consistent with the United States' NIH consensus statement for postmenopausal women not taking oestrogen, which could also include amenorrheic athletes. The current Australian RDI for calcium is 800 mg/d for adults and 1000 mg/d for postmenopausal women. During adolescence it is essential that athletes meet their calcium requirements, as this is the time when peak bone mass occurs.

- What can be done when counselling female athletes who are not consuming enough calcium? Expounding the long-term risk of osteoporosis usually has little impact. However, if an individual has seen the debilitating effects of osteoporosis in their family or friends, they are usually more receptive to preventative strategies. Start by suggesting an increase in calcium intake by dietary means, but if this strategy is not possible or feasible then a calcium supplement may be required. Referral to a sports physician for a bone density scan can be considered. An athlete with a low calcium intake together with a low bone density may be more receptive to change, once they have seen the results of their bone density scan.

- Female athletes consuming a low energy intake are at high risk of a low calcium intake. The sports dietitian can assist the athlete with practical ways of meeting their calcium requirements from dietary sources. Where this is not possible, a calcium supplement may be warranted. It is important to check the amount of elemental calcium contained in the supplement to ensure the most economical way of meeting the calcium requirements. To minimise interaction with food, calcium supplements are best taken at bedtime or between meals. The absorption of calcium is most effective when the supplement is taken in doses of 500 mg or less (Heaney et al. 1988). However, the timing of taking the supplement needs to be weighed up with the likelihood of compliance and whether the athlete is taking other supplements, such as iron. Although absorption may be higher by splitting a 500 mg supplement into two 250 mg doses, compliance with this regimen is often poor; a single dose taken at bedtime enhances compliance.

- Female athletes considered to be at high risk of osteopenia may need pharmacological intervention, biochemical measures of hormone status and bone density assessment. Situations where medical referrral is warranted include:
  1. being amenorrheic for longer than six months;
  2. a history of anorexia nervosa;
  3. occurrence of stress fractures;
  4. postmenopausal; and
  5. a strong family history of osteoporosis.

- Routine screening of female athletes is not recommended unless indicated, as there is a small radiation dose associated with bone density assessment by DXA.

- Women of all ages should be encouraged to participate in regular weight-bearing activity or weight training, as these types of activities have been shown to have a positive effect on bone density. Weight-bearing activities include jogging, tennis, aerobics and walking. Activities such as cycling and swimming, although excellent for aerobic fitness, are unlikely to have much effect on bone mass.

REFERENCES

Abraham S, Beaumont PJ, Fraser IF, Llewellyn Jones D. Body-weight exercise and menstrual states among ballet dancers in training. J Obstet Gynaecol 1982;99:507–10.

Abrams SA, Grusak MA, Stuff J, O'Brien KO. Calcium and magnesium balance in 9–14-year-old children. Am J Clin Nutr 1997;66:1172–7.

Albanese AA, Edelson AH, Lorenze AH, Woodhull MC, Wein EH. Problems of bone health in elderly. NY State J Med 1975;75:326–36.

Aloia JF, Cohn SH, Ostuni JA, Cane R, Ellis K. Prevention of involutional bone loss by exercise. Ann Intern Med 1978;89:356–8.

American College of Sports Medicine. The female athlete triad: disordered eating, amenorrhoea, osteoporosis (Conference Summary). Washington DC: 19 June 1992.

Avioli LV, Heaney RP. Calcium intake and bone health (editorial). Calcif Tissue Int 1991;48:221–3.

Bailey DA. The Saskatchewan bone mineral accrual study: bone mineral acquisition during the growing years. Int J Sports Med 1997;18(suppl)3:S191–S4.

Bailey DA, Martin AD, McKay HA et al. Calcium accretion in girls and boys during puberty. J Bone Miner Res 2000;15:2245–50.

Bailey DA, Wedgev JH, McCulloch RG, Martin AD, Bernhardson SC. Epidemiology of fractures at the distal end of the radius in children associated with growth. J Bone Joint Surg 1989;71-A:1225–31.

Ballard JE, McKeown BC, Graham HM, Zinkgraf SA. The effect of high level physical activity (8.5 METs or greater) and oestrogen replacement therapy upon bone mass in postmenopausal females, aged 50–68 years. Int J Sports Med 1990;11:208–14.

Baran D, Sorensen A, Grimes J, et al. Dietary modification with dairy products for preventing vertebral bone loss in premeopausal women: a three year prospective study. J Clin Endocrinol Metal 1989;70:264–70.

Barrow GW, Saha S. Menstrual irregularity and stress fractures in collegiate female distance runners. Am J Sports Med 1988;16:209–16.

Bassey EJ, Ramsdale SJ. Increase in femoral bone density in young women following high-impact exercise. Osteoporos Int 1994;4:72–5.

Bennell KL, Malcom SA, Thomas SA, et al. Risk factors for stress fractures in female track-and-field athletes: a retrospective analysis. Clin J Sports Med 1995;5:229–35.

Bennell KL, Malcolm SA, Thomas SA, Wark JD, Brukner PD. The incidence and distribution of stress fractures in competitive track and field athletes. Am J Sports Med 1996;24:211–17.

Bennell KL, Malcolm SA, Wark JD, Brukner PD. Skeletal effects of menstrual disturbances in athletes. Scan J Med Sci Sports 1997;7:261–73.

Bloomfield SA, Williams NI, Lamb DR, Jackson RD. Non-weight-bearing exercise may increase lumbar spine bone mineral density in healthy postmenopausal women. Am J Phys Med Rehab 1993;72:204–9.

Bonjour JP, Carrie AL, Ferrari S, et al. Calcium-enriched foods and bone mass growth in prepubertal girls: a randomized double-blind, placebo-controlled trial. J Clin Invest 1997;99:1287–94.

Brooks SM, Sanborn CF, Albrecht BH, Wagner WW. Diet in athletic amenorrhoea. Lancet 1984;2:559–60.

Bullen BA, Skinner GS, Beittens IZ, von Mering G, Turnball BA, McArthur JW. Induction of menstrual disorders by strenuous exercise in untrained women. N Engl J Med 1985;312:1349–53.

Cameron KR, Wark JD, Telford RD. Stress fractures and bone loss—the skeletal cost of intense athleticism. Excel 1992;8:39–55.

Cann CE, Martin MC, Genant HK, Jaffe RB. Decreased spinal mineral content in amenorrheic women. JAMA 1984;251:626–9.

Carbon R, Sambrook PN, Deakin V, et al. Bone density of elite female athletes with stress fractures. Med J Aust 1990;153:373–6.

Carlberg KA, Buckman MT, Peake GT, Reidesel ML. Body composition of oligo/amenorrheic athletes. Med Science Sports Exerc 1983;215–17.

Carter DR, Caler WE, Spengler DM, et al. Uniaxial fatigue of human cortical bone: the influence of tissue physical characteristics. J Biomech 1981;14:461–70.

Cavanaugh DJ, Cann CE. Brisk walking does not stop bone loss in postmenopausal women. Bone 1988;9:201–4.

Chen EC, Brzyski RG. Exercise and reproductive dysfunction. Fertil Steril 1999;71:1–6.

Chow RK, Harrison JE, Brown CF, Hajek V. Physical fitness effect on bone mass in postmenopausal women. Arch Phys Med Rehab 1986;67:231–4.

Cokkinades VE, Macera CA, Pate RR. Menstrual function among habitual runners. Women Health 1990;16:59–69.

Colletti LA, Edwards J, Gordon L, Shary J, Bell NH. The effects of muscle-building exercise on bone mineral density of the radius, spine and hip in young men. Calcif Tissue Int 1989;45:12–14.

Cumming RG. Calcium intake and bone mass: a quantitative review of the evidence. Calcif Tissue Int 1990;47:194–201.

Dalen N, Olsson KE. Bone mineral content and physical activity. Acta Orthopaedica Scandinavica 1974;45:170–4.

Dalsky GP. Effect of exercise on bone: permissive influence of oestrogen and calcium. Med Sci Sports Exerc 1990;22:281–4.

Davee AM, Rosen CJ, Adler RA. Exercise patterns and trabecular bone density in college women. J Bone Miner Res 1990;5:245–50.

Dawson-Hughes B, Dallal GE, Krall EA, Sadowski L, Sahyoun N, Tannenbaum S. A controlled trial of the effect of calcium supplementation on bone density in postmenopausal women. N Engl J Med 1990;323:878–83.

Deuster PA, Kyle SB, Moser PB, Vigersky RA, Schoomaker EB. Nutritional intakes and status of highly trained amenorrheic and eumenorrheic women runners. Fertil Steril 1986;46:636–43.

Drinkwater BL, Nilson K, Chesnut CH, Bremner WJ, Shainholtz S, Southworth MB. Bone mineral content of amenorrheic and eumenorrheic athletes. N Engl J Med 1984;311:277–81.

Drinkwater BL, Nilson K, Ott S, Chesnut CH. Bone mineral density after resumption of menses in amenorrheic athletes. JAMA 1986;256:380–2.

Drinkwater BL, Bruemner B, Chesnut CH. Menstrual history as a determinant of current bone density in young athletes. JAMA 1990;263:545–8.

Elders PJM, Netelenbos JC, Lips P, et al. Calcium supplementation reduces vertebral bone loss in perimenopausal women: a controlled trial in 248 women between 46 and 55 years of age. J Clin Endocrinol Metab 1991;73:533–40.

Elders PJM, Lips P, Netelenbos JC, et al. Long-term effect of calcium supplementation on bone loss in perimenopausal women. J Bone Miner Res 1994;9:963–70.

Epstein S. Serum and urinary markers of bone remodelling: assessment of bone turnover. Endo Rev 1988;9:437–49.

Ettinger B, Genant HK, Cann CE. Postmenopausal bone loss is prevented by treatment with low-dosage oestrogen with calcium. Ann Intern Med 1987;106:40–5.

Friedlander AL, Genant HK, Sadowsky S, Byl NN, Gluer C. A two-year program of aerobics and weight training enhances bone mineral density of young women. J Bone Miner Res 1995;10:574–85.

Frish RE, McArthur JW. Menstrual cycles: fatness as a determinant of minimum weight for height necessary for their maintenance or onset. Science 1974;185:949–51.

Frost HM. Skeletal adaptations to mechanical usage (SATMU): 2. Redefining Wolff's Law: the remodelling problem. Anat Rec 1990;226:403–22.

Frusztajer NT, Dhuper S, Warren MP, et al. Nutrition and the incidence of stress fractures in ballet dancers. Am J Clin Nutr 1990;51:779–83.

Gadpaille WJ, Sanborn CF, Wagner WW. Athletic amenorrhoea, major affective disorders and eating disorders. Am J Pysch 1987;144:939–42.

Gleeson PB, Protas EJ, LeBlanc AD, Schneider VS, Evans HJ. Effects of weight lifting on bone mineral density in premenopausal women. J Bone Miner Res 1990;5(2):153–8.

Grimston SK, Engsberg JR, Kloiber R, Hanley DA. Menstrual, calcium and training history: relationship to bone health in female runners. Clin Sports Med 1990;2:119–28.

Grinspoon S, Miller K, Coyle C, et al. Severity of osteopenia in oestrogen-deficient women with anorexia nervosa and hypothalamic amenorrhoea. J Clin Endocrinol Metab 1999;84:2049–55.

Halberg L. Does calcium interfere with iron absorption? Am J Clin Nutr 1998;68:3–4.

Harber VJ, Webber CE, Sutton JR, MacDougall JD. The effect of amenorrhoea on calcaneal bone density and total bone turnovers in runners. Int J Sports Med 1991;12:505–8.

Heaney RP. Oestrogen–calcium interactions in the post–menopause: a quantitative description. Bone and Mineral 1990;11:67–84.

Heaney RP. The bone-remodelling transient: implications for the interpretation of clinical studies of bone mass change. J Bone Miner Res 1994;9:1515–23.

Heaney RP, Recker RR, Saville PD. Menopausal changes in bone remodelling. J Lab Clin Med 1978;92:964–70.

Heaney RP, Weaver CM, Recker RR. Calcium absorption from spinach. Am J Clin Nutr 1988;47:707–9.

Heinrich CH, Going SB, Pamenter RW, Perry CD, Boyden TW, Lohman TG. Bone mineral content of cyclically menstruating female resistance and endurance trained athletes. Med Sci Sports Exerc 1990;22(5):558–63.

Hergenroeder AC. Bone mineralisation, hypothalamic amenorrhoea and sex steroid therapy in female adolescents and young adults. J Pediatr 1995;126:683–9.

Hetland ML, Haarbo J, Christiansen C, Larsen T. Running induces menstrual disturbances but bone mass is unaffected, except in amenorrheic women. Am J Med 1993;95:53–60.

Highet R. Athletic amenorrhoea: an update on aetiology, complications and management. Sports Med 1989;7:82–108.

Horsman A, Gallagher JC, Simpson M, Nordin BEC. Prospective trial of oestrogen and calcium in postmenopausal women. Br Med J 1977;2:789–92.

Huddleston AL, Rockwell D, Kulund DN, Harrison RB. Bone mass in lifetime tennis athletes. JAMA 1980;244:1107–9.

Johnston CC, Miller JZ, Slemenda CW, et al. Calcium supplementation and increases in bone mineral density in children. N Engl J Med 1992;327:82–7.

Jones HH, Priest JD, Hayes WC, Tichenor CC, Nagel DA. Humeral hypertrophy in response to exercise. J Bone Joint Surg 1977;59A:204–8.

Kadel NJ, Tietz CC, Kronmal RA. Stress fractures in ballet dancers. Am J Sports Med 1992;20:445–9.

Kaiserauer S, Snyder AC, Sleeper M, Zierath J. Nutritional, physiological, and menstrual status of distance runners. Med Science Sports Exerc 1989;21:120–5.

Kanis JA. Calcium nutrition and its implications for osteoporosis. Eur J Clin Nutr 1994;48:757–67, 833–41.

Kanis JA, Passmore R. Calcium supplementation of the diet. Br Med J 1989;298:137–40, 205–8.

Karlsson MK, Johnell O, Obrant KJ. Bone mineral density in weight lifters. Calcif Tissue Int 1993;52:212–15.

Keen AD, Drinkwater BL. Irreversible bone loss in former amenorrheic athletes. Osteoporos Int 1997;7:311–15.

Keizer HA, Rogol AD. Physical exercise and menstrual cycle alterations. What are the mechanisms? Sports Med 1990;10:218–35.

Kerr DA, Morton A, Dick I, Prince R. Exercise effects on bone mass in postmenopausal women are site specific and strain dependent. J Bone Miner Res 1996;11:218–25.

Krall EA, Dawson-Hughes B. Heritable and life-style determinants of bone mineral density. J Bone Miner Res 1993;8:1–9.

Krolner B, Toft B, Nielsen SP, Tondevold E. Physical exercise as prophylaxis against involutional vertebral bone loss: a controlled trial. Clin Sci 1983;64:541–6.

Lane NE, Bloch DA, Jones HH, et al. Long-distance running, bone density and osteoarthritis. JAMA 1986;255:1147–51.

Lee WTK, Leung SSF, Leung DMY, Tsang HSY, Lau J, Cheng JCY. A randomized double-blind controlled calcium supplementation trial, and bone and height acquisition in children. Brit J Nutr 1995;74:125–39.

Lee WTK, Leung SSF, Wang SH, et al. Double-blind controlled calcium supplementation and bone mineral accretion in children accustomed to a low-calcium diet. Am J Clin Nutr 1994;60:744–50.

Linberg JS, Fears WB, Hunt MM, et al. Exercise induced amenorrhoea and bone density. Ann Int Med 1984;101:647–8.

Linnell SL, Stager JM, Blue PW, Oyster N, Robertshaw D. Bone mineral content and menstrual regularity in female runners. Med Sci Sports Exerc 1984;16:343–8.

Lloyd T, Andon MB, Rollings N, et al. Calcium supplementation and bone mineral density in adolescent girls. JAMA 1993;270:841–4.

Lloyd T, Triantafyllou SJ, Baker ER, et al. Women athletes with menstrual irregularity have increased musculoskeletal injuries. Med Sci Sports Exerc 1986;18:374–9.

Lohman T, Going S, Pamenter R, et al. Effects of resistance training on regional and total bone mineral density in premenopausal women: a randomized prospective study. J Bone Miner Res 1995;10:1015–24.

Loucks AB, Horvath SM. Athletic amenorrhoea: a review. Med Sci Sports Exerc 1985;17:56–72.

Loucks AB, Horvath SM, Freedom PS. Menstruation and validation of body fat prediction in athletes. Hum Biol 1984;56:383–92.

Malina RM, Spirduso WW, Tate C, Baylor AM. Age at menarche and selected menstrual characteristics in athletes at different competitive levels and in different sports. Med Sci Sports Exerc 1978;10:218–22.

Marcus R, Cann C, Madvig P, et al. Menstrual function and bone mass in elite women distance runners. Ann Int Med 1985;102:158–63.

Marcus R, Carter DR. The role of physical activity in bone mass regulation. Adv Sports Med Fitness 1988;1:63–82.

Martin AD, Bailey DA, McKay HA, Whiting S. Bone mineral and calcium accretion during puberty. Am J Clin Nutr 1997;66:611–15.

Martin AD, McCulloch RG. Bone dynamics: stress, strain and fracture. J Sports Sci 1987;5:155–63.

Mazess RB, Barden HS. Bone density in premenopausal women: effects of age, dietary intake, physical activity, smoking and birth-control pills. Am J Clin Nutr 1991;53:132–42.

McBryde AM Jr. Stress fractures in runners. Clin Sports Med 1985;4:737–52.

Micklesfield LK, Lambert EV, Fataar AB, Noakes TD, Myburgh KH. Bone mineral density in mature premenopausal ultramarathon runners. Med Sci Sports Exerc 1995;27:688–96.

Micklesfield LK, Reyneke L, Fataar A, Myburgh KH. Long-term restoration of deficits in bone mineral density is inadequate in premenopausal women with prior menstrual irregularity. Clin J Sport Med 1998;8:155–63.

Moen SM, Sanborn CF, Dimarco NM, et al. Lumbar bone mineral density in adolescent female runners. J Sports Med Phys Fitness 1998;38:234–9.

Myburgh KH, Hutchins J, Fataar AB, Hough SF, Noakes TD. Low bone density is an etiology factor for stress fractures in athletes. Ann Int Med 1990;113:754–9.

National Health & Medical Research Council. Recommended dietary intakes for use in Australia. Canberra: Australian Government Publishing Service, 1991.

National Institute of Health. Optimal calcium intake. National Institute of Health consensus statement. 1994;12:1–31.

Nativ A, Armsey TD. Stress injury to bone in the female athlete. Clin Sports Med 1997;16:197–224.

Nelson ME, Clark N, Otradovec CL, et al. Elite women runners: association between menstrual status, weight history and stress fractures. Med Sci Sport Exerc 1987;19:S13.

Nelson ME, Fiatorone MA, Morganti CM, Trice I, Greenberg RA, Evans WJ. Effects of high-intensity strength training on multiple risk factors for osteoporotic fractures. JAMA 1994;272:1909–14.

Nelson ME, Fisher EC, Catsos PD, Meredith CN, Turksoy RN, Evans WJ. Diet and bone status in amenorrheic runners. Am J Clin Nutr 1986;43:910–16.

Nielsen HK, Brixen K, Kristensen LP, et al. Effects of different kinds of exercise on bone mass and bone metabolism in elderly women. Eur J Exp Musculoskel Res 1992;1:41–6.

Nilas L, Christiansen C, Rodbro P. Calcium supplementation and postmenopausal bone loss. Br Med J 1984;289:1103–6.

Nilsson BE, Westlin NE. Bone density in athletes. Clin Ortho Related Research 1971;77:179–82.

Nordin BEC. Calcium and osteoporosis. Nutr 1997;13:664–86.

Nordin BEC, Heaney RP. Calcium supplementation of the diet: justified by present evidence. Br Med J 1990;300:1056–60.

Nordin BE, Need AG, Morris HA, Horowitz M. The nature and significance of the relation between urine sodium and urine calcium in women. J Nutr 1993;123:1615–22.

Notelovitz M, Martin D, Tesar R, et al. Oestrogen therapy and variable-resistance weight training increase bone mineral in surgically menopausal women. J Bone Miner Res 1991;6:583–90.

Nowson CA, Green RM, Guest CS, et al. The effect of calcium supplementation on bone mass in adolescent female twins. In: Burkhardt P, Heaney RP, eds. Challenges of modern medicine. Ares-Serono Symposia Publications, 1995:169–75.

Nowson CA, Green RM, Hopper JL, et al. A co-twin study of the effect of calcium supplementation on bone density during adolescence. Osteoporos Int 1997;7:219–25.

Orwoll ES, Ferar J, Oviatt SK, McClung MR, Huntington K. The relationship of swimming exercise to bone mass in men and women. Arch Int Med 1989;149:2197–200.

Parfitt AM. The cellular basis of bone remodelling: the quantum concept reexamined in light of recent advances in the cell biology of bone. Calcif Tissue Int 1984;36:S37–S45.

Parfitt AM. The two faces of growth: benefits and risks to bone integrity. Osteopor Int 1994;4:382–98.

Peterson SE, Peterson MD, Raymond G, Gilligan C, Checovich MM, Smith EL. Muscular strength and bone density with weight training in middle-aged women. Med Sci Sports Exerc 1991;23:499–504.

Pettersson U, Stalnacke BM, Ahlenius GM, Henriksson-Larsen K, Lorentzon R. Low bone mass density at multiple skeletal sites, including the appendicular skeleton in amenorrheic runners. Calcif Tissue Int 1999;64:117–25.

Pocock NA, Eisman JA, Hopper JL, et al. Genetic determinants of bone mass in adults: a twin study. J Clin Invest 1987;80:706–10.

Prince R, Devine A, Dick I, et al. The effects of calcium supplementation (milk powder or tablets) and exercise on bone density in postmenopausal women. J Bone Miner Res 1995;10:1068–75.

Prince RL, Smith M, Dick IM, et al. Prevention of postmenopausal osteoporosis: a comparative study of exercise, calcium supplementation, and hormone-replacement therapy. N Engl J Med 1991;325:1189–95.

Recker RR, Davies KM, Hinders SM, et al. Bone gain in young adult women. JAMA 1992;268:2403–8.

Recker RR, Saville PD, Heaney RP. Effect of oestrogens and calcium carbonate on bone loss in postmenopausal women. Ann Intern Med 1977;87:649–55.

Reid IR, Ames RW, Evans MC, Gamble GD, Sharpe SJ. Effect of calcium supplementation on bone loss in postmenopausal women. N Engl J Med 1993;328:460–4.

Reid IR, Ames RW, Evans MC, Gamble GD, Sharpe SJ. Long-term effects of calcium supplementation on bone loss and fractures in postmenopausal women: a randomized controlled trial. Am J Med 1995;98:331–5.

Reid IR, Schooler BA, Hannon SF, Ibbertson HK. The acute biochemical effects of four proprietary calcium preparations. Aust NZ J Med 1986;16:193–7.

Rencken ML, Chesnut CH, Drinkwater BL. Bone density at multiple skeletal sites in amenorrheic athletes. JAMA 1996;276:238–40.

Riggs BL, Wahner HW, Melton LJ, Richelson LS, Judd HL, O'Fallon WM. Dietary calcium intake and rates of bone loss in women. J Clin Invest 1987;80:979–82.

Riis B, Thomsen K, Christiansen C. Does calcium supplementation prevent postmenopausal bone loss? N Engl J Med 1987;316:173–7.

Risser WL, Lee EJ, Leblanc A, Poindexter HB, Risser JMH, Schneider V. Bone density in eumenorrheic female college athletes. Med Sci Sports Exerc 1990;570–4.

Robinson TL, Snow-Harter C, Taaffe DR, Gillis D, Shaw J, Marcuss R. Gymnasts exhibit higher bone mass than runners despite similar prevalence of amenorrhoea and oligomenorrhoea. J Bone Miner Res 1995;10:26–35.

Rockwell JC, Sorenson AM, Baker S, Leahey D, Stock JL. Weight training decreases vertebral bone density in premenopausal women: a prospective study. J Clin Endocrinol Metab 1990;71:988–93.

Rubin LA, Hawker GA, Peltekova VD, Fielding LJ, Ridout R, Cole DEC. Determinants of peak bone mass: clinical and genetic analyses in a young female Canadian cohort. J Bone Miner Res 1999;14:633–43.

Rutherford OM. Spine and total body bone mineral density in amenorrheic endurance athletes. J Appl Physiol 1993;74:2904–8.

Sanborn CF, Albrecht BH, Wagner WW. Athletic amenorrhoea: lack of association with body fat. Med Sci Sports Exerc 1987;19:207–12.

Sandler RB, Cauley JA, Hom DL, Sashin D, Kriska AM. The effects of walking on the cross-sectional dimensions of the radius in postmenopausal women. Calcif Tissue Int 1987;41:65–9.

Scott EC, Johnston FE. Science nutrition, fat and policy: tests of the critical-fat hypothesis. Current Anthropol 1985;26:463–73.

Simkin A, Ayalon J, Leichter I. Increased trabecular bone density due to bone-loading exercises in postmenopausal osteoporotic women. Calcif Tissue Int 1987;40:59–63.

Sinning WE, Little KD, Wilson JR, Bowers BM. Body composition and menstrual function in women athletes. Abstract. Med Sci Sports Exerc 1985;17:214.

Slemenda C, Hui SL, Longcope C, Johnston CC. Sex steroids and bone mass: a study of changes about the time of menopause. J Clin Invest 1987;80(5):1261–9.

Slemenda CW, Peacock M, Hui SL, Zhou L, Johnston CC. Reduced rates of skeletal remodelling are associated with increased bone mineral density during the development of peak skeletal mass. J Bone Miner Res 1997;12:676–82.

Smith DA, Anderson JJB, Aitken JM, Shimmins J. The effects of calcium supplements of the diet on bone mass measurements. In: Kuhlencordt F, Kruse HP, eds. Calcium metabolism, bone and metabolic bone disease. Berlin: Springer, 1975:278–82.

Smith EL, Gilligan C, Smith PE, Sempos CT. Calcium supplementation and bone loss in middle-aged women. Am J Clin Nutr 1989;50:833–42.

Smith EL, Reddan W, Smith PE. Physical activity and calcium modalities for bone mineral increase in aged women. Med Sci Sports Exerc 1981;13:60–4.

Snead DB, Weltman A, Weltman JY, et al. Reproductive hormones and bone mineral density in women runners. J Appl Physiol 1992;72:2149–56.

Snow-Harter C, Bouxsein ML, Lewis BT, Carter DR, Marcus R. Effects of resistance and endurance exercise on bone mineral status of young women: a randomized exercise intervention trial. J Bone Miner Res 1992;7:761–9.

Stepan JJ, Pospichal J, Presl J, Pacovsky V. Bone loss and biochemical indices of bone remodelling in surgically induced postmenopausal women. Bone 1987;8:279–84.

Taaffe DR, Snow-Harter C, Connolly DA, Robinson TL, Brown MD, Marcus R. Differential effects of swimming versus weight-bearing activity on bone mineral status of eumenorrheic athletes. J Bone Miner Res 1995;10:586–93.

Vuori I, Heinonen A, Sievanen H, Kannus P, Pasanen M, Oja P. Effects of unilateral strength training and detraining on bone mineral density and content in young women: a study of mechanical loading and deloading on human bones. Calcif Tissue Int 1994;55:59–67.

Walberg JL, Johnston CS. Menstrual function and eating behaviour in female recreational weight lifters and competitive body builders. Med Sci Sports Exerc 1991;23:30–6.

Warren MP, Brooks-Gunn J, Fox RP, Lancelot C, Newman D, Hamilton WG. Lack of bone accretion and amenorrhoea: evidence for a relative osteopenia in weight-bearing bones. J Clin Endocrinol Metab 1991;72:847–53.

Warren MP, Brooks-Gunn J, Hamilton LH, Warren LF, Hamilton WG. Scoliosis and fractures in young ballet dancers. N Engl J Med 1986;314:1348–53.

Wolman RL, Clark P, McNally E, Harries M, Reeve J. Menstrual state and exercise as determinants of spinal trabecular bone density in female athletes. Brit Med J 1990;301:516–18.

Wolman RL, Clark P, McNally E, Harries MG, Reeve J. Dietary calcium as a statistical determinant of spinal trabecular bone density in amenorrheic and oestrogen-replete athletes. Bone Min 1992;17:415–23.

Wolman RL, Harries MG, Fyfe I. Slipped upper femoral epiphysis in an amenorrheic athlete. BMJ 1989;299(6701):720–1.

World Health Organization technical report series, No. 843. Assessment of fracture risk and its application to screening for postmenopausal osteoporosis. Geneva: World Health Organization, 1994.

Young N, Formica C, Szmukler G, Seeman E. Bone density at weight-bearing and non-weight-bearing sites in ballet dancers: the effects of exercise, hypogonadism and body weight. J Clin Endocrinol Metab 1994;78:449–54.

Zanker CL. Bone metabolism in exercise associated amenorrhoea: the importance of nutrition. Brit J Sports Med 1999;33:228–9.

Zanker CL, Swaine IL. Bone turnover in amenorrheic and eumenorrheic women distance runners. Scand J Med Sci Sports 1998;8:20–6.

CHAPTER 11

Iron depletion in athletes

Vicki Deakin

11.1 INTRODUCTION

Elite and recreational athletes undertaking hard training have a higher requirement and turnover of iron than less physically active people and quickly deplete iron stores. Female and adolescent athletes are at highest risk of iron depletion and often have difficulty meeting iron requirements. Although iron is widely distributed in foods, its absorption is influenced by the way foods are combined in meals and snacks. High-carbohydrate diets recommended for athletes may be high in compounds that inhibit iron absorption. While type of diet is a contributing factor to iron depletion in athletes, physiological and medical factors also play a role.

If untreated, iron depletion can ultimately lead to iron deficiency anaemia, which severely impairs aerobic performance. Although most scientific studies suggest there is no measurable impairment of aerobic performance when iron stores are low or when the athlete is iron-deficient (without anaemia), some iron-deficient athletes do experience physiological or psychological effects, which can affect training potential. Dietary strategies to help prevent iron depletion should be implemented early in the training program, where possible. Early detection of depleted iron stores and dietary intervention is warranted to prevent anaemia developing. Recovery from anaemia is slow; it can take months for athletes to reach previous condition and training levels.

11.2 FUNCTION OF IRON IN RELATION TO PERFORMANCE

A decrease in performance capacity and recovery is related to the function of iron and its role in oxygen transport and energy metabolism. Iron is essential:

- for the synthesis of the oxygen transport proteins, haemoglobin in the blood and myoglobin in the muscle;

- as a component of the electron transport system that controls the energy release from cells;
- as a component of an enzyme system (ribonucleotide reductase enzyme) required for the production of DNA;
- as a catalyst in the production of free radicals; and
- for erythropoiesis (red blood cell production).

The body cannot manufacture its own iron and is dependent on the diet for its supply. The largest component of iron in the body is found in the oxygen transport proteins—haemoglobin in the blood (60–70% of total iron) and myoglobin in the muscle tissue (10% of total iron) (Neilsen & Nachtigall 1998). Iron is transported through the plasma and extravascular fluids in protein carriers called transferrin. The rest is mainly stored as ferritin and haemosiderin in the liver, bone marrow and muscle ready for erythropoiesis, although a small component (around 2%) is used in metabolic systems.

Iron depletion affects performance capacity in two ways. Firstly, a lack of iron may limit haemoglobin production. In this instance, maximal oxygen uptake is decreased and, as a result, delivery of oxygen to the tissues will also decrease. Secondly, insufficient iron reduces the capacity of muscle to use oxygen for the oxidative production of energy—in the form of adenosine triphosphate (ATP). This oxidative process in the muscle mitochondria requires the iron-containing electron transport proteins, and iron–sulphur proteins and cytochromes. When muscles are iron-depleted, therefore, aerobic metabolism is impaired.

11.3 STAGES OF IRON DEPLETION, INCLUDING THE EFFECTS OF THESE STAGES ON PERFORMANCE CAPACITY IN ATHLETES

Although a continuous process, iron depletion has been categorised into three stages: depletion of iron stores, iron deficiency without anaemia, and iron deficiency anaemia. Sports anaemia is another iron status category that applies to a phenomenon seen in athletic populations. As iron is depleted progressively, all iron-containing compounds in the body eventually reduce in amount, although not all compounds become affected at the same time. Interpreting these values in an athletic population is described in detail in Section 11.6.1.

The effect on performance capacity varies between individuals and at each stage of the iron depletion process. Some individuals appear more susceptible to experiencing clinical symptoms than others (see Section 11.6.2).

11.3.1 *Depleted iron stores and iron deficiency without anaemia*

Many athletes, especially adolescents and females, present with biochemical measures that indicate depleted iron stores or iron deficiency without anaemia (Bergstrom et al. 1996, p.159–60). Biochemical measures that are collected on a

Table 11.1   *Cut-off population reference levels for iron status measures for detection of iron depletion at each category*

Stage	Changes in iron status measures	Serum ferritin (μg/L)	Haemoglobin (g/dL)	Transferrin saturation (%)
Normal iron storage	All iron status within population reference ranges	> 30 (F) > 110 (M)	> 12.0 (F) > 14.0 (M)	20–40 (M, F)
Depletion of iron stores	Low serum ferritin, normal to high serum transferrin saturation, normal haemoglobin and haematocrit	< 30 (M, F)	Normal range of haemoglobin	20–40 (M, F)
Iron deficiency	Low serum ferritin, low serum transferrin and serum iron, reduced transferrin saturation, free erythrocyte protoporhyrin increases, normal haemoglobin	< 12 (M, F)	Normal range of haemoglobin	< 16 (M, F)
Iron deficiency anaemia	Low haemoglobin, hypochromic, microcytic red blood cells, reduced mean corpuscular volume, low haematocrit, low serum iron, transferrin and transferrin saturation	< 10 (M, F)	< 12 (F) < 14 (M)	< 16 M, F)

M = male, F = female
Adapted from: Crosby and O'Neill (1984); Cook and Finch (1992); Cobiac and Baghurst (1993)

single occasion are difficult to interpret in individual athletes, and do not necessarily confirm an iron deficiency condition. Repeated measures in combination with other diagnostic protocol, including clinical symptoms and dietary assessment, are needed to confirm a genuine diagnosis (see Section 11.6.2). Even when clinical symptoms are evident, iron depletion or deficiency can easily be misdiagnosed in athletes using biochemical measures. Blood status measures below the reference ranges listed in Table 11.1 are often normal for individuals, especially adolescents, and are closely associated with maturational age, body mass, sex, genetic factors and physical activity (Rossander-Hulten & Hallberg 1996, p. 153–5). Interpretation of specific biochemical measures of iron status specific to an athletic population is described later in Section 11.6.1.

Most studies have found no improvement in aerobic capacity ($VO_{2\ max}$) in response to iron supplementation in athletes with depleted or exhausted iron stores without anaemia (Newhouse & Clement 1989; Fogelholm 1992; Neilsen & Nachtigall 1998; Ashenden et al. 1998). Although iron deficiency and iron depletion have been linked to higher than usual levels of lactic acid with exercise (Lukaski et al. 1991), only a few studies have supported a decrease in lactic acid levels after supplementation compared to levels before supplementation (Schoene et al. 1983; LaManca & Haymes 1993a). High levels of lactic acid inhibit physical activity. Symptoms of fatigue and lethargy may or may not be present in iron depletion. Whether these symptoms are related to the iron depletion or other factors, such as over-training, are difficult to determine. In summary, depleted and exhausted iron store levels do not necessarily limit performance when haemoglobin is in the normal range.

11.3.2 *Iron deficiency anaemia*

Iron deficiency anaemia is detected by blood iron status measures that are below population reference standards and also below the 'usual or normal' levels for an individual. In this condition, inadequate iron is available in the bone marrow and manufacture of haemoglobin and red blood cells is limited. Diagnosis is confirmed if red blood cells become small and pale, and clinical symptoms are present (see Section 11.6.2). Iron deficiency anaemia reduces ability to undertake aerobic activity, mainly because of insufficient haemoglobin (Newhouse & Clement 1988), but can also cause disturbances of brain metabolism, muscle metabolism, immunity and temperature control, depending on its severity (Bothwell 1995). Iron deficiency anaemia responds well to dietary intervention and iron supplements.

11.3.3 *Sports anaemia*

Sports anaemia has a similar profile of iron status measures to iron deficiency anaemia (see Table 11.1) but the red blood cells are normal in colour and size. A low iron status measure in an athletic population is not necessarily indicative of genuine iron depletion or deficiency. For some athletes, an expanded plasma volume resulting in a dilutional effect explains these apparently low iron status measurements in the blood. Increases in plasma volume are a 'normal' physiological response to hard exercise (Dressendorfer et al. 1991) with up to 20% increases reported in runners (Dill et al. 1974; Brotherhood et al. 1975).

Sports anaemia occurs in athletes early in the training program, especially after a rest period or injury, or after an endurance phase of training (Convertino 1991) but is unlikely to affect performance. Sports anaemia, therefore, is not considered genuine iron deficiency anaemia, in that iron is not limiting red blood cell production (Newhouse & Clement 1988). The phenomenon is usually transitory. Unlike iron deficiency anaemia and iron depletion, low iron status measures do not respond to iron supplements (Hegenauer et al. 1983; Magnusson et al. 1984). Weight and colleagues (1992) conclude that the term 'sports anaemia' is misleading and that its use should be discouraged.

As it is difficult to differentiate between sports anaemia and true iron depletion or iron deficiency from a single blood test using readily available iron status measures, Ashenden et al. (1998) suggest that low iron status measures from the first blood test of an athlete should be treated as a risk for developing anaemia.

11.4 PREVALENCE OF IRON DEPLETION IN ATHLETES

Although the prevalence of depleted iron stores in athletes is usually higher than control groups, the reported prevalence of iron deficiency anaemia is quite low (< 3%) and similar between athletes and untrained individuals (Fogelholm 1995).

11.4.1 *From biochemical studies*

The prevalence of iron depletion in athletes based on low serum ferritin levels varies according to type of sport, age of athletes and sex. Fogelholm (1995) has summarised serum ferritin values from iron studies of athletes since 1980, including only those studies with control groups. In these studies, the pooled mean prevalence of low serum ferritin was 37% (range 13–50%) in male and female athletes (n = 329) and 23% (range 10–46%) in controls (n = 286). The highest prevalence occurs in endurance sports, in female and adolescent athletes, irrespective of the type of sport and intensity of training (Diehl et al. 1982; Rowland & Kelleher 1989; Weight et al. 1992; Newhouse et al. 1993; Pate et al. 1993; Williford et al. 1993).

The prevalence of low ferritin levels in males is usually higher in runners, particularly distance runners, than cyclists and rowers (Dufaux et al. 1991; Fogelholm 1995) but often higher or no different than controls in other endurance sports (e.g. rowers) (Dufaux et al. 1981) and team sports (Fogelholm 1995).

11.4.2 *From dietary studies*

Athletes on low energy intakes are the most frequently reported groups of athletes whose diets contain less than recommended intakes of iron (Ellsworth et al. 1985; Barr 1987;

Risser & Risser 1990; Haymes 1992). Iron intakes of athletes are usually higher or no different to untrained controls (Resina et al. 1991; Fogelholm 1995). Under-reporting, a common problem in dietary surveys, however, can distort actual intakes and bias the interpretation of the results. In some studies, the control groups are also not meeting the RDI for iron and are under-reporting energy intake (see Chapter 3, Section 3.3.3.1).

Despite the potential bias from under-reporting in dietary surveys, females are still at greater risk of depleting iron stores than males because they generally eat less food and therefore have less total iron available in their diets.

11.5 *AETIOLOGY OF IRON DEPLETION IN ATHLETES*

A number of physiological and dietary factors are associated with iron deficiency in athletes. High iron requirements and losses of iron induced by strenuous exercise, maturational age and growth requirement, sub-optimal intakes and low bioavailability of dietary iron are all implicated.

11.5.1 *Physiological factors*

A 'normal' physiological response to strenuous exercise is an increase in vascularity accompanied by an increase in red cell mass and haemoglobin, all of which are dependent on dietary iron. Requirements for iron are higher in adolescents during a growth spurt although a higher absorption of iron usually compensates for this increase. Although iron requirements may be higher in athletes than sedentary people, exercise-induced iron loss is strongly implicated as a cause of iron deficiency. Athletes involved in strenuous exercise lose iron in several ways: through sweating (LaManca et al. 1988; Waller & Haymes 1996); from gastrointestinal bleeding (Lampe et al. 1987; Nachtigall et al. 1996); by the breakdown of red blood cells caused by mechanical and capillary trauma (Miller et al. 1988) or from injury associated with blood loss. No single theory of physiological factor has explained the magnitude of the decline in serum ferritin seen during training (Cook 1994).

Few studies have attempted to estimate accurately the extent of iron loss through sweat during prolonged exercise. However, losses are reported to be relatively greater in distance runners and greater in female than male runners (LaManca et al. 1988). Gastrointestinal blood loss of large magnitude has been documented in male and female distance runners (McMahon et al. 1984; Lampe et al. 1987), but the aetiology is not well understood. It may be caused by desquamation of cells from the intestinal wall or ischaemia of the stomach and intestinal lining. Some loss has been attributed to the habitual use of anti-inflammatory drugs.

The presence of blood or intact red blood cells in the urine reported by athletes after strenuous physical activity (Siegal et al. 1979) may be caused by trauma to the bladder wall. Mechanical trauma or weakening of the red cell membranes has been associated with footstrike haemolysis (destruction of red blood cells) during running (Miller et al. 1988).

Finally, women usually have a higher requirement for iron than men because of blood loss from menstruation. Of interest, however, is that many female athletes experience a reduction in severity and frequency of menses, so iron loss by menstruation is not a major contributing factor to iron depletion.

11.5.2 *Dietary factors*

Low intakes of iron-rich foods and/or foods with a low iron bioavailability (see Section 11.5.2.2), in combination with the physiological mechanisms related to high requirements in athletes, all contribute to iron depletion.

11.5.2.1 *Type of diets associated with a low iron intake*

Low-energy diets

Low-energy diets accompanied by iron intakes less than population recommendations have been reported in both male and female athletes from various sports (Haymes 1992), but especially in females maintaining a lean body mass. Athletes who habitually consume low-energy diets—below 8300 kJ (2000 kcal)—also usually have sub-optimal iron intakes, and low iron status (Clement & Sawchuk 1984).

Vegetarian diets

Athletes who follow vegetarian diets or who eat little red meat or meat products usually have lower iron status than meat-eaters, despite similar iron intakes (Seiler et al. 1989; Snyder et al. 1989). Iron derived from plant foods is poorly absorbed (see Section 11.5.2.2). Lacto-ovo-vegetarians who include large intakes of dairy foods, but exclude animal flesh, are at risk of developing iron deficiency, as milk and dairy products are poor sources of iron, and the high calcium present in these foods inhibits iron absorption from other sources, if eaten at the same time.

Natural food eaters

Athletes who avoid commercial or packaged foods such as breakfast cereals are missing out on products that are iron-fortified (have extra iron added). For example, one serve of porridge contains about half the iron content of most commercial breakfast cereals. Contrary to popular belief, bread, breakfast cereals and other cereal-based products contribute more iron in the western diet than meat and meat products (McLennan & Podger 1998).

Very high carbohydrate diets and athletes with a high energy expenditure

High-carbohydrate diets were associated with low iron stores in a study of 76 elite Australian Institute of Sport (AIS) athletes (24 males and 45 females) (Telford et al. 1993). Total iron intake of these athletes was considered satisfactory, therefore these low iron stores may be related to the low bioavailability of iron from some carbohydrate-rich foods (e.g. cereals and breads) in the diets of these athletes.

Those athletes with very high energy expenditure also had the lowest iron status measurements, despite high iron intakes (Telford et al. 1993). These low iron measures were likely to be the result of physiological factors unrelated to iron intake influencing iron loss and turnover (see Section 11.5.1).

Fad diets and weight-control products

Some fad or popular diets and sports products are marketed to athletes for performance-enhancement, weight gain or weight loss. Promoters often make exaggerated claims about the efficacy of these products and diets. In most cases, scientific theory and evidence does not support these claims. Some fad diets or formulations are detrimental if used for a long time, because of inadequate nutrient composition. For example, a diet based mainly on fruit is deficient in protein, iron, zinc, and many other important nutrients. The habitual use of beverages from formulated diets or protein supplements as a substitute for meals is not recommended for athletes as most formulations do not meet the energy or nutrient needs of hard training. Athletes who follow unusual eating regimens, consistently miss meals and have erratic eating patterns can also consume sub-optimal intakes of iron. These types of dietary habits are not atypical of adolescents, a high-risk group for iron deficiency (Abrahams et al. 1988; Bothwell 1995).

11.5.2.2 *Bioavailability of iron*

Bioavailability of iron is defined as the amount of ingested iron, which is absorbed and utilised for metabolic functions (Hurrell 1997). Bioavailability of iron is related to iron status (whether deficient or replete), the amount of total iron consumed, and other naturally occurring components in food that can inhibit or enhance iron uptake (Hulten et al. 1995).

Bioavailability and iron status

Iron status controls the absorption as well as the distribution and transport of iron to different tissues in the body. In an iron-replete individual, total iron absorption is around 5–15% from the total diet (Moore 1964). Whereas in people who are iron depleted, anaemic or have increased physiological requirements to support growth, pregnancy or lactation, absorption increases considerably and roughly parallels the change in iron requirements (Hallberg & Hulten 1996, p. 177; Fairweather-Tait 1996, p. 143). Athletes with low iron stores also show enhanced absorption of iron (Nachtigall et al. 1996). The actual mechanism responsible for this up-regulation of iron absorption is still unknown.

Bioavailability of iron from foods

Iron in foods exists in two forms: haem and non-haem iron. Meat, liver, seafoods and poultry contain both forms while plant sources, mainly cereals, legumes, vegetables and eggs contain only the non-haem form. Meat contains 30–70% of its total iron as haem iron (MacPhail et al. 1985; Rangan et al. 1997). In Australian meat, the iron content of cooked beef, lamb, pork and chicken is 60–65% of total iron as haem iron, whereas sausages, liver and fish contain lower amounts of haem iron (20–40%)(Rangan et al. 1997). Hallberg (1981) suggested that haem iron represented only around 10–15% of total daily iron intakes in diets of industrialised populations. This is based on the contribution of meat in the total diets of these populations. However, recent work from Australia, where meat is relatively inexpensive (compared to Europe and Asian countries), and consumed frequently in main meals, reveals haem iron intakes may be higher than Hallberg's earlier estimations (Rangan et al. 1997). Estimations of the amount of haem iron available for consumption in the food supply suggested a haem iron supply of 60% of total iron available (Rangan et al. 1997). This is higher than the estimated 40% contribution of haem iron available for consumption in the United States. In Australia, consumer preference for leaner meat, which has a higher iron density that fattier cuts, is likely to account for the apparent haem iron increase in the Australian food supply. Irrespective of these figures, an athlete consuming a high-carbohydrate diet is probably eating less meat and therefore less haem iron and a diet with low bioavailability.

11.5.2.3 *Components in foods affecting absorption of iron*

To date, studies of iron bioavailability using absorption methodology or radioactive labelling of iron in food have not been undertaken in an athletic population. In the absence of such data, the information presented here comes from absorption studies of iron in other population groups. There is no physiological evidence to indicate that the absorption of iron from healthy non-anaemic athletes would be any different to that of any other healthy population.

Based on a compilation of iron absorption studies, single plant foods containing non-haem iron have relatively low and variable absorption rates (2–8%), because of the presence of inhibitory or enhancing components in food (see Table 11.2). Absorption of haem iron from single foods, and when included in a mixed meal, is much greater (15–35%) (Monsen et al. 1978) and was believed, until recently, to be largely unaffected by enhancing or inhibiting components. However, recent research, using updated absorption methodology, has shown that haem iron absorption could also be inhibited by other components in meals, such as calcium content, and enhanced by peptides from partially digested muscle tissue (Hallberg et al. 1997).

Inhibitors and enhancers present in food (listed in Table 11.2) affect the bioavailability of iron, when they are consumed at the same time as iron-rich foods. Many iron-rich foods themselves, including cereal grains and spinach, contain substantial quantities of inhibiting components that bind iron and limit its absorption. Soy bean and its products contain several different inhibiting compounds.

Table 11.2 *Components in food that affect bioavailability of iron, mainly from non-haem food sources*

Iron enhancers	Iron inhibitors
Vitamin C–rich foods [1,2] *(salad, lightly cooked green vegetables, some fruits and citrus fruit juices or vitamin C fortified fruit juices)*	Phytate (myoinostol hexaphosphate) [8,6] *(cereal grains, wheat bran, legumes, nuts, peanut butter, seeds, bran, soy products, soy protein, spinach)*
Some fermented foods (with a low pH) [5,6] *(sauerkraut, misu, some types of soy sauce)*	Polyphenolic compounds [1,4,6] *(strong tea and coffee, herb tea, cocoa, red wine, some spices (e.g. oregano))*
Peptides from partially digested muscle tissue enhance both haem and non-haem iron [10] *(often called the Meat Enhancement Factor, beef, lamb, chicken, fish, pork, liver)*	Calcium inhibits both haem and non-haem iron [1,2,3] *(milk, cheese)*
Alcohol and some organic acids [6] *(very low pH foods containing citric acid, tartaric acid (e.g. citrus fruit))*	Peptides from partially digested plant proteins [7,4,9,12] *(soy protein isolates, soy products)*

[1]*Hallberg 1981;* [2]*Hallberg et al. 1993;* [3]*Cook et al. 1991b;* [4]*Hallberg and Rossander 1982b;* [5]*Baynes et al. 1990, 1992;* [6]*Gilooly et al. 1983;* [7]*Lynch et al. 1994;* [8]*Brune et al. 1992;* [9]*Hurrell 1997;* [10]*Layrisse et al. 1998;* [11]*Gilooly et al. 1984;* [12]*Hallberg and Rossander 1982a*

Inhibitors of non-haem iron bioavailability

Inhibiting compounds are thought to bind iron or make iron unavailable for absorption. Although fibre *per se* does not inhibit iron absorption (Brune et al. 1992), foods rich in fibre usually contain phytates, which are powerful inhibitors. Phytate, which can inhibit non-haem absorption by 50–80%, concentrates in the bran and germ of cereal grains and legumes and is often added as soy protein isolates to manufactured foods (Hurrell 1997). Vegetables and fruits are poor sources of phytate. High-bran cereals can have more than 3000 mg phytate/100 g wheat cereal compared to cornflakes with around 70 mg phytate/100 g cereal (Harland & Oberleas 1987).

Polyphenolic compounds found in plants include phenolic acid, flavonoids and their products. Tannic acid (or tannin—a flavonoid in food), for example, is highest in black tea compared with other types of tea (e.g. herbal or green teas) and is a potent inhibitor of non-haem iron absorption. In a western-style breakfast (toast and tea), the absorption of iron was reduced by 60% because of concurrent consumption with tea (Rossander et al. 1979). In another study, coffee reduced absorption of non-haem iron by 35% from a hamburger meal and tea reduced absorption of non-haem iron by 62% (Hallberg & Rossander 1982b). The inhibition of iron absorption by tannate salts (the insoluble salt in tea), and to a lesser extent in coffee, is strongly dose-related. Even at low tannate concentrations of 5 mg, absorption of iron was inhibited by 30%; at concentrations of 25 mg, by 67%, and at concentrations of 100 mg by 88% (Brune et al. 1989). Coffee/tea consumption and high carbohydrate intakes were significantly associated with low serum ferritin in 111 adult female runners (Pate et al. 1993). One glass of red wine (high in polyphenolic compounds) reduced iron absorption from a small bread meal by 75% (Cook et al. 1995).

The overall inhibitory effects on iron absorption from calcium in milk and dairy foods are less clear and appear weaker than other inhibitory components, although both the absorption of haem and non-haem iron from food can be impaired (Hurrell 1997). The relatively weak effect of calcium on iron absorption, from a total varied diet reported by Reddy and Cook (1997), does not justify avoidance of milk or dairy foods with iron-rich food (e.g. milk with breakfast cereal). Inadequate intakes of calcium are already a concern for female and adolescent athletes and removal of milk from breakfast foods would further decrease calcium intakes.

Peptides, from the partial digestion of proteins, can both inhibit or enhance non-haem iron absorption depending on their source (Hurrell 1997). As shown in Table 11.2, peptides derived from legume proteins are inhibitory and bind iron in the intestinal lumen while peptides from animal protein appear to enhance iron absorption with the exception of calcium peptides from dairy foods (MacFarlane et al. 1988; Hurrell 1997).

Enhancers of iron absorption

The most well defined enhancers of iron absorption are vitamin C–rich (ascorbic acid) foods, other low pH (acidic) foods and the quantity of animal muscle tissue present in each meal. The low pH of these enhancing compounds, and their potential to chelate iron, reduces ferric iron to the more soluble ferrous iron, which increases iron bioavailability for absorption (Hurrell 1997).

Ascorbic acid is the most potent iron-enhancer known. One glass of orange juice containing 110 mg ascorbic acid consumed with a hamburger meal increased absorption of non-haem iron by 85% (Hallberg & Rossander 1982b). Large amounts of ascorbic acid in doses up to 500 mg were needed to achieve significant effects on iron absorption from meals with high phytate and tannate content (Hallberg et al. 1986). The enhancing effects of ascorbic acid are dose-related and high intakes can reduce the negative effect on iron absorption exerted by phytate in cereals and other inhibitors (Hallberg et al. 1989). As a general guideline for enhancing iron absorption, Hallberg and colleagues (1989) suggested that foods containing about 50 mg of ascorbic acid should be included with each main meal. Table 11.7 provides examples of vitamin C-rich foods.

Muscle tissue in meat exerts a promoting effect on the absorption of both haem and non-haem iron, which appears to be related to the cysteine-containing peptides in these tissues (Layrisse et al. 1984). So not only is the haem iron in meat well-absorbed, but the peptides resulting from digestion of meat increase the absorption of iron from other iron-rich foods. This explains why people who eat meat every-day or most days have higher serum ferritin levels than non-meat eaters (Bothwell 1995).

Relevance of bioavailability studies to an athletic population

Most of the early studies of bioavailability of iron in the 1970s and 80s were conducted on single foods and then later on complete meals. In 1991, Cook and colleagues published a new technique to determine the total amount of iron absorbed from the whole diet over several days instead of just meals or single foods (Cook et al. 1991a). The follow-up studies investigating the iron bioavailability of the whole diet confirm the importance of combining foods in the total diet as a means to maximise iron absorption (Hulten et al. 1995; Hallberg et al. 1997). Athletes, however, are encouraged to consume total diets that may have a low iron bioavailability (high in cereals and phytates) and compromise iron status. Nutrition education about food combinations to enhance iron absorption, therefore, is essential. Section 11.10 describes such food combinations.

11.6 ASSESSMENT OF IRON STATUS OF AN ATHLETE: CLINICAL PERSPECTIVES

11.6.1 Biochemical measures of iron status: clinical and research perspectives

As a preventative measure in sports medicine practice, routine haematological measures of iron status are often conducted to detect iron depletion rather than to estimate its severity. Iron-depleted athletes can quickly develop iron deficiency if not detected early. An array of iron status measures are available to fully assess iron status; however, in most sports medicine practices, usually only serum iron, ferritin, transferrin, transferrin saturation and haemoglobin are routinely measured, together with a full blood count. The interpretation of these and other biochemical iron status measures, used mainly in research, are briefly described in this section. Further detailed information is found elsewhere (Smith & Roberts 1994; Pyne et al. 1997).

Most biochemical reference ranges for evaluating iron status in athletes are still based on population reference standards as mentioned earlier (see Section 11.3). There are differences in the range of some of these measures between athletes and the general population (as outlined in this section), so interpretation based on population or reference data can be distorted or erroneous. Although reference values may be inappropriate for athletes, they still serve as the main data for interpretation. Appendix 11, Table 11.11 summarises these population values in SI units (Systeme International d'Unites) with corresponding conversion to British units.

The extent of iron depletion is determined by examining several biochemical measures found in the three main iron-containing compartments of the body; storage iron, transport iron and red blood cells. Combinations of several of these parameters help confirm a diagnosis of iron depletion and its severity.

11.6.1.1   *Storage iron*

Serum ferritin

Storage iron comprises intra-cellular ferritin and haemosiderin which are found mainly in the liver, spleen and bone marrow, with small stores circulating in the blood as serum ferritin. Serum ferritin is the most commonly used single indicator of iron stores (Borch-Iohnsen 1995) and is closely associated with intra-cellular ferritin in the body, which parallels concentration of storage iron (Lipschitz et al. 1974). Small amounts of ferritin are normally present in the serum in concentrations between 15 and 300 µg/L in healthy non-athletic adults (Worwood 1991). The mean normal serum ferritin concentration in the absence of iron deficiency in non-athletic adults was reported to be 69.2 µg/L in 174 men and 34 µg/L in 152 women (Cook et al. 1974). Similar values are reported in elite adult athletes, although the data appears skewed toward the lower end of the range (Telford & Cunningham 1991; Ashenden et al. 1998).

In physically untrained adults, serum ferritin below 30 µg/L indicates iron depletion or iron deficiency (Crosby & O'Neill 1984) and 12 µg ferritin/L denotes exhaustion of iron stores (Cook et al. 1974). Early studies suggested that athletes had absent iron stores in the bone marrow when serum ferritin was around 20 µg/L (Clement & Asmundson 1982). However, a recent study, although based on a non-athletic population, suggested that the translation of serum ferritin into actual amounts of stored iron should be cautious (Hulten et al. 1995). Hulten and colleagues (1995) reported that the variation seen in serum ferritin in individuals is only partially explained by the variation in iron stores.

Serum ferritin levels and iron stores vary with age, sex and physical activity, and are low in young children and in adolescents during the growth phase (Baynes 1996). Often male adolescent athletes have low serum ferritin, despite high dietary iron intakes and iron supplements (Telford et al. 1993). Low serum ferritin may be physiologically 'normal' at this age as a slow increase in serum ferritin occurs through adolescence with a major rise in males in late adolescence and early adult years (Bothwell 1995; Bergstrom et al. 1996, p. 161). The reasons for a sharp increase in adolescent males and postmenopausal females have not been defined. Females do not show this late adolescent increase. Their levels tend to increase slowly to about the age of menopause and then increase relatively sharply. Adult reference values for serum ferritin cannot be applied reliably to children and adolescents (Bergstrom et al. 1996, p. 151). Reference ranges for children are available in most textbooks about biochemistry or haematology.

Serum ferritin declines in elite athletes during the training seasons. In 46 matched pairs of female AIS athletes serum ferritin declined by around 25% during training seasons, with greater declines seen in weight-bearing sports (i.e. netball and basketball) than non-weight-bearing sports (i.e. swimming and rowing) (Ashenden et al. 1998).

11.6.1.2 *Transport iron*

Serum iron and serum transferrin, by themselves, are of limited value in determining iron status. Instead, total serum iron-binding capacity is usually estimated at the same time so that the percentage saturation of transferrin can be calculated. Transferrin saturation and the recently introduced serum transferrin receptor measures are more useful to determine early stage iron depletion than serum iron and serum transferrin.

Serum iron

Serum iron is generally lower in females than males, and appears unaffected by the menstrual cycle but shows a large diurnal variation of around 20% (Beaton et al. 1989), the highest values being found in the mornings and the lowest in the latter part of the day (Jacobs 1974). Population reference ranges for serum iron are 14–32 μmol/L for males and 11–29 μmol/L for females (see Appendix 11, Table 11.11). There is a true sex difference in values for serum iron as there is for serum haemoglobin, irrespective of physical activity. However, the mean serum iron concentration is reported to be higher in untrained people than in athletes (Brotherhood et al. 1975).

Transferrin, transferrin saturation and transferrin receptor

Serum transferrin binds iron in the blood for transport to the tissue. Transferrin saturation is the ratio of serum iron to iron-binding capacity and is the most accurate indicator of iron supply to the bone marrow (Australian Iron Status Advisory Board 1999). In a non-athletic population, transferrin saturation is usually 20–40% saturated, with iron giving a serum iron concentration in the range of 14–32 μ/L (see Appendix 11, Table 11.11). A critical level of < 16% transferrin saturation has been established for an adult as a level at which red blood cell production is compromised (Bothwell et al. 1979; Finch & Cook 1984). Transferrin saturation levels > 50% are suspect of iron overload and possibly haemochromatosis (See Section 11.8.2.3). With early depletion of iron stores, transferrrin saturation increases to the upper end of the usual range or slightly higher. In iron deficiency, transferrin saturation decreases (see Appendix 11, Table 11.11).

Transferrin receptors control the entry of iron-bearing transferrin into cells and provide a sensitive, early and quantitative evaluation of the magnitude of iron deficiency in tissues. A description of the biochemistry and kinetics of transferrin receptor in iron depletion is outside the scope of this chapter and is reviewed elsewhere (Baynes 1996; Cook et al. 1996). When serum ferritin levels fall below 12 μg/L, transferrin receptor levels begin to rise and can be three to four times the normal physiological range in overt iron deficiency anaemia (Huebers et al. 1990).

Serum transferrin receptor is not subject to fluctuations associated with changes in plasma volume, so is likely to be valid for use in athletes and during periods of rapid growth, in pregnant women (Akesson et al. 1998), and in people with infection or inflammation where serum ferritin can be distorted (Baynes 1996). However, it is unreliable in people with anaemia, people with chronic diseases associated with hyperdestruction or hypoproliferation of red blood cells, or people with disorders in erythropoiesis (Beguin et al. 1993).

The combined use of serum ferritin and transferrin receptor allows a more reliable definition of iron status than ferritin alone. However, as transferrin receptor is a relatively new technique, its role as a diagnostic tool in population research studies and in athletes is still being defined.

11.6.1.3 *Red blood cell measures (full blood count, morphology, reticulocytes and free erythrocyte protoporphyrin concentration)*

Full red blood cell count

Red blood cells (RBC) undergo changes in number, size, density and composition in individuals developing iron deficiency. As iron becomes low, RBC numbers decrease and show a sub-normal haemoglobin concentration and abnormal morphology. The haematological and biochemistry laboratory at the AIS in Canberra has reported changes in red blood cells of individual athletes who are developing iron deficiency. These are listed in Table 11.3.

Table 11.3 *Changes in red blood cells in individuals developing iron deficiency*

- cellular haemoglobin content of reticulocytes is reduced
- % hypochromic and % microcytic cells are increased
- haemoglobin content of RBC is reduced (MCH)
- RBC mean cell volume (MCV) is reduced
- RBC haemoglobin concentration (MCHC) is reduced
- microcytic, hypochromic RBC may start to appear as the severity of iron depletion progresses

Adapted from Pyne et al. (1997)

The technology needed to perform all of the tests listed in Table 11.3 may not be readily available to sports medicine practices.

Haemoglobin and haematocrit

Haemoglobin and haematocrit values decrease only when severe iron depletion is present (Bothwell et al. 1979) (see Table 11.1). These measures are subject to wide individual variability in physiologically 'normal' levels as well as between 3–5% diurnal variation (Beaton et al. 1989).

Haemoglobin and haematocrit values are similar for boys and girls until puberty when they are higher in boys than girls and similar to adult values. In the absence of anaemia, however, haemoglobin and haematocrit values are usually higher in athletes than non-athletes (Brotherhood et al. 1975), higher in men than women (Sanborn & Jankowski 1994), and positively associated with a high body mass index (BMI) in athletes (Telford & Cunningham 1991).

Red cell morphology

With increasing severity of iron depletion, the number of red blood cells progressively decreases. Blood cells become microcytic and hypochromic with occasional rod-shaped cells and target cells appearing. Blood films are prepared and examined when haematology analyses flags abnormal results that may indicate iron deficiency. This allows a morphological examination to discriminate between diseases that induce similar changes in RBC morphology such as iron deficiency anaemia and Thalassemia minor (an inherited disorder of haemoglobin synthesis).

Reticulocytes

Reticulocytes are red blood cells recently released from the bone marrow. The number of reticulocytes provides a more direct indication of bone marrow status. Novel reticulocyte parameters appear to be valuable tools for predicting iron deficiency erythropoiesis and for assessing responses to iron therapy in intensely training athletes (Pyne et al. 1997). Researchers at the AIS are currently investigating the haemoglobin content of reticulocytes as an early indicator of iron depletion, rather than the traditional ferritin measurement. Low haemoglobin content in reticulocytes will result in low haemoglobin content in mature red blood cells as the developing cells lose haemoglobin. Iron supplements may be beneficial at this point to boost iron stores and to prevent further iron-deficient erythropoiesis (Ashenden et al. 1998).

Protoporphyrin

Protoporphyrin forms a part of the synthesis of haemoglobin and accumulates in the form of free protoporphyrin in the red blood cells (free erythrocyte protoporphyrin) in iron deficiency. Free erythrocyte protoporphyrin (FEP) does not normally exceed 40 μmol/L of red blood cells but may be increased in iron deficiency. An increase in concentration of FEP occurs just before the onset of anaemia and is more sensitive as an early sign of iron depletion than haemoglobin (Beaton et al. 1989). FEP is often used in population surveys but infrequently in clinical practice, despite its stability in individuals.

11.6.1.4 *Errors in interpretation of biochemical measures of iron status in athletes*

The use of blood measures to assist in interpreting iron status from a single or one-off biochemical test of iron status is often unreliable or misleading. Haematological tests are susceptible to fluctuations from physiological and pathological conditions that confound interpretation, as seen in Table 11.4. There is a spectrum of varied responses of these haematological parameters which vary with acute and intense, prolonged exercise, with trained and untrained subjects, and in different climatic conditions. Dehydration at the time of blood testing can result in haemoconcentration.

Table 11.4 *Reported directions of change of haematological measures in conditions encountered by athletes*

	Haemoglobin	% transferrin saturation	Serum iron	Ferritin*
Dehydration at the time of testing	↑	↑	↑	↑
Inflammation, malignancy	↓	↓	↓	↑*
Infection (URTI, flu, virus)	↓	↓	↓	↑*
Acute strenuous exercise (post 24 hr) in a trained person	↓	↓	↓	↑*
After intense prolonged exercise (post-marathon)*	↓	↓	↓	↑*

↑ = *increase (haemoconcentration),* ↓ = *decrease (haemodilution),* * = *acute phase reactant observed in acute trauma and stress, URTI = upper respiratory tract infection*
Adapted from Smith and Roberts (1994); Fallon et al. (1999)

As a guideline, all biochemical measurements of iron status should be taken on a rest day or prior to any strenuous exercise as exercise can falsify the results. Falsely elevated serum ferritin has been reported after intense endurance training (Lampe et al. 1986), and ultra-endurance events (Fallon et al. 1999). Ferritin levels rise during and after acute strenuous exercise and endurance events while serum iron decreases, which is indicative of an acute phase response (Fallon et al. 1999). Infection, inflammation or malignancy can also falsely elevate serum ferritin concentrations, particularly inflammation associated with liver damage, decreased haemoglobin, haematocrit, free erythrocyte protoporphyrin, serum iron and transferrin (Finch & Huebers 1982). Even minor infections can depress serum haemoglobin (Beaton et al. 1989).

11.6.1.5 *Summary*

The diagnosis of iron deficiency in athletes using biochemical measures is difficult and controversial, and likely to require the use of a number of diagnostic criteria.

Biochemistry alone does not confirm a diagnosis. Serum ferritin has been routinely in sports medicine practice and research for initial assessment and prospective monitoring of iron stores in elite athletes. Iron status measures may also include transferrin receptor when the technique becomes widely available in the near future. Haemoglobin and haematocrit have limited use in early detection of iron depletion as significant decreases are only observed in iron deficiency anaemia. Transferrin saturation and red cell protoporphyrin identify approximately twice as many individuals with iron deficiency as does haemoglobin determination. Measuring and monitoring changes in red blood cells, particularly immature red blood cells (reticulocytes), as suggested by the Australian Institute of Sport (See Table 11.3), is useful for evaluating relative changes in iron status in individual athletes. Beaton et al. (1989) have reviewed the uses and limitations of the commonly used measures of iron status in fieldwork for epidemiological studies. Similar methodological considerations described by Beaton and colleagues (1989) could be applied to an athletic population.

11.6.2 *Clinical symptoms*

Iron deficiency anaemia is associated with symptoms of fatigue, weakness, breathlessness and impaired aerobic capacity. Even in mild anaemia or iron depletion without anaemia, sufferers often look pale, may have a slightly elevated resting pulse rate, feel 'run-down' or 'washed out', exhibit changes in mood state or have a diminished appetite. These types of symptoms are often non-specific and may be confused with over-training, with glandular fever or an infection, or may even be considered 'normal' in an athlete or teenager. Conversely, many athletes with low ferritin levels have no apparent or overt symptoms. Despite an absence of clinical symptoms of iron deficiency, one study reported that 100 intercollegiate female athletes considered their performance to be worse when iron-depleted (Risser et al. 1988). Experienced elite athletes are often overly concerned about ferritin levels, routinely request blood tests and self-supplement with iron when iron depletion is absent. Several reasons given for these concerns include, as a preventative measure, fear of performance decrements (Deakin 1995, unpublished). In anxious elite athletes with a history of iron depletion, any sign of fatigue or lethargy is usually perceived as iron depletion.

11.6.3 *Dietary assessment*

Dietary assessment usually involves a complete dietary history with or without other dietary survey methods to assess factors that influence food intake, iron intake and availability of non-haem iron. Estimating the potential effect of physiological, training and medical factors on iron losses is a crucial component of the dietary interview. Techniques for assessing iron status are found in the Practice tips in Section 11.10.

A habitual low intake and poor bioavailability of dietary iron, together with clinical symptoms and several iron status measures below reference values, confirm a diagnosis of iron depletion or iron deficiency anaemia.

11.7 DIETARY INTERVENTION FOR IRON DEPLETION AND IRON DEFICIENCY

11.7.1 Recommended iron intakes for athletes

Daily iron requirements for different sports have not been established and are likely to be highly variable. The RDI for iron for healthy adults in Australia is 7 mg/d for men and 12–16 mg/d for women (National Health and Medical Research Council 1991). Table 11.8 in Section 11.10 provides two examples of a day's food intake with high and low bioavailability of iron that meets these levels. Daily iron losses in endurance runners have been estimated at 1.5–1.7 mg iron/d in men and 2.2–2.3 mg iron/d in women (Haymes & Lamanca 1989), although there is still debate about whether endurance athletes have truly low iron stores (Ashenden et al. 1998). Basal or obligatory iron losses in untrained adults is only 0.9–1.0 mg/d in males and 0.7 to 0.8 mg/d in women (excluding menstrual losses) (Bothwell 1996, p. 6). To meet iron losses in endurance athletes, Haymes and Lamanca (1989) recommended iron intakes for distance runners of 17.5 mg/d for men and around 23 mg/d in normally menstruating women, assuming iron absorption to be 10% of dietary iron from the total diet.

Studies of the dietary intakes of athletes in various sports have shown that male, but not female, athletes easily achieve the RDIs for iron. The RDIs/RDAs may not be applicable to endurance athletes in hard training programs.

11.7.2 Increase the total consumption of dietary iron and iron bioavailability

Female athletes involved in endurance sports should have diets that are high in total iron and that have a high iron bioavailability. Section 11.10 provides practical dietary strategies to achieve high iron intakes and high bioavailability of iron from food combinations.

11.8 MEDICAL INTERVENTION: IRON SUPPLEMENTS

11.8.1 Do iron supplements enhance performance?

It is well established that iron supplementation enhances performance in athletes with iron deficiency. In non-anaemic iron-depleted and iron-deficient athletes, performance was not affected by iron supplementation of athletes involved in team sports (Telford et al. 1992), or in aerobic activity (Weight et al. 1988; Weight et al. 1992; Fogelholm et al. 1992).

Many athletes are self-administering iron supplements daily or intermittently as an ergogenic aid or as a preventive measure without being diagnosed as iron depleted. In a large cross-sectional survey of drug use in 658 Australian athletes, nearly 70% of respondents in numerous team sports reported taking iron supplements regularly (Australian Sports Commission 1983). Whether the iron supplements were self-administered or given under medical supervision was not assessed.

The safety of, and necessity for taking, daily iron supplements, as a prophylaxis is questionable. Some studies have used high doses of iron supplements (up to 300 mg iron/d) as a prophylaxis during regular rigorous training to prevent iron depletion in non-depleted athletes (Yoshida et al. 1990; Magazanik et al. 1991). Such supplementation may impose adverse side-effects (see Section 11.8.2.2), although side-effects were not investigated in these studies.

11.8.2 *Iron supplements for clinical treatment of iron depletion*

Decisions about supplementing iron are usually clinically made on an individual case-by-case basis. To treat iron deficiency anaemia, an iron-rich diet, in combination with high doses of iron supplementation (> 100 mg/d), is needed to replete exhausted iron stores. Recovery of iron stores takes around three months (Neilsen & Nachtigall 1998). Diet intervention alone is incapable of repleting iron stores in three months. Using diet therapy alone, Hallberg and colleagues (1998) have recently devised predictive equations to determine the rate of increase of iron stores in untrained adults with different iron requirements from a state of no iron stores. These equations suggest that it takes about two to three years to attain around 80% of iron stores in men and women by dietary means alone.

Supplements may be warranted in athletes with low or exhausted iron stores without anaemia. Nielson and Nachtigall (1998) suggest that there are sufficient results, from studies using controls, that support iron supplementation in all athletes with low iron stores. In practice, athletes diagnosed with low iron stores may never reach maximum iron stores. Therefore, iron supplements are important at least for short-term recovery.

In most cases, supplements are discontinued when serum ferritin returns to an acceptable range for the individual athlete, and diet therapy is maintained. The importance of habitually consuming a diet with a high bioavailability of iron is crucial to continued recovery.

11.8.2.1 *Dosage and duration of oral iron supplementation*

To treat iron deficiency anaemia, a high dosage of around 100 mg elemental iron/d is necessary, and doses of up to 300 mg of elemental iron per day have been used in severe cases (Balaban 1992). These doses are well above normal physiological levels. Ashenden and colleagues (1998) recommend a prolonged treatment period (greater than or equal to three months) with a dosage of elemental iron of 100 mg/day, taken on an empty stomach. Pharmaceutical iron supplements available in Australia are listed in Table 11.10 (see Practice tips).

It is of interest that recent studies on non-athletes have found that iron supplements taken two to three times a week are just as effective in increasing serum ferritin and haemoglobin (Schultink et al. 1993) as supplements taken daily (Tee et al. 1999). In one study of 624 adolescent females in Malaysia with mild, moderate and borderline anaemia, 120 mg taken once a week was found to be as effective in increasing haemoglobin and ferritin levels as 60 mg of elemental iron taken once a day (Tee et al. 1999). Research is needed to determine whether similar regimens are effective in athletes. Hallberg and colleagues (1998), however, are more in favour of daily iron supplementation which is known to increase depleted iron more rapidly because of higher daily absorption than weekly doses. Current practice also favours daily supplement use in athletes as rapid recovery is important.

11.8.2.2 *Side-effects of iron supplementation*

Intolerance, risk of iron overload and other drug interactions are often associated with high dose iron supplementation. Diarrhoea or constipation, abdominal discomfort, nausea, and an increased risk of infection have been reported (Finch & Huebers 1982). Habitual intakes of iron as supplements can interfere with zinc and copper absorption and possibly induce deficiencies in these minerals (Solomons 1986; Keen & Hackman 1986; Yadrick et al. 1989). Intakes as low as 18 mg of elemental iron depressed serum zinc levels in the short term (Dawson et al. 1989) as well as after discontinuing iron supplements (Newhouse et al. 1993). The reasons for this are unclear. The possibility that iron supplements induce deficiencies of other trace minerals, such as copper and zinc, or induce iron overload in susceptible people with haemochromatosis cannot be ignored.

11.8.2.3 *The long-term safety of iron supplements: the risk of iron overload*

In Australia, the gene responsible for hereditary haemochromatosis (iron overload) occurs in 10% of the Caucasian population; three in one thousand people are homozygous for haemochromatosis and therefore express the condition (Bothwell 1995). In people with haemochromatosis, iron slowly accumulates in tissues leading to irreversible tissue damage and disease. Haemochromatosis is often detected during routine haematological screening of athletes or during investigation of persistent fatigue. Haemochromatosis highlights the need for correct diagnosis of iron deficiency in athletes prior to recommendation of iron supplementation. Iron supplements are contraindicated in haemochromatosis.

11.8.3 *Intramuscular iron therapy*

Of concern is anecdotal evidence of elite athletes being given regular iron injections often in combination with high dosage iron supplements, presumably to enhance performance or prevent iron depletion. Problems with iron overload could be an outcome (see Section 11.8.2.3). Although iron injection leads to a rapid increase in iron stores (Ashenden et al. 1996), it carries a risk of anaphylactic shock, which can be fatal.

11.9 SUMMARY

Short-term sports anaemia is unlikely to be a sign of iron deficiency and may be attributed to a dilutional effect caused by an increased plasma volume. However, long-term sports anaemia associated with reduced ferritin and/or low haemoglobin levels, as well as changes in other biochemical indicators, may be diagnosed as iron depletion. The evidence linking inadequate dietary iron intake (particularly in female athletes) and gastrointestinal blood loss (in both male and female runners) to iron deficiency is convincing. Nutrition counselling to maximise iron intake and bioavailability is warranted in those athletes identified as anaemic, iron-deficient or at risk of developing iron deficiency. Iron depletion and iron deficiency can be prevented by recognition of risk groups of athletes, early detection using biochemical indicators, and early nutrition intervention. Iron deficiency anaemia in athletes in the absence of any disease is treated by nutrition intervention and oral iron supplements.

11.10 PRACTICE TIPS

Vicki Deakin and Fiona Pelly

Overview

- Athletes involved in regular intensive training programs are at risk of depleting iron stores, which can, if not detected and treated, develop into iron deficiency anaemia. Athletes are at risk of iron depletion for several reasons: high iron requirements and increased losses of iron in response to hard physical activity; sub-optimal total dietary iron intakes; and low bioavailability of dietary iron. Physiological factors associated with iron loss in athletes include excessive sweating, gastrointestinal bleeding, breakdown of red blood cells caused by mechanical trauma and blood loss through injury (see Section 11.5.1). Female athletes may have higher iron requirements than males because of menstrual blood losses. Sub-optimal intakes of iron are evident in athletes who follow low-energy diets, very high carbohydrate diets, fad diets, vegetarian diets or are natural food eaters (see Section 11.5.2.1). As athletes are encouraged to consume diets high in starchy carbohydrate, there is a risk that iron inhibitors in cereals and legumes will reduce iron bioavailability (see Section 11.5.2.3). Therefore, those athletes at risk of iron depletion need practical strategies for maintaining a high carbohydrate intake without compromising iron status. Food combinations that enhance iron absorption are important to achieve this outcome (see Section 11.11.7.2)

Biochemical detection of iron deficiency

- Detection of early biochemical signs of iron deficiency is difficult, as low iron status blood measures may be indicative of either an expanded plasma volume in response to training (i.e. 'sports anaemia') or true iron depletion or iron deficiency. Sports anaemia is not a true iron deficiency condition and will not respond to supplementation. Symptoms of iron deficiency anaemia may or may not be present even if serum ferritin or haemoglobin measures are low. All low iron status measures should be treated as potential iron depletion (Section 11.3.3).

Medical/physiological causes of iron deficiency

- On presentation or referral for treatment of iron deficiency, medical and physiological factors influencing iron status should be evaluated by a dietitian. These include:
  1. an increased requirement (e.g. a recent pregnancy or growth spurt);
  2. medications that influence an increase in gut pH, including habitual use of antacids (gastric reflux is not uncommon in athletes involved in high-intensity workouts);
  3. factors associated with excessive blood loss or turnover (e.g. frequent nose bleeds, blood donor, menorrhagia, recent pregnancy, gastrointestinal blood loss due to bleeding from ulcers, chronic use of anti-inflammatory drugs); and/or
  4. malabsorption of iron (e.g. ulcerative colitis, Crohn's disease, and infestation of parasites such as giardia lamblia, or worms).

Influence of training on iron depletion

- Assessment of the type, intensity and timing of an athlete's training and competition program requires investigation. Training schedules can interfere with meal patterns or time for food preparation, as well as imposing high physiological stress on iron reserves. Some athletes lose their appetites after a hard training session and eat poorly. Inquiries on sweat rate (which can be crudely measured by weight loss before and after training) are useful, as iron is lost through heavy sweating. Possible signs of blood loss after competition or heavy training is also important (e.g. discoloured urine, diarrhoea).

Dietary assessment of iron deficiency

- A complete dietary assessment should aim to reveal any beliefs and attitudes which might lead to low iron status and poor food choices. Some athletes eliminate or minimise meat consumption in an effort to enhance their carbohydrate intake. Female athletes and those involved in weight-category sports often eliminate meat in the mistaken belief that it is fattening. Some athletes report that meat is 'heavy' and fatty and tends to sit in their stomachs for a long time. Athletes involved in rigorous training schedules have limited time to prepare foods, and often resort to frequent snacking of readily accessible convenience foods. Typical choices are high in energy value but are usually not iron-dense. In summary, in a dietary assessment a dietitian should look for food beliefs and habits known to be associated with low iron status. These include:

1. elimination or very low intakes of meat, chicken, and fish;
2. vegetarianism;
3. irregular or erratic eating patterns;
4. prolonged loss of appetite after physical activity;
5. low intake of bread and breakfast cereal (a major source of iron in the diet);
6. low intakes of energy and total dietary iron, fad diets, inappropriate food combinations or poor variety in the diet (Section 11.5.2.1);
7. poor intake of foods rich in vitamin C (some fruits and vegetables) consumed with meals; and
8. excessive consumption of tea or coffee with meals (Section 11.5.2.3).

Dietary treatment: reference standards

- The Australian RDIs for iron may be inappropriate for some athletes. Some data suggest that losses of iron may be as high as 1.5–1.7 mg/d in male and 2.2–2.3 mg/d in female distance runners (Section 11.7.1). However, these high levels are not applicable to most athletes. As iron requirements are highly variable among individual athletes, it may be more appropriate to increase the RDIs to a slightly higher level than recommended for those athletes involved in endurance training programs.

Increasing iron supply from the diet

- Iron supply is the sum of total dietary iron intake and its bioavailability.

Increase total dietary iron intake

- Iron is found in a wide range of foods as shown in Table 11.5. Meat, especially liver and red meat, has a high total iron content (haem + non-haem). Red meat, including beef and lamb, has a higher haem and total iron content than chicken and fish. The colour of meat is largely determined by its iron content; the 'redder' the meat, the higher the myoglobin (the iron containing pigment) and hence iron content. Liver has the highest iron content because it stores iron. Meat is an important iron source in the diet although not the major contributor of iron in the national Australian diet. Iron-enriched breakfast cereal and bread are important contributors. Most commercial breakfast cereals are iron-fortified although the grains from which they are made, especially wheat- and corn-based breakfast cereals, are good natural sources of iron. When eaten regularly, breakfast cereals provide a substantial portion of iron in the diet. One bowl of iron-enriched breakfast cereal has four times the iron content of a bowl of porridge (see Table 11.5).

* Wholemeal bread has nearly twice the iron content of white bread (see Table 11.5), although the higher phytate content in wholemeal bread reduces its bioavailability. Legumes (e.g. lentils, baked beans, soy beans) are good sources of iron, but high in inhibitory components (phytate and soy peptides). Dried fruit, sweet corn, green leafy vegetables including broccoli, silverbeet, spinach, and Chinese green vegetables are also excellent sources of iron with a low phytate content.

Table 11.5   *Iron content of foods (mg/serve)*

ANIMAL SOURCES (good sources of haem and non-haem iron)		
	Serving size	Amount of total iron per serve (mg/serve)
Liver, cooked	(75 g)	8.3
Lean, cooked beef	2 slices (75 g)	2.3
Lean, cooked lamb	2 slices (75 g)	1.0
Eggs	1 boiled egg (55 g)	1.0
Tuna, dark flesh	75 g	0.7
Lean, cooked pork, ham	2 slices (75 g)	0.6
Lean, cooked chicken (no skin)	1 small breast (75 g)	0.5
Fish, white flesh	1 average piece (75 g)	0.3
PLANT SOURCES (good sources of non-haem iron)		
Commercial breakfast cereal (iron-enriched)	average serve (60 g)	5.6
Nuts (cashews, almonds)	50 g	1.6–3.1
Sweet corn	½ cup (120 g)	2.1
Lentils, cooked	½ cup (120 g)	2.0
Baked beans in sauce	½ cup (120 g)	1.8
Porridge, cooked oats	1 cup	1.6
Bread (wholemeal)	2 sandwich slices (60 g)	1.4
Potato	1 medium	1.4
Green leafy vegetables (broccoli, spinach, silverbeet, cabbage)	½ cup (120 g)	0.8–1.2
Milk chocolate	50 g block	0.7
Bread (white)	2 sandwich slices (60 g)	0.7
Dried fruit (prunes, apricots)	5–6 (50 g)	0.6
Fruit (fresh)	1 average piece	0.3–0.5

Source: Lewis et al. (1995) NUTTAB95

Increase the bioavailability of non-haem iron

- Although iron appears to be present in a wide range of different foods as seen in Table 11.5, it is not easily absorbed and only a small proportion of iron consumed is actually bioavailable (see Section 11.5.2.2). To maximise iron absorption from iron-rich plant foods, avoid concurrent consumption with foods that inhibit iron absorption such as tea, coffee and excessive intakes of bran (which contains high levels of phytate). A list of the phytate content of foods is found in Table 11.6.

Table 11.6 *Phytate content in foods*

Foods high in phytate		Foods low in phytate	
Food	Phytate content mg/100 g edible portion	Food	Phytate content mg/100 g edible portion
Wheat bran cereal (ready-to-eat) and wheatgerm	3168 (bran), 4071 (germ)	*Most fruits and vegetables have a low phytate content*	
Cashew nuts (most nuts are high in phytate)	1866	Rye bread	155
		Rice cereal (e.g. *Kelloggs' Rice Bubbles*™)	136
Seeds (sesame, poppy—all high in phytate)	1616–2189	Oatmeal, porridge (cooked)	111
		Sweet corn	129
Wheat cereal (ready-to-eat) (e.g. *Wheaties*™)	1467	Potato, boiled in skin	100
		Kelloggs' Cornflakes™	70
Soy flour	1398	White bread (not fibre-enriched)	69
Soy-based TVP, beef	1265		
Peanut butter	1252	Apples (raw)	63
Oatmeal, dry	943	Green peas, boiled	28
Lentils (raw)	434	Broccoli	18
Wholemeal bread (wheat)	390	Strawberries and other berries	6
Mixed grain breakfast cereal (e.g. *Kelloggs' Special K*™)	272		

TVP = *textured vegetable protein, a soy product*
Source: Harland and Oberlas (1987)

- Including a small serve of meat or vitamin C–rich foods with meals (for example, meat and salad on a sandwich, orange juice or fruit with breakfast) enhances iron absorption substantially from non-haem foods. Table 11.7 lists

Table 11.7 *Food sources of vitamin C–rich foods*

Food (mg/serve)	Serving size	Vitamin C
Fruits and fruit juices		
Fresh orange juice	1 glass (200 mL)	138
Commercial orange juice	1 glass (200 mL)	108
Cordial, blackcurrant	1 cup, 40 mL concentrate made up to 200 mL	116
Pawpaw	1 cup, diced	90
Orange and mango fruit juice drink	1 glass (200 mL)	64
Juice, apple (if fortified with vitamin C)	1 glass (200 mL)	31
Orange (navel) peeled	1 orange (160 g)	84
Kiwifruit	1 kiwifruit (50 g)	57
Strawberry	1 cup (100 g)	45
Rockmelon	1 cup, diced (165 g)	34
Vegetables, including salad vegetables		
Capsicum (red or green) raw	½ cup, chopped	102
Brussel sprouts (boiled, steamed, microwaved)	5 sprouts (85 g)	88
Cabbage (boiled, steamed, microwaved)	1 cup (135 g)	67
Cauliflower (boiled, steamed, microwaved)	1 floweret (90 g)	50
Broccoli (boiled, steamed, microwaved)	1 floweret (50 g)	43
Potato (boiled)	1 medium (145 g)	21
Tomato	1 medium (130 g)	18

Source: Lewis et al. (1995) NUTTAB95

examples of vitamin C–rich foods. Vitamin C, a water-soluble vitamin, can be easily lost from foods under certain environmental conditions. The vitamin C content of most fruits is stable and largely unaffected by light, heat or cooking. The vitamin C content of vegetables is less stable to heat and light and easily leaches into the cooking water. The longer the cooking time, the greater the losses of vitamin C from these foods. Therefore, vegetables cooked in little water (i.e. steamed) or for a short time (i.e. microwaved) retain more vitamin C than boiling for a long time. Most fruit juices have added vitamin C which not only fortifies the food but also helps reduce oxidation of the vitamin C present.

- The presence of other acids in citrus fruit (grapefruit, lemon, lime), in addition to vitamin C (ascorbic acid), also enhances absorption from non-haem foods.

- Foods fortified with iron may be a useful way of increasing total iron intake provided the iron has a high bioavailability. For example, iron-fortified breakfast cereals can contribute significantly to non-haem iron intake and are a good source of carbohydrate for the athlete. In contrast, iron-fortified cows milk and soy milk will contribute little to total iron intake due to poor bioavailability of iron. Special attention needs to be directed to enhancing bioavailability of non-haem iron for vegetarian athletes and others at risk of iron depletion. Table 11.8 shows two examples of diets with low and high bioavailability of iron but a similar total dietary iron content.

- A summary of dietary strategies for treating and preventing iron deficiency are outlined in Table 11.9.

Treatment with iron supplements

- Where iron deficiency and iron deficiency anaemia is diagnosed (i.e. serum ferritin < 30 g/L), an iron-rich diet alone is insufficient to restore iron levels quickly. Iron supplements are necessary but should not be given routinely to athletes without medical supervision. In addition to the possibility of inducing deficiencies of other trace minerals such as zinc and copper, habitual use of iron supplements can produce iron overload in people with haemochromatosis. Table 11.10 outlines the trade and generic names and elemental iron content of pharmaceutical iron supplements available in Australia. These supplements are in the form or iron salts (non-haem iron), which, if taken with foods, are affected by the inhibitory or enhancing components present in those foods.

Table 11.8   Example of foods of similar iron content with high and low bioavailability of iron

High bioavailability of iron			Low bioavailability of iron		
Food item	Serve size	Iron (mg)	Food item	Serve size	Iron (mg)
Iron-fortified breakfast cereal	60 g for ½ cup	5.6	Muesli mixed with wheatgerm & bran	¾ cup (60 g)	5.7
Cows milk	1 cup (250 mL)	0.2	Soy milk, fortified	1 cup (250 mL)	1.3
Fruit juice	1 cup	0	Tea	1 cup (250 mL)	0
Ham and salad sandwich on white bread (30g ham)	2 sandwiches	3.2	Peanut butter sandwich on white bread	2 sandwiches	1.9
Orange	1 medium	0.4	Apple	1 medium	0.3
Fruit juice, fortified with vitamin C	1 cup (250 mL)	0	Soy milk, fortified	1 cup (250 mL)	1.3
Pasta with lean ground beef (100 g ground beef)	1 cup (260 g)	3.3	Pasta with tomato-based sauce	1 cup (260 g)	1.9
Salad with lettuce, tomato, capsicum & carrot	1 cup (50 g)	1.0	Mixed lettuce	1 cup (50 g)	0.3
½ cup fruit salad	½ cup (110 g)	0.3	100 g carton fruit yoghurt or 2 scoops (60 g) ice cream		0.1
			Dried fruit	10 dried apricots	1.2
TOTAL		14.0	TOTAL		14.0

Source: Lewis et al. (1995) NUTTAB95

Table 11.9	*Dietary strategies for enhancing iron supply*

- Include at least small amounts of meat in main meals at least three to four times a week. This adds readily available iron to a meal and enhances absorption of iron from plant sources. Add meat to high-carbohydrate meals to enhance non-haem absorption (e.g. in a pasta sauce, in a stir-fry with rice or noodles, meat and vegetable kebabs with rice, hamburger or chicken burger).
- Use meat (e.g. liver pate, ham, beef, lamb, pork, chicken or salmon) on sandwiches as often as you can (at least 3–4 times a week).
- Regularly include shellfish and some dark cuts of meat or fish (e.g. beef, lamb, pork and chicken thigh have higher iron contents than chicken breast or salmon).
- Eat plant foods with high iron contents most days of the week (e.g. iron-fortified cereal, bread, some fruits (see Table 11.12), green leafy vegetables, and legumes).
- Combine plant foods containing a high phytate content (e.g. cereal grains, breads, breakfast cereal, soy products) with those rich in vitamin C (e.g. fruit juice with cereal, salad on sandwiches) and/or with meat.
- If diagnosed iron depleted or deficient, avoid or limit adding bran and wheatgerm to meals.
- If diagnosed iron depleted or deficient, avoid drinking strong tea and coffee with meals.

Dosage of iron supplements

- If a supplement is required, iron supplements containing 100 mg of elemental iron per day are usually prescribed with up to 300 mg iron per day for severe cases of iron deficiency anaemia. Ferrous sulfate (Ferrogradumet™) contains 100 mg of elemental iron and is usually prescribed on a once-per-day regimen. Ferrous gluconate (Fergon™) contains 33 mg of elemental iron and is often better tolerated. One tablet is usually prescribed three times a day. As most iron supplements are in the non-haem or inorganic form, concurrent consumption of a vitamin C–rich food or supplement is often recommended to enhance absorption. If supplements are taken on an empty stomach, further elimination of interference from inhibitory factors in food is possible. Iron supplements should be taken separately to calcium supplements to prevent any potential inhibitory effect. Side-effects such as constipation or gut irritation associated with chronic use of iron supplements are infrequently reported in athletes.

- Iron supplementation may be necessary for up to or greater than three months to treat iron deficiency anaemia, however, some athletes may return to normal biochemical values within a much shorter time, depending on the severity of the iron depletion.

Table 11.10 *Iron supplements available in Australia*

Trade name™	Iron salt (generic name)	Size of supplement	Elemental iron content/tablet	Other components
Blackmores iron compound	Ferrous phosphate	15 mg	5 mg	Sodium sulphate, potassium chloride
Blackmores for Women Bio iron*	Ferrous fumarate	15 mg	5 mg	Ascorbic acid, cyanocobalamin, folic acid, urtica dioica
FGF	Ferrous sulfate	270 mg	80 mg	Folic acid 300 µg
FGF 500	Ferrous sulfate	250 mg	80 mg	Folic acid 500 µg
Ferro-Gradumet	Ferrous sulfate	325 mg	105 mg	Nil
Ferro-Gradumet C	Ferrous sulfate	325 mg	105 mg	Ascorbic acid 500 mg
Fergon	Ferrous gluconate	300 mg	33 mg	Nil
Fefol	Ferrous sulfate	300 mg	80 mg	Folic acid
Nature's Way Iron-All	Ferrous fumarate	15 mg	5 mg	Ascorbic acid, cyanocobalamin, folic acid

* = as this supplement contains herbal products which contain unspecified ingredients, it cannot be guaranteed as permitted in sport (MIMS, 1999)

Source: MIMS 1999

Follow-up

- Athletes should be discouraged from self-administering iron supplements, as this may induce deficiencies of copper and zinc. Iron supplements are contraindicated in haemochromatosis (Section 11.8.2.3). Biochemical measures of iron status should be reviewed at 10–12 weeks or earlier in athletes on supplements and discontinued when iron status measurements are within usual or reference ranges.

Failure to respond to intervention

- Reasons for failure to respond to dietary iron intervention and iron supplements may relate to:
  1. poor compliance;
  2. insufficient dosage of oral iron (< 50 mg iron is associated with little improvement of haemoglobin and iron status (Haymes & Lamanca 1989);
  3. inadequate iron density in the diet to meet the demands of training (iron intakes may need to be set at higher than previous levels);
  4. excessive intake of unprocessed bran, or other cereal or soy products, because of high phytate content;
  5. a recent increase in training intensity and the likelihood of a corresponding increase in plasma volume (iron status levels may be falsely low due to a haemodilutional effect);
  6. an underlying chronic medical condition or parasite infestation that was previously undetected; or a recent illness that affects food intake; and
  7. consistently low biochemical measures of iron status, which may be usual or normal levels for an individual athlete.

- Individual biochemical parameters may need to be monitored over a number of months to give a more realistic indication of usual or baseline levels. Large fluctuations in these measures are indicative of dietary, physiological and training influences.

Further intervention

- If medical influences and poor compliance have been excluded:
  1. continue with dietary intervention for a further 6–10 weeks;
  2. for some athletes, a further increase in dosage or change in iron supplement may be considered; and
  3. regular monitoring of high-risk athletes is recommended to ensure optimal performance ability. This should include routine examination of serum ferritin and haemoglobin and regular dietary assessment.

REFERENCES

Abrahams SF, Mira M, Beumont PJV, Sowerbutts TD, Llewellyn-Jones D. Eating behaviours among young women. Med J Aust 1988;2:225–8.

Akesson A, Bjellerup P, Berglund M, Bremme K, Vahter M. Serum transferrin receptor: a specific marker of iron deficiency in pregnancy. Am J Clin Nutr 1998;68:1241–6.

Ashenden MJ, Martin DT, Boston T, et al. Iron injection increases serum ferritin concentration in female athletes—abstract. In: Australian Conference of Science and Medicine in Sport. National Convention Centre, Canberra: October, 1996:66–7.

Ashenden MJ, Martin DT, Dobson GP, McIntosh C, Hahn AG. Serum ferritin and anaemia in trained female athletes. Int J Sport Nutr 1998;8:223–9.

Australian Institute of Sport. Biochemistry Department, Canberra: 2000

Australian Iron Status Advisory Board. Melbourne: 1999.

Australian Sports Commission Survey of drug use in Australian Sport. Canberra: Australian Sports Medicine Federation, 1983.

Balaban EP. Sports anaemia. Clin Sports Med 1992;11:313–25.

Barr SI. Women, nutrition and exercise: a review of athletes, intakes and a discussion of energy balance in active women. Prog Food Nutr Sc 1987;11:307–61.

Baynes RD. Assessment of iron status. Clin Biochem 1996;29:209–15.

Baynes RD, Macfarlane BJ, Bothwell TH, et al. The promotive effect of soy sauce on iron absorption in human subjects. Eur J Clin Nutr 1990;44:419–24.

Beaton GH, Corey PN, Steele C. Conceptual and methodological issues regarding the epidemiology of iron deficiency and their implications for studies of the functional consequences of iron deficiency. Am J Clin Nutr 1989;50:575–88.

Beguin Y, Clemons GK, Pootrakul P, Fillet G. Quantitative assessment of erythropoiesis and functional characteristics of anemia based on measurements of serum transferrin receptor and erythropoietin. Blood 1993;81:1067–76.

Bergstrom E, Hernell O, Lonnerdal B, Persson LA. Sex differences in iron stores in adolescence. In: Hallberg L, Asp NG, eds. Iron nutrition in health and disease. London: John Libbey, 1996:157–63.

Borch-Iohnsen B. Determination of iron status: brief review of physiological effects on iron measures. Analyst 1995;8:891–3.

Bothwell TH. Iron balance and the capacity of regulatory systems to prevent the development of iron deficiency and overload. In: Hallberg L, Asp NG, eds. Iron nutrition in health and disease. London: John Libbey, 1996:3–16.

Bothwell T. Iron deficiency in teenagers: new directions in management. Canberra: Australian Iron status Advisory Panel, Symposium, November, 1995.

Bothwell TH, Charlton RW, Cook JD, and Finch CA. In: Iron Metabolism in Man. London, Oxford: Blackwell Scientific Publications, 1979:88–104.

Brotherhood J, Brozovic B, Pugh LGC. Haematological status of middle- and long-distance runners. Clinical Science and Molecular Medicine 1975;48:139–45.

Brune M, Rossander L, Hallberg L. Iron absorption and phenolic compounds: the importance of different phenolic structures. Eur J Clin Nutr 1989;43:547–8.

Brune M, Rossander-Hultén L, Hallberg L, Gleerup A, Sandberg AS. Iron absorption from bread in humans: inhibiting effects of cereal fiber, phytate and inositol phosphates with different numbers of phosphate groups. J Nutr 1992;122:442–9.

Clement DB, Asmundson RC. Nutritional intake and hematological parameters in endurance runners. Phys Sports Med 1982;10:37–43.

Clement DB, Sawchuk LL. Iron status and sports performance. Sports Med 1984;1:65–74.

Cobiac L, Baghurst K. Iron status and dietary iron intakes of Australians. Food Aust (suppl) April, 1993;S1–S23.

Convertino VA. Blood volume: its adaptation to endurance training. Med Sci Sports Exerc 1991;23:1338–48.

Cook JD. The effect of endurance training on iron metabolism. Sem Hemat 1994;3:146–54.

Cook JD, Dassenko SA, Lynch SR. Assessment of the role of nonheme iron availability in iron balance. Am J Clin Nutr 1991a;54:717–22.

Cook JD, Dassenko SA, Whittaker P. Calcium supplementation: effect on iron absorption. Am J Clin Nutr 1991b;53:106–11.

Cook JD, Lipschitz DA, Laughton EMM, Finch CA. Serum ferritin as a measure of iron stores in normal subjects. Am J Clin Nutr 1974;27:681–7.

Cook JD, Reddy MB, Hurrell RF. The effect of red and white wine on non-heme iron absorption in humans. Am J Clin Nutr 1995;61:800–4.

Cook JD, Skikne B, Baynes R. The use of serum transferrin receptor for the assessment of iron status. In: Hallberg L, Asp NG, eds. Iron nutrition in health and disease. London: John Libbey, 1996:49–58.

Crosby WH, O'Neill MA. A small dose iron tolerance test as an indicator of mild iron deficiency. J Am Med Assoc 1984;251:1986–7.

Dawson EB, Albers J, McGarrity W. Serum zinc changes due to iron supplementation in teen-age pregnancy. Am J Clin Nutr 1989;50:848–52.

Diehl DM, Lohmann TG, Smith SC, Kertzer RJ. Effects of physical training and competition on the iron status of female field hockey players. Int J Sports Med 1982;7:264–70.

Dill DB, Braithwaite K, Adams WC. Blood volume of middle-distance runners: effect of 2,300m altitude and comparison with non athletes. Med Sc Sports Exerc 1974;6:1–7.

Dressendorfer RH, Keen CL, Wade CE, Claybaugh R, Timmis GC. Development of runner's anaemia during a 20-day road race: effects of iron supplementation. Int J Sport Nutr 1991;12:332–6.

Dufaux B, Hoegerath A, Streitberger W, Hollmann W, Assmann G. Serum ferritin, transferrin, haptoglobin and iron in middle-distance and long-distance runners, elite rowers, and professional racing cyclists. Int J Sports Med 1981;2:43–6.

Ellsworth NM, Hewitt BF, Haskell WL. Nutrient intake of elite male and female nordic skiers. Phys Sports Med 1985;13:78–92.

Fairweather-Tait SJ. Iron requirements and prevalence of iron deficiency in adolescents: an overview. In: Hallberg L, Asp NG, eds. Iron nutrition in health and disease. London: John Libbey, 1996:137–48.

Fallon KE, Sivyer G, Sivyer K, Dare A. Changes in the haematological parameters and iron metabolism associated with a 1600 kilometre ultramarathon. Br J Sports Med 1999;33:27–32.

Finch CA, Cook JD. Iron deficiency. Am J Clin Nutr 1984;39:471–7.

Finch CA, Huebers H. Perspectives in iron metabolism. N Eng J Med 1982;306:1520–8.

Fogelholm M. Estimated energy expenditure, diet and iron status of male Finnish endurance athletes: a cross-sectional study. Scan J Sports Sc 1989;11:59–63.

Fogelholm M. Indicators of vitamin and mineral status in athletes' blood: a review. Int J Sports Nutr 1995;5:267–84.

Fogelholm M, Jaakkola L, Lammpisjaervi T. Effect of iron supplementation in female athletes with low serum ferritin concentration. Int J Sports Med 1992;13:158–62.

Gillooly M, Bothwell TH, Torrance JD, MacPhail AP, Derman DP, Bezwoda WR, Mills W, Charlton RW. The effects of organic acids, phytates and polyphenols on the absorption of iron from vegetables. Br J Nutr 1983;49:331–42.

Gillooly M, Torrance JD, Bothwell TH, et al. The relative effect of ascorbic acid on iron absorption from soy-based and milk-based infant formulas. Am J Clin Nutr 1984;40:522–7.

Hallberg L. Bioavailability of dietary iron in man. Annu Rev Nutr 1981;1:123–47.

Hallberg L, Brune M, Rossander L. Effect of ascorbic acid on iron absorption from different types of meals: studies with ascorbate rich foods and synthetic ascorbic acid given in different amounts with different meals. Hum Nutr: Appl Nutr 1986;40:97–113.

Hallberg L, Brune M, Rossander L. Iron absorption in man: ascorbic acid and dose-dependent inhibition by phytate. Am J Clin Nutr 1989;49:140–4.

Hallberg L, Hulten L. Iron requirements, iron balance and iron deficiency in menstruating and pregnant women. In: Hallberg L, Asp NG, eds. Iron nutrition in health and disease. London: John Libbey, 1996:165–81.

Hallberg L, Hulten L, Garby L. Iron stores in man in relation to diet and iron requirements. Eur J Clin Nutr 1998;52:623–31.

Hallberg L, Hulten L, Gramatkovski E. Iron absorption from the whole diet in men: how effective is the regulation of iron absorption? Am J Clin Nutr 1997;66:347–56.

Hallberg L, Rossander, L. Effect of different drinks on the absorption of non-haem iron from composite meals. Hum Nutr: Appl Nutr 1982b;36A:116–23.

Hallberg L, Rossander L. Effect of soy protein on nonheme iron absorption in man. Am J Clin Nutr 1982a;36:514–20.

Hallberg L, Rossander-Hulten L, Brune M, Gleerup A. Inhibition of haem-iron absorption in man by calcium. Br J Nutr 1993;69:533–40.

Harland BF, Oberleas D. Phytate in food. Wld Rev Nutr Diet 1987;52:235–59.

Haymes EM. Nutrition and the physically active female. Women Sport Phys Act 1992;1:35–47.

Haymes EM, Lamanca JF. Iron loss in runners during exercise: implications and recommendations. Sports Med 1989;7:277–85.

Hegenauer J, Strause L, Saltman P, Dann D, White J, Green R. Transitory hematologic effects of moderate exercise are not influenced by iron supplements. Eur J Appl Physiol 1983;52:57–61.

Huebers HA, Beguin Y, Pootrakul P, Einspar D, Finch CA. Intact transferrin receptors in human plasma and their relation to erythropoiesis. Blood 1990;75:102–7.

Hulten L, Gramatkovski E, Gleerup A, Hallberg L. Iron absorption from the whole diet: relation to meal composition, iron requirements and iron stores. Eur J Clin Nutr 1995;49:794–808.

Hurrell RF. Bioavailability of iron. Eur J Clin Nutr 1997;51:S4–S8.

Jacobs A. Erythropoiesis and iron deficiency anaemia. In: Jacobs A, Worwood M, eds. Iron in biochemistry and medicine. London and New York: Academic Press, 1974.

Keen CL, Hackman RM. Trace elements in athletic performance. In: Katch FL, ed. Sport, health and nutrition: 1984 Olympic Scientific Congress Proceedings, Vol 2. Champaign: Human Kinetics, 1986.

LaManca JJ, Haymes EM. Effects of low ferritin concentration on endurance performance. Int J Sport Nutr 1992;2:376–85.

LaManca JJ, Haymes EM. Effects of iron repletion on $VO_{2\ max}$, endurance and blood lactate in women. Med Sci Sports Exerc 1993;25:1386–92.

LaManca JJ, Haymes EM, Daly JA, Moffatt RJ, Waller MF. Sweat iron loss of male and female runners during exercise. Int J Sports Med 1988;9:52–5.

Lampe J, Ellefson M, Slavin J, Schwartz S, Apple F. The effect of marathon running on gastrointestinal transit time and fecal blood loss in women runners. Med Sc Sport Exerc 1987;19:S21.

Lampe JW, Slavin JL, Apple FS. Elevated serum ferritin concentrations in master runners after a marathon race. Int J Vit Nutr Res 1986;56:395–8.

Layrisse M, Martinez-Torres C, Leets I, Taylor P, Ramirez J. Effect of histidine, cysteine, glutathione or beef on iron absorption in humans. J Nutr 1984;114:217–23.

Lewis J, Milligan G, Hunt A. NUTTAB95 Nutrient table for use in Australia. Canberra: National Food Authority, 1995.

Lipschitz DA, Cook JD, Finch CA. A clinical evaluation of serum ferritin as an index of iron stores. N Eng J Med 1974;290:846–7.

Lukaski HC, Hall CB, Siders WA. Altered metabolic response of iron-deficient women during graded, maximal exercise. Eur J Appl Physiol 1991;63:130–45.

Lynch SR, Dassenko SA, Cook JD, Juillerat MA, Hurrell RF. Inhibitory effect of a soybean-protein related moiety on iron absorption in humans. Am J Clin Nutr 1994:60:567–72.

MacFarlane BJ, Baynes RD, Bothwell TH, Schmidt U, Mayet F, Friedman BM. Effect of lupines, a protein–rich legume on iron absorption. Eur J Clin Nutr 1988;42:683–7.

MacPhail AP, Charlton R, Bothwell TH, Bezwoda WR. Experimental fortificants. In: Clydesdale FM, Weimer KL, eds. Iron fortification of foods. New York: Academic Press, 1985:55–75.

Magazanik A, Weinstein Y, Abarbanek J, et al. Effect of an iron supplement on body iron status and aerobic capacity of young training women. Eur J Appl Physiol Occ Ther 1991;62:317–23.

Magnusson B, Hallberg L, Rossander L, Swolin B. Iron metabolism and sports anaemia: 11. A hematological comparison of elite runners and control subjects. Acta Med Scand 1984;216:157–64.

McLennan W, Podger A. National Nutrition Survey: nutrient intakes and physical measurements, Australia 1995. ABS cat no. 4805.0. Canberra: Australian Bureau of Statistics, 1998:80.

McMahon LF, Ryan MJ, Larson D, Fisher RL. Occult gastrointestinal blood loss in marathon runners. Ann Int Med 1984;100:846–7.

Miller BJ, Pate RR, Burgess W. Foot impact force and intravascular haemolysis during distance running. Int J Sports Med 1988;9:56–60.

MIMS Australia. MIMS Annual 1999. Sydney, NSW: Medi Media, 1999.

Monsen ER, Hallberg L, Layrisse M, Hegsted DM, Cook JD, Mertz W, Finch CA. Estimation of available dietary iron. Am J Clin Nutr 1978;31:134–41.

Moore CV. Iron Nutrition. In: Gross F, ed. Iron metabolism. Berlin: Springer-Verlaag, 1964:241–55.

Nachtigall DP, Neilsen R, Fischer R, Engelhardt R, Gabbe EE. Iron deficiency in distance runners: a reinvestigation [99]Fe-labeling and non invasive liver iron quantification. Int J Sports Med 1996;17:473–9.

National Health & Medical Research Council. Recommended Dietary Intakes for use in Australia. Canberra: Australian Government Publishing Service, 1991.

Newhouse IJ.Clement DB. Iron status in athletes: an update. Sports Med 1988;5:337–52.

Newhouse IJ, Clement DB, Lai C. Effects of iron supplementation and discontinuation on serum copper, zinc, calcium and magnesium levels in women. Med Sc Sports Exerc 1993;25:562–71.

Newhouse IJ, Clement DB, Taunton JE, McKenzie DC. The effects of prelatent/latent iron deficiency on physical work capacity. Med Sc Sports Exerc 1989;21:263–8.

Nielsen P, Natchtigall D. Iron supplementation in athletes: current recommendations. Sports Med 1998;26:207–16.

Pate RR, Miller BJ, Davis JM, Slentz CA, Klingshirn LA. Iron status of female runners. Int J Sports Nutr 1993;3:222–31.

Pyne D, Parisotto, R, Ashenden M. Iron status in highly trained swimmers: guidelines for interpretation and supplementation. Aust Swim Coach 1997;13:45–50.

Rangan AM, Ho RWL, Blight GD, Binns CW. Haem iron content of Australian meats and fish. Food Aust 1997;49:508–11.

Reddy MB, Cook JD. Effect of calcium intake on nonheme-iron absorption from a complete diet. Am J Clin Nutr 1997;65:1820–5.

Resina A, Gatteschi L, Giamberardino MA, Imreh F, Rubenni MG, Vecchiet L. Hematological comparison of iron status in trained top-level soccer players and control subjects. Int J Sports Med 1991;12:453–6.

Risser WL, Lee EJ, Poindexter HBW, et al. Iron deficiency in female athletes: its prevalence and impact on performance. Med Sc Sports Exerc 1988;20:16–21.

Risser WL, Risser JMH. Iron deficiency in adolescents and young adults. Phys Sportsmed 1990;18:87-8, 91, 94, 96-8, 101.

Rossander L, Hallberg L, Bjorn-Rasmussen E. Absorption of iron from breakfast meals. Am J Clin Nutr 1979;31:106–11.

Rossander-Hulten L, Hallberg L. Prevalence of iron deficiency in adolescents. In: Hallberg L, Asp NG, eds. Iron nutrition in health and disease. London: John Libbey, 1996:149–94.

Rowland TW, Kelleher JF. Iron deficiency in athletes. Sports Med 1989;143:197–200.

Sanborn CF, Jankowski CM. Physiologic considerations for women in sport. Clin Sports Med 1994;13:315–27.

Schoener RB, Esciourrou P, Robertson HT, Nilson KL, Robinson-Parsons J, Smith NJ. Iron repletion decreases maximal exercise lactate concentration in female athletes with minimal iron-deficiency anaemia. J Lab Clin Med 1983;102:306–12.

Seiler D, Nager D, Franz H, Hellstern P, Leitzman P, Jung K. Effects of long-distance running on iron metabolism and hematological parameters. Int J Sports Med 1989;10:357–62.

Siegal AJ, Hennekens CH, Solomon HS, Van Boeckel B. Exercise-related haematuria: findings in a group of marathon runners. J Am Med Ass 1979;241:391–2.

Smith DJ, Roberts D. Effects of high volume and/or intense exercise on selected blood chemistry parameters. 1994;27:435–40.

Snyder AC, Dvorak LL, Roepke JB. Influence of dietary iron source on measures of iron status among female runners. Med Sc Sports Exer 1989;21:7–10.

Solomons NW. Competitive interaction of iron and zinc in the diet: consequences for human nutrition. J Nutr 1986;116:927–35.

Tee ES, Kandiah M, Awin N, et al. School-administered weekly iron-folate supplements improve haemoglobin and ferritin concentrations in Malaysian adolescent girls. Am J Clin Nutr 1999;69:1249–56.

Telford RD, Bunney CJ, Catchpole EA, et al. Plasma ferritin concentration and physical work capacity in athletes. Int J Sport Nutr 1992;2:335–42.

Telford RD, Cunningham RB. Sex, sport and body-size dependency of hematology in highly trained athletes. Med Sc Sports Exerc 1991;23:778–94.

Telford RD, Cunningham RB, Deakin V, Kerr DA. Iron status and diet in athletes. Med Sc Sports Exerc 1993;25:796–800.

Waller MF, Haymes EM. The effects of heat and exercise on sweat iron loss. Med Sc Sports Exerc 1996;28:197–203.

Weight LM, Klein M, Noakes TD, Jacobs P. Sports anaemia—a real or apparent phenomenon in endurance trained athletes. Int J Sports Med 1992;13:344–7.

Weight LM, Myburgh KH, Noakes TD. Vitamin and mineral supplementation: effect on running performance in trained athletes. Am J Clin Nutr 1988;47:192–5.

Williford HN, Scharff-Olsen M, Keith RE, et al. Iron status in women dance instructors. Int J Sports Nutr 1993;3:387–97.

Worwood M. State of the art—Ferritin. Blood Rev 1991;4:259–69.

Yadrick MK, Kenny MA, Winterfeldt EA. Iron, copper, and zinc status: response to supplementation with zinc and iron in adult females. Am J Clin Nutr 1989;49:145–50.

Yoshida T, Udo M, Chida M, Ichioka M, Makigichi K. Dietary iron supplement during severe physical training in competitive female distance runners. Sports Training Med Rehab 1990;1:279–85.

APPENDIX: *Chapter 11*

Table 11.11 *Clinical laboratory values for measuring iron status*

Iron status measure	Diagnostic range for iron deficiency	Reference ranges for adults (SI units)	SI units	Conversion factor to British units	Reference range to British units	British units
Haemoglobin						
Females	< 12.0	120–160	g/L	0.1	12.0–16.0	g/dL
Males	< 13.0	140–175			14.0–17.5	
Haematocrit						
Females		0.33–0.43	1	0.01	33–43	%
Males		0.39–0.49			39–49	
Mean cell (corpuscular) volume (a)	< 80	76–100	L	1	76–100	µm³
Reticulocyte count (a)	NA	10–75	10⁹/L	100	10 000–75 000	mm³
Serum ferritin (a)	< 12	15–300	µg/L	1	15–300	ng/mL
Serum iron						
Females	17.9	11–29	µmol/L	5.5	60–160	µg/dL
Males		14–32			80–180	
Serum transferrin (a)	< than reference range	1.7–3.7	g/L	100	170–370	mg/dL
Total iron binding capacity (TIBC) (a)	< than reference range	45–82	µmol/L	5.5	250–460	µg/dL
Transferrin saturation serum Fe/TIBC (a)	< than reference range	20–40	%	1.00	20–40	%
Transferrin receptor	> 8.8 depletion > 18 iron deficiency	NA	NA	NA	3–9	mg/L
Free erythrocyte protoporphyrin (FEP)	> 70	NA	µmol/L		30	µg/dL

(a) = no data available on male and female reference intervals for some measures. For these measures, reference intervals can be satisfactorily applied to both sexes; NA = not available, SI = Systeme International d'Unites, British units = Imperial units, L = litres

Source: Data derived from Monsen (1987); Worwood (1990); Cook and Finch (1992); Cook et al. (1996), and based on a non-athletic population

CHAPTER 12

Vitamin, mineral and antioxidant needs of athletes

Mikael Fogelholm

12.1 VITAMINS AND MINERALS, AND SPORTS—AN INTRODUCTION TO THE TOPIC

Vitamins are organic compounds required in very small amounts (from a few micrograms to a few milligrams daily) to prevent clinical deficiency, and deterioration in health, growth and reproduction. A distinct feature of vitamins is that the human body is not able to synthesise them. Classification of vitamins is based on their relative solubility: fat-soluble vitamins (A, D, E and K) are more soluble in organic solvents, and water-soluble vitamins (B complex and C) in water.

Most vitamins participate in processes related to muscle contractions and energy expenditure (see Table 12.1). Vitamins of the B complex group (e.g. thiamin, riboflavin, vitamin B6, niacin, biotin and pantothenic acid) act as cofactors for enzymes regulating glycolysis, citric acid cycle, oxidative phosphorylation, β-oxidation (breakdown of fatty acids) and amino acid degradation. Folic acid and vitamin B12 are needed for haem synthesis. Ascorbic acid activates an enzyme regulating biosynthesis of carnitine which is necessary for fatty acid transportation from cell cytosol into mitochondria. Finally, antioxidant vitamins (mainly vitamins C and E) participate in the buffer system against free radicals, which are produced by increased energy turnover.

Minerals are inorganic substances found naturally on the earth. Based on their daily requirements, minerals are usually classified as macrominerals (e.g. sodium, potassium, calcium, phosphorus and magnesium), or trace elements (e.g. iron, zinc, copper, chromium and selenium). The daily dietary allowance for macrominerals is more than 100 mg/d, whereas trace elements are needed in much smaller quantities (less than 20 mg/d).

Table 12.1 Summary of the most important effects of vitamins on body functions related to athletic training and performance

	Cofactors and activators for energy metabolism	Nervous function, muscle contraction	Haemoglobin synthesis	Immune function	Antioxidant function	Bone metabolism
Water-soluble vitamins						
Thiamin	X	X				
Riboflavin	X	X				
Vitamin B6	X	X	X			
Folic acid		X	X	X		
Vitamin B12		X	X			
Niacin	X	X				
Pantothenic acid	X					
Biotin	X					
Vitamin C				X	X	
Fat-soluble vitamins						
Vitamin A				X	X	
Vitamin D						X
Vitamin E				X	X	

Several minerals and trace elements, such as magnesium, iron, zinc and copper, act as enzyme activators in glycolysis, oxidative phosphorylation and in the system responsible for maintenance of acid-base equilibrium (Table 12.2). Iron is needed for haem synthesis. Minerals (electrolytes) also affect muscle contraction.

As evident from the above introduction, micronutrients (i.e. vitamins and minerals) are essential for life. A well-balanced diet is generally believed to cover the needs for all micronutrients in healthy humans (National Research Council 1989; National Health and Medical Research Council 1991). Nevertheless, vitamin and mineral supplements, including vitamin C (especially), the B-complex vitamins, vitamin E and iron, are frequently used by athletes (Fogelholm et al. 1992a; Sobal & Marquart 1994; Ronsen et al. 1999). The common motivation for vitamin supplementation is to enhance recovery and improve sports performance.

The widespread use of vitamin and mineral supplements is justified and necessary: if a normal diet is unable to maintain an athlete's micronutrient status; if micronutrient supplements improve nutritional status and physiological functions of an athlete; and—most importantly—if supplements enhance athletic performance directly or indirectly (e.g. by enhancing recovery or by preventing infectious diseases). This chapter aims to answer the following questions:

- Are micronutrient requirements increased in athletes?
- Are there any significant differences between indices of micronutrient status between athletes and untrained controls?
- If the supply of one or several micronutrients is marginal, would an athlete's functional capacity be less than optimal?
- If micronutrients are given in excess of daily dietary allowances, would this improve indices of micronutrient status, body functions and athletic performance?

Reviews on micronutrients and sports are addressed in chapters on measuring nutritional status of athletes (Chapter 3), calcium (Chapter 10) and iron (Chapter 11). Therefore, the above issues are not covered in the present chapter. Chapter 17 provides additional information on the supplementation practices of athletes.

12.2 MEASURING VITAMIN AND MINERAL STATUS IN ATHLETES

12.2.1 What is nutritional status?

An organism has an adequate nutritional status of its cells, tissue, organs and anatomical systems; working together can undertake all nutrient-dependent functions. The relationship between micronutrient supply and functional capacity is 'bell-shaped' (see Figure 12.1) (Brubacher 1989). The core in the above relationship is that the output (functional capacity) is not improved after the 'minimal requirement for maximal output' is reached. In contrast, too high an intake may in some cases reduce the output below the maximal level.

Table 12.2   Summary of the most important effects of minerals on body functions related to athletic training and performance

	Cofactors and activators for energy metabolism	Nervous function, muscle contraction	Haemoglobin synthesis	Immune function	Antioxidant function	Bone metabolism
Macrominerals						
Sodium		X				
Potassium		X				
Calcium		X				X
Magnesium	X	X		X		X
Trace elements						
Iron	X		X		X	
Zinc	X			X	X	
Copper	X				X	
Chromium	X					
Selenium					X	

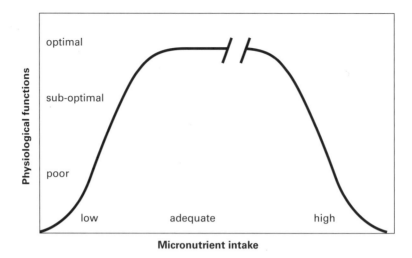

Figure 12.1 *The relation between micronutrient supply and functional capacity (Adapted from Brubacher 1989)*

Different body functions (single biochemical reactions, metabolic pathways, function of anatomical systems, and function of the host themselves) reach their maximal output at different levels of supply. In other words, the supply (intake) needed for optimal function of an anatomical system (e.g. the muscle) may be quite different from the supply needed to maximise the activity of a single enzyme (Solomons & Allen 1983).

Short-term inadequacy of vitamin and mineral intake is characterised by lowering of nutrient concentrations in different tissues and lowering of certain enzyme activities (see Figure 12.2). However, functional disturbances (such as decreased physical performance capacity) may appear later (Solomons & Allen 1983; Fogelholm 1995). In the opposite case, very large intakes increase the body pool and activity of some enzymes, but do not necessarily improve functional capacity (Fogelholm 1995).

12.2.2 *Assessment of nutritional status*

Ideally, nutritional status should be assessed by combining the information obtained from different (clinical, anthropometric, dietary, biochemical) markers (see Chapter 3, Section 3.1). Gross, clinical deficiency of nutrients cause detectable changes in, for instance, the skin or eyes. Anthropometric and body composition data are indicators of energy balance. Chronic negative energy balance is likely also to be associated with inadequate micronutrient intake. Assessment of dietary intakes in free-living people provide only estimates of 'usual' intakes of foods or nutrients and are not accurate measures (see Chapter 3, Section 3.2.1). Uncertainty about an individual's nutritional requirements and inaccuracies related to dietary assessment, therefore, preclude the use of dietary intakes as a sole indicator of nutritional status (Aggett 1990).

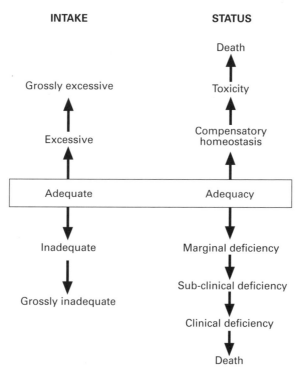

INTAKE   **STATUS**

Figure 12.2 *Dietary micronutrient intake and stages of micronutrient status*

Serum and plasma specimens are easy to collect and analyse, and therefore suitable for use with large numbers of people. Some water-soluble vitamins respond quickly to dietary intake (Singh et al. 1992b), and positive correlations between dietary intake and plasma concentration of ascorbic acid have been reported (Payette & Gray-Donald 1991). The concentrations of minerals or trace elements in blood, serum or plasma are under strong homeostatic control (Solomons & Allen 1983), which make them quite insensitive to marginal nutrient deficiency. In addition, factors unrelated to nutritional status, such as haemoconcentration, haemodilution or diurnal variation, may also affect blood chemistry. Therefore, a single measurement of serum concentrations of micronutrients should be interpreted with great caution.

Because serum and plasma concentrations are rather insensitive to marginal micronutrient deficiency, substantial research has been undertaken to identify other body compartments that would better represent the body's micronutrient status. Mononuclear leucocytes appear to be more sensitive indicators of vitamin C (Jacob 1990), magnesium (Weller et al. 1998) and zinc (Dolev et al. 1995) status, compared to the respective indicators in serum or plasma. Unfortunately, these interesting methods are still not used routinely and hardly anything is known about micronutrient concentrations in the leucocytes of athletes.

Erythrocyte enzyme activation co-efficients (E-AC) are used as indicators for the status of thiamin (enzyme: transketolase (TK)), riboflavin (glutathione reductase (GR)) and vitamin B6 (aspartate aminotransferase (AST), also called glutamate oxalacetate transaminase, (GOT)). In these methods, the activity of an enzyme is measured with and without in vitro cofactor (vitamin B) saturation. The activation co-efficient (AC) is calculated by dividing saturated activity by basal activity (Bayomi & Rosalki 1976). High ACs indicate inadequate nutritional status. These techniques are extremely interesting, because they are truly functional rather than static, as is the case of nutrient concentrations in plasma and serum (Solomons & Allen 1983).

Both physiological and analytical factors affect the sensitivity and specificity of blood tests as indicators of vitamin status. These factors lead to a notable analytical variation between laboratories. Ideally, each laboratory should make its own reference interval, or ascertain that the chosen reference interval is made by precisely comparable methods. Otherwise, the reported number of athletes with 'sub-clinical deficiency' could be wrong (Fogelholm et al. 1993b).

The enzymes that are used for assessment of thiamin, riboflavin and vitamin B6 status represent one metabolic pathway in the erythrocytes. Therefore, they do not necessarily indicate the function of other metabolic pathways in other tissues, e.g. glycolysis or the Kreb's cycle in the muscles. Moreover, when people follow a typical western mixed diet, erythrocyte concentrations of TK, GR and AST are not saturated *in vivo* by their cofactor. Consequently, after supplementation, their basal activity increases and activation co-efficient decreases (Guilland et al. 1989; Fogelholm et al. 1993b). However, these changes are not necessarily associated with improved physical performance (see Section 12.6.1).

Recently, the relationships among exercise, free radicals and lipid peroxidation have raised considerable interest. Breath pentane, thiobarbituric acid reactive substances (TBARS) and malondialdehyde (MDA) are indicators of lipid peroxidation caused by free radicals in humans. Unfortunately, these markers neither indicate the source or timing of lipid peroxidation (Alessio 1993), nor do they permit quantitative correlation of peroxidation (Weber 1990). MDA and TBARS, for instance, may arise from other pathways besides lipid peroxidation (Weber 1990). Moreover, during sleep and light daily activities, products of lipid peroxidation may be produced and remain in regions where blood-flow is limited (Weber 1990). When blood-flow during exercise is increased and blood is redistributed to new regions, these products may then be 'washed out'.

12.3 EFFECTS OF EXERCISE ON VITAMIN AND MINERAL REQUIREMENTS OF ATHLETES

12.3.1 *Requirements of water-soluble vitamins and antioxidants*

Physical activity increases energy expenditure. In his review, van der Beek (1991) proposed that high metabolic activity might increase the turnover of several vitamins of the B-complex group. Indeed, some old data support the above view. For example, Sauberlich et al. (1979) found that thiamin requirements in male subjects were 30% higher when daily energy intake was 15.1 MJ (3600 kcal), compared with 11.7 MJ (2600 kcal). However, an energy-related requirement for thiamin has also been questioned (Caster & Mickelsen 1991). Vitamin losses through sweat are minimal, even in physically active people (Brotherhood 1984).

Energy production involves reduction of molecular oxygen (O_2) in the mitochondria. The reduction is not always complete, and about 2–5% of the molecular oxygen turns into a free radical (superoxide radical, O_2^-) (Sjödin et al. 1990). The free radicals are unstable, reactive and potentially harmful chemical substances with unpaired electrons in their outer orbitals (Sen 1995). An excessive production of free radicals, or an insufficient protection against them, has been linked to cell and mitochondria membrane damage, deterioration of the immune defence system, ageing, cancer and atherosclerosis (Jacob & Burri 1996).

In humans, indirect evidence of lipid peroxidation during physical exertion includes increased pentane exhalation in the breath (Dillard et al. 1978; Simon-Schnass & Pabst 1988; Dekkers et al. 1996; Leaf et al. 1997), and elevated MDA in serum and erythrocytes (Lovlin et al. 1987; Sumida et al. 1989; Dekkers et al. 1996; McBride et al. 1998). Not all studies show an exercise-induced increase in indices of lipid peroxidation (Laaksonen et al. 1995; Margaritis et al. 1997). It is, however, apparent that lipid peroxidation is increased, if the preceding exercise is intense and strenuous enough (Leaf et al. 1997).

Scavenger enzymes and antioxidant vitamins (mainly vitamins C and E and β-carotene) build up a protection system against free radical attack. Mena et al. (1991) showed that highly trained athletes have higher activities of several scavenger enzymes, but the effects of moderate training are apparently much smaller (Tiidus et al. 1996). An increased need for endogenous defence against free radicals may, nevertheless, increase the requirement for antioxidant vitamins (Sen 1995; Dekkers et al. 1996; Jacob & Burri 1996).

12.3.2 *Requirements of minerals*

The losses of magnesium and zinc through sweat may be important. The exercise-induced concentration of magnesium in sweat has varied between 3–36 mg/L in different studies (Beller et al. 1975; Costill et al. 1976; Costill et al. 1982; Verde et al. 1982; Wenk et al. 1989). Each litre of sweat would thus increase the daily magnesium needs by 3–34%, given a dietary bioavailability of 30% (Anon. 1984) and a daily dietary allowance of 350 mg (National Research Council 1989). Similarly, the zinc concentration in sweat has varied between 0.6–1.5 mg/L (Beller et al. 1975; Aruoma et al. 1988) which would mean a 17–42% increase in the daily needs for each additional litre of sweat. Unfortunately, the interpretation of these data is difficult, because of several problems in sweat analyses. For instance, the composition of sweat varies with the collection site (Gutteridge et al. 1985; Aruoma et al.

1988). Moreover, it is uncertain whether a short sampling period represents long-term conditions (Brune et al. 1986). The variation between different studies reflects the above-mentioned methodological problems.

In addition to sweating, micronutrients may be lost in urine or faeces. On one day of physical exercise, Deuster et al. (1987) found elevated (22%) magnesium excretion. Similarly, higher excretion of magnesium (21–76%) (Singh 1990a; Nuviala et al. 1999) and zinc (Lichton et al. 1988; Deuster et al. 1989) has been found in trained athletes compared with controls. Results are not without contradiction: Nuviala et al. (1999) reported similar urinary zinc excretion in female athletes and untrained controls, and Zorbas et al. (1999) found increased copper excretion in trained subjects only when their activity was markedly restricted. Finally, because of an increase in free radical formation during strenuous exercise, the requirements for zinc and copper (in $Zn_2 Cu_2$-superoxide dismutase enzyme) and selenium (in glutathione peroxidase) may also be greater than normal in physically active people.

In summary, it is biologically plausible to conjecture that athletic training, especially if it leads to very high energy expenditure, increases the requirements of micronutrients (at least through losses in sweat, urine and perhaps in faeces), and through increased free radical production. Nevertheless, the data to date are insufficient to allow any quantification of micronutrient requirements in athletes. Because of a wide safety margin, the RDIs/RDAs for vitamins and minerals (Table 12.3) may still be used for athletes, although with caution.

12.4 BIOCHEMICAL INDICATORS OF VITAMIN AND MINERAL STATUS IN ATHLETES

Most biochemical measures that are indices of nutrient status in individuals are markers for risk and do not usually confirm a true diagnosis of nutrient overload or deficiency without other clinical and dietary assessment measures (see Chapter 3). One-off biochemical measures in individuals, although below usual population measures, may be normal for an individual. Biochemical measures of vitamins and minerals only become diagnostic in individuals in moderate to severe nutrient depletion states, which is unusual in an athletic population. Biochemical measures of vitamins and mineral status in athletes are useful in research to compare relative differences between athletes and untrained controls, and allow an evaluation of nutrient requirements of groups of athletes involved in varying types of physical activity.

12.4.1 *Biochemical indicators of water-soluble vitamin status*
12.4.1.1 *Vitamin B group*
Cross-sectional studies comparing vitamin B status in athletes and untrained controls give inconclusive results. Guilland et al. (1989) found higher erythrocyte

Table 12.3 *Examples of recommended daily allowances: Recommended Dietary Intakes (RDIs) for vitamins and minerals for use in Australia by adults*

	Men	Women	Pregnancy	Lactation
Vitamin A				
(µg retinol equivalents)	750	750	+0	+450
Thiamin (mg)	1.1	0.8	+0.2	+0.4
Riboflavin (mg)	1.7	1.2	+0.3	+0.5
Niacin (mg)	19	13	+2	+5
Vitamin B6 (mg)	1.3–1.9	0.9–1.4	+0.1	+0.7–0.8
Folate (µg)	200	200	+200	+150
Vitamin B12 (µg)	2.0	2.0	+1.0	+0.5
Vitamin C (mg)	40	30	+30	+45
Vitamin E (mg α equiv)	10.0	7.0	+0	+2.5
Zinc (mg)	12	12	+4	+6
Iron (mg)	7	12–16	+10–20	+0
Iodine (mg)	150	120	+30	+50
Magnesium (mg)	320	270	+30	+70
Calcium (mg)	800	800	+300	+400
Phosphorus (mg)	1000	100	+200	+200
Selenium (µg)	85	70	+10	+15
Sodium (mg)	920–2300	920–2300	+0	+0
Potassium (mg)	1950–5460	1950–5460	+0	+0

Source: National Health & Medical Research Council (1991)

transketolase activation co-efficient (E-TKAC) in athletes than in untrained controls, whereas Fogelholm et al. (1992a, 1992b) found both lower and comparable E-TKAC in athletes. Keith and Alt (1991) found higher erythrocyte glutathione reductase activation co-efficient (E-GRAC) in female athletes, but Guilland et al. (1989) reported levels comparable to the controls. Only Guilland et al. (1989) have reported erythrocyte aspartate amino transferase activation co-efficient (E-ASTAC) values for both athletes and untrained controls; no difference was observed. All differences reported in the above studies were small, however, and most probably without any functional significance.

The effects of a 24-week fitness-type exercise program on micronutrient status in previously untrained female students have been studied (Fogelholm 1992). Indicators for thiamin and riboflavin status were unchanged throughout the study. E-ASTAC increased in exercise and decreased in control groups, which may indicate marginally impaired vitamin B6 status in the exercise group. However, the magnitude of the change (from 2.02 to 2.11) is not likely to affect functional capacity (Fogelholm et al. 1993a, 1993b).

The effects of varying the training volume on E-TKAC have also been studied in Finnish cross-country skiers (Fogelholm et al. 1992b). Despite very strenuous training in August and November, and clearly lighter training in February and in May, E-TKAC showed no seasonal variation.

12.4.1.2   *Vitamin C*

Reported data on vitamin C status in physically active people and untrained individuals are scarce. Serum ascorbic acid concentrations were the same (Guilland et al. 1989; Fogelholm et al. 1992a; Rokitzki et al. 1994a) or higher (Fishbaine & Butterfield 1984) in athletes than in controls. The pooled mean concentrations for serum or plasma ascorbic acid in the above studies were 59 and 56 µmol/L for athletes (n = 533) and controls (n = 193), respectively.

12.4.2   *Biochemical indicators of fat-soluble vitamin status*
12.4.2.1   *Vitamin A*

Serum concentration for ß-carotene, the provitamin for retinol, is more responsive to marginal changes in status than retinol. Takatsuka et al. (1995) reported that hard physical activity was associated with lower β-carotene concentrations in Japanese men and women. The results in this cross-sectional study were adjusted for age, BMI, diet, smoking, serum cholesterol and serum triglycerides. Guilland et al. (1989) found comparable β-carotene concentrations in athletes and controls.

12.4.2.2   *Vitamin E*

Moderate physical activity has not been shown to have any negative effects on vitamin E (α-tocopherol) concentration in plasma (Kitamura et al. 1997; Thomas et al. 1998) or in the muscle (Tiidus et al. 1996). Only a few studies have compared plasma α-tocopherol levels between competitive athletes and controls. Guilland et al. (1989) reported similar results, but Karlsson et al. (1992) found lower levels in athletes than in controls. Nevertheless, in the latter study, the ratio between athletes' and controls' α-tocopherol concentration was precisely the same as the ratio between athletes' and controls' free cholesterol concentration in plasma. Because α-tocopherol is transported in lipoproteins together with cholesterol, dissimilar blood lipid profiles in athletes and controls might explain the difference found by Karlsson et al. (1992).

12.4.3   *Biochemical indicators of mineral status*
12.4.3.1   *Iron*

Biochemical indicators of iron status in athletes have been studied extensively and are reviewed in Chapter 11, Section 11.6.1.

12.4.3.2   *Magnesium*

The data on mineral status in athletes and controls, published between 1980 and 1994, have been pooled in an analytical review (Fogelholm 1995). The mean serum magnesium concentration in athletes (n = 516 in seven studies) was 0.84 mmol/L, and in controls (n = 251) 0.85 mmol/L. More recent studies reported that athletes had similar (Crespo et al. 1995; Nuviala et al. 1999) or even higher (Nuviala et al. 1999) serum magnesium concentration, as compared to sedentary controls. Lower (Casoni et al. 1990) or similar (Fogelholm et al. 1991) erythrocyte magnesium concentrations were found in athletes, compared with untrained controls. In a controlled intervention, a 24-week fitness-type exercise program did not affect serum or erythrocyte magnesium content in previously untrained young women (Fogelholm 1992).

12.4.3.3 *Zinc*

The mean serum zinc concentration, pooled from studies published between 1980 and 1994, was 13.5 µmol/L in athletes (n = 587 in 11 studies) and 13.7 µmol/L in controls (n = 244) (Fogelholm 1995). More recent studies have also found similar serum zinc levels in athletes and sedentary controls (Crespo et al. 1995; Nuviala et al. 1999). Following increased physical activity, three longitudinal studies found a negative time-trend for serum or plasma zinc (Miyamura et al. 1987; Lichton et al. 1988; Couzy et al. 1990). In contrast, serum zinc increased in competitive sailors during a three-week transatlantic race (Fogelholm & Lahtinen 1991). Other studies have not found any associations between training volume and serum zinc concentration (Lukaski et al. 1990; Ohno et al. 1990; Fogelholm 1992; Fogelholm et al. 1992b; Dolev et al. 1995).

Data on zinc levels in other body compartments are scarce, but the few findings are interesting. Several studies have reported a positive association between high or increased physical activity and erythrocyte zinc concentration (Ohno et al. 1990; Singh et al. 1990b; Fogelholm et al. 1991; Fogelholm 1992). Dolev et al. (1995) reported maintenance of zinc concentration in erythrocytes, but an increased concentration in mononuclear leucocytes, in male military recruits during a 12-week training program. The increase in erythrocyte and leucocyte zinc level might be related to increased amounts of intra-cellular zinc-dependent enzymes, such as superoxide dismutase.

12.4.3.4 *Copper, chromium and selenium*

In studies published between 1980 and 1994, the pooled mean results of plasma copper concentration tended to be higher for females and for athletes: 16.3 and 15.1 µmol/L for female athletes and controls, and 14.7 and 14.1 µmol/L for male athletes and controls, respectively (Fogelholm 1995). Data on other trace elements are even scarcer. Anderson et al. (1988) reported similar plasma chromium concentrations in athletes and untrained controls. A competitive sailing crew had lower serum selenium concentration than controls (Fogelholm & Lahtinen 1991). Nevertheless, even the sailing crew's results were clearly within the reference range for selenium.

In summary, the available indices of magnesium, zinc, copper, chromium and selenium do not suggest compromised status in physically active people. Because of the lack of sensitivity of these indices, this interpretation must be taken with caution.

12.5 DOES MARGINAL DEFICIENCY OF VITAMINS AND MINERALS AFFECT PHYSICAL PERFORMANCE?

Studies involving marginal deficiency of vitamins and minerals test the hypothesis that physical performance is impaired already when the status of one or several micronutrients is indicative of marginal deficiency.

12.5.1 Vitamins

12.5.1.1 Thiamin

Earlier studies have shown that sub-clinical thiamin deficiency is associated with increased exercise-induced blood lactate concentrations, especially after a pre-exercise glucose load (Sauberlich 1967). The deterioration of physical capacity in marginal deficiency, however, is less evident. Despite a five-week thiamin-depleted diet, Wood et al. (1980) did not find decreased working capacity in male students. E-TKAC decreased significantly, showing that the activity of this enzyme was affected faster than the activity of the enzymes of glycolysis and the citric acid cycle in working muscles.

12.5.1.2 Riboflavin

Significant changes in riboflavin supply affect both muscle metabolism and neuro-muscular function. Data on the effects of marginal riboflavin supply are, however, scarce. In three studies (Belko et al. 1984, 1985; Trebler Winters et al. 1992), a four- to five-week marginal riboflavin intake lowered E-GRAC, but no relation between vitamin status and aerobic capacity was found. Similarly, Soares et al. (1993) did not find changes in muscular efficiency during moderate-intensity exercise after a seven-week period of riboflavin-restricted diet. Decreased urinary riboflavin excretion might be one mechanism to conserve riboflavin and prevent changes in riboflavin-dependent body functions during marginal depletion, which may explain the outcome of these studies.

12.5.1.3 Vitamin B6

In male wrestlers and judo athletes, a decrease in E-ASTAC indicated deteriorated vitamin B6 supply during a three-week weight-loss regimen (Fogelholm et al. 1993a). Maximal anaerobic capacity, speed or strength were, however, not affected. Also, Coburn et al. (1991) showed that the muscle tissue was quite resistant to a six-week vitamin B6 depletion.

12.5.1.4 *Vitamin C*

In one study (van der Beek et al. 1990), a vitamin C-restricted diet reduced whole blood ascorbic acid concentration. Nevertheless, the marginal vitamin supply in the blood did not produce any significant effects on maximal aerobic capacity or lactate threshold in healthy volunteers. In contrast to the above study, Johnston et al. (1999) reported that a three-week experimental vitamin C depletion was associated with reduced work efficiency during sub-maximal exercise and that work performance increased after repletion with vitamin C supplements (two weeks, 500 mg/d).

12.5.1.5 *Multivitamins*

Finally, a combined depletion of thiamin, riboflavin, vitamin B6 and ascorbic acid has been found to affect both E-TKAC and aerobic working capacity (van der Beek et al. 1988). Because of the multiple depletion, the independent role of the single vitamins could not be demonstrated.

12.5.2 *Minerals*

Even mild iron deficiency anaemia has a negative impact on endurance performance (see Chapter 11). The effects of marginal status of other minerals on physical performance in healthy volunteers have been studied only rarely. Van Loan et al. (1999) investigated the effects of induced zinc depletion on muscle function in eight male subjects who were fed a formula diet (< 0.5 mg Zn/d for 33 or 41 days). The mean serum zinc concentration decreased from an initial 11.0 µmol/L to 3.4 µmol/L at the end of depletion. Muscle endurance (total work capacity in isokinetic exercise tests) declined, but peak force was not affected. The authors speculated that the effects observed could have been related to decreased activity of lactate dehydrogenase, a zinc-dependent enzyme, and a concomitant increase in blood lactate concentration.

12.6 EFFECTS OF SUPPLEMENTATION ON BIOCHEMICAL INDICES OF MICRONUTRIENT STATUS AND PHYSICAL PERFORMANCE

Depletion studies show that even marginal micronutrient deficiency conditions may impair physical performance. Nevertheless, the available data suggest that micronutrient deficiencies in athletes are rare and no more common than in untrained subjects. These findings lead to two questions with considerable practical importance:

- Are the observed indicators of micronutrient status compatible with optimal athletic performance?
- Would a nutrient intake beyond the daily dietary recommendations (i.e. supplementation) improve physical capacity?

12.6.1 *Effects of water-soluble vitamin supplementation on performance*

12.6.1.1 *Thiamin*

Thiamin supplementation (> 7.5 mg/d) improves the activity of erythrocyte TK (van Dam 1978; Guilland et al. 1989; Fogelholm et al. 1993b). Nevertheless, despite improved indicators of thiamin status, several studies have shown that thiamin supplementation did not improve functional capacity in athletes who were not deficient (Telford et al. 1992a, 1992b; Webster 1998) or in young, moderately trained adults (Singh et al. 1992a, 1992b; Fogelholm et al. 1993b).

12.6.1.2 *Riboflavin*

Riboflavin supplementation improves the activity of erythrocyte GR (van Dam 1978; Weight et al. 1988b; Guilland et al. 1989; Fogelholm et al. 1993b) in athletes or trained students, even without indications of impaired vitamin status (Weight et al. 1988b). One early study suggested that supplementation and improved riboflavin status was related to improved neuromuscular function (Haralambie 1976). In contrast, later studies did not find any beneficial effects of riboflavin supplementation on maximal oxygen uptake (Weight et al. 1988a, 1988b; Singh et al. 1992a, 1992b) or exercise-induced lactate appearance in the blood (Weight et al. 1988a, 1988b; Fogelholm et al. 1993b).

12.6.1.3 *Vitamin B6*

Chronic supplementation of vitamin B6 increases the erythrocyte ASAT activity (van Dam 1978; Guilland et al. 1989; Fogelholm et al. 1993b) and plasma pyridoxal-5-phosphate (PLP) concentration (Weight et al. 1988a; Coburn et al. 1991) even in healthy subjects. Supplementation of vitamin B6, in combination with other B-complex vitamins (van Dam 1978; Bonke & Nickel 1989), has improved shooting target performance (Bonke & Nickel 1989) and improved muscle irritability (van Dam 1978) in male athletes. In contrast, a number of other studies did not find any association between improved indicators of vitamin B6 status and maximal oxygen uptake (Weight et al. 1988a, 1988b), exercise-induced lactate appearance in blood (Manore & Leklem 1988; Weight et al. 1988a, 1988b; Fogelholm et al. 1993b) or other tests of physical performance (Telford et al. 1992a, 1992b; Virk et al. 1999). In fact, an increase in the biochemical indicators of vitamin B6 status is not necessarily associated with a change in intramuscular vitamin B6 content (Coburn et al. 1991).

It appears that vitamin B6, either as an infusion (Moretti et al. 1982) or given orally as a 20 mg/d supplement (Dunton et al. 1993), stimulates growth hormone production during exercise. The hypothetical mechanism behind this effect is that PLP acts as the coenzyme for dopa decarboxylase, and high concentrations might promote the conversion of L-dopa to dopamine (Manore 1994). The physiological significance of the above effect on muscle growth and strength is not known.

12.6.1.4   *Folate and vitamin B12*

There are only a few studies linking folic acid or vitamin B12 supply to sports-related functional capacity. Folate supplementation and increased serum folate concentration did not affect maximal oxygen uptake (Matter et al. 1987), anaerobic threshold (Matter et al. 1987) or other measures of physical performance (Telford et al. 1992a, 1992b). Together with thiamin and vitamin B6 supplementation, elevated intake of vitamin B12 was, however, associated with improved target shooting performance (Bonke & Nickel 1989).

12.6.1.5   *Other B vitamins (e.g. thiamin and pantothenic acid)*

Data on supplementation of other B-vitamins and performance are even scarcer. Recently, Webster et al. (1998) reported no effect of a combined thiamin and pantothenic acid supplementation on a 2000 m time trial by cycle ergometer.

12.6.1.6   *Vitamin C*

In a review, Gerster (1989) concluded that a vast majority of studies have not shown any measurable effects of vitamin C supplementation on maximal oxygen uptake, lactate threshold or exercise-induced heart rate in well-nourished subjects. However, an interesting aspect of interaction between vitamin C and physical activity is related to the proposed connection with upper respiratory tract infections (URTIs). Strenuous physical activity seems to increase the risk for URTI during the first week or two after exercise (Nieman & Pedersen 1999). In his meta-analysis, Hemilä (1995) identified three placebo-controlled studies that examined the effects of vitamin C supplementation on URTI in subjects during and after physical stress. The pooled rate ratio of URTI was 0.50 (95% confidence interval 0.35–0.69) in favour of the group receiving vitamin C (600–1000 mg/d). Hence, these studies suggest a positive effect of vitamin C supplementation during and after strenuous physical activity. Nevertheless, these data do not prove that supplementary vitamin C would be beneficial also during moderate training. Moreover, it is not known whether the potential effect of vitamin C supplementation on the common cold in athletes has any significant long-term effects on performance.

12.6.2   **Effects of fat-soluble vitamin supplementation on performance**

There are no data on the effects of retinol, vitamin D or vitamin K supplementation on athletes' performances or other parameters. On the other hand, several studies have shown that α-tocopherol supplementation (typical dose > 100 mg/d) reduces breath pentane excretion (Simon-Schnass & Pabst 1988) and serum MDA concentration (determined as TBARs) (Simon-Schnass & Pabst 1988; Sumida et al. 1989; Meydani et al. 1993; Rokitzki et al. 1994) during exercise. Both breath pentane and serum MDA were used as indicators of lipid peroxidation. Despite the association between vitamin E supplementation and indices of lipid peroxidation, most studies have not supported the hypothesis that vitamin E attenuates exercise-induced muscle damage (Dekkers et al. 1996; Kaikkonen et al. 1998).

In one controlled trial (Simon-Schnass & Pabst 1988), vitamin E supplementation maintained aerobic working capacity at very high altitude (> 5000 m). More recent studies have not proven that vitamin E intake exceeding daily recommendations would have any beneficial effects on athletic performance (Rokitzki et al. 1994b; Kanter & Williams 1995; Tiidus & Houston 1995; Buchman et al. 1999).

12.6.3 *Effects of mineral supplementation on performance*

Iron supplementation does not improve performance in athletes with low iron stores (i.e. low ferritin) (see Chapter 11, Section 11.3). However, the benefit of iron supplementation to performance in athletes with diagnosed iron deficiency anaemia is well established. Data on supplementation of other minerals than iron are scarce. In two studies (Terblanche et al. 1992; Weller et al. 1998), oral magnesium (365–500 mg/d for three weeks) neither increased serum magnesium levels nor improved physical performance. Similarly, in other studies (Singh et al. 1992b; Telford et al. 1992a), a supplement containing several minerals and trace elements failed to affect indicators of nutritional status and athletic performance.

Chromium supplementation, mainly as chromium picolinate, during training has been proposed to stimulate insulin function and to promote muscle growth. In an earlier controlled trial, chromium (200 µg/d) or placebo was given to healthy, previously untrained students, during a 12-week weight lifting program (Hasten et al. 1992). Supplementation was associated with greater body weight gain in women, but not in men. Strength was not affected. Despite this preliminary finding, more recent studies with athletes have not found any significant effects of chromium on weight, body composition or strength (Clancy et al. 1994; Trent & Thieding-Cancel 1995; Lukaski et al. 1996; Walker et al. 1998). Hence, it seems that short-term (4–12 weeks) chromium supplementation with doses varying from 200–800 µg/d does not promote muscle growth or strength in weight-trained individuals (see also Chapter 17).

12.7 *POTENTIAL RISKS OF VITAMIN AND MINERAL SUPPLEMENTS*

12.7.1 *Risks related to high intake of water-soluble vitamins*

Although the scientific data do not support the hypothesis that high vitamin and mineral intake enhance performance in well-nourished athletes, the use of supplements is very common (Sobal & Marquart 1994). Many athletes use supplements as a precaution, 'just in case'. Nevertheless, very high, chronic intake of one or several micronutrients may involve risks. Therefore, any precautionary use of supplements should remain well within the safe levels of intake.

12.7.1.1 *Thiamin, riboflavin and B6*

Adverse reactions of chronic, elevated oral administration of thiamin are virtually unknown (Marks 1989). For chronic oral use, the safe dose is at least 50–100 times the recommended daily intake, that is, above 100 mg daily. Riboflavin in large doses may cause a yellow discoloration of the urine, which might cause concern in people not aware of the origin of the colour (Alhadeff et al. 1984). However, there is no evidence of any harmful effects even with oral riboflavin doses exceeding 100 times the recommended daily intake (Marks 1989). In contrast to thiamin and riboflavin, megadoses of vitamin B6 may have toxic and possibly permanent effects. The most common disorder is sensory neuropathy (Bässler 1989). Long-term supplementation should not exceed 200 mg/d, that is, 100 times the recommended allowance (Marks 1989).

12.7.1.2 *Folate and B12*

The effects of high doses of folate have not been widely studied, but some results indicate a possible interference with zinc metabolism (Marks 1989; Reynolds 1994). The current estimate of the safety dose is between 50 and 100 times the daily recommended intake (Marks 1989). The safety margin for vitamin B12 appears to be much larger, because even doses as high as 30 mg/d (i.e. 10 000 times the recommended intake) have been used without noticeable toxic effects (Marks 1989).

12.7.1.3 *Other B vitamins (e.g. nicotinic acid, biotin and pantothenic acid)*

Acute oral intake of at least 100 mg of nicotinic acid per day (i.e. at least five times the recommended daily allowance) causes vasodilatation and flushing, which is a rather harmless effect (Marks 1989). The safe chronic dose appears to be at least 50 times the recommended allowance or 1 g/d. There are no reported toxic effects of biotin and pantothenic acid intake up to 100 times the recommended allowance (Alhadeff et al. 1984; Marks 1989).

12.7.1.4 *Vitamin C*

Very high (> 1 g/d), chronic doses of vitamin C may lead to formation of oxalate stones, increased uric acid excretion, diarrhoea, vitamin B12 destruction and iron overload (Alhadeff et al. 1984). However, excluding diarrhoea, the risk for the above toxic effects is likely to be very low in healthy individuals, even with intake of several grams daily (Rivers 1989).

12.7.2 *Risks related to high intake of fat-soluble vitamins*
12.7.2.1 *Vitamin A*

Chronic toxic intake of pre-formed retinol (vitamin A) will cause joint or bone pain, hair loss, anorexia and liver damage. The safety level for chronic use is estimated to be ten times the recommended allowance, that is 10 g retinol daily (Marks

1989). Because of an increased risk of spontaneous abortion and birth-defects, the safe level during pregnancy may be only four to five times the daily recommendation. β-carotene, a water-soluble form of vitamin A, in contrast to pre-formed retinol, is not toxic. This provitamin is stored under the skin and is converted to active retinol only when needed.

12.7.2.2 *Vitamin D and vitamin E*

Vitamin D is potentially toxic, causing hypercalcaemia, hypercalciuria, soft-tissue calcification, anorexia and constipation, and eventually irreversible renal and cardiovascular damage (Davies 1989). Intakes of ten times the recommendation should not be exceeded. High calcium intakes may enhance the toxicity of vitamin D. Vitamin E, in contrast to vitamins A and D, is apparently not toxic for healthy individuals (Machlin 1989). The safety factor for long-term administration is at least 100 times the recommended daily intake, that is, at least 1 g/d in oral use.

12.7.3 *Risks related to high intake of minerals*

The body pool of macrominerals, and especially of trace elements, is under strong homeostatic control. Therefore, toxicity by dietary means or supplements is rare. If, however, toxic symptoms appear, they are severe and can even be fatal. Intakes needed for toxic effects are, luckily, extremely high. For instance, the first toxic symptoms (vomiting, diarrhoea) of zinc overload are seen after a huge intake of at least 4 g (normal dietary intake is 10–15 mg/d). Extremely high intakes of copper can lead to liver cirrhosis or hepatic necrosis, and too much selenium causes changes in skin and hair, and neurological abnormalities. The threshold between the daily allowance and toxicity level of selenium is relatively small.

Although severe toxicity is very rare, high mineral intake may interfere with nutrient absorption at the intestinal mucosa (O'Dell 1985). Chronic zinc intake of 50 mg/d decreases both iron and copper bioavailability. Analogously, high intake of either iron or copper interferes with zinc absorption. Therefore, a surplus of one trace element may cause marginal deficiency of another trace element, especially when the intake of the latter is marginal (see Chapter 11, Section 11.8.2.2). Because intestinal interactions are observed with rather low dosages, precautionary use of mineral supplements (i.e. not specifically to treat a diagnosed deficiency) that does not exceed three times the RDI/RDA is warranted.

12.8 *SUMMARY*

The daily requirement of at least some vitamins and minerals is increased beyond normal levels in highly physically active people. The potential reasons for this increased requirement are excretion through sweating, urine and perhaps faeces, and through increased free radical production. Unfortunately, it is not possible to quantify micronutrient requirements of athletes. Measures on micronutrient status and supplementation trials are needed to evaluate whether or not normal dietary intakes in athletes are sufficient to cover the increased requirements.

Most studies have not revealed any significant differences between athletes' and controls' indices of micronutrient status. The results suggest that athletic training, *per se*, does not lead to micronutrient deficiency. These data should, however, be interpreted very carefully. Because of the insensitivity of most indices to marginal deficiency, the results do not exclude the possibility of minor differences between the athletes and controls. In addition, the data do not exclude the possibility that some individual athletes (and controls) have inadequate status.

Physical performance can be affected even when micronutrient deficiency is only marginal. In depletion experiments, changes in one or more biochemical indices of micronutrient status were seen before or together with impairments in physical work capacity. Despite the associations between indices of micronutrient status and performance in depletion studies, the rationality of routine laboratory assessment of water-soluble vitamin, magnesium or trace element (excluding iron) status in athletes seems doubtful. Because the prevalence of even marginal deficiency is low, routine assessment would lead to numerous false positive diagnoses.

Supplementation of water-soluble vitamins is associated with improved corresponding indicators in blood. Moreover, supplementation of vitamin C may decrease the incidence of URTIs after very strenuous physical exercise, and vitamin E has a lowering effect on indices of lipid peroxidation during exercise. However, studies do not conclusively show that micronutrient supplementation would increase physical performance. Consequently, the levels of indicators of vitamin and mineral status seen in athletes are apparently compatible with optimal physical functions.

The evidence for benefits of vitamin and mineral supplements on athletic performance is extremely limited. In addition, high intake of single micronutrients may lead to physiological disturbances, especially if the diet is inadequate. Hence, an athlete should try to ensure adequate vitamin and mineral status mainly by a well-balanced diet. If, for any reason, an athlete wants to use micronutrient supplements as a precaution, a multivitamin-mineral supplement with amounts not exceeding two times the RDA is likely to be both safe and adequate for optimal sports performance.

12.9 PRACTICE TIPS

Julie Tatnell

- In the absence of clear proof that athletes have special requirements for vitamins and minerals, it is appropriate to use population RDIs/RDAs as a guideline for dietary intake goals for athletes. However, some caution is needed in the case of some minerals, such as iron and calcium, where the requirements of individuals are increased by special circumstances. These minerals are covered in more detail in Chapters 10 and 11.

- In general, athletes who consume a variety of nutrient-rich foods and enjoy a high energy to balance the energy cost of their training should be able to consume vitamins and minerals in amounts that exceed population RDIs/RDAs. Athletes who consume restricted energy intakes over prolonged periods, or who restrict the range of foods commonly eaten, may be at risk of sub-optimal intakes of some micronutrients.

- Assessment of the micronutrient status of an athlete is complex and requires information from a variety of sources, including the assessment of dietary intake, clinical history and some biochemical and haematological measurements. Further details are supplied in Chapter 3, Chapter 10 and Chapter 11. In assessing an athlete's dietary patterns, dietary records, dietary histories, food frequency questionnaires and self-assessment checklists are all useful, but must be interpreted in light of the inaccuracies of self-reported dietary intake data. Food checklists and food frequency questionnaires are useful for targeting the usual intake of certain groups of foods, and may help to pinpoint the risk of sub-optimal intake of specific nutrients.

- Creative menu planning can promote an increased dietary range for fussy eaters or athletes with limited food availability. It is often possible to find alternative dietary sources or different food forms to boost the intake of nutrients that appear to be 'at risk'. For example, fortified soy products can provide a calcium exchange for dairy products, berries and tropical fruits might provide a more exotic choice for athletes who claim to dislike fruit, and salads can be exchanged for cooked vegetables. Some athletes who do not like plain cooked vegetables served with a meal will enjoy vegetables served on a pizza or in soup. Athletes who are travelling to third-world countries with poor food range, or a high risk of gastrointestinal upsets due to contamination of uncooked foods, may be temporarily without their usual intake of fruits and vegetables. A supply of tetra-pack or dehydrated fruit juices, dried fruit and snack packs of tinned fruit can help to improve dietary variety and nutrient intake (see Practice tips for Chapter 24: Nutrition for the travelling athlete).

- In the case of the inability or unwillingness of an athlete to improve their dietary intake, the use of a specific micronutrient supplement may be warranted. A low dose (< 2–3 × RDI/RDA), broad range multivitamin/mineral supplement is the best option for general dietary support. Dietary supplementation may also be needed in the case of a diagnosed micronutrient deficiency, however, steps should also be taken to improve the dietary intake, so that long-term supplementation can be avoided. Chapters 10 and 11 provide more detail on the management of inadequate intake of these specific nutrients.

- To date, there is no sound evidence to confirm that the consumption of additional vitamin, mineral and antioxidants over and above the known requirements of an athlete improves performance. In preference, athletes should be encouraged to consume a diet containing a wide variety of nutrient-rich foods. Athletes must be given guidelines regarding shopping, preparation of quick, easy meals and suitable snack ideas, and should be educated regarding time management to ensure that good eating is not disregarded due to training and other commitments.

- Many athletes are not able to translate nutrient needs into food choices, and are swayed by the advertisements for vitamin and mineral supplements that claim that our food supply is unable to supply us with our dietary requirements. The sports dietitian should provide athletes with practical examples of food sources of vitamins and minerals, showing how requirements can be met via diet. In the case of antioxidants it is valuable for the athlete to be aware that the combination of antioxidants and other phytochemicals found in food provide greater benefits than isolated nutrients found in the supplement.

- Since there is an ever-increasing number of vitamin, mineral and antioxidant supplements on the market, it is important that the sports dietitian stay in touch with what is available. While it is time consuming, it is valuable to meet with sales representatives of the companies selling the supplement, obtain samples and, if possible, attend information sessions regarding the product. Gather as much information as possible so that your athletes have the benefit of your informed, unbiased opinion. However, be wary that your interest and attendance may be misinterpreted by multi-level marketing companies as a sign of endorsement of their product (see Practice tips in Chapter 17: Dietary supplements and nutritional ergogenic aids in sport).

- It is important that the sports dietitian stay in touch with research regarding vitamin, mineral and antioxidant supplementation. Journals, libraries, the Internet, researchers and other sports dietitians are all invaluable resources. Attend any education sessions where possible.

- It is important that the sports dietitian take into consideration the psychology behind the use of any type of supplement (see Chapter 17: Dietary supplements and nutritional ergogenic aids in sport). Most athletes are under constant pressure to improve their performance and are often prepared to take unproven, potentially harmful, or even banned substances in order to do so. Athletes should recognise the value of a sports dietitian to maximise their diet to reach their sporting potential, rather than spending time and money on factors that more than likely just distract them from the task at hand.

- Even if advised not to, an athlete may still decide to take a vitamin, mineral or antioxidant supplement providing nutrient intakes in considerable excess of their individual requirements. It is important that the athlete is made aware of the potential disadvantages of this action; including the cost, the potential distraction from good eating patterns, risk of toxicity (particularly in the case of vitamin A), and the possibility of the product containing a banned substance (see Chapter 17, Section 17.4). The latter is becoming a significant issue particularly with products being purchased from other countries via the Internet. It is vital that the risk of doping be considered before athletes take any supplement.

- If an athlete makes a public testimonial about their use of vitamin, mineral or antioxidant supplements, they must take responsibility for the fact that many junior or less talented athletes may follow their actions in the hope that it will narrow the gap between them and the 'elite'. High profile athletes should be invited to consider their social responsibilities and should take care when considering using their talent to promote an unproven product.

REFERENCES

Aggett P. Scientific considerations in the formulation of RDI. Eur J Clin Nutr 1990;44:37–43.

Alessio HM. Exercise-induced oxidative stress. Med Sci Sports Exerc 1993;25:218–24.

Alhadeff L, Gualtieri T, Lipton M. Toxic effects of water-soluble vitamins. Nutr Rev 1984;42:33–40.

Anderson RA, Bryden NA, Polansky MM, Deuster PA. Exercise effects on chromium excretion of trained and untrained men consuming a constant diet. J Appl Physiol 1988;64:249–52.

Anonymous. Recommended daily amounts of vitamins and minerals in Europe. Nutr Abstr Rev (Series A) 1990;60:827–42.

Aruoma OI, Reilly T, MacLaren D, Halliwell B. Iron, copper and zinc concentrations in human sweat and plasma: the effects of exercise. Clin Chem Acta 1988;177:81–8.

Bässler KH. Use and abuse of high dosages of vitamin B6. In: Walter P, Stähelin H, Brubacher G, eds. Elevated dosages of vitamins. Stuttgart: Hans Huber Publishers, 1989:120–6.

Bayomi RA, Rosalki SB. Evaluation of methods of coenzyme activation of erythrocyte enzymes for detection of deficiency of vitamins B1, B2, and B6. Clin Chem 1976;22:327–35.

Belko AZ, Meredith MP, Kalkwarf HJ, et al. Effects of exercise on riboflavin requirements: biological validation in weight reducing women. Am J Clin Nutr 1985;41:270–7.

Belko AZ, Obarzanec E, Roach R, et al. Effects of aerobic exercise and weight loss on riboflavin requirements of moderately obese, marginally deficient young women. Am J Clin Nutr 1984;40:553–61.

Beller GA, Maher JT, Hartley LH, Bass DE, Wacker WEC. Changes in serum and sweat magnesium levels during work in the heat. Aviat Space Anvironm Med 1975;46:709–12.

Bonke D, Nickel B. Improvement of fine motoric movement control by elevated dosages of vitamin B1, B6, and B12 in target shooting. In: Walter P, Stähelin H, Brubacher G, eds. Elevated dosages of vitamins. Stuttgart: Hans Huber Publishers, 1989:198–204

Brotherhood JR. Nutrition and sports performance. Sports Med 1984;1:350–89.

Brubacher GB. Scientific basis for the estimation of the daily requirements for vitamins. In: Walter P, Stähelin H, Brubacher G, eds. Elevated dosages of vitamins. Stuttgart: Hans Huber Publishers, 1989:3–11.

Brune M, Magnusson B, Persson H, Hallberg L. Iron losses in sweat. Am J Clin Nutr 1986;43:438–43.

Buchman AL, Killip D, Ou CN, et al. Short-term vitamin E supplementation before marathon running: a placebo-controlled trial. Nutrition 1999;15:278–83.

Casoni I, Guglielmini C, Graziano L, et al. Changes of magnesium concentrations in endurance athletes. Int J Sports Med 1990;11:234–7.

Caster WO, Mickelsen O. Effect of diet and stress on the thiamin and pyramin excretion of normal young men maintained on controlled intakes of thiamin. Nutr Res 1991;11:549–58.

Clancy SP, Clarkson PM, DeCheke ME, et al. Effects of chromium picolinate supplementation on body composition, strength, and urinary chromium loss in football players. Int J Sport Nutr 1994;42:142–53.

Coburn SP, Ziegler PJ, Costill DL, et al. Response of vitamin B6 content of muscle to changes in vitamin B6 intake in men. Am J Clin Nutr 1991;53:1436–42.

Costill DL, Cote R, Fink W. Muscle water and electrolytes following varied levels of dehydration in man. J Appl Physiol 1976;40:6–11.

Costill DL, Cote R, Fink WJ. Dietary potassium and heavy exercise: effects on muscle water and electrolytes. Am J Clin Nutr 1982;36:266–75.

Couzy F, Lafargue P, Guezennec CY. Zinc metabolism in the athlete: influence of training, nutrition and other factors. Int J Sports Med 1990;11:263–6.

Crespo R, Releca P, Lozano D, et al. Biochemical markers of nutrition in elite-marathon runners. J Sports Med Phys Fitness 1995;35:268–72.

Davies M. High-dose vitamin D therapy: indications, benefits and hazards. In: Walter P, Stähelin H, Brubacher G, eds. Elevated dosages of vitamins. Stuttgart: Hans Huber Publishers, 1989:81–6.

Dekkers JC, van Doornen JP, Kemper HCG. The role of antioxidant vitamins and enzymes in the prevention of exercise-induced muscle damage. Sports Med 1996;21:213–38.

Deuster PA, Day BA, Singh A, Douglass L, Moser-Veillon PB. Zinc status of highly trained women runners and untrained women. Am J Clin Nutr 1989;49:1295–301.

Deuster PA, Dolev E, Kyle SB, Anderson RA, Schoomaker EB. Magnesium homeostasis during high-intensity aerobic exercise in men. J Appl Physiol 1987;62:545–50.

Dillard CJ, Litov RE, Savin WM, Dumelin EE, Tappel AL. Effects of exercise, vitamin E, and ozone on pulmonary function and lipid peroxidation. J Appl Physiol 1978;45:927–32.

Dolev E, Burstein R, Lubin F, et al. Interpretation of zinc status indicators in a strenuously exercising population. J Am Diet Assoc 1995;95:482–4.

Dunton N, Virk R, Young J, Leklem J. The influence of vitamin B6 supplementation and exercise on vitamin B6 metabolism and growth hormone. FASEB Journal 1993;7:A727.

Fishbaine B, Butterfield G. Ascorbic acid status of running and sedentary men. Int J Vit Nutr Res 1984;54:273.

Fogelholm M. Micronutrient status in females during a 24-week fitness-type exercise program. Ann Nutr Metab 1992;36:209–18.

Fogelholm M. Indicators of vitamin and mineral status in athletes' blood: a review. Int J Sport Nutr 1995;5:267–86.

Fogelholm M, Himberg J-J, Alopaeus K, et al. Dietary and biochemical indices of nutritional status in male athletes and controls. J Am Coll Nutr 1992a;11:181–91.

Fogelholm GM, Koskinen R, Laakso J, Rankinen T, Ruokonen I. Gradual and rapid weight loss: effects on nutrition and performance in male athletes. Med Sci Sports Exerc 1993a;25:371–7.

Fogelholm M, Laakso J, Lehto J, Ruokonen I. Dietary intake and indicators of magnesium and zinc status in male athletes. Nutr Res 1991;11:1111–18.

Fogelholm M, Lahtinen P. Nutritional evaluation of a sailing crew during a transatlantic race. Scand J Med Sci Sports 1991;1:99–103.

Fogelholm M, Rehunen S, Gref CG, et al. Dietary intake and thiamin, iron and zinc status in elite Nordic skiers during different training periods. Int J Sport Nutr 1992b;2:351–65.

Fogelholm M, Ruokonen I, Laakso J, VuorimaaT, Himberg J-J. Lack of association between indices of vitamin B1, B2, and B6 status and exercise-induced blood lactate in young adults. Int J Sport Nutr 1993b;3:165–76.

Gerster H. The role of vitamin C in athletic performance. J Am Coll Nutr 1989;8:636–43.

Guilland J-C, Penaranda T, Gallet C, et al. Vitamin status of young athletes including the effects of supplementation. Med Sci Sports Exerc 1989;21:441–4.

Gutteridge JMC, Rowley DA, Halliwell B, Cooper DF, Heeley DM. Copper and iron complexes catalytic for oxygen radical reactions in sweat from human athletes. Clin Chem Acta 1985;145:267–74.

Haralambie G. Vitamin B2 status in athletes and the influence of riboflavin administration on neuromuscular irritability. Nutr Metab 1976;20:1–8.

Hasten DL, Rome EP, Franks BD, Hegstedt M. Effects of chromium picolinate on beginning weight training students. Int J Sport Nutr 1992;2:343–50.

Hemilä H. Vitamin C and common cold incidence: a review of studies with subjects under heavy physical stress. Int J Sports Med 1995;17:379–83.

Jacob RA. Assessment of human vitamin C status. J Nutr 1990;120:1480–5.

Jacob RA, Burri BJ. Oxidative damage and defence. Am J Clin Nutr 1996;63:S985–S90.

Johnston CS, Swan PD, Corte C. Substrate utilization and work efficiency during submaximal exercise in vitamin C depleted-repleted adults. Int J Vitam Nutr Res 1999;69:41–4.

Kaikkonen J, Kosonen L, Nyyssönen K, et al. Effect of combined coenzyme Q10 and d-alpha-tocopheryl acetate supplementation on exercise-induced lipid peroxidation and muscular damage: a placebo-controlled double-blind study in marathon runners. Free Radic Res 1998;29:85–92.

Kanter MM, Williams MH. Antioxidants, carnitine, and choline as putative ergogenic aids. Int J Sport Nutr 1995;5:S120–S31.

Karlsson J, Diamant B, Edlund PO, et al. Plasma ubiquinone, alpha-tocopherol and cholesterol in man. Int J Vit Nutr Res 1992;62:160–4.

Keith RE, Alt LA. Riboflavin status of female athletes consuming normal diets. Nutr Res 1991;11:727–34.

Kitamura Y, Tanaka K, Kiyohara C, et al. Relationship of alcohol use, physical activity and dietary habits with serum carotenoids, retinol and alpha-tocopherol among male Japanese smokers. Int J Epidemiol 1997;26:307–14.

Laaksonen R, Fogelholm M, Himberg JJ, Laakso J, Salorinne Y. Ubiquinone supplementation and exercise capacity in trained young and older men. Eur J Appl Physiol 1995;72:95–100.

Leaf DA, Kleinman MT, Hamilton M, Barstow TJ. The effect of exercise intensity on lipid peroxidation. Med Sci Sports Exerc 1997;29:1036–9.

Lichton IJ, Miyamura JB, McNutt SW. Nutritional evaluation of soldiers subsisting on meal, ready-to-eat operational rations for an extended period: body measurements, hydration, and blood nutrients. Am J Clin Nutr 1988;48:30–7.

Lovlin R, Cottle W, Pyke I, Kavanagh M, Belcastro AN. Are indices of free radical damage related to exercise intensity? Eur J Appl Physiol 1987;56:313–16.

Lukaski HC, Bolonchuk WW, Siders WA, Milne DB. Chromium supplementation and resistance training: effects on body composition, strength, and trace element status of men. Am J Clin Nutr 1996;63:954–65.

Lukaski HC, Hoverson BS, Gallagher SK, Bolonchuk WW. Physical training and copper, iron, and zinc status of swimmers. Am J Clin Nutr 1990;51:1093–9.

Machlin LJ. Use and safety of elevated dosages of vitamin E in adults. In: Walter P, Stähelin H, Brubacher G, eds. Elevated dosages of vitamins. Stuttgart: Hans Huber Publishers, 1989:56–68.

Manore M. Vitamin B6 and exercise. Int J Sport Nutr 1994;4:89–103.

Manore M, Leklem JE. Effects of carbohydrate and vitamin B6 on fuel substrates during exercise in women. Med Sci Sports Exerc 1988;20:233–41.

Margaritis I, Tessier F, Richard M-J, Marconnet P. No evidence of oxidative stress after a triathlon race in highly trained competitors. Int J Sports Med 1997;18:186–90.

Marks J. The safety of the vitamins: an overview. In: Walter P, Stähelin H, Brubacher G, eds. Elevated dosages of vitamins. Stuttgart: Hans Huber Publishers, 1989:12–20.

Matter M, Stittfall T, Graves J, et al. The effect of iron and folate therapy on maximal exercise performance in female marathon runners with iron and folate deficiency. Clin Sci 1987;72:415–22.

McBride JF, Kraemer WJ, Triplett-McBride T, Sebastianelli W. Effect of resistance exercise on free radical production. Med Sci Sports Exerc 1998;30:67–72.

Mena P, Maynar M, Gutierrez JM, et al. Erythrocyte free radical scavenger enzymes in bicycle professional racers: adaptation to training. Int J Sports Med 1991;12:563–6.

Meydani M, Evans WJ, Handelman G, et al. Protective effect of vitamin E on exercise-induced oxidative damage in young and older adults. Am J Physiol 1993;25:218–24.

Miyamura JB, McNutt SW, Lichton IJ, Wenkam NS. Altered zinc status of soldiers under field conditions. J Am Diet Assoc 1987;87:595–7.

Moretti C, Fabbri A, Gnessi L, et al. Pyridoxine (B6) suppresses the rise in prolactin and increases the rise in growth hormone induced by exercise. N Engl J Med 1982;307:444–5.

National Health & Medical Research Council. Recommended Dietary Intakes for use in Australia. Canberra: Australian Government Publishing Service, 1991.

National Research Council. Recommended Dietary Allowances. Washington, DC: National Academy Press, 1989.

Nieman DC, Pedersen BK. Exercise and immune function: recent developments. Sports Med 1999;27:73–80.

Nuviala RJ, Lapieza MG, Bernal E. Magnesium, zinc, and copper status in women involved in different sports. Int J Sport Nutr 1999;9:295–309.

O'Dell BL. Bioavailability of and interactions among trace elements. In: Chandra RK, ed. Trace elements in nutrition of children. New York: Nestlé Nutrition Vevey/Raven Press, 1985:41–59.

Ohno H, Sato Y, Ishikawa M, et al. Training effects on blood zinc levels in humans. J Sports Med Phys Fitness 1990;30:247–53.

Payette H, Gray-Donald K. Dietary intake and biochemical indices of nutritional status in an elderly population, with estimates of the precision of the 7-d food record. Am J Clin Nutr 1991;54:478–88.

Reynolds RD. Vitamin supplements: current controversies. J Am Coll Nutr 1994;13:118–26.

Rivers JM. Safety of high-level vitamin C ingestion. In: Walter P, Stähelin H, Brubacher G, eds. Elevated dosages of vitamins. Stuttgart: Hans Huber Publishers, 1989:95–102.

Rokitzki L, Hinkel S, Klemp C, Cufi D, Keul J. Dietary, serum and urine ascorbic acid status in male athletes. Int J Sports Med 1994a;5:435–40.

Rokitzki L, Logemann E, Huber G, Keck E, Keul J. α-Tocopherol supplementation in racing cyclists during extreme endurance training. Int J Sports Nutr 1994b;4:253–64.

Ronsen O, Sundgot-Borgen J, Maehlum S. Supplement use and nutritional habits in Norwegian elite athletes. Scand J Med Sci Sports 1999;9:28–35.

Sauberlich HE. Biochemical alterations in thiamin deficiency—their interpretation. Am J Clin Nutr 1967;20:528–42.

Sauberlich HE, Herman YF, Stevens CO, Herman RH. Thiamin requirement of the adult human. Am J Clin Nutr 1979;32:2237–48.

Sen CK. Oxidants and antioxidants in exercise. J Appl Physiol 1995;79:675–86.

Simon-Schnass I, Pabst H. Influence of vitamin E on physical performance. Int J Vit Nutr Res 1988;58:49–54.

Singh A, Deuster PA, Day BA, Moser-Veillon PB. Dietary intakes and biochemical markers of selected minerals: comparison of highly trained runners and untrained women. J Am Coll Nutr 1990a;9:65–75.

Singh A, Deuster PA, Moser PB. Zinc and copper status of women by physical activity and menstrual status. J Sports Med Phys Fitness 1990b;30:29–36.

Singh A, Moses FM, Deuster PA. Chronic multivitamin-mineral supplementation does not enhance physical performance. Med Sci Sports Exerc 1992a;24:726–32.

Singh A, Moses FM, Deuster PA. Vitamin and mineral status in physically active men: effects of high-potency supplement. Am J Clin Nutr 1992b;55:1–7.

Sjödin B, Hellsten Westing Y, Apple FS. Biochemical mechanisms for oxygen free radical formation during exercise. Sports Med 1990;10:236–54.

Soares MJ, Satyanarayana K, Bamji MS, et al. The effects of exercise on the riboflavin status of adult men. Br J Nutr 1993;69:541–51.

Sobal J, Marquart LF. Vitamin/mineral supplement use among athletes: a review of the literature. Int J Sport Nutr 1994;4:320–34.

Solomons NW, Allen LH. The functional assessment of nutritional status: principles, practise and potential. Nutr Rev 1983;41:33–50.

Sumida S, Tanaka K, Kitao H, Nakadomo F. Exercise-induced lipid peroxidation and leakage of enzymes before and after vitamin E supplementation. Int J Biochem 1989;21:835–8.

Takatsuka N, Kawakami N, Ohwaki A, et al. Frequent hard physical activity lowered serum beta-carotene level in a population study of a rural city of Japan. Tohoku J Exp Med 1995;176:131–5.

Telford RD, Catchpole EA, Deakin V, Hahn AG, Plank AW. The effects of 7 to 8 months of vitamin/mineral supplementation on the vitamin and mineral status of athletes. Int J Sport Nutr 1992a;2:123–34.

Telford RD, Catchpole EA, Deakin V, Hahn AG, Plank AW. The effects of 7 to 8 months of vitamin/mineral supplementation on athletic performance. Int J Sport Nutr 1992b;2:135–53.

Terblanche S, Noakes TD, Dennis SC, Marais DW, Eckert M. Failure of magnesium supplementation to influence marathon running performance or recovery in magnesium-replete subjects. Int J Sport Nutr 1992;2:154–64.

Thomas TR, Ziogas G, Yan P, Schmitz D, LaFontaine T. Influence of activity level on vitamin E status in healthy mean and women and cardiac patients. J Cardiopulm Rehabil 1998;18:52–9.

Tiidus PM, Houston ME. Vitamin E status and response to exercise training. Sports Med 1995;20:12–23.

Tiidus PM, Pushkarenko J, Houston ME. Lack of antioxidant adaptation to short-term aerobic training in human muscle. Am J Physiol 1996;271:R832–R6.

Trebler Winters LR, Yoon J-S, Kalkwarf HJ, et al. Riboflavin requirements and exercise adaptation in older women. Am J Clin Nutr 1992;56:526–32.

Trent LK, Thieding-Cancel D. Effects of chromium picolinate on body composition. J Sports Med Phys Fitness 1995;35:273–80.

van Dam B. Vitamins and sport. Br J Sports Med 1978;12:74–9.

van der Beek EJ. Vitamin supplementation and physical exercise performance. J Sports Sci 1991;9:77–89.

van der Beek EJ, van Dokkum W, Schrijver J, et al. Thiamin, riboflavin, and vitamins B6 and C: impact of combined restricted intake on functional performance in man. Am J Clin Nutr 1988;48:1451–62.

van der Beek EJ, van Dokkum W, Schriver J, et al. Controlled vitamin C restriction and physical performance in volunteers. J Am Coll Nutr 1990;9:332–9.

Van Loan MD, Sutherland B, Lowe NM, Turnlund JR, King JC. The effects of zinc depletion on peak force and total work of knee and shoulder extensor and flexor muscles. Int J Sport Nutr 1999;9:125–35.

Verde T, Shephard RJ, Corey P, Moore R. Sweat composition in exercise and in heat. J Appl Physiol 1982;53:1540–5.

Virk RS, Dunton NJ, Young JC, Leklem JE. Effect of vitamin B6 supplementation on fuels, catecholamines, and amino acids during exercise in men. Med Sci Sports Exerc 1999;31:400–8.

Walker LS, Bemben MG, Bemben DA, Knehans AW. Chromium picolinate effects on body composition and muscular performance in wrestlers. Med Sci Sports Exerc 1998;30:1730–7.

Weber GF. The measurement of oxygen-derived free radicals and related substances in medicine. J Clin Chem Clin Biochem 1990;28:569–603.

Webster MJ. Physiological and performance responses to supplementation with thiamin and pantothenic acid derivatives. Eur J Appl Physiol 1998;77:486–91.

Weight LM, Myburgh KH, Noakes TD. Vitamin and mineral supplementation: effect on the running performance of trained athletes. Am J Clin Nutr 1988a;47:192–5.

Weight LM, Noakes TD, Labadarios D, et al. Vitamin and mineral status of trained athletes including the effects of supplementation. Am J Clin Nutr 1988b;47:186–91.

Weller E, Bachert P, Meinck H-M, et al. Lack of effect of oral Mg-supplementation on MG in serum, blood cells, and calf muscle. Med Sci Sports Exerc 1998;30:1584–91.

Wenk C, Steiner G, Kunz P. Evaluation of the losses of water and minerals: description of the method with the example of a 10 000 m race. Int J Vit Nutr Res 1989;59:425.

Wood B, Gijsbers A, Goode A, Davis S, Mulholland J, Breen K. A study of partial thiamin restriction in human volunteers. Am J Clin Nutr 1980;33:848–61.

Zorbas YG, Charapakin KP, Kakurin VJ. Daily copper supplement effects on copper balance in trained subjects during prolonged restriction of muscular activity. Biol Trace Elem Res 1999;69:81–98.

Preparation for competition

Louise Burke

INTRODUCTION

An athlete's goals during competition are to perform to their optimum level. A range of factors can impair performance, including issues related to nutrition. Competition eating is based on the principle of implementing nutritional strategies that can reduce or delay the onset of factors that cause fatigue or performance impairment. Of course, practical issues must also be considered, particularly in light of the frequency with which athletes are required to travel interstate or overseas to compete in their target events. Competition nutrition includes special eating strategies undertaken before, during and in the recovery from the event. In this chapter we will review the strategies undertaken in the hours or days prior to competition, to prepare the athlete to perform at their best.

NUTRITIONAL FACTORS CAUSING FATIGUE DURING PERFORMANCE

A variety of nutritional factors can reduce an athlete's ability to perform at their best during exercise (see Table 13.1). The risk and severity of an encounter during competition depends on issues including:

- the duration and intensity of the exercise involved;
- the environmental conditions—for example, temperature and humidity;
- the training status of the athlete;
- individual characteristics of the athlete; and
- the success of nutritional strategies before and during the event.

It is relatively easy to investigate the physiological factors limiting the performance of simple exercise tasks (e.g. running or cycling) undertaken in an exercise physiology laboratory. Furthermore, factors identified in laboratory simulations of

Table 13.1 *Nutritional factors associated with fatigue or a decline in performance*

Depletion of glycogen stores in the active muscle
Hypoglycaemia
Other mechanisms of 'central fatigue' involving neurotransmitters
Dehydration
Hyponatraemia
Gastrointestinal discomfort and upset

simple competitive events such as these, may well apply to the real-life performances of athletes. However, it is more complicated to measure or predict factors limiting the performance of complex sporting events, particularly ball games and racquet sports in which competition demands have a high degree of inter- and intra-athlete variability. Sports scientists try to pinpoint the likely risk that various factors will cause fatigue in a given sport or event, based on the available applied sports research, as well as accounts of past competition experiences of the athletes involved. With this knowledge, athletes can then be guided to undertake specific competition nutrition strategies that will minimise or delay the onset of these problems.

13.2.1 *Setting a competition nutrition plan to combat factors causing fatigue*

Competition nutrition strategies should target the specific physiological challenges that affect the performance of the athlete's sport. According to the characteristics of the event, strategies might aim to minimise fluid deficits, ensure fuel availability or prevent gastrointestinal discomfort. Ideally, an athlete should combat these challenges by undertaking a combination of nutrition strategies before, during and even in the recovery period of an event. Although further systematic studies are needed to investigate the benefits of combining two or more strategies, it is logical that a multi-tasked approach would be superior to a single strategy. For example, it appears that the combination of carbohydrate (CHO) intake before, as well as during, an endurance event is superior to the performance benefits gained from undertaking each of these strategies in isolation (Wright et al. 1991; Burke et al. 1995; Chryssanthopoulos & Williams 1997). However, in practice, the athlete may not always be able to exploit each opportunity for a nutritional intervention. When one opportunity is missed or under-utilised, greater emphasis on tactics at another opportunity may help to compensate. For example, an athlete who has not been able to refuel muscle CHO stores before a prolonged event should place greater emphasis on consuming CHO during the event. Conversely, in events where opportunities to drink during exercise are limited and large fluid deficits occur, the athlete should pay extra attention to hydration before the event starts, and perhaps even experiment with hyperhydration (fluid overload). In any case, the athlete should set a complete plan for competition eating, using nutritional strategies that complement and enhance each other.

Pre-competition nutrition strategies include dietary interventions that are implemented during the week prior to an event, as well as special tactics that are undertaken in the minutes or hours before the event begins. An athlete's plan must balance the physiological challenges that are likely to be experienced during the event, with the practicality of undertaking preventative action via nutritional interventions. For example, an athlete undertaking an event involving prolonged moderate or intermittent high-intensity activity may identify that pre-event fuelling-up may help to delay the onset of the fatigue that would be expected with the depletion of muscle glycogen stores. Studies show that it may require 72 hours of exercise taper and high CHO intake to maximise muscle glycogen stores (i.e. to CHO load) in preparation for such an endurance event (Costill et al. 1981; Sherman et al. 1981). This pre-event activity is justifiable and compatible with the training program of an athlete who competes in one or two important events each year. However, if the event is just one of a series of closely held competitions, for example, part of a weekly race schedule or team game fixture, a complete CHO loading preparation would be deemed impractical and overstated. Athletes who compete frequently in endurance events often choose to undertake an abridged dietary preparation before less important events, or between events that are sandwiched in a tournament or weekly competition schedule. Meanwhile, the full preparation of CHO loading is saved for single events or the most important competitions. In the world of competitive sport, 'optimal' must make way for 'most practical' on many occasions.

13.3 *PRE-EVENT FUELLING*

The depletion of body CHO stores is a major cause of fatigue during exercise (see Chapter 2 for review). Optimising CHO status in the muscle and liver is a primary goal of competition preparation. The key ingredients for glycogen storage are dietary CHO intake and, in the case of muscle stores, tapered exercise or rest (for review see Friedman et al. 1991; Ivy 1991; Robergs 1991). The duration of pre-event fuelling will depend on the balance between the anticipated fuel needs of the event and the preparation time that can be devoted to the event.

13.3.1 *Muscle glycogen storage*

Since the 1960s, when the biopsy technique was first used to measure exercise metabolism, sports scientists have been able to directly measure the glycogen content in isolated muscle samples, and thus determine the factors that enhance or impair storage. More recently, indirect techniques of muscle glycogen measurement involving nuclear magnetic resonance spectroscopy (Roden & Shulman 1999) have increased the practical opportunities to study such factors.

Studies of glycogen synthesis describe a biphasic response, consisting of a rapid early phase for the first 24 hours (non-insulin-dependent) followed by a slow phase (insulin-dependent) lasting several days (Piehl 1974; Ivy & Kuo 1998). Early studies proposed that activity of the glycogen synthase enzyme plays a key role in determining the rates of glycogen synthesis (GS) in the muscle (Danforth 1965) although this relationship does not totally explain all observations of glycogen synthesis. For example, differences in post-exercise glycogen storage have been found in the absence of differences in GS activity (Ivy et al. 1988; Griewe et al. 1999), and the increased GS activity observed immediately after glycogen-depleting exercise returns to normal in advance of the glycogen supercompensation that can be observed in trained muscle exposed to several days of high CHO intake (see Ivy & Kuo 1998). Insulin- or exercise-stimulated translocation of GLUT-4 protein transporter to the muscle membrane increases muscle glucose uptake and is also a determinant of glycogen resynthesis (McCoy et al. 1996). Factors affecting post-exercise resynthesis of glycogen exercise will be discussed in greater detail in Chapter 15.

Recently, investigators have reported that there are two separate glycogen pools within muscle. This adds a new dimension to our understanding of glycogen synthesis and utilisation. Research has identified a primer for glycogen synthesis, the protein glycogenin, which acts both as the core of the glycogen molecule and the enzyme stimulating self-glycosylation (Alonso et al. 1995). The initial accumulation of glucose units to glycogenin forms a glycogen type now known as proglycogen, which is of relatively smaller size. The storage of proglycogen is most prominent during the first phase of recovery and is sensitive to the provision of dietary CHO (Adamo et al. 1998). During the second phase of glycogen recovery, glycogen storage occurs mainly in the pool of macroglycogen: a glycogen molecule with greater amounts of glucose for each glycogenin core. It is an increase in the macroglycogen pool that appears to account for glycogen supercompensation in the muscle following two to three days of high CHO intake (Adamo et al. 1998).

Research indicates that the pools of proglycogen and macroglycogen are metabolically distinct. It is speculated that proglycogen is the small and dynamic intermediate form of glycogen, whereas macroglycogen is the larger storage form that increases on a relative basis as total glycogen increases (Adamo & Graham 1998). Adamo and Graham suggest that when the proglycogen pool has reached a critical limit in a favourable CHO environment, a portion is then synthesised into macroglycogen. Conversely, a study of a marathon race has shown that the pools of glycogen are utilised at separate rates (Asp et al. 1999). Future studies may allow us to exploit this information, and determine new factors and strategies that enhance the metabolic availability of glycogen pools or increase storage.

13.3.2 *Fuelling-up for non-endurance events*

In the absence of muscle damage, muscle glycogen stores can be normalised by 24 hours of rest and an adequate CHO intake (7–10 g/kg body mass (BM) per day)

(Costill et al. 1981; Burke et al. 1995). Such stores appear adequate for the muscle fuel needs of events of less than 60–90 minutes in duration; at least, CHO loading to achieve supercompensated glycogen levels does not enhance the performance of these events (for review, see Hawley et al. 1997a).

Typically, the resting values for muscle glycogen in trained muscle is 100–120 mmol/kg wet weight (ww). Allowing for a typical rate of glycogen synthesis at ~5 mmol/kg ww/h, the athlete should set aside 24–36 hours, following their last training session, to normalise fuel stores prior to non-endurance events. For many athletes this might be as simple as scheduling a day of rest or light training before the event, while continuing to follow high-CHO eating patterns. However, not all athletes eat sufficient CHO in their typical or everyday diets to maximise glycogen storage, particularly females who restrict their total energy intake to control body-fat levels (Burke 1995). These athletes may need education or encouragement to temporarily remove their energy restriction and prioritise refuelling as the dietary goal on the day before competition. Similarly, some athletes may need to reorganise their training programs to allow a lighter training day or rest on the day prior to their event. At minimum, the athlete should avoid training sessions that cause significant muscle damage on the day before competition since such damage interferes with glycogen storage (O'Reilly et al. 1987; Costill et al. 1990).

13.3.3 *CHO loading for endurance events*

The term 'CHO loading' is used to describe anything from fuelling-up for an endurance event, to rationalising a food binge of great quantity and dubious quality. Strictly speaking, CHO loading should refer to practices that aim to maximise or supercompensate muscle glycogen stores prior to a competitive event that would otherwise deplete these fuel reserves. CHO-loading protocols may elevate muscle glycogen stores to ~150–250 mmol/kg ww. This will be an important strategy for events lasting more than 90 minutes, which would otherwise be limited by the depletion of muscle glycogen stores (for review, see Hawley et al. 1997a).

CHO-loading protocols were an outcome of the first studies undertaken in the late 1960s by Scandinavian sports scientists using muscle biopsy techniques. In a series of studies (Bergstrom & Hultman 1966; Ahlborg et al. 1967; Bergstrom et al. 1967; Hermanssen et al. 1967), these researchers found that endurance, or capacity for prolonged moderate-intensity exercise, was determined by pre-exercise muscle glycogen stores. Several days of a low-CHO diet depleted muscle glycogen stores and reduced cycling endurance compared with a normal CHO diet. However, the subsequent high CHO intake over several days caused a supercompensation of glycogen stores and prolonged the cycling time to exhaustion. A clever research design involving one-legged cycling showed that glycogen supercompensation was localised to the muscle that had been previously depleted, and studies identified the activity of glycogen synthase enzyme as an important factor in glycogen synthesis. These pioneering studies produced the classical seven-day model of CHO loading, involving a three to four day depletion phase of hard training and low CHO intake, and finishing with a three to four day loading phase of high CHO eating and exercise taper. Early field studies of prolonged running events showed that CHO loading might enhance sports performance, not by allowing the athlete to run faster, but by prolonging the time that race pace could be maintained (Karlsson & Saltin 1971).

Studies extended to trained subjects produced a modified CHO-loading strategy. Sherman and colleagues showed that well-trained athletes were able to supercompensate muscle glycogen stores without a depletion or glycogen-stripping phase (Sherman et al. 1981). The runners in this study elevated their muscle glycogen stores with three days of taper and high CHO intake, regardless of whether this was preceded by a depletion phase or a more typical diet and training preparation. For well-trained athletes at least, CHO loading may be seen as an extension of fuelling-up (rest and high CHO intake) over three to four days. The modified CHO-loading protocol offers a more practical strategy for competition preparation by avoiding the fatigue and complexity of extreme diet and training requirements associated with the previous depletion phase. However, although CHO loading is so well known that it has entered everyday language, even in its simplified form it seems difficult for athletes to master. At least one study has shown that in real life, athletes may not have the knowledge to plan a suitable exercise taper; furthermore they fail to reach the daily CHO intake targets of 7–10 g/kg BM needed to maximise glycogen storage (Burke & Read 1987).

13.3.3.1 *Gender and CHO loading*

Most studies of glycogen storage have been conducted with male subjects, with the assumption that the results also apply to female athletes. However, one study has reported that female athletes were less responsive to a CHO-loading protocol (i.e. failed to supercompensate muscle glycogen stores compared to male subjects) and failed to show a performance benefit following this dietary strategy (Tarnopolsky et al. 1995). It is difficult to undertake gender comparison studies due to problems in matching males and females for important parameters such as aerobic capacity (relative versus absolute values). Furthermore, CHO-loading studies such as the one undertaken by Tarnopolsky and colleagues have been criticised for the failure to control for, or the selection of a particular phase of, the menstrual cycle, or for the intake of smaller amounts of dietary CHO as a result of restricted energy intake by females. Although females may increase CHO intake to achieve a similar relative energy contribution, total CHO intake will be restricted if total energy intake is low. Without a substantial increase in the intake of substrate, a female athlete could not expect to increase muscle fuel stores nor gain the potential performance enhancement arising from increased fuel availability.

Gender differences in substrate utilisation and storage are still being investigated and explained (for review, see Tarnopolsky 1999). There is some evidence that the menstrual status of female athletes affects glycogen storage, with greater storage occurring during the luteal phase rather than the follicular phase (Nicklas et al. 1989; Hackney 1990). With this in mind, a CHO-loading study was recently undertaken with well-trained female athletes who were in the luteal phase of their menstrual cycle (Walker et al. in press). A modified loading protocol was utilised with the focus on an exercise taper and increased CHO intake over the final four days. This program achieved a 13% increase in muscle glycogen stores compared with storage on a moderate CHO intake, and increased time to exhaustion during sub-maximal cycling. This study showed that when sufficient CHO is consumed in a favourable hormonal environment, female athletes can increase their glycogen stores and improve exercise endurance (Walker et al. in press). However, although male subjects were not included in this study to allow a direct comparison, the researchers noted that the supercompensation achieved by the females was of a lower magnitude than commonly reported in studies of male athletes. The existence and practical significance of physiological limitations to glycogen storage in female athletes remain to be further investigated. In the meantime, it is likely that inadequate CHO intake is a common cause of sub-optimal fuel stores in athletes who are driven by body fat and BM concerns.

13.3.3.2 *CHO loading and performance of endurance events*

Theoretically, CHO loading could enhance the performance of exercise or sporting events that would otherwise be limited by glycogen depletion. An increase in pre-event glycogen stores can prolong the duration for which moderate-intensity exercise can be undertaken before fatiguing. It may also enhance the performance of a set amount of work (i.e. a set distance) by preventing the decline in pace or work output that would otherwise occur as glycogen stores decline towards the end of the task. In a recent review of CHO loading studies, Hawley et al. (1997a) summarised that supercompensation of glycogen stores is beneficial for the performance of exercise of greater than 90 minutes' duration, with the majority of studies investigating exercise protocols involving cycling or running. Typically, CHO loading will postpone fatigue and extend the duration of steady-state exercise by ~20%, and improve performance over a set distance or workload by 2–3% (Hawley et al. 1997a). Such an intervention would provide a substantial improvement in most simple endurance events such as marathons, prolonged cycling and triathlon races and cross-country skiing events. The literature typically shows that shorter events of 45–90 minute duration do not show significant performance benefits from CHO loading (Sherman et al. 1981; Hawley et al. 1997b).

Of course, many athletes undertake prolonged events of a less predictable nature—for example, tennis matches or football games that extend for at least 60–90 minutes of playing time. The interaction of prolonged duration and intermittent high-intensity exercise, which is associated with an increased rate of glycogen utilisation, might be expected to result in muscle glycogen depletion during the event. While it is intuitive that performance in such sports would be enhanced by supercompensation of muscle glycogen stores, it is extremely difficult to undertake studies that measure the performance of complex and variable sports such as these. Whereas some studies have shown that pre-event enhancement of fuel stores is of benefit to the performance of the movement patterns in a soccer-simulated trial (Bangsbo et al. 1992), an indoor soccer game (Balsom et al. 1999), and a real-life ice hockey game (Akermark et al. 1996), other studies have failed to show significant improvement in the performance of skill-based tasks in a simulation of a soccer match (Abt et al. 1998). Decisions about the benefits of CHO loading may be specific not only to the sport, but to the individual athlete, depending on the requirements of their position or style of play. Of course, the logistics of competition in many of these sports, where games may be played daily to twice a week, would prevent a full CHO-loading preparation before each event. Nevertheless, athletes in these sports should fuel up prior to each competition as well as is practical, and perhaps experiment with an extended preparation before the most important games, such as the final of the tournament.

It is of note that the majority of studies of CHO loading have failed to employ a placebo in their design: most studies have used a cross-over design in which subjects are fed a high-CHO preparation on one occasion, and a low-moderate CHO diet as a control. Since the benefits of CHO loading are well-known, it might be argued that the responses to the high-CHO preparation will be psychologically as well as physiologically driven. Indeed, it is interesting to note that the two studies that have employed a placebo design, masking the true diets, failed to find benefits from CHO loading (Hawley et al. 1997b; Burke et al. 2000). Although this probably reflects that the exercise and dietary protocols used in the studies are such that moderately enhanced glycogen stores do not provide additional benefits, it may also be a result of the removal of the placebo effect.

Finally, the interaction of various dietary strategies with CHO loading deserves systematic research. There is evidence that the benefits from supercompensation of glycogen stores persist, or are additive to the effects of consuming CHO during a prolonged exercise task (Widrick et al. 1993; Rauch et al. 1995). Such studies need to be conducted over a greater range of exercise events.

13.4 *THE PRE-EVENT MEAL (1–4 HOURS PRE-EVENT)*

Foods and drinks consumed in the four hours prior to exercise have a role in fine-tuning competition preparation. The pre-event menu can be eaten largely for comfort or confidence, or it may play an active role in preparation by contributing to refuelling and rehydrating goals. There has been much undeserved publicity about the negative effects of eating CHO-rich foods in the hour before exercise, an issue that will be discussed separately (in Section 13.4.1).

The goals of the pre-event meal are to (Hawley & Burke 1998):

- continue to fuel muscle glycogen stores if they have not fully restored or loaded since the last exercise session;
- restore liver glycogen content, especially for events undertaken in the morning where liver stores are depleted from an overnight fast;
- ensure that the athlete is well hydrated;
- prevent hunger, yet avoid the gastrointestinal discomfort and upset often experienced during exercise; and
- include foods and practices that are important to the athlete's psychology or superstitions.

The pre-event meal menu should include CHO-rich foods and drinks, especially in the case where body CHO stores are sub-optimal, or where the event is of the duration and intensity to challenge these stores. A CHO-rich meal consumed four hours before exercise significantly increases the glycogen content of muscle and liver which have been depleted by previous exercise or an overnight fast (Coyle et al. 1985). Compared to results achieved after an overnight fast, the intake of a substantial amount of CHO (~200–300 g) in the two to four hours before exercise has been shown to prolong cycling endurance (Wright et al. 1991) and enhance performance of an exercise test undertaken at the end of a standardised cycling task (Neufer et al. 1987; Sherman et al. 1989). CHO availability is enhanced by increasing muscle and liver glycogen stores, as well as by the storage of glucose in the gastrointestinal space for later release. Since liver glycogen stores are labile and may be substantially depleted by an overnight fast, pre-exercise CHO intake on the morning of an event may be important for maintaining blood glucose levels via hepatic glucose output during the latter stages of prolonged exercise.

Despite these benefits, the issue of CHO intake prior to exercise is not straightforward. In fact, the elevation of plasma insulin concentrations following pre-exercise CHO feedings could be a potential disadvantage to exercise metabolism and performance. A rise in insulin suppresses lipolysis and fat utilisation, concomitantly accelerating CHO oxidation and causing a decline in plasma glucose concentrations at the onset of exercise. These metabolic alterations have been observed even when CHO was consumed four hours before exercise, and persisted despite the normalisation of plasma glucose and insulin concentrations at the onset of exercise (Coyle et al. 1985). However, such metabolic perturbations do not appear detrimental to performance. One safeguard is to ensure that the amount of CHO in the pre-event meal is substantial rather than minor; thus, any increase in CHO utilisation during exercise will be more than offset by the large increase in CHO availability.

In the field it is not always practical to consume a substantial CHO-rich meal or snack in the four hours before a sporting event. For example, it is unlikely that an athlete will want to sacrifice sleep to eat heartily before an early morning race start.

Most will settle for a lighter meal or snack before the event, and consume CHO throughout the event to balance missed fuelling opportunities. A smaller pre-event meal may also make sense for events or athletes predisposed to gastrointestinal discomfort. Foods with a low-fat, low-fibre and low-moderate protein content are the preferred choice for the pre-event menu since they are less prone to cause gastrointestinal upsets (Rehrer et al. 1992). Liquid meal supplements or CHO-containing drinks and bars are useful for athletes who suffer from pre-event nerves or an uncertain pre-event timetable. Above all, the individual athlete should choose a strategy that suits their situation and their past experiences, and can be fine-tuned with further experimentation.

13.4.1 *CHO consumed in the hour before exercise*

In 1979, a study published by Foster et al. created panic and confusion among athletes and sports scientists (Foster et al. 1979). The study found, compared to exercise in the fasted state, feeding 75 g of glucose 30 minutes prior to exercise impaired cycle time to exhaustion at 80% of $VO_{2\ max}$. The pre-event feeding did not alter the length of time subjects were able to ride during more intense (100% of $VO_{2\ max}$) exercise. The investigators observed a rapid drop in blood glucose concentration during the first ten minutes of exercise after subjects had been fed CHO, but noted that this response was transient and was not associated with fatigue. Although muscle glycogen content was not determined, the reduction in endurance following CHO feeding was attributed to an accelerated muscle glycogenolysis (Foster et al. 1979).

Unfortunately the results of this study have been so widely reported and publicised that warnings to avoid CHO intake during the hour prior to endurance exercise have become part of sports nutrition dogma (Inge & Brukner 1986, p. 94–5; Wilmore & Costill 1994, p. 353). However, reviews of the literature reveal that this is the only study to find a reduction in performance capacity after the ingestion of CHO in the hour before exercise (Coyle 1991; Hawley & Burke 1995). These reviews summarise that the findings of other investigations of pre-exercise CHO feeding range from no detrimental effect to improvements in performance in the order of 7–20% (Coyle 1991; Hawley & Burke 1995). In most cases, the decline in blood glucose observed during the first 20 minutes of exercise is self-corrected with no apparent effects on the athlete.

Nevertheless, there seems to be a small percentage of athletes who respond negatively to CHO feedings in the hour before exercise. These athletes experience an exaggerated CHO oxidation and decrease in blood glucose concentrations at the start of exercise, suffering a rapid onset of fatigue and symptoms of hypoglycaemia. Why some athletes experience such an extreme reaction is not known. One study has suggested that risk factors include the intake of small amounts of CHO (< 50 g), increased sensitivity to insulin, a lower sympathetic-induced counter-regulation, and exercise intensity of low-moderate workload (Kuipers et al. 1999). Not all athletes who experience a major decline in blood glucose concentrations experience hypoglycaemic symptoms; there is preliminary evidence that sensitisation to low glucose levels may adapt the athlete to an increased threshold before symptoms are reported (Kuipers et al. 1999). Nevertheless, these effects are so clear-cut that at-risk athletes will be easily identified. Preventative action for this group includes a number of options:

- experiment to find the critical time before exercise that CHO intake should be avoided;
- consume a substantial amount of CHO in the pre-event snack and/or meal (> 70 g);
- choose low glycaemic index (GI) CHO-rich intakes (which have an attenuated and sustained blood glucose and insulin response) in the pre-event menu;
- include some high-intensity sprints during the warm-up to the event to stimulate hepatic glucose output; and
- consume CHO during the event.

13.4.2 *Pre-exercise CHO and the glycaemic index*

CHO-rich foods and drinks do not produce identical blood glucose and insulin responses; neither do they respond according to the dogma that simple CHO types produce rapid and short-lived rises in blood glucose concentrations while complex CHO-rich foods produce a flatter and sustained blood glucose rise. The GI offers a means to measure and utilise the individual blood glucose profiles achieved by consuming various CHO-rich foods and drinks. The GI provides a ranking of CHO foods based on the measured post-prandial blood glucose response compared to that of a reference food, either glucose or white bread. It has been shown to provide a reliable and consistent measure of relative blood glucose response to CHO-rich foods and meals. Furthermore, GI values have been used to manipulate meals and diets to produce a desired metabolic or clinical outcome, which is useful for the treatment of diabetes, hyperlipidemias and, potentially, obesity (for review see Wolever 1990; Brand Miller 1994).

Early studies of pre-exercise CHO feedings showed different outcomes according to the type of sugar ingested. In particular, studies showed that fructose, a low-GI saccharide, could be consumed before exercise without producing the metabolic impairments seen with glucose feedings (Hargreaves et al. 1985). Thomas and co-workers (1991) were the first to suggest the potential of the GI in the arena of sports nutrition, by undertaking a manipulation of the glycaemic response to pre-exercise CHO-rich meals (Thomas et al. 1991). A meal providing one gram of CHO per kilogram BM in the form of a low-GI food (lentils), eaten one hour prior to cycling at 67% of $VO_{2\ max}$, was found to prolong time to exhaustion compared with the ingestion of an equal amount of CHO eaten in the form of a high-GI food (potatoes). These results were attributed to lower glycaemic and insulinemic responses to the low-GI trial compared with the high-GI meal, promoting more stable blood glucose levels during exercise and increased free fatty acid (FFA) concentrations. Reduced values for exercise respiratory exchange ratio (RER) were observed in the low-GI trial, indicating reduced rates of CHO oxidation. Although muscle glycogen was not measured, the authors suggested that glycogen sparing may have occurred with the low-GI CHO trial (Thomas et al. 1991).

This study revived the prejudices about the metabolic perturbations caused by CHO feedings prior to exercise, and suggested an alternative way to increase or sustain CHO availability during exercise while attenuating any harmful responses of pre-exercise CHO feedings. The concept of a sustained carbohydrate supply is supported by Guezennec and colleagues who observed a delayed oxidation of the CHO coming from low-GI pre-exercise feedings during a subsequent exercise bout, although the effect on exercise performance was not measured (Guezennec et al. 1993). The results of the Thomas study have been widely publicised and are largely responsible for the general advice that athletes should choose pre-exercise meals based on low-GI CHO-rich foods and drinks (Brand Miller et al. 1998). However, other studies have failed to find performance benefits following the intake of a low-GI pre-exercise meal. The literature pertaining to the GI of pre-exercise CHO feedings has been summarised in Table 13.2.

This literature shows that CHO meals based on low-GI foods achieve a lower post-prandial blood glucose response, and a generally attenuated decline in blood glucose concentrations at the onset of exercise. There is also general, but not complete, agreement on the degree to which these differences translate into sustained metabolic effects during longer-term exercise. A second study by Thomas and co-workers (1994) repeated the protocol in which subjects consumed one gram of CHO per kilogram BM, from meals of varying GI, 60 minutes prior to steady-state cycling. There was a correlation between the GI of the meal and the decline in blood glucose and FFA concentrations during exercise; the low-GI meals were associated with higher glucose and FFA concentrations after 90 minutes of exercise than the high-GI meals. They concluded that low-GI meals appeared to provide a sustained source of CHO throughout the exercise and later recovery. Meanwhile, others who have provided high- or low-CHO meals 45 minutes to three hours prior to the onset of steady-state cycling or running also found a greater decline in blood glucose levels with higher-GI meals, and greater CHO oxidation throughout 50–120 minutes of exercise compared with meals with lower GI (Sparks et al. 1998; DeMarco et al. 1999; Wee et al. 1999). In contrast, Febbraio and Stewart found that differences in the pre-exercise glucose and insulin responses to the high- and low-GI meals, consumed 45 minutes before steady-state cycling, disappeared shortly after the onset of exercise (Febbraio & Stewart 1996). They observed no differences in total CHO oxidation over two hours of exercise between the two CHO treatments, and similar muscle glycogen utilisation in both CHO trials and a water trial. Further investigation is needed to see whether short-term differences in glycogen

Table 13.2 Studies of GI index and pre-exercise CHO intake

Study	Subjects	Exercise protocol	CHO feedings	Enhanced performance	Findings
Thomas et al. 1991	8 trained M cyclists	Cycling to exhaustion @ 67% $VO_{2\,max}$	Water or 1 g/kg BM CHO High-GI meal (potatoes) Low-GI meal (lentils) Glucose 60 min pre-exercise	Yes (low GI vs high GI) No difference between low GI and glucose	Compared with high-GI food, low-GI food reduced blood glucose changes (rise pre-exercise and decline during exercise) Decrease in suppression of FFA also CHO sparing/sustained CHO availability suggested as explanation for increased endurance (~20%) with low GI compared with high GI Strange that no difference between low GI and glucose
Thomas et al. 1994	6 trained M cyclists	Cycling to exhaustion @ 67% $VO_{2\,max}$	1 g/kg CHO Low-GI powdered food High-GI powdered food Low-GI breakfast cereal High-GI cereal 60 min pre-exercise	No	Inverse correlation between GI and decline in blood glucose, or suppression of FFA during exercise No differences in performance times No correlation between GI and endurance
Febbraio & Stewart 1996	6 well-trained M cyclists	120 min cycling @ 70% $VO_{2\,max}$ + 15 min TT	Placebo (low joule jelly) or 1 g/kg CHO High-GI meal (potatoes) Low-GI meal (lentils) 45 min pre-exercise	No	Low-GI food reduced pre-exercise rise in blood glucose compared with high-GI food, however no differences in glucose or insulin during steady-state exercise No differences in total CHO oxidation between the two CHO treatments, and similar muscle glycogen utilisation over 120 min No differences in TT performance between 3 trials
Sparks et al. 1998	8 well-trained M cyclists	50 min cycling @ 67% $VO_{2\,max}$ + 15 min TT	Placebo (low-joule soft drink) or 1 g/kg CHO High-GI meal (potatoes) Low-GI meal (lentils) 45 min pre-exercise	No	Low-GI food reduced pre-exercise rise in blood glucose and decline during exercise compared with high-GI food Higher CHO oxidation during exercise with high-GI trial No differences in work completed in 15 min TT between trials

(continues)

(continued)

Study	Subjects	Exercise protocol	CHO feedings	Enhanced performance	Findings
Burke et al. 1998	6 well-trained M cyclists	120 min cycling @ 70% $VO_{2\,max}$ + 15 min TT	Placebo (low joule jelly) or 2 g/kg CHO Low-GI meal (pasta) High-GI meal (potatoes) 120 min pre-exercise Note: 10% CHO solution consumed during exercise to provide ~1 g/kg CHO	No	Low-GI food reduced rise in pre-exercise blood glucose compared with high-GI food CHO fed during exercise minimised all differences in glucose, insulin, FFA during exercise No difference in substrate oxidation or performance of TT between trials
DeMarco et al. 1999	10 trained cyclists	Cycling for 120 min @ 70% $VO_{2\,max}$, followed by time to exhaustion @ 100% $VO_{2\,max}$	Water or 1.5 g/kg CHO Low-GI meal High-GI meal 30 min pre-exercise	Yes	Low-GI meal maintained glucose during exercise and reduced CHO oxidation compared with high-GI meal Time to exhaustion at maximal effort prolonged by 59%
Wee et al. 1999	8 active M & F	Running to exhaustion @ 70% $VO_{2\,max}$	2 g/kg CHO Low-GI meal High-GI meal 3 hours pre-exercise	No	High-GI meal caused a decline in blood glucose at the onset of exercise Low-GI meal attenuated this response and reduced CHO oxidation during first 80 min of exercise No differences in endurance

utilisation occur during the early stages of exercise, in line with the typical time course of differences in blood glucose concentrations. However, this study suggests that any glycaemic differences at the onset of exercise are short-lived and of transient consequence to metabolism.

Perhaps the greatest conflicts in the pre-event menu debate lie with the effect on exercise performance. As summarised in Table 13.2, most studies fail to show performance benefits arising from the consumption of a low-GI pre-event meal, even when metabolism has been altered throughout the exercise. An important factor in the interpretation of these studies, as with many areas of sports nutrition research, lies in the issue of defining and measuring 'performance'. It should be noted that both studies that report a beneficial exercise outcome following the lowering of the GI of the pre-event meal have measured time to exhaustion at a fixed work rate as their interpretation of performance; however, not all studies using this protocol show performance differences resulting from differences in the pre-exercise meal. It has been observed that 'time to exhaustion' protocols have a high co-efficient of variation with respect to time (McClellan et al. 1995). In addition, they are not readily applied to the world of competitive sport where a successful performance is determined by being able to complete a set amount of work or set distance in the shortest possible time, and where the athlete is free to choose and vary their work rate. One outcome of choosing a dependent variable with a low degree of reliability is that it increases the risk of achieving a type II error (failing to detect a real change). Thus, a possible explanation for the failure of studies to find an improvement in endurance associated with improved metabolic characteristics during prolonged exercise, is that small changes are masked by the inherent variability of the exercise task.

Nevertheless, whether changes in endurance, if they exist, translate into improvements in competitive performance must also be questioned. It is important if the results of studies are to be translated into practical advice for competitive athletes that the study design and variables should be chosen to mimic the situation of sport as closely as possible. It is interesting to note that none of the studies that have used a time-trial outcome to measure performance have shown enhancements as a result of lowering the GI of the pre-event meal.

Finally, a central issue that is overlooked in the debate is the overall importance of pre-exercise feedings in determining CHO availability during prolonged exercise. In endurance exercise events a typical and effective strategy used by athletes to promote CHO availability is to ingest CHO-rich drinks or foods during the event. Yet, in the typical pre-event meal study, athletes are expected to perform prolonged exercise while consuming water or no intake at all. The final and practical message to the athlete can only be considered when the interaction of pre-exercise and during-exercise CHO intake has been studied. We feel that it is important to investigate whether the GI of pre-exercise CHO intake has any remaining impact when large amounts of CHO are consumed during the session. We tested six well-trained cyclists who ate three different pre-event meals on separate occasions before cycling for 120 minutes at 70% $VO_{2\,max}$, followed by a time trial to complete a set amount of work (Burke et al. 1998). Meals were fed two hours before exercise and consisted of two grams of CHO per kilogram BM of either high-GI food (potato) or low-GI food (pasta), or a placebo (low-energy jelly). During exercise subjects ingested a 10% solution of glucose labelled with a tracer, providing an intake of ~1 g CHO/kg/h. Despite pre-exercise differences in glucose, insulin and FFA concentrations between trials, there were no differences during exercise. Furthermore, there were no differences between any of the trials with regard to total CHO oxidation over the 120 minutes of steady-state exercise, or the oxidation of the CHO consumed from the glucose drink. There were no differences in the time to complete the performance ride. This study showed that when CHO is consumed during exercise according to sports nutrition guidelines, any effects of pre-exercise CHO intake on both metabolism and cycling performance are diminished. Further investigation is needed to support this finding.

Each athlete must judge the benefits and the practical issues associated with pre-exercise feedings in their particular situation. In cases where an athlete may not be able to consume CHO during a prolonged event or workout, they may find it useful to choose a menu based on low-GI CHO foods to promote a more sustained release of CHO throughout exercise. However, there is no evidence of universal benefits from such menu choices, particularly where the athlete is able to refuel during their session, or where their favoured and familiar food choices happen to have a high GI. In the overall scheme, pre-event eating needs to balance a number of factors including the athlete's food likes, availability of choices, and gastrointestinal comfort.

13.5 *PRE-EXERCISE HYDRATION*

Dehydration poses one of the most common nutritional problems occurring in sport. Chapter 14 details strategies to enhance fluid balance during training and competition sessions. Since on most occasions, fluid intake during exercise will be unable to match the rate of sweat loss, it is critical for the athlete to start the session well-hydrated. Special attention is needed to ensure full restoration of fluid balance after previous exercise bouts, particularly if unusually large fluid losses have become a sudden way of life, leading to chronic dehydration. Chapter 15 deals with strategies to promote rapid restoration of fluid deficits.

13.5.1 *Pre-exercise hyperhydration*

Many athletes undertake events in which significant dehydration is inevitable, and poses a challenge to both their health and their performance. Such dehydration can occur when an athlete's sweat rate is extremely high, when there is little opportunity to drink during the event, or when these factors are combined. Some athletes have experimented with hyperhydration (or fluid overloading) in the hours prior to the event to attempt to reduce the total fluid deficit incurred. This practice has been shown to increase total body water, expand plasma volume and ultimately enhance performance in a subsequent exercise trial (Moroff & Bass 1965). However, there are some shortcomings and possible disadvantages to simple fluid overloading techniques. Firstly, much of the fluid is excreted via urination. Since the body has a well-developed system to regulate the volume and concentration of its fluid content both at rest and during exercise, fluid overloading may have a detrimental effect on performance if it causes the significant interruption of having to urinate immediately before or in the early stages of the event. The discomfort of excess fluid in the gut has also been shown to impair performance of moderate-high intensity exercise (Robinson et al. 1995). On rare occasions, if taken to extreme levels and in susceptible individuals, excessive fluid intake may lead to hyponatraemia or 'water intoxication'. Clearly, fluid overloading just before an event is a strategy that needs to be researched before any firm recommendations can be made to athletes.

A recent study by Kristal-Boneh and colleagues (1995) examined the effect of chronic periods of fluid overloading. Heat-acclimatised subjects were required to double their usual fluid intake for a week, from a mean intake of 1980 mL/d to 4085 mL/d. This was found to reset normal fluid balance to retain an extra 600 mL of fluid. Several experimental trials in the heat found that superior hydration status increased heat tolerance and enhanced duration of work in the heat; increased achievement of maximal aerobic workload at a lower heart rate; and improved performance in a time trial (Kristal-Boneh et al. 1995). More work is needed to confirm these results, however, they support the advice often given to athletes competing in a hot climate, to increase their fluid intake over the days leading up to the event. Whether this advice merely ensures fluid balance rather than promoting fluid overload has not been adequately tested prior to this study. Of course, the impact of any gain in BM as a result of increased fluid retention might need to be taken into account in sports that are weight restricted (e.g. light-weight rowing) or weight-sensitive (e.g. running, uphill riding). In many sports an increase in BM may increase the energy cost of the activity, impede the speed of acceleration and change of direction, and decrease the power to weight (BM) ratio. Whether this occurs, and whether the small impairments in performance are more than offset by the improvement in fluid balance, needs to be individually studied.

13.5.1.1 *Glycerol hyperhydration*

A method of hyperhydration under current study involves the consumption of a small amount of glycerol (1–1.2 g/kg BM) along with a large fluid bolus (25–35 mL/kg) in the hours prior to exercise. Glycerol, a three-carbon alcohol, provides the backbone to triglyceride molecules and is released during lipolysis (see Chapter 16, Sections 16.2 and 16.5). Within the body it is evenly distributed throughout fluid compartments and exerts an osmotic pressure. When consumed orally, it is rapidly absorbed and distributed among body fluid compartments before being slowly metabolised via the liver and kidneys. When consumed in combination with a substantial fluid intake, the osmotic pressure will enhance the retention of this fluid and the expansion of the various body fluid spaces. Typically, this allows a fluid expansion or retention of ~600 mL above a fluid bolus alone, by reducing urinary volume. Further information on glycerol as an hyperhydrating agent is found in Chapter 17, Section 17.7.3, and a thorough review of glycerol is provided by Robergs & Griffin (1998).

The effect of glycerol hyperhydration strategies on thermoregulation and exercise performance is at present unclear. Studies investigating the effects on sports performance have been summarised in Chapter 17 (Appendix, Table 17.11). This summary shows that at least some of the inconsistencies in the literature are due to differences in study methodologies. However, the most promising scenario involves the use of glycerol to maximise the retention of fluid bolus just prior to an event in which a substantial fluid deficit cannot be prevented. In some but not all studies of this type, glycerol hyperhydration has been associated with performance benefits. Of particular interest are two recent studies undertaken with competitive athletes (see Chapter 17, Table 17.11). In both studies competitive cyclists were able to do more work in a time trial undertaken in the heat, following hyperhydration with glycerol, compared with a trial using a fluid·overload with a placebo drink (Hitchins et al. 1999; Anderson et al. 2000). The study by Anderson and colleagues is reviewed in more detail in Chapter 25. Even if future studies confirm the beneficial effects of glycerol hyperhydration strategies, it may require careful research to determine the mechanisms behind the effect. At present the theoretical advantages of increased sweat losses and greater capacity for heat dissipation, and attenuation of cardiac and thermoregulatory challenges, are not consistently seen (see Table 17.11).

Finally, glycerol hyperhydration strategies need to be fine-tuned, and perhaps individualised for specific situations. As previously discussed, the cost of a gain in BM might need to be considered in some sports. Other side-effects from the use of glycerol include nausea, gastrointestinal distress, and headaches resulting from increased intracranial pressure. These problems have been reported among some but not all subjects in the current studies. Fine-tuning of protocols may reduce the risk of these problems, however some individuals may remain at a greater risk than others. At the present time, glycerol hyperhydration should remain an activity that is supervised and monitored by appropriate sports science/medicine professionals, and only used in competition situations after adequate experimentation and fine-tuning has occurred.

13.5.2   *Priming the stomach with a fluid bolus*

Even if the athlete is not aiming to fluid overload, there can be good reasons to have a drink just before exercise. Effective rehydration during exercise depends on maximising the rate of fluid delivery from the stomach to the intestine for absorption. One of the factors affecting gastric emptying is gastric distension due to the volume of stomach contents. According to Noakes et al., optimal delivery of fluid from the stomach can be achieved by beginning exercise with a comfortable volume of fluid in the stomach, and adopting a pattern of periodic fluid intake during the exercise. This method is designed to top up gastric contents as they partially empty (Noakes et al. 1991). Obviously the athlete will need to experiment to determine what is a comfortable volume with which to prime gastric volume, and in particular how comfortable this feels once exercise has commenced. However, as a general rule of thumb, most athletes can tolerate a bolus of about 5 mL/kg BM (i.e. 300–400 mL) of fluid immediately before the event starts. This may provide a useful start to fluid intake tactics during exercise (see Chapter 14).

13.6 SUMMARY

The outcomes of pre-event nutrition strategies range from psychological well-being and confidence to optimal fluid and fuel status. The importance of these strategies will depend on the range and severity of physiological challenges that are likely to limit performance in the athlete's individual event. This may be determined by characteristics of the event itself, as well as the degree to which the athlete has been able to recover since their last workout or competition event. Nutrition strategies may include increased CHO intake during the day(s) prior to the event, as well as the extended fuelling-up known as CHO loading, which has been shown to enhance endurance and the performance of prolonged exercise events. The pre-event meal also provides an opportunity to refuel muscle and liver glycogen stores. There is some concern that pre-exercise CHO feedings may increase CHO utilisation during exercise, but the intake of substantial amounts of CHO can offset the increased rate of substrate use. The choice of low-GI CHO-rich foods in the pre-event menu may also sustain the delivery of CHO during exercise, however this does not provide a guaranteed performance advantage, especially when additional CHO is consumed during the event. Pre-event preparation should also consider fluid balance, with strategies to rehydrate from previous dehydration associated with exercise or weight-making activities, as well as the potential for hyperhydration in preparation for events in which a large fluid deficit is unavoidable. A variety of eating practices can be chosen by the athlete to meet their competition preparation goals. These need to consider the practical aspects of nutrition such as gastrointestinal comfort, the athlete's likes and dislikes, and food availability. Above all, the athlete should experiment with their pre-event nutrition practices to find and fine-tune strategies that are successful. These may be individual to the athlete and their specific event. Pre-event nutrition practices should be undertaken as part of an integrated competition nutrition plan. Ideally, an athlete should combat these challenges of competition by undertaking a systematic plan of nutrition strategies before, during and even in the recovery after an event.

13.7 PRACTICE TIPS

Lorna Garden

Fuelling for competition

- It is important for the sports dietitian to have an extensive understanding of the individual athlete's competition plan in order to advise on appropriate dietary preparation. Interview questions should help determine the usual pre-competition dietary habits of the athlete, the timing and place of competition, food and fluids available, support people, recovery time between events (if appropriate), and the athlete's competition goals.

- The decision to CHO load needs to be made based on consideration of the physiological requirements of the athlete's event (see Table 13.3). The athlete needs to have a good comprehension of the rationale for loading; and the requirements, side-effects, and practical difficulties associated with achieving an exercise taper and high CHO intake.

- Where an athlete presents with medical problems such as diabetes or other endocrine disorders or gastrointestinal issues it is important that the athlete, sports dietitian and physician work together in preparing the athlete for competition.

- It is useful for the athlete to know that CHO loading is likely to be associated with a body-mass gain of ~2 kg. This needs to be viewed as positive rein-forcement that they have significantly increased glycogen stores. Encouraging the athlete to weigh-in each morning, unclothed and after voiding, can help determine how the loading is progressing.

- For most athletes a CHO-loading regime will involve 3–5 days of a CHO intake between 7–10 g/kg BM/d or 70–85% of energy. Since this may repre-sent an unusual dietary pattern for many athletes, help will be needed to devise suitable food choices and meal plans. Useful resources for the athlete include CHO ready-reckoners and an individualised CHO loading plan (see sample in Table 13.4).

- Some athletes will find it difficult to tolerate the higher fibre content of a high-CHO diet, particularly if wholegrain and wholemeal breads and cereals and large quantities of fruit are consumed. To avoid gastrointestinal symptoms such as flatulence, diarrhoea and gut discomfort, the sports dietitian may need to advise on low-fibre/residue alternatives such as white bread, plain cereals, tinned and peeled fruit and liquid forms of CHO.

- Athletes who struggle to meet higher CHO needs may need to include refined CHOs such as glucose confectionery, jelly, jam, honey, and soft drinks to supplement more nutritious but bulkier forms of CHO. Liquid meal supplements and high-CHO supplements are also useful as low-bulk, CHO-rich drinks.

- Fluid consumption is increased during the loading period. The sports dietitian should indicate that copious volumes of clear urine is a sign of being well hydrated. Monitoring fluid intake using a marked water bottle or a record of drinks consumed can assist the athlete to meet increased fluid goals. Juice, cordials, soft drink, sports drinks and other CHO/liquid-meal supplements may be useful in helping meet both CHO and fluid needs.

- Athletes should be encouraged to practise their CHO-loading regimen well before important competitions to ensure they are familiar and comfortable with food choices and quantities. This may be appropriate before a long training session or a minor event.

- Athletes should be reassured that although their nutritional goals for some vitamins and minerals may not be met during CHO loading, this is not a problem as a balanced diet will be resumed after competition.

Table 13.3 *Factors affecting the decision to CHO load*

CHO loading should be considered if:	CHO loading is not necessary if:
The exercise is moderate intensity, endurance activity where heavy demands are placed on glycogen stores (e.g. marathon, triathlon, cross-country skiing)	The exercise is not an endurance activity and normal glycogen stores will be adequate to fuel the event
The activity is likely to involve more than 90 minutes of continuous exercise	The event will last less than 60–80 minutes
The athlete is currently eating less than 8–9 g CHO/kg BM/d and is motivated to follow a loading regimen	The activity is high intensity for a short duration and will be adversely affected by the weight gain associated with loading (e.g. sprint events, field events)
There are no medical reasons contraindicating a very high CHO diet for a 3–5 day period	The athlete is already eating a very high CHO diet (> 8–9 g/kg BM/d or more than 800 g CHO/d)
	The athlete has unstable diabetes, or is hyperlipidemic, and a very high CHO diet is contraindicated

Pre-event meal

- Athletes need an understanding of the role of the pre-event meal in topping up liver glycogen levels and the relative importance of a high-CHO diet in the days leading up to competition.

- The psychological role of the pre-event meal and the athlete's likes and dislikes need to be carefully considered when planning appropriate foods and

Table 13.4 *Example of a CHO-loading menu for one day*

This plan for a 70 kg athlete provides approximately: **600 g CHO (74% E or 8.5 g CHO/kg BM), 30 g fat (8% E), 115 g protein (15% E)**   **and 13 MJ**

BREAKFAST
2 cups plain breakfast cereal with low-fat milk
1 piece fresh fruit
2 slices wholemeal toast with jam
1 glass fruit juice

SNACK
1 muesli bar, low fat
1 piece fresh fruit

LUNCH
2 rolls or bagels, 1 filled with tuna and salad, 1 filled with sliced banana and honey
1 cup canned fruit
1 tub low-fat fruit yoghurt or light fromage frais
Water

SNACK
1 low-fat smoothie (blend ½ cup fruit salad with 1 cup low-fat milk and 2 scoops
  low-fat ice-cream)

DINNER
2 cups hokkein or egg noodles stir-fried with Asian vegetables and 1–2 tbsp black
  bean or sweet and sour sauce
200 g low-fat creamed rice with 1 diced mango or other seasonal fruit
1 can soft drink

fluids before competition. The psychological value of ingesting foods that are familiar and 'tried and true' should not be underestimated.

- The pre-event meal should be based on high-CHO foods that are low in fat and protein to decrease the risk of gastrointestinal problems during the event (see Table 13.5). Athletes who are prone to gastric discomfort during competition may also benefit from reducing dietary fibre or choosing liquid meals prior to exercise.

- Where an athlete is nervous pre-event and unable to eat or tolerate solid foods, the sports dietitian may need to advise on appropriate liquid meal supplements such as home-made smoothies or commercial beverages.

- Commercial liquid meal supplements may also be a useful pre-event meal when travelling for competition to countries where familiar foods are unlikely to be available.

- Athletes should be encouraged to experiment with pre–exercise eating before training sessions to find foods and drinks they are comfortable with. The timing of pre-event eating will be individual to the athlete and their event, however, a general schedule of two to four hours before the event should be suitable for most athletes.

- Athletes involved in endurance events may wish to trial low-GI foods such as porridge, pasta, baked beans, multigrain bread, oranges and yoghurt prior to competition. There is no evidence that low-GI foods provide universal benefits to performance, however they are most likely to be useful before prolonged workouts where a sustained release of fuel can't be provided by intake during the session itself.

- The response to eating high-GI foods immediately prior to exercise is likely to be individual and should be trialled and monitored during training, well before competition days. In most cases, where an athlete is eating 30–90 minutes before an event, practical issues such as convenience and tolerance will become more crucial than the GI in deciding the pre-event menu.

- Athletes who have dehydrated or fluid restricted to make weight will need an individualised plan to promote rapid rehydration between weighing-in and commencing competition. If time is very limited, liquid meal supplements may be a preferable option to solid food prior to the event.

- Liquid meal supplements may also be useful as a pre-event meal for athletes who compete in sports where aesthetic requirements such as a 'flat stomach' are important (e.g. gymnasts, dancers, divers).

Table 13.5 *Suggestions for pre-event food and fluid intake*

Pre-event foods and fluids
Plain breakfast cereal with low-fat milk and fruit
Porridge with low-fat milk and fruit juice
Pancakes/pikelets with maple syrup, honey or golden syrup
Toast, muffins, or crumpets with honey/jam/syrup
Baked beans on toast
Creamed rice (with low-fat milk) and tinned fruit
Spaghetti with low-fat tomato-based sauce
Jacket potato with creamed corn
Low-fat breakfast bar or muesli bar and banana
Roll or sandwich with banana and honey
Fresh fruit salad with low-fat yoghurt or fromage frais
Smoothie based on low-fat milk or soy milk, low-fat yoghurt and mango/banana/berries

Hydration: prior to the event

- Athletes should be encouraged to begin their events well hydrated by consuming extra fluids in the days leading up to competition.

- When the athlete has several events or races scheduled, a plan should be made to ensure that fluid losses are recovered after each exercise session.

- Hydration prior to competition should be carefully planned, especially before events carried out in hot and humid weather. Fluid intake before an event should include at least 300–600 mL fluid with the pre-event meal and then 150–300 mL fluid every 15–20 minutes up until about 45 minutes to one hour before the event, leaving time for a toilet stop prior to exercise beginning.

- Athletes who are likely to dehydrate significantly during their event (e.g. situations where sweat rate is high and/or there are limited drinking opportunities) may benefit from hyperhydration. However, before this process is used in the competition setting, it should be carefully trialled prior to a long training session to check for benefits and side-effects. Athletes will need to approximately double their usual fluid intake for the week prior to the event, and may expect to see an overall fluid gain of over 500 mL. The use of drinks containing sodium (e.g. sports drinks) may assist with fluid retention.

- Hyperhydrating with glycerol in the hours prior to the event may be beneficial to some athletes, however, this should also be carefully trialled, preferably under the supervision of a qualified sports scientist.

- Effective rehydration during exercise can be enhanced by priming the stomach with a bolus of fluid prior to the event, to take advantage of the effect of gastric distension on gastric emptying. Athletes will need to experiment to determine the maximum volume that can be tolerated without stomach discomfort during the event. Most athletes will tolerate around 300–400 mL of fluid immediately before the event.

- Whilst water is adequate for hydration before shorter events, the use of CHO–electrolyte beverages (sports drinks) prior to exercise can assist in meeting both fluid and CHO needs, particularly before endurance events. Beverages containing sodium, such as sports drinks, may also be useful in assisting with fluid retention prior to and during the event and can reduce the need for frequent urination.

REFERENCES

Abt G, Zhou S, Weatherby R. The effect of a high-carbohydrate diet on the skill performance of midfield soccer players after intermittent treadmill exercise. J Sci Med Sport 1998;1:203–12.

Adamo KB, Graham TE. Comparison of traditional measurements with macroglycogen and proglycogen analysis of muscle glycogen. J Appl Physiol 1998;84:908–13.

Adamo KB, Tarnopolsky MA, Graham TE. Dietary carbohydrate and postexercise synthesis of proglycogen and macroglycogen in human skeletal muscle. Am J Physiol 1998;275:E229–E34.

Ahlborg B, Bergstrom J, Brohult J. Human muscle glycogen content and capacity for prolonged exercise after difference diets. Foersvarsmedicin 1967;85–99.

Akermark C, Jacobs I, Rasmusson M, Karlsson, J. Diet and muscle glycogen concentration in relation to physical performance in Swedish elite ice hockey players. Int J Sport Nutr 1996;6:272–84.

Alonso MD, Lomako J, Lomako WM, Whelan WJ. A new look at the biogenesis of glycogen. FASEB J 1995;9:1126–37.

Anderson MJ, Cotter JD, Garnham AP, Casley DJ, Febbraio MA. Effect of glycerol-induced hyperhydration on thermoregulation and metabolism during exercise in the heat. Int J Sport Nutr Exerc Metab 2001;11:315–33.

Asp S, Daugaard JR, Rohde T, Adamo KB, Graham T. Muscle glycogen accumulation after a marathon: roles of fiber type and pro- and macroglycogen. J Appl Physiol 1999;86:474–8.

Balsom PB, Wood K, Olsson P, Ekblom B. Carbohydrate intake and multiple sprint sports: with special reference to football (soccer). Int J Sports Med 1999;20:48–52.

Bangsbo J, Norregaard L, Thorsoe F. The effect of carbohydrate diet on intermittent exercise performance. Int J Sports Med 1992;13:152–7.

Bergstrom J, Hermansen L, Hultman E, Saltin B. Diet, muscle glycogen and physical performance. Acta Physiol Scand 1967;71:140–50.

Bergstrom J, Hultman E. Muscle glycogen synthesis after exercise: an enhancing factor localised to the muscle cells in man. Nature 1966;210:309–10.

Brand Miller JC. Importance of glycemic index in diabetes. Am J Clin Nutr 1994;59(suppl):S747–S52.

Brand Miller J, Foster-Powell, Colagiuri S, Leeds A. The G.I. Factor, 2nd edn. Sydney: Hodder & Stoughton, 1998.

Burke LM. Nutrition for the female athlete. In: Krummel D, Kris-Etherton P, eds. Nutrition in women's health. Maryland: Aspen Publishers, 1995:263–98.

Burke LM, Claassen A, Hawley JA, Noakes TD. Carbohydrate intake during prolonged cycling minimizes effect of glycemic index of preexercise meal. J Appl Physiol 1998;85:2220–6.

Burke LM, Collier GR, Beasley SK, et al. Effect of coingestion of fat and protein with carbohydrate feedings on muscle glycogen storage. J Appl Physiol 1995;87:2187–92.

Burke LM, Hawley JA, Schabort EJ, St. Clair Gibson A, Mujika I, Noakes TD. Carbohydrate loading failed to improve 100-km cycling performance in a placebo-controlled trial. J Appl Physiol 2000;80:1284–90.

Burke LM, Read RSD. A study of carbohydrate loading techniques used by marathon runners. Can J Sports Sci 1987;12:6–10.

Chryssanthopoulos C, Williams C. Pre-exercise carbohydrate meal and endurance running capacity when carbohydrates are ingested during exercise. Int J Sports Med 1997;18:543–8.

Costill DL, Sherman WM, Fink WJ, Maresh C, Witten M, Miller JM. The role of dietary carbohydrates in muscle glycogen resynthesis after strenuous running. Am J Clin Nutr 1981;34:1831–6.

Costill DL, Pascoe DD, Fink WJ, Robergs RA, Barr SI, Pearson D. Impaired muscle glycogen resynthesis after eccentric exercise. J Appl Physiol 1990;69:46–50.

Coyle EF. Timing and method of increased carbohydrate intake to cope with heavy training, competition and recovery. J Sports Sci. 1991;9(suppl):29–52.

Coyle EF, Coggan AR, Hemmert MK, Lowe RC, Walters TJ. Substrate usage during prolonged exercise following a pre-exercise meal. J Appl Physiol 1985;59:429–33.

Danforth W. Glycogen synthase activity in skeletal muscle. J Biol Chem 1965;240:588–93.

DeMarco HM, Sucher KP, Cisar CJ, Butterfield GE. Pre-exercise carbohydrate meals: application of glycemic index. Med Sci Sports Exercise 1999;31:164–70.

Febbraio MA, Stewart KL. CHO feeding before prolonged exercise: effect of glycemic index on muscle glycogenolysis and exercise performance. J Appl Physiol 1996;81:1115–20.

Foster C, Costill DL, Fink WJ. Effects of pre-exercise feedings on endurance performance. Med Sci Sports 1979;11:1–5.

Friedman JE, Neufer PD, Dohm GL. Regulation of glycogen resynthesis following exercise. Sports Med 1991;11:232–43.

Griewe JS, Hickner RC, Hansen PA, Racette AB, Chen MM, Holloszy JO. Effects of endurance exercise training on muscle glycogen accumulation in humans. J Appl Physiol 1999;87:222–6.

Guezennec CY, Sabatin P, Duforez F, Koziet J, Antoine JM. The role of type and structure of complex carbohydrate response to physical exercise. Int J Sports Med 1993;14:224–31.

Hackney AC. Effects of the menstrual cycle on resting muscle glycogen content. Horm Metab Res 1990;22:647.

Hargreaves M, Costill DL, Katz A, Fink WJ. Effects of fructose ingestion on muscle glycogen usage during exercise. Med Sci Sports Exerc 1985;17:360–3.

Hawley JA, Burke LM. Effect of meal frequency and timing on physical performance. Brit J Nutr 1997;77(suppl):S91–S103.

Hawley J, Burke L. Peak performance. Sydney: Allen & Unwin, 1998.

Hawley JA, Palmer G, Noakes TD. Effects of 3 days of carbohydrate supplementation on muscle glycogen content and utilisation during a 1-h cycling. Eur J Appl Physiol 1997b;76:407–12.

Hawley JA, Schabort EJ, Noakes TD, Dennis SC. Carbohydrate-loading and exercise performance: an update. Sports Med 1997a;24:73–81.

Hermanssen L, Hultman E, Saltin B. Muscle glycogen during prolonged severe exercise. Acta Physiol Scand 1967;129–39.

Hitchins S, Martin DT, Burke LM, et al. Glycerol hyperhydration improves cycle time trial performance in hot humid conditions. Eur J Appl Physiol 1999;80:494–501.

Inge K, Brukner P. Food for sport. Australia: William Heinemann, 1986.

Ivy JL. Muscle glycogen synthesis before and after exercise. Sports Medicine 1991;11:6–19.

Ivy JL, Katz AL, Cutler CL, Sherman WM, Coyle EF. Muscle glycogen storage after exercise: effect of time of carbohydrate ingestion. J Appl Physiol 1988;65:1480–5.

Ivy JL, Kuo CH. Regulation of GLUT4 protein and glycogen synthase during muscle glycogen synthesis after exercise. Acta Physiol Scand 1998;162:295–304.

Karlsson J, Saltin B. Diet, muscle glycogen, and endurance performance. J Appl Physiol 1971;31:203–6.

Kristal-Boneh E, Glusman JG, Shitrit R, Chaemovitz C, Cassuto Y. Physical performance and heat tolerance after chronic water loading and heat acclimation. Aviat Space Environ Med 1995;66:733–8.

Kuipers H, Fransen EJ, Keizer HA. Pre-exercise ingestion of carbohydrate and transient hypoglycemia during exercise. Int J Sports Med 1999;20:227–31.

McClellan TM, Cheung SS, Jacobs I. Variability of time to exhaustion during submaximal exercise. Can J Appl Physiol 1995;20:39–51.

McCoy M, Proietto J, Hargreaves M. Skeletal muscle GLUT-4 and post-exercise muscle glycogen storage. J Appl Physiol 1996;80:411–16.

Moroff SV, Bass DE. Effects of over-hydration on man's physiological responses to work in the heat. J Appl Physiol 1965; 20:267–70.

Neufer PD, Costill DL, Flynn MG, Kirwan JP, Mitchell JB, Houmard J. Improvements in exercise performance: effects of carbohydrate feedings and diet. J Appl Physiol 1987;62:983–8.

Nicklas BJ, Hackney AC, Sharp RL. The menstrual cycle and exercise: performance, muscle glycogen, and substrate responses. Int J Sports Med 1989;10:264–9.

Noakes TD, Rehrer NJ, Maughan RJ. The importance of volume in regulating gastric emptying. Med Sci Sports Exerc 1991;23:307–13.

O'Reilly KP, Warhol MJ, Fielding RA, Frontera WR, Meredith CN, Evans WJ. Eccentric exercise-induced muscle damage impairs muscle glycogen repletion. J Appl Physiol 1987;63:252–7.

Piehl K. Time course for refilling of glycogen stores in human muscle fibres following exercise-induced glycogen depletion. Acta Physiol Scand 1974;90:297–302.

Rauch LH, Rodger I, Wilson GR, et al. The effects of carbohydrate loading on muscle glycogen content and cycling performance. Int J Sports Nutr 1995;5:25–36.

Rehrer NJ, Van Kemenade M, Meester W, Brouns F, Saris WHM. Gastrointestinal complaints in relation to dietary intake in triathletes. Int J Sport Nutr 1992;2:48–59.

Robergs RA. Nutrition and exercise determinants of postexercise glycogen synthesis. Int J Sport Nutr 1991;1:307–37.

Robergs RA, Griffin SE. Glycerol: biochemistry, pharmacokinetics and clinical and practical applications. Sports Med 1998;26:145–67.

Robinson TA, Hawley JA, Palmer GS, et al. Water ingestion does not improve 1-h cycling performance in moderate ambient temperatures. Eur J Appl Physiol 1995;14:153–60.

Roden M, Shulman GI. Applications of NMR spectroscopy to study muscle glycogen metabolism in man. Ann Rev Med 1999;50:277–90.

Sherman WM, Brodowicz G, Wright DA, Allen WK, Simonsen J, Dernbach A. Effects of 4-hour pre-exercise carbohydrate feedings on cycling performance. Med Sci Sports Exerc 1989;21:598–604.

Sherman WM, Costill DL, Fink WJ, Miller JM. Effect of exercise-diet manipulation on muscle glycogen and its subsequent utilisation during performance. Int J Sports Med 1981;2:114–18.

Sparks MJ, Selig SS, Febbraio MA. Pre-exercise carbohydrate ingestion: effect of the glycemic index on endurance exercise performance. Med Sci Sports Exerc 1998;30:844–9.

Tarnopolsky MA, Atkinson SA, Phillips SM, MacDougall JD. Carbohydrate loading and metabolism during exercise in men and women. J Appl Physiol 1995;75:2134–41.

Tarnopolsky MA. Gender differences in metabolism. New York: CRC Press, 1999.

Thomas DE, Brotherhood JE, Brand JC. Carbohydrate feeding before exercise: effect of glycemic index. Int J Sports Med 1991;12:180–6.

Thomas DE, Brotherhood JR, Brand Miller J. Plasma glucose levels after prolonged strenuous exercise correlate inversely with glycemic response to food consumed before exercise. Int J Sport Nutr 1994;4:361–73.

Walker JL, Heigenhauser GFJ, Hultman E, Spriet LL. Dietary carbohydrate, muscle glycogen content and endurance performance in well-trained women. In press.

Wee SL, Williams C, Gray S, Horabin J. Influence of high and low glycemic index meals on endurance running capacity. Med Sci Sports Exerc 1999;31:393–9.

Widrick JJ, Costill DL, Fink WJ, Hickey MS, McConell GK, Tanaka H. Carbohydrate feedings and exercise performance: effect of initial muscle glycogen concentration. J Appl Physiol 1993;74:2998–3005.

Wilmore J, Costill DL. Physiology of sport and exercise. Champaign, Illinois: Human Kinetics, 1994.

Wolever TMS. The glycemic index. World Rev Nutr Diet 1990;62:120–85.

Wright DA, Sherman WM, Dernbach AR. Carbohydrate feedings before, during, or in combination improve cycling endurance performance. J Appl Physiol 1991;71:1082–8.

Fluid and carbohydrate intake during exercise

Ron Maughan

14.1 INTRODUCTION

In any sports competition lasting longer than about 30 minutes, there is scope for intake of food and fluid during the event, and the choice of intake has the potential to influence the outcome. Indeed, in recent major track championships, drinks have been available—and have been taken by competitors—in races over distances of 5000 and 10 000 metres. Certainly in the former event, and possibly also in the latter, any benefit is likely to be psychological rather than purely physiological. Hard physical effort is associated with an increased body temperature, a decrease in body water content due to sweat loss, a fall in the body's carbohydrate (CHO) stores in the liver and in the muscles, and, perhaps, a fall in the blood glucose concentration. All of these factors can impair performance by reducing exercise capacity and, in some circumstances, by bringing about an impairment of skilled movements and of decision making. In extreme situations, all of these factors, with the sole exception of muscle glycogen depletion, have the potential to cause collapse, which may progress to irreversible harm. Such medical emergencies can almost always be avoided, and, with proper attention to food and fluid intake, the athlete should be able to achieve a performance that reflects a combination of genetic potential and training status.

Although ingestion of CHO and fluids can improve performance, this is not necessarily true for all individuals in all situations. Athletes prone to gastrointestinal problems often avoid any solid or liquid intake for some hours before, and also during, competition. The choice of food and fluids will also be influenced by a variety of factors, including the nature and duration of the event, the climatic conditions, the pre-event nutritional status, and the physiological and biochemical character-istics of the individual. The circumstances of each athlete, each sport and each competition must therefore be considered when making recommendations.

It must also be recognised that food and fluid consumed during competition are part of a specific short-term nutritional strategy aimed at maximising performance at that particular time. When choosing foods and fluids to be consumed during competition, there is no need to take account of long-term nutritional goals, except perhaps, and even then to a limited extent, in extreme endurance events such as the Tour de France or in multi-day running events. In the Tour de France, prolonged exercise is performed on a daily basis over a long period and the food consumed during each day's competition may account for about one half of the total daily intake (Saris et al. 1989), but even this extreme event lasts for only 22 days. A balanced diet is therefore not necessary and intake is targeted at minimis-ing the impact of those factors that are responsible for fatigue and impaired performance.

14.2 *FATIGUE DURING EXERCISE*

In the exercise physiology laboratory, fatigue and the nutritional interventions that influence the fatigue process are studied intensively. The subjects used in these studies are often relatively sedentary, and although club level athletes may some-times participate, it is seldom possible to recruit a population of elite athletes willing to take part in such investigations. The experimental models used in labo-ratory studies also differ from the competitive situation, usually involving exercise at a constant power output that has to be continued for as long as possible. Even where intermittent exercise or time trial models are used, subjects exercise alone in an artificial environment without many of the stresses that accompany competi-tion. Advice given to those elite athletes is therefore based on extrapolations from the limited available information.

The role of carbohydrate (CHO) in muscle metabolism and in exercise perform-ance is discussed in detail in Chapters 2, 13 and 15. The extensive literature makes it clear that CHO metabolism is central to the athlete's ability to sustain an inten-sive training load and to perform well in competition. In warm environments, however, fatigue occurs while substantial CHO stores remain (Parkin et al. 1999), and performance is limited more by thermoregulatory failure and dehydration. These observations, which are not new, point clearly to the nutritional strategies that the athlete should adopt to improve performance.

14.3 *CHO SUPPLEMENTATION DURING EXERCISE*

The ingestion of CHO during exercise provides a number of benefits for metabo-lism and performance. These effects are well described in relation to prolonged bouts of moderate-intensity and intermittent-intensity exercise, but recent studies suggest that CHO ingestion may also be useful for the performance of high-intensity exercise of about one hour duration. This section will discuss these various benefits.

14.3.1 *Prevention of hypoglycaemia*

The blood glucose concentration is normally maintained within a very narrow range by regulation of the addition of glucose to the circulation and its removal by peripheral tissues. Glucose can be added from the gastrointestinal tract after food intake or from the liver, which stores about 80–100 g of glycogen in the fully fed state and can also synthesise glucose from non-CHO sources. The primary hormones regulating the blood glucose concentration are insulin and glucagon, but it is increasingly recognised that a large number of other peptide hormones also play key roles in this process, either directly or by influencing the circulating insulin and glucagon levels. Important hormones in this respect are growth hormone, cortisol, somatostatin and the catecholamines. Because of the obvious difficulties in making the measurements, there is a limited amount of data on the changes in liver glycogen content during prolonged exercise, but it is clear that a progressive fall occurs, with low levels being reached when subjects are exhausted (Hultman & Nilsson 1971).

It is important to maintain the circulating blood glucose concentration above about 2.5 mmol/L. The cells of the central nervous system have an absolute requirement for glucose as a fuel, and when the blood glucose concentration falls below this level, the rate of uptake by the brain may not be sufficient to meet its metabolic needs. Hypoglycaemia leads to a variety of symptoms, including dizziness, nausea and disorientation. Hypoglycaemia was one of the earliest medical problems identified in marathon runners suffering from fatigue and collapse at the end of a race. Levine et al. (1924) obtained blood samples from runners at the end of the 1923 Boston marathon race and observed that three of the 12 runners studied finished the race in a very poor condition and had a blood glucose concentration of less than 2.8 mmol/L. These same authors recognised that CHO feeding during the race could prevent the onset of hypoglycaemic symptoms. In the following year's race, this was shown to be the case, and an improvement in performance was also reported when CHO was consumed (Gordon et al. 1925). CHO ingested during exercise will enter the blood glucose pool at a rate that will be dictated by the rates of gastric emptying and absorption from the intestine; if this exogenous CHO can substitute for the body's limited endogenous glycogen stores, then exercise capacity should be increased in situations where liver or muscle glycogen availability limits endurance.

Several studies have shown that the ingestion of even modest amounts of glucose during prolonged exercise will maintain or raise the circulating glucose concentration (Costill et al. 1973; Pirnay et al. 1982; Erickson et al. 1987). Glucose can be replaced by a variety of other sugars, including sucrose, glucose polymers and mixtures of sugars, without markedly affecting this response. Ingestion of large amounts of fructose can also maintain or elevate the blood glucose concentration at the end of prolonged exhausting exercise (Maughan et al. 1989), although some studies have not reported a marked effect (Erickson et al. 1987). Fructose is relatively slowly absorbed in the intestine, and must be converted by the liver to glucose before it can be oxidised by muscle. Tracer studies show that the maximum rate of oxidation of orally ingested fructose is less than that for glucose, sucrose or oligosaccharides (Wagenmakers et al. 1993). Perhaps for this reason, the ingestion of solutions containing only fructose is not generally effective in improving performance of prolonged exercise (Maughan et al. 1989; Murray et al. 1989). Fructose in combination with other sugars seems to be well tolerated, and can result in improved performance (Murray et al. 1987).

14.3.2 *Additional fuel to the exercising muscle during prolonged exercise*

The muscle glycogen store is large relative to that of the liver, amounting to about 300–400 g in the average 70 kg well-fed sedentary individual. The addition of those qualifications indicates the influence of body size, especially muscle mass, nutritional status and training status on muscle glycogen storage. The requirement for CHO to be available as a fuel to support muscle metabolism during intense exercise is well known. In well-trained marathon runners running at racing pace, the rate of CHO oxidation can be about 3–4 g per minute, but if this was sustained, the available CHO stores would be depleted long before the finish line was reached. Certainly in cycling (Hermansen et al. 1967) and perhaps also in running (Williams 1998), the point of fatigue in prolonged exercise coincides closely with the depletion of glycogen in the exercising muscles. Increasing muscle glycogen stores prior to exercise can also improve performance in both cycling (Ahlborg et al. 1967) and running (Karlsson & Saltin 1971).

Where performance is limited by the size of the body's endogenous liver or muscle glycogen stores, exercise capacity should be improved when CHO is consumed. Several studies have shown that the ingestion of glucose during prolonged intense exercise will prevent the development of hypoglycaemia by maintaining or raising the circulating glucose concentration (Costill et al. 1973; Pirnay et al. 1982; Erickson et al. 1987). In prolonged exercise, performance, which was measured in most of the early studies as the time for which a fixed power output could be sustained, is improved by the addition of an energy source in the form of CHO. More recent studies have used a variety of different experimental models and have confirmed that this improvement in performance seems to apply also to other exercise models. Beneficial effects of CHO ingestion are seen during constant-effort cycling (Coggan & Coyle 1991) as well as during running (Tsintzas et al. 1993). Improvements in performance have also been reported in cycling time trials carried out in the laboratory, and in a variety of running models, including intermittent shuttle running tests. Williams (1989) and Williams et al. (1990) have used an experimental model in which the subject is able to adjust the treadmill speed while running; the subject can then be encouraged either to cover the maximum distance possible in a fixed time or to complete a fixed distance in the fastest time possible. They showed that ingestion of one litre of a glucose polymer-sucrose (50 g/L) solution did not significantly increase the total distance covered in a two-hour run, but that the running speed was greater over the last 30 minutes of exercise when CHO was given compared with a placebo trial (Williams 1989). They observed a similar effect when a CHO solution (50 g of glucose–glucose polymer, or 50 g of fructose–glucose polymer) or water was given in a 30 km treadmill time trial (Williams et al. 1990). The running speed decreased over the last 10 km of the water trial, but was maintained in the other two runs; there was no significant difference between the three trials in the time taken to cover the total distance. As with the cycling exercise, the conclusion must be that ingestion of CHO-containing drinks is generally effective in improving performance.

This ergogenic effect was initially attributed to a sparing of the body's limited muscle glycogen stores by the oxidation of the ingested CHO (Hargreaves et al. 1984; Erickson et al. 1987), but other studies have failed to show a glycogen-sparing effect of CHO ingested during prolonged exercise (Coyle 1991). The current consensus view seems to be that there is probably little or no sparing of muscle glycogen utilisation, although liver glucose release is slowed (Bosch et al. 1994; McConnell et al. 1994). The primary benefit of ingested CHO is probably its role in supplementing the endogenous stores in the later stages of exercise (Coyle 1997).

14.3.2.1 *Amount and timing of CHO intake*

It is clear from tracer studies that a substantial part of the CHO ingested during exercise is available for oxidation, but there appears to be an upper limit of about one gram per minute to the rate at which ingested CHO can be oxidised, even when much larger amounts are ingested (Wagenmakers et al. 1993). This has been used as an argument to suggest that CHO should not be ingested at rates of more than one gram per minute, but these high rates of oxidation will not be achieved if the amount ingested is not in excess of this. In prolonged exercise, ingested CHO can account for something between about 10% and 30% of the total amount of CHO oxidised (Hawley et al. 1992). Gastric emptying and intestinal absorption rates should allow for a faster rate of CHO supply, and the fate of that fraction of the ingested CHO that is not oxidised is not clear at the present time (Rehrer et al. 1992).

Based on the feeding protocols used in studies that show performance enhancements, it has been suggested that carbohydrate should be ingested at a rate of about 30–60 g/h (Coyle 1991; ACSM 1996). Of course, this is meant as a general guideline that must be adapted to the needs of each sport and each athlete. As suggested above, full benefits may not be seen in some situations unless intakes in excess of this recommendation are achieved. In many sports these general guidelines appear adequate and can be met simultaneously with fluid needs by consuming commercial CHO–electrolyte drinks (see Section 14.4).

Although tracer studies show that little of the ingested CHO is oxidised during the first 60 minutes of exercise (Hawley et al. 1992), there are several studies which suggest that CHO intake should begin early in exercise, or at least well in advance of the onset of fatigue. For example, McConell et al. (1996) studied eight well-trained men who rode for two hours at 70% of VO_2 max, followed immediately by a 15-minute time trial. Subjects ingested either 250 mL of a 7 g/100 mL CHO solution every 15 minutes throughout exercise, or a placebo for 90 minutes followed by a 21 g/100 mL CHO beverage at 91, 105 and 120 minutes. Despite starting the time trial with significantly elevated plasma glucose concentrations when CHO was ingested late in exercise, subjects completed a greater amount of work during the 15 minutes when they had been fed CHO throughout exercise. These results suggest that CHO ingestion improves performance through mechanisms other than, or in addition to, an increased CHO availability to the contracting muscles.

Of course, in most sports, practical considerations dictate the timing and frequency of CHO (and fluid) intake during the event. During many endurance events (e.g. running and cycling), energy replacement occurs while the athlete is literally 'on the run'. Saris et al. (1989) reported that about half of the daily energy intake of Tour de France cyclists was ingested during each day's cycling stage. Intake is generally much less in running events of comparable duration, as few runners are able to tolerate solid food, even when the exercise intensity is low. Intake during competition may be limited by consideration of the time lost in stopping or slowing down to consume food or fluid, or the impact of such ingestion on gastrointestinal discomfort. In other events, such as team sports, there are formal and informal pauses in play, and these may provide an opportunity to consume CHO/fluid. Athletes should be encouraged to make use of the opportunities provided in their sport to consume fluid and additional CHO. Experimentation and practice in training and in minor competitions will help to determine the best strategies for each situation.

14.3.2.2 *Type of CHO*

In most of the early studies, CHO ingested during exercise was in the form of glucose, but the type of CHO does not appear to be critical, and glucose, sucrose and oligosaccharides have all been shown to be effective in maintaining the blood glucose concentration, and in improving endurance capacity when ingested during prolonged exercise (Maughan 1994). There are theoretical advantages in the use of sugars other than glucose. Substitution of glucose polymers for glucose will allow an increased CHO content without an increased osmolality, and may also have taste advantages, but the available evidence suggests that the use of glucose polymers rather than free glucose does not alter the blood glucose response or the effect on exercise performance (Ivy et al. 1979; Coyle et al. 1983, 1986; Maughan et al. 1987; Coggan & Coyle 1988; Hargreaves & Briggs 1988). Similar effects are seen with the feeding of sucrose (Sasaki et al. 1987) or mixtures of sugars (Murray et al. 1987; Mitchell et al. 1988; Carter & Gisolfi 1989).

Some studies have suggested that long-chain glucose polymer solutions are more readily used by the muscles during exercise than are glucose or fructose solutions (Noakes 1990), but others have found no difference in the oxidation rates of ingested glucose or glucose polymer (Massicote et al. 1989; Rehrer 1990). Massicote et al. (1989) also found that ingested fructose was less readily oxidised than glucose or glucose polymers. Mixtures of glucose and fructose in equal amounts seem to have some advantages: when ingested in combination there is an increased total exogenous CHO oxidation (Adopo et al. 1994). Fructose in high concentrations is generally best avoided on account of the risk of gastrointestinal upset. The argument advanced in favour of the ingestion of fructose during exercise, namely that it provides a readily available energy source but does not stimulate insulin release and consequent inhibition of fatty acid mobilisation, is in any case not well founded; insulin secretion is suppressed during exercise. These studies have been reviewed by Maughan (1994). There may be benefits in including a number of different CHOs, for example, free glucose, sucrose and maltodextrin. Such combinations have taste implications, which may influence the amount consumed, and, by limiting the osmolality and providing a number of transportable solutes, may maximise the rate of sugar and water absorption in the small intestine (Shi et al. 1995).

14.3.3 *Effects on performance of other exercise events*

Although most studies of the beneficial effects of CHO ingestion in exercise have concerned prolonged moderate-intensity or intermittent high-intensity exercise, recent studies have identified other situations of potential benefit. Studies in field situations, or in laboratory settings simulating competition, have shown that CHO ingestion during team and racquet games, sometimes (Vergauwen et al. 1998) but not always (Zeederberg et al. 1996) enhances measures of mental and physical skill by reducing the impairment seen with fatigue. Of considerable interest are the growing number of studies to report benefits of CHO ingestion during performance of high-intensity exercise lasting about one hour (Below et al. 1995; Jeukendrup et al. 1997; Millard-Stafford et al. 1997). In these situations, the intake of a CHO drink was shown to enhance the performance of cycling time trials lasting one hour or running and cycling time trials (of ~10 minutes) undertaken at the end of ~50 minutes of exercise. CHO availability to the muscle is not considered to be limiting in the performance of such exercise, and further research is needed to confirm and explain the effects. It is possible that benefits to 'central performance', involving the brain and nervous system, are involved.

14.3.4 *Other effects of CHO ingestion*

Athletes in hard training are anxious to avoid any illness or injury that might interrupt training. These athletes may, however, be more susceptible to minor opportunistic infections than the sedentary individual, particularly those affecting the upper respiratory tract (Nieman & Pedersen 1999). While not serious in themselves, the disruption to training can have negative physical and psychological effects. Several reviews of the literature (for example, Shephard 1997) suggest that exercise-induced increases in the release of catecholamines and glucocorticoids may be responsible for the reduced effectiveness of the immune system. Ingestion of CHO during exercise is effective in attenuating the rise in circulating catecholamine and cortisol concentrations that is normally observed during prolonged strenuous exercise, and has also been reported to reduce some of the immunosuppressive effects of exercise (Nieman et al. 1997). In contrast to this finding, Bishop et al. (1999) have recently reported that ingestion of a CHO drink before and during 90 minutes of an exercise session designed to simulate soccer match play had no effect on circulating cortisol concentration or on a number of markers of immune function. Notwithstanding the lack of an effect observed in this last study, it does seem that benefits may accrue to the athlete in hard training from the ingestion of CHO-containing drinks during each prolonged training session.

Another recent piece of evidence suggests that CHO ingestion during exercise may promote recovery of muscle glycogen stores in the post-exercise period (Kuo et al. 1999). In this study, rats performed two three-hour swimming bouts, separated by 45 minutes of rest, to deplete muscle glycogen stores. A 50% glucose solution was administered by stomach tube at the end of each of the exercise bouts. CHO feeding resulted in glycogen supercompensation at 16 hours after exercise, an effect attributed to a stimulation of GLUT-4 protein expression in response to CHO. This suggests another reason for ingestion of CHO during exercise that is likely to result in substantial depletion of the muscle glycogen stores: this effect will be of particular significance when a second exercise bout—whether training or another competition—must follow after a short interval.

14.4 EFFECTS OF HYPERTHERMIA AND DEHYDRATION ON PERFORMANCE

It is a matter of common experience that the perception of effort is increased, and exercise capacity reduced, in hot climates. This was recognised by the early pedestrians: in a challenge race held in Curacao in August, 1808, the local man chose to start the race at the hottest time of day to gain an advantage over his European opponent, Lieutenant Fairman. Notwithstanding his disadvantage, Fairman won, but declared the event to be much more stressful than any other event he participated in (Thom 1813). More recently, the effects of increasing ambient temperature were quantified when Galloway and Maughan (1997) showed that exercise capacity at a fixed power output was greatly reduced at 31°C (55 min) compared to the same exercise performed at 11°C (93 min). They also observed that the exercise time was already reduced (to 81 min) at the comparatively modest temperature of 21°C. Parkin et al. (1999) have shown similar effects and also showed that there remained a substantial amount of muscle glycogen at the point of fatigue when the ambient temperature was high (40°C).

When the ambient temperature is higher than skin temperature, the only mechanism by which heat can be lost from the body is evaporation of water from the skin and respiratory tract. Complete evaporation of one litre of water from the skin will remove 2.4 MJ (580 kcal) of heat from the body, and sweat losses are determined primarily by the intensity and duration of exercise and by the ambient temperature and humidity. Data for typical sweat losses in a range of sports activities have been compiled by Rehrer and Burke (1996). However, sweat rates vary greatly between individuals, even when the metabolic rate is apparently similar, and high sweat rates are sometimes necessary even at low ambient temperatures if an excessive rise in body temperature is to be prevented (Maughan 1985).

Water losses are derived in varying proportions from plasma, extracellular water, and intracellular water. Any decrease in plasma volume is likely to adversely affect thermal regulation and exercise capacity. When the metabolic rate is high, blood flow to the muscles must be maintained at a high level to supply oxygen and substrates, but a high blood flow to the skin is also necessary for the convection of heat to the body surface where it can be dissipated (Nadel 1990). When the ambient temperature is high and blood volume has been decreased by sweat loss during prolonged exercise, there may be difficulty in meeting the requirement for a high blood flow to both these tissues. In this situation, skin blood-flow is likely to be compromised, allowing body temperature to rise but preventing a catastrophic fall in central venous pressure (Rowell 1986). Muscle blood flow is also reduced, but oxygen extraction is increased to maintain oxidative energy metabolism (Gonzalez-Alonso et al. 1999).

Coyle and colleagues have also investigated these factors and found that increases in core temperature and heart rate during prolonged exercise are graded according to the level of hypohydration achieved (Montain & Coyle 1992a). They also showed that the ingestion of fluid during exercise increases skin blood-flow, and therefore thermoregulatory capacity, independent of increases in the circulating blood volume (Montain & Coyle 1992b). Plasma volume expansion using dextran/saline infusion was less effective in preventing a rise in core temperature than was the ingestion of sufficient volumes of a CHO–electrolyte drink to maintain plasma volume at a similar level. This suggests that oral intake achieves beneficial effects other than the maintenance of blood volume.

It is often reported that exercise performance is impaired when an individual is dehydrated by as little as 2% of body weight, and that losses in excess of 5% of body weight can decrease the capacity for work by about 30% (Saltin & Costill 1988).

Although this observation has been broadly confirmed by later studies, the original data on which it is based are obscure. Dehydration can compromise performance in high-intensity exercise as well as endurance activities (Nielsen et al. 1982; Armstrong et al. 1985). Although sweat losses during brief exercise are small, prior dehydration (by as much as 10% of body mass) is common in weight category sports where participants are often hypohydrated during competition. Nielsen et al. (1982) showed that prolonged exercise, which resulted in a loss of fluid corresponding to 2.5% of body weight, resulted in a 45% fall in the capacity to perform high intensity exercise. It may be that even very small fluid deficits impair performance but the methods used are not sufficiently sensitive to detect small changes. Walsh et al. (1994) have reported that a fluid deficit of less than 2% of body mass results in impaired performance of a time trial task.

The mechanisms responsible for the reduced exercise performance in the heat are not entirely clear, but Nielsen et al. (1993) have proposed that the high core temperature itself is involved. This proposition was based on the observation that a period of acclimatisation was successful in delaying the point of fatigue, but that this occurred at the same core temperature. The primary effect of acclimatisation was to lower the resting core temperature, and the rate of rise of temperature was the same on all trials. This observation is further supported by numerous studies which show that manipulation of the body heat content prior to exercise can alter exercise capacity: performance is extended by prior immersion in cold water and reduced by prior immersion in hot water (Gonzalez-Alonso et al. 1999).

14.4.1 *Electrolyte balance*

The sweat loss that accompanies prolonged exercise leads to a loss of electrolytes and water from the body. Although the volume loss is easily estimated from changes in body mass after correction for substrate oxidation and respiratory water loss, electrolyte loss is rather more difficult to quantify and the extent of these losses has been the subject of much debate. The values for sweat electrolyte content in Table 14.1 show the great inter-individual variability in the concentration of the major electrolytes.

Table 14.1 *Concentration of the major electrolytes present in sweat, plasma and intracellular (muscle) water in humans*

	Plasma (mmol/L)	Sweat (mmol/L)	Intracellular (mmol/L)
Sodium	137–144	40–80	10
Potassium	3.5–4.9	4–8	148
Calcium	4.4–5.2	3–4	0–2
Magnesium	1.5–2.1	1–4	30–40
Chloride	100–108	30–70	2

These values are collated from a variety of sources [see Maughan (1994) for further details]

Sodium, the most abundant cation of the extracellular space, is the major electrolyte lost in plasma: chloride, which is also mainly located in the extracellular space, is the major anion. This ensures that the greatest fraction of fluid loss is derived from the extracellular space, including the plasma. Although the composition of sweat is highly variable, sweat is always hypotonic with regard to body fluids, and the net effect of sweat loss is an increase in plasma osmolality. The plasma concentration of sodium and potassium also generally increases, suggesting that replacement of these electrolytes during exercise may not be necessary.

When the exercise duration is very prolonged and when excessively large volumes of low-sodium drinks (such as plain water or cola drinks) are taken during exercise, hyponatraemia has been reported to occur. Hyperthermia and hypernatraemia associated with dehydration are commonly encountered in athletes requiring medical attention at the end of long-distance races, and the symptoms usually resolve on treatment with oral rehydration solutions. Intravenous rehydration with saline, and sometimes with added glucose, is commonly used at some marathon medical facilities, but there is little evidence that this is generally more effective than the oral route. However, it has become clear that a small number of individuals at the end of very prolonged events may be suffering from hyponatraemia in conjunction with either hyperhydration (Noakes et al. 1985, 1990) or dehydration (Hiller 1989). All the reported cases have been associated with ultramarathon or prolonged triathlon events. Most of the cases have occurred in events lasting in excess of eight hours, and there are few reports of cases where the exercise duration is less than four hours. Noakes et al. (1985) reported four cases of exercise-induced hyponatraemia; race times were between seven and ten hours, and post-race serum sodium concentrations were 115–125 mmol/L. Estimated fluid intakes were 6–12 L, and consisted of water or drinks containing low levels of electrolytes. Estimated total sodium chloride intake during the race was 20–40 mmol. Frizell et al. (1986) reported even more astonishing fluid intakes of 20–24 L of fluids (an intake of almost 2.5 L/h sustained for a period of many hours, which is in excess of the maximum gastric emptying rate that has been reported) with a mean sodium content of only 5–10 mmol/L in two runners who collapsed after an ultramarathon run and who were found to be hyponatraemic (serum sodium concentration 118–123 mmol/L). These reports indicate that some supplementation with sodium salts may be required in extremely prolonged events where large sweat losses can be expected and where it is possible to consume large volumes of fluid. They also suggest that medical staff should be alert to the possibility of hyponatraemia occurring in this situation, but this should not divert attention from the fact that most competitors will be hypohydrated and hypernatraemic.

14.4.2 *Fluid replacement and exercise performance*

Most of the early studies carried out to investigate the effects of dehydration and rehydration on exercise in a military setting used very prolonged walking exercise as an experimental model and water as the fluid replacement. More recent studies have used a variety of exercise models more relevant to competitive sports situations, and most have investigated the effects of CHO–electrolyte drinks rather than of plain water. There have, however, been a few studies where the effects of plain water or of CHO-free electrolyte solutions have been investigated. In prolonged exercise at low intensity, water may be as effective as dilute saline solutions (Barr et al. 1991) or nutrient–electrolyte solutions (Levine et al. 1991) in maintaining cardiovascular and thermoregulatory function. Maughan et al. (1996) had 12 male subjects exercise to fatigue at about 70% of VO_2 max on four occasions after appropriate familiarisation tests. When subjects ingested plain water (100 mL every 10 minutes) median exercise time was longer (93 minutes) than when no drink was given (81 minutes). Subjects also completed trials where dilute CHO–electrolyte drinks were given and these also extended exercise time compared to the no-drink trial. In a prolonged (90 minute) intermittent high-intensity shuttle running test designed to simulate the demands of competitive soccer, McGregor et al. (1999) found that ingestion of flavoured water (5 mL/kg before the test and 2 mL/kg at 15-minute intervals) was effective in preventing a decline in performance of a soccer-specific skilled task. When no fluid was given, performance deteriorated.

It is clear that the addition of CHO has a number of potential benefits, including a reduction in the rate of decline of muscle glycogen concentration, which may be important for performance. The separate effects of providing fluid and CHO were investigated by Below et al. (1995), who used an experimental model where subjects performed 50 minutes of exercise at about 80% of VO_2 max followed by a time trial where a set amount of work had to be completed as fast as possible. During the initial 50 minutes of exercise, subjects were given either a small volume (200 mL) of water, a small volume of water with added CHO (40% solution, 79 g of maltodextrin), a large volume (1330 mL) of flavoured water, or a large volume of water with the same amount of CHO as in the other CHO trial (as a 6% solution). They found water ingestion to be effective in improving performance; exercise time was 11.34 minutes on the placebo trial and 10.51 minutes on the water trial. Exercise time on the CHO trial was 10.55 minutes, indicating that CHO provision during exercise acted independently to improve performance, and the effects were found to be additive, with the shortest time (9.93 minutes) when the 6% CHO drink was given.

The results of these and other studies (see Maughan and Shirreffs (1998) for a review) suggest that fluid replacement is effective in improving exercise performance in a variety of different situations, and that an additional benefit is gained by the addition of CHO, and possibly also of electrolytes, to fluids ingested during exercise. The optimum formulation of drinks for use in different exercise situations has not, however, been clearly established at the present time.

14.5 GUIDELINES FOR REPLACING FLUID AND CHO DURING EXERCISE

The major components of the sports drink that can be manipulated to alter its functional properties are shown in Table 14.2. To some extent these factors can be manipulated independently, although addition of increasing amounts of CHO or electrolyte will generally be accompanied by an increase in osmolality, and alterations in the solute content will have an impact on taste characteristics, mouth feel and palatability.

Table 14.2 *Variables that can be manipulated to alter the functional characteristics of a sports drink*

CHO concentration
Type of CHO
Osmolality
Electrolyte composition and concentration
Flavouring components
Other active ingredients

As well as providing an energy substrate for the working muscles, the addition of CHO to ingested drinks will promote water absorption in the small intestine, provided the concentration is not too high. Because of the role of sugars and sodium in promoting water uptake in the small intestine, it is sometimes difficult to separate the effects of water replacement from those of substrate and electrolyte replacement when CHO–electrolyte solutions are ingested. Below et al. (1995) have shown that ingestion of CHO and water had separate and additive effects on exercise performance, and concluded that ingestion of dilute CHO solutions would optimise performance. Most reviews of the available literature have come to the same conclusion (Lamb & Brodowicz 1986; Murray 1987; Coyle & Hamilton 1990; Maughan & Shirreffs 1998).

14.5.1 CHO content

The optimum concentration of CHO to be added to a sports drink will depend on individual circumstances. High CHO concentrations will delay gastric emptying, thus reducing the amount of fluid that is available for absorption, but will increase the rate of CHO delivery. If the concentration is high enough to result in a markedly hypertonic solution, net secretion of water into the intestine will result, and this will actually increase the danger of dehydration. High concentrations of sugars (> 10%) may also result in gastrointestinal disturbances (Davis et al. 1988). Where the primary need is to supply an energy source during exercise, increasing the sugar content of drinks will increase the delivery of CHO to the site of absorption in the small intestine. Beyond a certain limit, however, simply increasing CHO intake will not continue to increase the rate of oxidation of exogenous CHO

(Wagenmakers et al. 1993). Dilute glucose–electrolyte solutions may also be as effective, or even more effective, in improving performance as more concentrated solutions (Davis et al. 1988), and adding as little as 90 mmol/L (about 16 g/L) glucose may improve endurance performance (Maughan et al. 1996).

The consequences of severe dehydration and hyperthermia are potentially fatal, but the symptoms of CHO depletion are usually nothing more than severe fatigue. It seems sensible, therefore, to favour more dilute solutions, especially when training or competing in warm weather.

14.5.2 *Osmolality*

It has become common to refer to CHO–electrolyte sports drinks as isotonic drinks, as though the tonicity was their most important characteristic. The osmolality of ingested fluids is important as this can influence both the rates of gastric emptying and of intestinal water flux: both of these processes together will determine the effectiveness of rehydration fluids at delivering water for rehydration and substrate for oxidation (Schedl et al. 1994). Ingestion of strongly hypertonic drinks will promote net secretion of water into the intestine, and, although this effect is transient, it will result in a temporary exacerbation of the extent of dehydration. The composition of the drinks and the nature of the solutes is, however, of greater importance than the osmolality itself (Maughan 1994).

Osmolality is identified as an important factor influencing the rate of gastric emptying of liquid meals, but there seems to be rather little effect of variations in the concentration of electrolytes on the emptying rate, even when this substantially changes the test meal osmolality (Rehrer 1990). The effect of increasing osmolality seems to be important only when nutrient-containing solutions are examined, and energy density is undoubtedly the most significant factor influencing the rate of gastric emptying (Brener et al. 1983; Vist & Maughan 1994). There is some evidence that substitution of glucose polymers for free glucose, which will result in a decreased osmolality for the same CHO content, may be effective in increasing the volume of fluid and the amount of substrate delivered to the intestine. This is one reason for the inclusion of glucose polymers of varying chain length in the formulation of sports drinks. Vist and Maughan (1995) have shown that there is an acceleration of emptying when glucose polymer solutions are substituted for free glucose solutions with the same energy density. At low (about 40 g/L) concentrations, this effect is small, but it becomes appreciable at higher (180 g/L) concentrations; where the osmolality is the same (as in the 40 g/L glucose solution and 180 g/L polymer solution), the energy density is of far greater significance in determining the rate of gastric emptying. This effect may therefore be important when large amounts of energy must be replaced after exercise, but is unlikely to be a major factor during exercise where more dilute drinks are taken.

Water absorption occurs largely in the proximal segment of the small intestine, and, although water movement is itself a passive process driven by local osmotic gradients, it is closely linked to the active transport of solute (Schedl et al. 1994). Net flux is determined largely by the osmotic gradient between the luminal contents and intracellular fluid of the cells lining the intestine. Absorption of glucose is an active, energy-consuming process linked to the transport of sodium. The rate of glucose uptake is dependent on the luminal concentrations of glucose and sodium, and dilute glucose–electrolyte solutions with an osmolality which is slightly hypotonic with respect to plasma will maximise the rate of water uptake (Wapnir & Lifshitz 1985). Solutions with a very high glucose concentration will not necessarily promote an increased glucose uptake relative to more dilute solutions, but, because of their high osmolality, will cause a net movement of fluid into the intestinal lumen (Gisolfi et al. 1990). This results in an effective loss of body water and will exacerbate any pre-existing dehydration. Other sugars, such as sucrose (Spiller et al. 1982) or glucose polymers (Jones et al. 1983, 1987) can be substituted for glucose without impairing glucose or water uptake, and may help by increasing the total transportable substrate without increasing osmolality. In contrast, iso-energetic solutions of fructose and glucose are isosmotic, and the absorption of fructose is not an active process in humans: it is absorbed less rapidly than glucose and promotes less water uptake (Fordtran 1975). The use of different sugars which are absorbed by different mechanisms and which might thus promote increased water uptake is supported by recent evidence from an intestinal perfusion study (Shi et al. 1995).

Although most of the popular sports drinks are formulated to have an osmolality close to that of body fluids (Maughan 1994), and are promoted as isotonic drinks, there is good evidence that hypotonic solutions are more effective when rapid rehydration is desired (Wapnir & Lifshitz 1985). Although it is argued that a higher osmolality is inevitable when adequate amounts of CHO are to be included in sports drinks, the optimum amount of CHO necessary to improve exercise performance has not been clearly established.

14.5.3   *Electrolyte composition and concentration*

The available evidence indicates that the only electrolyte that should be added to drinks consumed during exercise is sodium, which is usually added in the form of sodium chloride (Maughan 1994). Sodium will stimulate sugar and water uptake in the small intestine and will help to maintain extracellular fluid volume. There is much debate as to the optimum sodium concentration, and it has been argued that equilibration occurs so rapidly in the upper part of the small intestine that addition of high concentrations of sodium is not necessary (Schedl et al. 1994). Although most soft drinks of the cola or lemonade variety contain virtually no sodium (1–2 mmol/L), sports drinks commonly contain about 10–30 mmol/L sodium, and oral rehydration solutions intended for use in the treatment of diarrhoea-induced dehydration, which may be fatal, have higher sodium concentrations, in the range 30–90 mmol/L. A high sodium content, although it may stimulate jejunal absorption of glucose and water, tends to make drinks unpalatable, and it is important that drinks intended for ingestion during or after exercise should have a pleasant taste in order to stimulate consumption. Specialist sports drinks are generally formulated to strike a balance between the twin aims of efficacy and palatability, although it must be admitted that not all achieve either of these aims.

14.5.4 *Taste*

Taste is an important factor influencing the consumption of fluids, and the choice of anion to accompany sodium may be important in this regard. The thirst mechanism is rather insensitive and will not stimulate drinking behaviour until some degree of dehydration has been incurred (Hubbard et al. 1990). This absence of a drive to drink is reflected in the rather small volumes of fluid that are typically consumed during exercise. In endurance running events, voluntary intake seldom exceeds about 0.5 L/h (Noakes 1993), and seems to be largely unrelated to the sweating rate. Because the sweat losses normally exceed this, even in cool conditions, a fluid deficit is almost inevitable whenever prolonged exercise is performed. Anything that stimulates drinking behaviour is therefore likely to be advantageous, and palatability is clearly important. Several factors will influence palatability, and the addition of a variety of flavours has been shown to increase fluid intake relative to that ingested when only plain water is available. Hubbard et al. (1984) and Szlyk et al. (1989) found that the addition of flavourings resulted in an increased consumption (by about 50%) of fluid during prolonged exercise. More recently, Bar-Or and Wilk (1996) have shown that the fluid intake during exercise of children presented with a variety of flavoured drinks is very much influenced by taste preference: under the conditions of this study, sufficient fluid to offset sweat losses was ingested only when a grape-flavoured beverage was available. In many of these studies, the addition of CHOs and/or electrolytes accompanied the flavouring agent, and the results must be interpreted with some degree of caution.

Given the need to add electrolytes to fluids intended to maximise the effectiveness of rehydration, there are clearly palatability issues that influence the formulation. Effective post-exercise rehydration requires replacement of electrolyte losses as well as the ingestion of a volume of fluid in excess of the volume of sweat loss (Shirreffs et al. 1996) (see Chapter 15, Section 15.4.2). When sweat electrolyte losses are high, replacement with drinks with a high sodium content can result in an unpalatable product. This can be alleviated to a large degree by substituting other anions for the chloride that is normally added. The addition of CHO has a major impact on taste and mouth feel, and a variety of different sugars with different taste characteristics can be added.

14.6 *SUMMARY*

The intake of fluid and CHO offers benefits to the performance of a number of sports events and exercise activities. The effects of dehydration on performance are now well known, with the penalties ranging from subtle, but often important, decrements in performance at low levels of fluid deficit to the severe health risks associated with substantial fluid losses during exercise in the heat. Although evidence of the beneficial effects of CHO intake during exercise has existed for over 70 years, sports scientists are still to discover all the situations in which benefits occur and to explain the mechanisms involved. Optimal strategies for CHO and fluid intake during exercise are yet to be fine-tuned, and ultimately will be determined by practical issues such as the opportunity to eat or drink during an event, and gastrointestinal comfort.

14.7 *PRACTICE TIPS*

Michelle Minehan

Non-endurance sports: events of less than 30 minutes duration

Primary concern: minimal interference to competition

Recommendations:

1. Begin exercise in a well-hydrated condition.

2. Replace fluid losses as completely as possible between competition sessions.

- Athletes commonly approach competition in a hypohydrated condition as a result of failing to replace daily body fluid losses, or as a result of deliberate dehydration strategies which are undertaken to 'make weight' in weight-limited sports (see Chapter 8). Exercising in a hypohydrated condition increases the risk of thermal injury and may reduce performance.

- Fluid ingested during exercise of less than 30 minutes duration will not benefit performance, as it will not become available to the body within the time frame of the competition. However, the ingestion of fluid may offer some advantages such as to alleviate dry mouth and improve perceived exertion. Athletes must weigh up any perceived benefits of drinking during exercise against potential disadvantages such as increased body mass (BM) and having to slow down to drink.

- Athletes competing in tournament situations or multiple events should aim to rehydrate between sessions to avoid a progressive dehydration over the competition.

Events of 30–60 minutes duration

Primary concerns: fluid intake, some support for CHO provision

Recommendations:

1. Begin exercise in a well-hydrated condition.

2. Use a fluid replacement plan that has been practised in training; drink as much as is practical and comfortable in attempting to match sweat losses.

3. Use a beverage which is cool (15–20°C), palatable and provides CHO.

4. Ingest beverage regularly to maintain gastric volume and increase fluid availability.

5. Make the most of opportunities to drink within the confines of the sport.

6. Replace fluid losses as completely as possible between competition sessions.

- Theoretically, athletes should aim to drink enough to offset fluid losses. In practical terms, athletes should aim to drink as much as is comfortable and practical. Generally, athletes will tolerate 150–300 mL every 15–20 minutes. However, individuals vary enormously in their rates of gastric emptying, sweat loss and tolerance of fluid volume. Each athlete must devise an individualised drinking schedule that is the best compromise between minimising gastrointestinal discomfort and the time lost in taking a drink, while reducing fluid deficits. Fluid requirements can be estimated by having the athlete weigh themselves before and after exercise sessions (see Table 14.3). A fluid replacement plan can then be developed, and fine-tuned during training. With experimentation and practice, it is possible for athletes to train themselves to tolerate greater volumes and learn to drink at a rate that matches sweat losses as closely as possible. Hydration regimens should always be practised in training before trying them in competitive situations.

- The volume of fluid ingested is more important than the timing, however, drinking regularly will help to maintain a high rate of gastric emptying as fluids leave the stomach faster when gastric volume is high. It also makes sense to begin drinking early in competition to minimise dehydration rather than trying to reverse a severe deficit later in the event.

- A supplementary source of CHO during exercise has been shown to improve performance in some events of as little as one hour in duration. A general recommendation of 30–60 g CHO per hour is suggested. Most sports drinks contain 60–80 g/L, making these rates of CHO ingestion easy to achieve. Gastric emptying slows as the energy density and osmolality of the fluid increase but solutions of up to 8% CHO can generally be tolerated, especially if a high gastric volume is maintained. Beverages that contain more than 8% CHO are more likely to cause gastrointestinal distress.

- Sodium chloride replacement is not necessary in short exercise periods, however, the inclusion of sodium chloride in a sports drink may promote fluid retention in the extracellular compartment, help maintain the osmotic drive to drink and improve the palatability of the drink. Fluids will be consumed in greater amounts when they are palatable during exercise, are kept cool (15–20°C), are served in a user-friendly container and are readily accessible.

- Combinations of sucrose, glucose, fructose and maltodextrins are all acceptable forms of CHO for ingestion provided that fructose does not predominate.

- The rules and conditions of some sports place restrictions on the opportunity to drink. Each athlete needs to identify opportunities to drink and practise strategies to utilise each opportunity. Sports such as netball, basketball and soccer restrict fluid intake to breaks in play, and drinks can only be taken from the sidelines. Players need to practise getting to the sidelines and distributing water bottles quickly. Other codes of football allow additional fluid to be provided by trainers on the field. Trainers need to monitor players and ensure fluids are distributed to all players. Players must make the effort to look for trainers and communicate their fluid needs. Opportunities for fluid intake in team sports are reviewed by Burke and Hawley (1997). Athletes competing in individual sports need to practise skills such as drinking on the run and grabbing drinks from aid stations.

Table 14.3 *Quick method for determining sweat loss*

1. Weigh athletes before and after training in minimal clothing and after towel drying
2. Monitor volume of fluid consumed during training
3. Determine change in body mass before and after any toilet stops
4. Sweat loss (mL) = Change in body mass (g) + Fluid intake (mL) − Urine losses (g)

Endurance sports: events of 1–3 hours duration

Primary concerns: fluid replacement plus CHO provision

Recommendations:

1. Begin exercise in a well hydrated state.

2. Use a fluid replacement plan that has been practised in training; drink as much as is practical and comfortable in attempting to match sweat losses.

3. Choose a beverage that is cool (15–20°C), palatable and provides CHO.

4. Begin ingesting fluid early in the exercise and continue to ingest beverage regularly to maintain gastric volume and increase fluid availability.

5. Plan to consume 30–60 g CHO/hour of exercise.

6. Note the recommendations for CHO intake that have been discussed in the tips for events of 30–60 minutes duration. Some additional comments are provided below:

- Sports drinks are intended to cater for the masses and suit the average sports event. For some individuals in some situations it may be desirable to vary the standard sports drink formula. On occasions when CHO needs take priority over fluid needs (for example, in prolonged events carried out in cold conditions), a more concentrated solution might be useful. Alternatively, a more dilute preparation (for example, 4%) might be appropriate for exercise in extremely hot conditions when fluid needs are of greatest priority.

- Athletes use a variety of foods, fluids and gels during competition. Some provide a more concentrated source of CHO and will slow gastric emptying. However, solids can be desirable during prolonged competition as they increase the flavour options available, provide different textures and help to relieve hunger. Solids and gels also have the advantage of being a compact form of CHO, reducing the amount of sports drink an athlete must carry to enable refuelling. This is particularly useful for training sessions or events conducted without the support of handlers or an intricate network of aid stations. Table 14.4 describes various food and fluids, which may be used in competition.

Table 14.4 *Food and fluid choices for endurance events*

Description	Amount to provide 50 g CHO	Comments
Water		Does not assist with fuel needs, but may be drunk in addition to sports drinks or solid food to make up total fluid needs.
Sports drinks (5–8% CHO + electrolytes)	600–1000 mL	Best option for meeting fluid and CHO requirements simultaneously. Has a good taste profile to encourage voluntary intake. Provides small amounts of electrolytes.
Soft drink (11% CHO)	500 mL	May be more slowly absorbed due to CHO content. Negligible source of electrolytes. Provides alternative flavour during long events. Cola drinks provide a small amount of caffeine.
Fruit juices (8–12% CHO)	500 mL	May be more slowly absorbed due to CHO content. Negligible source of electrolytes. Possible risk of gastrointestinal upset if juice is high in fructose.
Sports gel (60–70% CHO)	1½–2 gels	Concentrated CHO source. Suitable for large fuel boost. Experiment to avoid gastrointestinal discomfort. Fluid requirements will need separate attention.

Description	Amount to provide 50 g CHO	Comments
Banana	2–3 medium	Solid foods, especially those containing fibre, may cause gastrointestinal concerns in some individuals, but may help to relieve hunger during long events. Several portions are needed to provide substantial amounts of CHO. Fluid needs will need separate attention.
Jelly beans	50 g	Compact CHO source. Large amounts may cause diarrhoea. Fluid needs will need separate attention.
Jam sandwich	2 thick slices + 4 teaspoons of jam	Avoid adding fat sources to sandwich (peanut butter, margarine). See comments for bananas.
Chocolate bar	1½ bars	Portable and well-liked snack. May help relieve hunger. High in fat therefore may be more slowly absorbed. Fluid needs will need separate attention.
Muesli bar	2 bars	Solid foods, especially those containing fibre, may cause gastrointestinal concerns in some individuals, but may help to relieve hunger during long events. Several bars are needed to provide substantial amounts of CHO, and some bars may be high in fat. Fluid needs will need separate attention.
Breakfast bar	1½ bars	Lower fat content than muesli bars. See other comments for muesli bars.
Sports bars	1–1½ bars	Compact source of CHO. Varying levels of fat. May have various herbal additives of unknown function.

Adapted from Burke L. In: Burke L, Deakin V, eds. Clinical Sports Nutrition. Sydney: McGraw-Hill, 1994:359–62

Events of greater than three hours duration

Primary concerns: fluid and CHO, with some attention to sodium losses

Recommendations:

1. Begin exercise in a well hydrated condition.

2. Use a fluid replacement plan that has been practised in training; drink as much as is practical and comfortable in attempting to match sweat losses.

3. Choose a beverage which is cool (15–20°C), palatable and provides CHO and sodium. It may be useful to change flavours to avoid 'flavour fatigue'.

4. Begin ingesting fluid early in the exercise and continue to ingest beverage regularly to maintain gastric volume and increase fluid availability.

5. Plan to consume 30–60 g CHO/hour of exercise, although larger amounts may be needed as the duration of exercise increases.

6. Plan for replacement of sodium losses. Sports drinks provide small but useful amounts of sodium chloride.

See comments on fluid and CHO intake above. Additional comments are provided below:

- Hyponatraemia is a possibility in ultra-endurance events. A beverage containing sodium chloride, such as a sports drink, should be considered. Athletes who use alternative CHO sources such as cola drinks, gels and fruit should recognise that these are low in sodium. Hence additional sources of sodium may be required.

Prolonged, skill-based sports (e.g. archery, golf)

Primary concerns: fluid plus CHO provision

Recommendations:

- Begin exercise in a well hydrated condition.

- Use a fluid replacement plan that has been practised in training; drink as much as is practical and comfortable in attempting to match sweat losses.

- Use a beverage which is cool (15–20°C) and palatable.

- Plan to consume CHO drinks or foods in amounts similar to usual daily intake or training practices.

- Sports such as archery, shooting and bowling can involve prolonged periods of competition, however, the aerobic requirements of the sport are quite low. Drinking a fluid that is cool and palatable will encourage fluid intake. The athlete will also need to consume CHO over the day's competition, using a variety of snacks and drinks that are enjoyable and practical to consume. Athletes need to plan fluid and fuel replacement strategies which suit competition schedules or rules.

REFERENCES

Adopo E, Perronet F, Massicote D, Brisson G, Hilaire-Marcel C. Respective oxidation of exogenous glucose and fructose given in the same drink during exercise. J Appl Physiol 1994;76:1014–19.

Ahlborg B, Bergstrom J, Brohult J, Ekelund L-G, Hultman E, Maschio G. Human muscle glycogen content and capacity for prolonged exercise after different diets. Forsvarsmedicin 1967;3:85–99.

American College of Sports Medicine. Position stand: exercise and fluid replacement. Med Sci Sports Exerc 1996;28:i–vii.

Armstrong LE, Costill DL, Fink WJ. Influence of diuretic-induced dehydration on competitive running performance. Med Sci Sports Exerc 1985;17:456–61

Bar-Or O, Wilk B. Water and electrolyte replenishment in the exercising child. Int J Sport Nutr 1996;6:93–9.

Barr, SI, Costill DL, Fink WJ. Fluid replacement during prolonged exercise: effects of water, saline or no fluid. Med Sci Sports Exerc 1991;23:811–17.

Below P, Mora-Rodriguez R, Gonzalez-Alonso J, Coyle EF. Fluid and carbohydrate ingestion independently improve performance during 1 h of intense cycling. Med Sci Sports Exerc 1995;27:200–10.

Bishop NC, Blannin AK, Robson PJ, Walsh NP, Gleeson M. The effects of carbohydrate supplementation on immune responses to a soccer-specific exercise protocol. J Sports Sci 1999;17:787–96.

Bosch AN, Dennis SC, Noakes TD. Influence of carbohydrate ingestion on fuel substrate turnover and oxidation during prolonged exercise. J Appl Physiol 1994;76:2364–72.

Brener W, Hendrix TR, McHugh PR. Regulation of the gastric emptying of glucose. Gastroenterol 1983;85:76–82.

Burke LM, Hawley JA. Fluid balance in team sports: guidelines for optimal practices. Sports Med 1997;24:38–54.

Carter JE, Gisolfi CV. Fluid replacement during and after exercise in the heat. Med Sci Sports Exerc 1989;21:532–9.

Coggan AR, Coyle EF. Effect of carbohydrate feedings during high-intensity exercise. J Appl Physiol 1988;65:1703–9

Coggan AR, Coyle EF. Carbohydrate ingestion during prolonged exercise: effects on metabolism and performance. Ex Sport Sci Rev 1991;19:1–40

Costill DL, Bennett A, Branam G, Eddy D. Glucose ingestion at rest and during prolonged exercise. J Appl Physiol 1973;34:764–9

Coyle EF. Fuels for sport performance. In: Lamb DR, Murray R, eds. Perspectives in exercise science and sports medicine. Vol 10: Optimising sport performance. Carmel: Benchmark Press, 1997:95–138.

Coyle EF. Timing and method of increased carbohydrate intake to cope with heavy training, competition and recovery. J Sports Sci 1991;9(suppl):1–40.

Coyle EF, Coggan AR, Hemmert MK, Ivy JL. Muscle glycogen utilization during strenuous exercise when fed carbohydrate. J Appl Physiol 1986;61:165–72.

Coyle EF, Hagberg JM, Hurley BF, Martin WH, Ehsani AH, Holloszy JO. Carbohydrate feeding during prolonged strenuous exercise can delay fatigue. J Appl Physiol 1983;55:230–5.

Coyle EF, Hamilton M. Fluid replacement during exercise: effects on physiological homeostasis and performance. In: Gisolfi CV, Lamb DR, eds. Perspectives in exercise science and sports medicine. Vol 3: Fluid homeostasis during exercise. Carmel: Benchmark Press, 1990:281–8.

Davis JM, Burgess WA, Slentz CA, Bartoli WA, Pate RR. Effects of ingesting 6% and 12% glucose/electrolyte beverages during prolonged intermittent cycling in the heat. Eur J Appl Physiol 1988;57:563–9.

Erickson MA, Schwartzkopf RJ, McKenzie RD. Effects of caffeine, fructose, and glucose ingestion on muscle glycogen utilisation during exercise. Med Sci Sports Exerc 1987;19:579–83.

Fordtran JS. Stimulation of active and passive sodium absorption by sugars in the human jejunum. J Clin Invest 1975;55:728–37

Frizell RT, Lang GH, Lowance DC, Lathan SR. Hyponatraemia and ultramarathon running. JAMA 1986;255:772–4.

Galloway SD, Maughan RJ. Effects of ambient temperature on the capacity to perform cycle exercise in man. Med Sci Sports Exerc 1997;29:1240–9.

Gisolfi CV, Summers RW, Schedl HP. Intestinal absorption of fluids during rest and exercise. In: CV Gisolfi, Lamb DR, eds. Perspectives in exercise science and sports medicine. Vol 3: Fluid homeostasis during exercise. Carmel: Benchmark Press, 1990:129–80.

Gonzalez-Alonso J, Teller C, Andersen CL, Jensen FB, Hyldig T, Nielsen B. Influence of body temperature on the development of fatigue during prolonged exercise in the heat. J Appl Physiol 1999;86:1032–9.

Gordon B, Cohn LA, Levine SA, Matton M, Scriver WDM, Whiting WB. Sugar content of the blood in runners following a marathon race. JAMA 1925;185:508–9.

Hargreaves M, Briggs CA. Effect of carbohydrate ingestion on exercise metabolism. J Appl Physiol 1988;65:1553–5.

Hargreaves M, Costill DL, Coggan A, Fink WJ, Nishibata I. Effect of carbohydrate feedings on muscle glycogen utilisation and exercise performance. Med Sci Sports Exerc 1984;16:219–22.

Hawley JA, Dennis SC, Noakes TD. Oxidation of carbohydrate ingested during prolonged endurance exercise. Sports Med 1992;14:27–42.

Hermansen L, Hultman E, Saltin B. Muscle glycogen during prolonged severe exercise. Acta Physiol Scand 1967;71:129–39.

Hiller WDB. Dehydration and hyponatraemia during triathlons. Med Sci Sports Exerc 1989;21:S219–S21.

Hubbard RW, Sandick BL, Matthew WT, et al. Voluntary dehydration and alliesthesia for water. J Appl Physiol 1984;57:868–75.

Hubbard RW, Szlyk PC, Armstrong LE. Influence of thirst and fluid palatability on fluid ingestion during exercise. In: Gisolfi CV, Lamb DR, eds. Perspectives in exercise science and sports medicine. Vol 3: Fluid homeostasis during exercise. Carmel: Benchmark Press, 1990:39–95.

Hultman E, Nilsson LH. Liver glycogen in man: effect of different diets and muscular exercise. Adv Exp Biol Med 1971;11:143–51

Ivy J, Costill DL, Fink WJ, Lower RW. Influence of caffeine and carbohydrate feedings on endurance performance. Med Sci Sports Exerc 1979;11:6–11.

Jeukendrup A, Brouns F, Wagenmakers AJM, Saris WHM. Carbohydrate–electrolyte feedings improve 1 h time trial performance. Int J Sports Med 1997;18:125–9.

Jones BJM, Brown BE, Loran JS, Edgerton D, Kennedy JF. Glucose absorption from starch hydrolysates in the human jejunum. Gut 1983;24:1152–60.

Jones BJM, Higgins BE, Silk DBA. Glucose absorption from maltotriose and glucose oligomers in the human jejunum. Clin Sci 1987;72:409–14.

Karlsson J, Saltin B. Diet, muscle glycogen and endurance performance. J Appl Physiol 1971;31:203–6.

Kuo C-K, Hunt DG, Ding Z, Ivy JL. Effect of carbohydrate supplementation on post-exercise GLUT-4 protein expression in skeletal muscle. J Appl Physiol 1999;87:2290–6.

Lamb DR, Brodowicz GR. Optimal use of fluids of varying formulations to minimize exercise-induced disturbances in homeostasis. Sports Med 1986;3:247–74.

Levine L, Rose MS, Francesconi RP, Neufer PD, Sawka MN. Fluid replacement during sustained activity: nutrient solution vs. water. Aviat Space Env Med 1991;62:559–64.

Levine SA, Gordon B, Derick CL. Some changes in the chemical constituents of the blood following a marathon race. JAMA 1924;82:1778–9.

McConnell G, Fabris S, Proietto J, Hargreaves M. Effect of carbohydrate ingestion on glucose kinetics during exercise. J Appl Physiol 1994;77:1537–41.

McConell G, Kloot K, Hargreaves M. Effect of timing of carbohydrate ingestion on endurance exercise performance. Med Sci Sports Exerc 1996;28:1300–4

McGregor SJ, Nicholas CW, Lakomy HKA, Williams C. The influence of intermittent high-intensity shuttle running and fluid ingestion on the performance of a soccer skill. J Sports Sci 1999;17:895–903.

Massicotte D, Péronnet F, Brisson G, Bakkouch K, Hilaire-Marcel C. Oxidation of a glucose polymer during exercise: comparison with glucose and fructose. J Appl Physiol 1989;66:179–83.

Maughan RJ. Thermoregulation and fluid balance in marathon competition at low ambient temperature. Int J Sports Med 1985;6:15–19.

Maughan RJ, Fenn CE, Gleeson M, Leiper JB. Metabolic and circulatory responses to the ingestion of glucose polymer and glucose/electrolyte solutions during exercise in man. Eur J Appl Physiol 1987;56:356–62.

Maughan RJ, Fenn CE, Leiper JB. Effects of fluid, electrolyte and substrate ingestion on endurance capacity. Eur J Appl Physiol 1989;58:481–6.

Maughan RJ. Fluid and electrolyte loss and replacement in exercise. In: Harries M, Williams C, Stanish WD, Micheli LL, eds. Oxford textbook of sports medicine. Oxford: Oxford University Press, 1994:82–93.

Maughan RJ, Bethell L, Leiper JB. Effects of ingested fluids on homeostasis and exercise performance in man. Exp Physiol 1996;81:847–59.

Maughan RJ, Shirreffs SM. Fluid and electrolyte loss and replacement in exercise. In: Harries M, Williams C, Stanish WD, Micheli LL, eds. Oxford textbook of sports medicine, 2nd edn. New York: Oxford university Press, 1998:97–113.

Mitchell JB, Costill DL, Houmard JA, Flynn MG, Fink WJ, Beltz JD. Effects of carbohydrate ingestion on gastric emptying and exercise performance. Med Sci Sports Exerc 1988;20:110–15.

Montain SJ, Coyle EF. Influence of graded dehydration on hyperthermia and cardiovascular drift during exercise. J Appl Physiol 1992a;73:1340–50.

Montain SJ, Coyle EF. Fluid ingestion during exercise increases skin blood flow independent of increases in blood volume. J Appl Physiol 1992b;73:903–10.

Murray, R. The effects of consuming carbohydrate–electrolyte beverages on gastric emptying and fluid absorption during and following exercise. Sports Med 1987;4:322–51.

Murray R, Eddy DE, Murray TW, Seifert JG, Paul GL, Halaby GA. The effect of fluid and carbohydrate feedings during intermittent cycling exercise. Med Sci Sports Exerc 1987;19:597–604.

Murray R, Seifert JG, Eddy DE, Halaby GA. Carbohydrate feeding and exercise: effect of beverage carbohydrate content. Eur J Appl Physiol 1989;59:152–8.

Nadel ER, Mack GW, Nose H. Influence of fluid replacement beverages on body fluid homeostasis during exercise and recovery. In: Gisolfi CV, Lamb DR, eds. Perspectives in exercise science and sports medicine. Vol 3: Fluid homeostasis during exercise. Carmel: Benchmark Press, 1990:181–5.

Nielsen B, Hales JRS, Strange S, Christensen NJ, Warberg J, Saltin B. Human circulatory and thermoregulatory adaptations with heat acclimation and exercise in a hot, dry environment. J Physiol 1993;460:467–86.

Nielsen B, Kubica R, Bonnesen A, Rasmussen IB, Stoklosa J, Wilk B. Physical work capacity after dehydration and hyperthermia. Scand J of Sports Sci 1982;3:2–10.

Nieman DC, Henson DA, Garner EB, et al. Carbohydrate affects natural killer cell redistribution but not function after running. Med Sci Sports Exerc 1997;29:1318–24.

Nieman DC, Pedersen BK. Exercise and immune function: recent developments. Sports Med 1999;27:73–80.

Noakes TD. The dehydration myth and carbohydrate replacement during prolonged exercise. Cycling Science 1990;1:23–9.

Noakes, TD. Fluid replacement during exercise. In: Holloszy JO, ed. Exercise and sports science reviews. Vol 21. Baltimore: Williams & Wilkins. 1993:297–330.

Noakes TD, Goodwin N, Rayner BL, Branken T, Taylor RKN. Water intoxication: a possible complication during endurance exercise. Med Sci Sports Exerc 1985;17:370–5.

Noakes TD, Norman RJ, Buck RH, Godlonton J, Stevenson K, Pittaway D. The incidence of hyponatraemia during prolonged ultraendurance exercise. Med Sci Sports Exerc 1990;22:165–70.

Parkin JM, Carey MF, Zhao S, Febbraio MA. Effect of ambient temperature on human skeletal muscle metabolism during fatiguing submaximal exercise. J Appl Physiol 1999;86:902–8.

Pirnay F, Crielaard JM, Pallikarakis N, et al. Fate of exogenous glucose during exercise of different intensities in humans. J Appl Physiol 1982;53:1620–4.

Rehrer NJ. Limits to fluid availability during exercise. De Vriesebosch: Haarlem, 1990.

Rehrer NJ, Burke LM. Sweat losses during various sports. Aust J Nutr Diet 1996;53:S13–S16.

Rehrer NJ, Wagenmakers AJM, Beckers EJ, et al. Limits to liquid carbohydrate supplementation during exercise: gastric emptying, intestinal absorption and oxidation. J Appl Physiol 1992;72:468–75.

Rowell LB. Human Circulation. New York: Oxford University Press, 1986.

Saltin B, Costill DL. Fluid and electrolyte balance during prolonged exercise. In: Horton ES, Terjung RL, eds. Exercise, Nutrition, and Metabolism. New York: Macmillan, 1988:150–8.

Saris WHM, van Erp-Baart MA, Brouns F, Westerterp KR, ten Hoor F. Study on food intake and energy expenditure during extreme sustained exercise: the Tour de France. Int J Sports Med 1989;10:S26–S31.

Sasaki H, Maeda J, Usui S, Ishiko T. Effect of sucrose and caffeine ingestion on performance of prolonged strenuous running. Int J Sports Med 1987;8:261–5.

Schedl HP, Maughan RJ, Gisolfi CV. Intestinal absorption during rest and exercise: implications for formulating oral rehydration beverages. Med Sci Sports Exerc 1994;26:267–80.

Shephard RJ. Physical activity, training, and the immune response. Carmel: Cooper Publishing, 1997.

Shi X, Summers RW, Schedl HP. Effect of carbohydrate type and concentration and solution osmolality on water absorption. J Appl Physiol 1995;27:1607–15.

Shirreffs SM, Taylor AJ, Leiper JB, Maughan RJ. Post-exercise rehydration in man: effects of volume consumed and sodium content of ingested fluids. Med Sci Sports Exerc 1996;28:1260–71.

Spiller RC, Jones BJM, Brown BE, Silk DBA. Enhancement of carbohydrate absorption by the addition of sucrose to enteric diets. J Parent Ent Nut 1982;6:321.

Stafford-Millard M, Rosskopf LB, Snow TK, Hinson BT. Water versus carbohydrate–electrolyte ingestion before and during a 15 km run in the heat. Int J Sport Nutr 1997;7:26–38.

Szlyk PC, Sils IV, Francesconi RP, Hubbard RW, Armstrong LE. Effects of water temperature and flavoring on voluntary dehydration in men. Physiol Behav 1989;45:639–47.

Thom W. Pedestrianism, or an account of the performance of celebrated pedestrians. Aberdeen: Chalmers, 1813.

Tsintzas OK, Liu R, Williams C, Campbell I, Gaitanos G. The effect of carbohydrate ingestion on performance during a 30 km race. Int J Sport Nutr 1993;3:127–39.

Vergauwen L, Brouns F, Hespel P. Carbohydrate supplementation improves stroke performance in tennis. Med Sci Sports Exerc 1998;30:1289–95.

Vist GE, Maughan RJ. The effect of increasing glucose concentration on the rate of gastric emptying in man. Med Sci Sports Exerc 1994;26:1269–73.

Vist GE, Maughan RJ. The effect of osmolality and carbohydrate content on the rate of gastric emptying of liquids in man. J Physiol 1995;486:523–31.

Wagenmakers AJM, Brouns F, Saris WH, Halliday D. Oxidation rates of orally ingested carbohydrates during prolonged exercise in men. J Appl Physiol 1993;75:2774–80.

Walsh RM, Noakes TD, Hawley JA, Dennis SC. Impaired high-intensity cycling performance time at low levels of dehydration. Int J Sports Med 1994;15:392–8.

Wapnir RA, Lifshitz F. Osmolality and solute concentration—their relationship with oral rehydration solution effectiveness: an experimental assessment. Pediatric Research 1985;19:894–8.

Williams C. Diet and endurance fitness. Am J Clin Nutr 1989;49:1077–83.

Williams C. Diet and sports performance. In: Harries M, Williams C, Stanish WD, Micheli LL, eds. Oxford textbook of sports medicine, 2nd edn. Oxford: Oxford University Press, 1998:77–97.

Williams C, Nute MG, Broadbank L, Vinall S. Influence of fluid intake on endurance running performance: a comparison between water, glucose and fructose solutions. Eur J Appl Physiol 1990;60:112–19.

Zeederberg C, Leach L, Lambert EV, Noakes TD, Dennis SC, Hawley JA. The effect of carbohydrate ingestion on the motor skill of soccer players. Int J Sport Nutr 1996;6:348–55.

CHAPTER 15

Nutrition for recovery after competition and training

Louise Burke

15.1 INTRODUCTION

Recovery after exercise poses an important challenge to the modern athlete. Athletes commonly undertake strenuous training programs involving one or more prolonged high-intensity exercise sessions each day, typically allowing 6–24 hours for recovery between workouts. In some sports, competition is conducted as a series of events or stages. In sports such as swimming or track and field, athletes are scheduled to compete in a number of brief races, or in a series involving heats, semi-finals and finals, often performing more than once each day. In tennis and team-sport tournaments, or cycle stage races, competitors may be required to undertake one or more lengthy events each day, with the competition extending for one to three weeks. Even where athletes compete in a weekly fixture, optimal recovery is desired to allow the athlete to train between matches or races.

Recovery involves a complex array of desirable processes of adaptation to physiological stress. In the training situation, with correct planning of the workload and the recovery time, adaptation allows the body to become fitter, stronger or faster. In the competition scenario, however, there may be less control over the work to recovery ratio. A simpler but more realistic goal for the athlete may be to face the next opponent, or the next round or stage in a competition, as well prepared as possible.

Recovery encompasses a complex range of nutrition-related issues including:

a. restoration of muscle and liver glycogen stores;
b. replacement of fluid and electrolytes lost in sweat;
c. regeneration, repair and adaptation processes following the catabolic stress and damage caused by the exercise.

This last issue remains somewhat nebulous and involves many processes ranging from protein synthesis to the activities of the immune and antioxidant defence systems. This chapter will focus on the more well-defined and well-studied issues of restoration of fluid balance and glycogen stores, summarising the current guidelines on strategies for post-exercise fluid and food intake to enhance these processes. Discussion of issues related to post-exercise protein metabolism and recovery are provided in Chapter 5. While this review and the resulting guidelines will focus on fluid and carbohydrate (CHO) goals, some attention should be paid to the simultaneous intake of other nutrients. Future research may elucidate how the quantity and timing of intake of protein and some micronutrients may be crucial in promoting optimal function of the repair and adaptation processes.

In many situations, optimal recovery after training or competition will only occur with a specially organised nutrition plan. After all, thirst and voluntary fluid intake are unlikely to keep pace with large sweat losses. In addition, typical Western eating patterns are unlikely to provide CHO intakes that reach the threshold of daily glycogen storage. These plans must be made in recognition of the practical factors that interfere with an athlete's post-exercise fluid and food intake plans (see Table 15.1). This is particularly important for the travelling athlete, who may be challenged by an inaccessible and foreign food supply. Special recognition of the needs of the travelling athlete is found in greater detail in Chapter 24.

Table 15.1 *Practical factors interfering with post-exercise fluid and food intake (Burke 1997)*

Fatigue—interfering with ability/interest to obtain or eat food
Loss of appetite following high-intensity exercise
Limited access to (suitable) foods at exercise venue
Other post-exercise commitments and priorities (e.g. coaches' meetings, drug tests, equipment maintenance, warm-down activities)
Traditional post-competition activities (e.g. excessive alcohol intake)

15.2 ISSUES IN POST-EXERCISE REFUELLING

The depletion of muscle glycogen provides a strong drive for its own resynthesis (Zachwieja et al. 1991). Muscle glycogen resynthesis takes precedence over restoration of liver glycogen, and even in the absence of a dietary supply of CHO after exercise it occurs at a low rate (1–2 mmol/kg wet weight (ww) of muscle per hour), with some of the substrate being provided through gluconeogenesis (Maehlum & Hermansen 1978). High-intensity exercise that results in high post-exercise levels of lactate appears to be associated with rapid recovery of glycogen stores in the absence of additional CHO feeding (Hermansen & Vaage 1977). After moderate-intensity exercise, muscle glycogen synthesis is dependent on provision of exogenous CHO. The rate of glycogen storage is affected by factors regulating glucose transport into the cell, such as the insulin- or exercise-stimulated translocation of GLUT-4 protein transporter to the muscle membrane (McCoy et al. 1996). It is also determined by factors regulating glucose disposal, such as the activity of glycogen synthase enzyme (Danforth 1965; McCoy et al. 1996). Changes in these factors are responsible for a biphasic muscle glycogen storage pattern, or a decline in glycogen storage rate over time (Ivy & Kuo 1998). Glycogen storage is impaired by damage to the muscle fibre such as that caused by eccentric exercise or direct contact injury (Costill et al. 1988, 1991).

Liver glycogen stores are more labile than muscle glycogen stores, and may be depleted by an overnight fast or by a prolonged bout of exercise. Strategies to enhance the restoration of liver glycogen stores have been less well studied due to practical problems in obtaining liver biopsy samples. Nevertheless, it is considered that liver glycogen is restored by a single CHO-rich meal, and that fructose ingestion may cause a greater rate of liver glycogen synthesis than glucose intake (Blom et al. 1987).

Maximal rates of post-exercise muscle glycogen storage reported during the first 12 hours of recovery are within the range of 5–10 mmol/kg ww/h (Blom et al. 1987; Ivy et al. 1988a; Reed et al. 1989). Coyle (1991) has commented that with a mean glycogen storage rate of 5–6 mmol/kg ww/h, 20–24 hours of recovery are required for normalisation of muscle glycogen levels following exercise depletion. In real life the training and competition schedules of many athletes often provide considerably less time than this. Since performance in subsequent exercise sessions may depend on the success of muscle CHO restoration strategies, many athletes may compromise subsequent performance by beginning with inadequate muscle fuel stores. Several controllable factors can enhance or impair the rate of muscle glycogen storage (see Table 15.2). Some of these dietary factors will be discussed in greater detail in this chapter.

15.2.1 *Amount of CHO intake*

The most important dietary factor affecting muscle glycogen storage is the amount of CHO consumed. There is a direct relationship between the quantity of dietary CHO and post-exercise glycogen storage, at least until the muscle storage capacity or threshold has been reached. Costill and co-workers (1981) reported that incremental increases in CHO intake from 188 g through to 648 g per day resulted in increasing amounts of glycogen storage during 24 hours of recovery from prolonged exercise. However, a threshold seemed to occur at a CHO intake of between 525–648 g per 24 hours, approximately 7–9 g CHO/kg body mass (BM) of subjects. In terms of acute post-exercise recovery (e.g. zero to six hours post-exercise), Blom et al. (1987) reported that a glucose intake equal to 0.7 g/kg BM every two hours after a depletion trial produced a faster rate of muscle glycogen synthesis than an intake of 0.35 g/kg BM every two hours; however, the rate was not increased by a CHO intake of 1.4 g/kg BM every two hours. Ivy et al. (1988a) also described a glycogen storage threshold. They reported that an intake of 1.5 g CHO/kg BM at

| **Table 15.2** | *Factors affecting restoration of muscle glycogen stores* |

Factors that enhance the rate of restoration
- Depleted stores—the lower the stores, the faster the rate of recovery
- Immediate intake of CHO after exercise
- Adequate amounts of CHO:
  - 1–1.5 g CHO/kg body mass, immediately after exercise
    7–10 g CHO/kg body mass, per 24 hours
  - Focus on CHO-rich foods with a high–glycaemic index

Factors that have minimal effect on rate of restoration
- Gentle exercise during recovery
- Spacing of meals and snacks (provided total amount of CHO is adequate)
- Other food at meals (e.g. fat- or protein-rich foods) provided that total amount of CHO is adequate

Factors that reduce the rate of restoration
- Damage to the muscle (contact injury or delayed-onset muscle-soreness caused by eccentric exercise)
- Delay in intake of CHO after exercise
- Inadequate amounts of CHO
- Reliance on CHO-rich foods with a low–glycaemic index
- Prolonged and high-intensity exercise during recovery

two-hourly intervals resulted in similar glycogen storage in depleted muscles during four hours of recovery as an intake of 3.0 g/kg BM every two hours.

Taken together, it appears that the optimal rate of glycogen storage is achieved when 0.7–1.0 g of CHO is consumed every two hours in the early stages of recovery, leading to a total CHO intake of 7–10 g/kg BM over 24 hours (Costill 1988; Coyle 1991). These figures form the basis of CHO intake guidelines for athletes who desire to optimise muscle glycogen recovery within a busy training or competition schedule. However, total CHO intake recommendations or requirements may be higher in some situations. For example, athletes who undertake strenuous daily competition may need to meet the fuel requirements of their continued exercise in addition to post-exercise recovery needs. In the Tour de France, cyclists riding at least six hours each day have been reported to consume 12–13 g CHO/kg BM/d (Saris et al. 1989). In fact, the ingestion of substantial amounts of CHO during low- to moderate-intensity exercise has been reported to increase net glycogen storage during the session, particularly within non-active muscle fibres that have been previously depleted (Kuipers et al. 1987). Increased CHO intake may also be useful in the case of muscle damage (e.g. following eccentric exercise), which typically impairs the rate of post-exercise glycogen resynthesis. Costill et al. (1990) reported that low rates of glycogen restoration in damaged muscles may be partially overcome by increased CHO intake during the first 24 hours of recovery.

15.2.2 *Timing of CHO intake*

Storage of glycogen is rapid during the first 24 hours of recovery, followed by a slower rate of synthesis thereafter. The highest storage rates occur during the first few hours post-exercise. In addition to the activation of glycogen synthase, early post-exercise recovery is marked by an exercise-induced permeability of the muscle cell membrane to glucose and increased muscle insulin sensitivity. CHO feeding during these early stages appears to accentuate these effects by increasing blood glucose and insulin concentrations. Ivy et al. (1988b) reported that the immediate intake of CHO after prolonged exercise resulted in higher rates of glycogen storage (7.7 mmol/kg ww/h) during the first two hours of recovery, slowing thereafter to the more typical rates of storage (4.3 mmol/kg ww/h).

Although this study has been interpreted to highlight the significantly higher rates of glycogen synthesis in early recovery, it is unlikely that these differences (7.7 versus 4.3 mmol/kg ww/h) are of physiological importance. The most important finding of this study is that failure to consume CHO in the immediate phase of post-exercise recovery leads to very low rates of glycogen restoration until feeding occurs. Thus the importance of early intake of CHO following strenuous exercise is to avoid delaying the provision of substrate to the muscle cell, more than to take advantage of a period of moderately enhanced glycogen synthesis. This strategy is most important when there is only four to eight hours of recovery between exercise sessions, but may be of less impact when there is a longer recovery time (12 or more hours). For example, Parkin et al. investigated glycogen storage over eight hours and 24 hours of recovery when high-GI CHO meals were begun immediately after exercise, or delayed for two hours. They found no difference in glycogen restoration at either of these time points as a result of delaying the first CHO meal (Parkin et al. 1997). The results of these studies are summarised in Figure 15.1. Overall it appears that when the interval between exercise sessions is short, the athlete should maximise the effective recovery time by beginning CHO intake as soon as possible. However, when longer recovery periods are available, the athlete can choose their preferred meal schedule as long as total CHO intake goals are achieved. It is not always practical or enjoyable to consume substantial meals or snacks immediately after a strenuous workout.

Whether CHO is best consumed in large meals or as a series of snacks has also been studied. Studies by Costill and co-workers (1981) and our own group have reported that as long as total CHO is adequate, long-term (24-hour) recovery of muscle glycogen synthesis appears unaffected by the frequency of intake. Muscle glycogen storage over 24 hours was similar when 525 g of CHO was fed as two meals or seven meals (Costill et al. 1981), and when 10 g CHO/kg BM was consumed as four large meals or 16 hourly snacks (Burke et al. 1996). Similar muscle glycogen storage was achieved despite marked differences in blood glucose and insulin profiles over 24 hours (Burke et al. 1996). By contrast, Doyle et al. (1993) reported very high rates of glycogen synthesis during four hours of recovery when a high intake of CHO was fed at 15-minute intervals, and suggested that higher, sustained

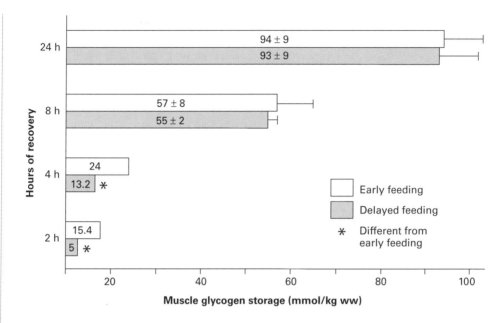

Figure 15.1 *Effect of delaying the post-exercise snack or meal on restoration of muscle glycogen. Immediate intake of CHO increases effective recovery time, and permits greater glycogen storage when recovery period is < 8 hours (* = p < 0.05), than when first meal is delayed for 2 hours. This strategy is less important when longer recovery time is available. Data taken from Ivy et al. 1988 and Parkin et al. 1997*

insulin and glucose profiles were responsible for this effect. However, these rates were compared with literature values of post-exercise glycogen restoration and were not tested against a control amount of CHO fed in less frequent meals. It is possible that enhanced insulin and glucose concentrations permit greater glycogen storage during the first hours of recovery, or when total CHO intake is restricted. However, during longer periods of recovery, when total CHO intake is optimal and able to achieve threshold storage levels, manipulations of plasma substrates and hormones within physiological ranges do not add a further benefit.

In summary, it appears that meeting total CHO requirements is more important than the pattern of intake, and that the athlete is advised to choose a food schedule that is practical and comfortable. One benefit of small frequent meals may be in overcoming the gastric discomfort often associated with eating large amounts of bulky high-CHO foods.

15.2.3 *Type of CHO intake*

Different types of CHO and CHO foods appear to have different effects on muscle glycogen synthesis rates. Since glycogen storage is influenced by both insulin and a rapid supply of glucose substrate, it has been proposed that CHO sources of high GI might enhance post-exercise refuelling. Glucose and sucrose feedings after prolonged exercise have been reported to produce similar rates of muscle glycogen recovery, whereas the intake of fructose produces a lower rate of glycogen storage (Blom et al. 1987). However, such studies of single nutrient feedings of mono- or di-saccharides during zero to six hours of recovery do not deal with the more relevant issues of food intake and everyday nutrition goals.

Older studies of the type of CHO-rich foods and glycogen storage failed to find consistent results, most probably because they used the confusing 'simple' and 'complex' CHO classification to determine their food choices. For example, Costill and co-workers reported that a diet of simple CHOs (sucrose, glucose and fructose) was equal to a diet composed of complex CHOs (starchy foods) in restoring muscle glycogen levels 24 hours after glycogen depletion. However, after 48 hours the complex CHO diet resulted in greater muscle glycogen gains (Costill et al. 1981). Conversely, Roberts found that simple and complex CHO diets produced similar glycogen restoration following 72 hours of refuelling after exercise depletion (Roberts et al. 1988). Because both studies failed to measure glucose and insulin profiles, or to provide full description of the foods used in their recovery diets, it is difficult to judge the results critically. However, the use of structural classification of CHO-rich foods to determine meal choices is unlikely to guarantee that the diets were truly different in glycaemic response. Table 15.3 provides information about the GI of some CHO-rich foods. Kiens and colleagues (1990) appear to be the first to attempt to study CHO foods and muscle glycogen storage based on actual rather than assumed glycaemic responses. In a brief summary they reported that a high-CHO diet based on foods with a high GI produced greater storage of glycogen during six hours of recovery than a diet based on low-GI, CHO-rich foods (Kiens et al. 1990). However, at 20, 32 and 44 hours of recovery there were no differences in muscle glycogen levels between diets. Plasma insulin levels during the first six hours were greater with the high-GI diet, but glucose and insulin concentrations were similar at all other time points. Because of the absence of descriptions of the foods provided to subjects, and because the diets were described interchangeably as high GI/simple and complex/low GI, there is some confusion interpreting the results of this study (Kiens et al. 1990).

A more recent study from our group (Burke et al. 1993) supports the benefits of refuelling with high-GI, CHO-rich foods. We observed greater glycogen storage during 24 hours of recovery from a depletion trial when cyclists consumed a high-CHO diet based on high-GI sources, compared to glycogen storage following an identical amount of CHO eaten in the form of low-GI, CHO-rich foods (Burke et al. 1993). However, the magnitude of increase in glycogen storage (~30%) with the high-GI CHO trial was greater than the increase in 24-hour blood glucose and insulin concentrations. In other words, while the outcome of the study was as predicted, we were not able to completely explain these findings in terms of alteration of glucose and insulin responses.

Table 15.3 *The glycaemic index (GI) of foods and sugars*

High (GI > 85)	Moderate (GI = 60–85)	Low (GI < 60)
White bread	Pasta/noodles	Apples/pears
Wholemeal bread	Popcorn	Cherries
Nutrigrain™	Porridge	Peaches
Cornflakes™	Potato chips/crisps	Apple juice (unsweetened)
Weetbix™	Special K™	All-bran™
Potato	White rice (boiled)	Baked beans
Rockmelon	Sweetcorn	Lentils
Raisins	Sponge cake	Ice cream
Bananas	Oranges	Yoghurt
Cornchips	Orange juice	Fructose
Sugar (sucrose)	Chocolate	Brown rice (boiled)
Honey		Milk (all types)
Cordial/sports drinks		Peas, green
Glucose		Peanuts

Adapted from Foster-Powell and Brand Miller 1995, where white bread is standard reference food

We attempted to explore this issue further in another study involving the frequency of CHO intake (Burke et al. 1996). In this study we simulated the flattened glucose and insulin responses of a low-GI diet by feeding our original high-GI recovery diet in a 'nibbling' pattern. In other areas of nutrition research, a pattern of small frequent snacks has been used to mimic the delayed absorption of low-GI foods, and has been able to produce the metabolic advantages associated with low-GI diets (Jenkins et al. 1994). In our study, subjects received identical diets composed of high-GI CHO-rich foods during 24 hours of post-exercise recovery; on one occasion this was consumed in four large meals and on the other, as 16 small snacks. Despite marked difference in glucose and insulin responses over the 24-hour recovery period, there was no difference in glycogen storage between the 'nibbling' diet and the conventional high-GI meals ('gorging' trial) (Burke et al. 1996). It is possible that the diets may have caused different rates of glycogen storage in the early phases of recovery (zero to eight hours). Since a low glycogen level provides a stimulus for glycogen storage, a slower rate of synthesis in one diet during early recovery may have been masked by a faster catch-up phase during the later hours. Equally it is possible that both diets, providing 10 g CHO/kg BM/d, reached or exceeded the threshold for glycogen storage in our subjects. These data support the concept that when total CHO intake is adequate, manipulations of glucose and insulin levels within physiological ranges are not critical in long-term or daily glycogen storage. The importance of adequate CHO intake is further reinforced.

Thus the cause of the reduced glycogen storage with low-GI, CHO-rich foods is unclear, and may involve a combination of factors. Studies measuring the absorption of food by indirect methods (e.g. breath hydrogen methods) or direct techniques (ileostomy output in ileostomates) have reported that a considerable amount of the CHO in low-GI foods is not absorbed (Wolever et al. 1986; Jenkins et al. 1987). This may provide an additional mechanism to explain less efficient glycogen storage with some CHO-rich foods. Indeed, Joszi and co-workers (1996) commented that the poor digestibility of a high-amylose starch mixture (lower GI) provided a likely explanation for the lower muscle glycogen storage observed during 13 hours of recovery after exercise compared with glycogen storage during trials in which subjects consumed solutions of glucose, maltodextrins and a high-amylopectin starch (all high GI) (Joszi et al. 1996). They observed that indigestible CHO forms provide a poor substrate for muscle glycogen resynthesis and overestimate the available CHO consumed by subjects. This issue needs to be further studied in relation to real foods.

Nevertheless, data from a study of chronic exposure to a lower GI diet support the observations of the reduced muscle glycogen storage with low-GI, CHO-rich foods. This study from the laboratory of Kiens and Richter (1996) investigated the effect of 30 days of a high- or low-GI diet on insulin action and muscle substrates in recreationally active subjects. They found evidence of some adaptations over the duration of the trial; by the end of the period the initial differences in the daily profile of blood glucose and insulin concentrations between diets was diminished. However, muscle glycogen concentrations declined over the 30 days on the low-GI diet, so that at day 30 muscle stores were significantly reduced from pre-trial values and lower than at the completion of the high-GI trial (Kiens & Richter 1996). Further work is required to elucidate the mechanism of lower glycogen storage with low-GI foods and diets, and to confirm whether this occurs in the diets of free-living subjects.

Finally, a recent study by Piehl Aulin et al. (2000) found that post-exercise ingestion of a CHO solution containing glucose polymers was associated with greater glycogen storage over the first four hours of recovery than an isocaloric glucose solution. They suggested that the low osmolality of the drink led to greater gastric emptying rates and faster delivery of substrate to the depleted muscle. There were no differences in blood glucose and insulin profiles during the recovery period. However, it was postulated that if a greater delivery of glucose to the intestine were combined with a greater non-insulin dependent uptake of glucose in the early post-exercise period, true differences in glucose kinetics would be masked by apparently minor differences in blood glucose concentrations. This hypothesis merits further investigation, and may explain differences in glycogen storage from different types of CHO sources.

15.2.4 *Forms of CHO feeding*

Both solid and liquid forms of CHO appear to be equally efficient in providing substrate for muscle glycogen synthesis (Keizer et al. 1986; Reed et al. 1989). Practical issues such as compactness and appetite appeal may be important in choosing CHO foods and fluids to meet the athlete's total CHO intake goals. Liquid forms of CHO or CHO foods with a high fluid content may be particularly appealing to fatigued athletes.

15.2.5 *Infusion of CHO*

Intravenous (IV) delivery of CHO might be a practical way to ensure intake of recovery substrates when an athlete has impaired gastrointestinal function and/or limited time between workouts during which sleep and other activities compete with eating time. Such a situation can be found in events such as the Tour de France where competitors need to recover overnight to tackle stages lasting five to eight hours, and may finish each stage in a state of extreme fatigue and substantial dehydration. Certainly the expense and risks involved with CHO infusion mean that it might only be considered in extreme circumstances. Nevertheless, the mystique of IV feeding has led to ideas that it might provide a superior method of restoration, promoting faster and higher levels of glycogen storage compared with the oral intake of similar amounts of CHO. Several studies argue against this idea. Firstly, when oral CHO intake has been compared with infusion of matched amounts of CHO (i.e. infusion adjusted to match blood glucose concentrations achieved by eating CHO), it was observed that the IV feeding route produced significantly lower insulin concentrations. Despite this, rates of glycogen storage were similar between treatments (Blom et al. 1989).

Recently, Hansen et al. studied the effects of supraphysiological levels of blood glucose and insulin, achieved by infusions of both glucose and insulin (Hansen et al. 1999). IV delivery of glucose was undertaken to maintain glucose concentrations at ~20 mmol/L, while insulin infusion kept this hormone at its maximal effective concentration. After eight hours, muscle glycogen had risen to the levels normally associated with glycogen supercompensation. Therefore, it was concluded that infusion techniques can achieve glycogen storage at a faster rate. However, the IV feedings did not produce greater glycogen levels than that which could be achieved by dietary means, albeit over a longer time period. Most importantly, the study was terminated for ethical reasons after only two subjects completed it. Both became ill at the end of the study period, complaining of nausea and vomiting (Hansen et al. 1999). In summary, maximal provision of glucose and insulin via infusion can increase the rate of glycogen storage over a period of eight hours; however, similar total recovery can be achieved by dietary means given sufficient time, and with far less cost in terms of side-effects, risks and expense.

15.2.6 *Co-ingestion of other nutrients*

It is possible that the presence of other macronutrients in CHO foods, or simultaneously ingested at a meal, may influence muscle glycogen storage. While this hypothesis has not been systematically tested, it might be speculated that effects on digestion, insulin secretion or the satiety of meals are potentially important. For example, Zawadzki and co-workers (1992) reported that the co-ingestion of protein (40 g) with CHO feedings (112 g) every two hours increased the rate of muscle glycogen storage during four hours of recovery in glycogen-depleted subjects. An enhanced insulin response was suggested to explain this response, although other studies have shown that alterations in insulin response have not been associated with changes in muscle glycogen storage when total CHO intake was adequate (Burke et al. 1995). Unfortunately the Zawadzki study did not include an energy control; therefore it is unclear whether the addition of protein provided a special mechanism for enhanced glycogen synthesis, or whether supplementary energy or CHO would have achieved the same effect.

A more recent study by Roy et al. (1998) compared acute post-exercise storage of glycogen synthesis following CHO intake, an isocaloric protein and CHO combination, and a placebo feeding. There was no difference in glycogen storage between the CHO-only feeding and the CHO–protein feedings, but both treatments produced greater storage compared with the placebo.

Our laboratory has observed that the addition of fat (1.6 g/kg BM/d) and protein (1.2 g/kg BM/d) to a high-CHO diet (7 g/kg BM/d) did not alter muscle glycogen storage during 24 hours of recovery from strenuous exercise, despite alterations in glucose and insulin ratios (Burke et al. 1995). Since an isocaloric diet with additional CHO (12 g/kg BM/d) also failed to produce increased CHO storage, it appears that CHO intake in the first diet already reached the threshold of glycogen storage for our subjects. Thus it was concluded that the presence of other macronutrients does not alter muscle glycogen synthesis when total CHO intake is adequate. However, it was noted that the consumption of large amounts of protein and fat (particularly the latter) may displace CHO foods within the athlete's energy requirements and gastric comfort, thereby indirectly interfering with glycogen storage by promoting inadequate CHO intake.

15.3 *CHO INTAKE GUIDELINES FOR TRAINING AND RECOVERY*

Chapters 13, 14 and 15 summarise the abundant literature describing beneficial effects of CHO feeding strategies, singly or in combination, on the performance of a single exercise session. These results can be summarised into specific guidelines (see Table 15.4). Since the primary goal of CHO intake is to provide fuel for the working muscle, it makes sense to describe CHO needs relative to the BM of the athlete. While this does not entirely account for differences in the amount of muscle actively involved in an exercise task, it at least recognises the considerable variability in the body size of athletes—for example, the 45 kg marathon runner and the 100 kg football player (Burke et al. in press).

It has proved difficult to extrapolate these guidelines into recommendations for the everyday diet of the athlete. This is partly due to misunderstandings arising from the terminology used to describe CHO intake (Burke et al. in press). Since the

Table 15.4 *Guidelines for CHO intake for athletes (Burke et al. in press)*

Situation	Recommended CHO intake
A. Acute/single event	
Optimal daily muscle glycogen storage (e.g. for post-exercise recovery, or to fuel-up or CHO-load prior to an event)	7–10 g/kg BM/d
Rapid post-exercise recovery of muscle glycogen, where recovery between session is < 8 h	1 g/kg BM immediately after exercise, repeated after 2 h
Pre-event meal to increase CHO availability prior to prolonged exercise session	1–4 g/kg BM eaten 1–4 h pre-exercise
CHO intake during moderate-intensity or intermittent exercise of > 1 h	0.5–1.0 g/kg/h (30–60 g/h)
B. Chronic or everyday situation	
Daily recovery/fuel needs for athlete with moderate exercise program (i.e. < 1 h of exercise of low intensity)	5–7 g/kg/d
Daily recovery/fuel needs for endurance athlete (i.e. 1–3 h of moderate- to high-intensity exercise)	7–10g/kg BM/d
Daily recovery/fuel needs for athlete undertaking extreme exercise program (i.e. > 4–5 h of moderate- to high-intensity exercise such as Tour de France)	10–12+ g/kg BM/d

1960s, population dietary guidelines have expressed recommendations for the intake of macronutrients in terms of the ratio of dietary energy that they should typically contribute. CHO has been considered an 'energy filler'; the energy ratio left after protein requirements have been met, and health benefits of moderating fat intake to a lower, 'healthier' level have been taken into account. Population guidelines in Westernised countries typically recommend an increased CHO intake, particularly from nutritious CHO-rich foods, to provide at least 50–55% of total dietary energy (United States Department of Agriculture and Health and Human Services 1990; National Health and Medical Research Council 1992). These generic guidelines promote the health benefits of a relative decrease in fat intake and increase in CHO intake across a population, but may be unable to address specific needs of special subgroups. Athletes who have specific CHO needs to fuel their daily training programs and a wider range of energy requirements than found in the general population represent one such subgroup (Burke et al. in press).

Typically, dietary guidelines specially prepared for athletes have followed the tradition of describing ideal CHO intake in terms of an energy ratio. For example, athletes are advised by the American and Canadian Dietetic Associations (1995) to consume diets providing '60–65% of energy from CHO' or, according to the 1994 position statement prepared for FIFA, the international governing body of soccer (Ekblom & Williams 1994), 'at least 55% of energy from CHO'. In the case of endurance or endurance-training athletes, who undertake prolonged daily exercise sessions with increased fuel requirements, CHO intake recommendations have been set variously at '> 60% of energy' (in the 1995 position statement prepared for IAAF, the international governing body of athletics) (Maughan & Horton 1995), or '65–70% of dietary energy' (American and Canadian Dietetic Associations 1995). It should be noted that dietary guidelines or position statements have a different focus from individual studies in which CHO intake is manipulated to achieve an acute effect such as glycogen supercompensation. In such studies, where extreme or atypical diets are often used to ensure that the desired effect is produced, subjects may be fed CHO intakes of > 70% of energy. However, in setting guidelines for chronic intakes of CHO, nutrition experts must take into account the practicality of planning meals, and long-term nutritional issues such as requirements for energy, and other macronutrients and micronutrients. Thus the CHO intake goal is moderated (lower than 70% of energy) to ensure that other nutritional goals can be met simultaneously (Burke et al. 2001).

As discussed in our recent review, the rigid interpretation of guidelines based on energy ratios can prove unnecessary and unfeasible for some athletes (Burke et al. 2001). Athletes who have very high energy intakes (e.g. > 4000–5000 kcal/d or 16–20 MJ/d) will achieve absolute CHO intakes of over 650–900 g CHO/d with a dietary prescription of 65–70% energy. This may exceed their combined requirement for daily glycogen storage and training fuel, and furthermore, may be bulky and impractical to consume. Athletes with such large energy intakes may be able to meet their daily needs for glycogen recovery with a CHO intake providing 45–60% of energy. By contrast, other athletes report lower energy intakes than might be expected. These athletes may need to devote a greater proportion of their dietary intake (e.g. up to 65–70% of energy) to CHO intake, and even then may fail to meet the absolute CHO intakes suggested for optimal daily glycogen recovery. This is particularly true of female athletes (for review, see Burke 1995). In practice, CHO and energy needs of athletes are not always well synchronised. Our review of the self-reported intakes of athletes found in dietary surveys failed to find a significant relationship between the grams of CHO consumed (g/kg BM) and the percentage of dietary energy provided by CHO (Burke et al. 2001).

Therefore, we prefer to provide recommendations for everyday CHO intake in grams (relative to the BM of the athlete) and allow flexibility for the athlete to meet these intakes within the context of their energy needs and other dietary goals (Burke et al. 2001). Guidelines, interpolated from studies of acute fuel needs for training, are provided in Table 15.3. We propose that such guidelines are not only more specific to the muscle's fuel needs, but are more user-friendly. The athlete can use food composition information or ready-reckoners of the CHO content of food to plan or assess their food intake against these target ranges (Burke et al. 2001). The ranges are quite generous, to allow for individual variability in fuel needs and the opportunity to achieve these. With the specialised and individualised advice of a sports nutrition expert, an athlete should be able to fine-tune their daily CHO intake goals. This approach is in agreement with a more recent position paper on nutrition for athletes and physically active people by the New Zealand Dietetic Association (1998), whereby the daily CHO intake requirements were set at 6–10 g/kg BM.

15.3.1 *Success of guidelines in promoting recovery*

It is relatively easy to find research literature that supports the acute benefits of a high-CHO diet in promoting recovery between exercise sessions. Numerous studies show that strategies to enhance glycogen stores between or before a prolonged exercise bout results in enhanced endurance and performance (for review see Chapter 13 and Hargreaves 1999). More specifically, Fallowfield and Williams (1993) reported that a high-CHO diet restored endurance capacity within 22.5 hours of recovery between running sessions, whereas an isocaloric diet of lower CHO content was associated with decreased endurance. Glycogen stores were not measured in this study, but the high-CHO recovery diet was presumed to promote greater resynthesis of glycogen in preparation for the second exercise trial (Fallowfield & Williams 1993).

While a high-CHO intake has been shown to benefit acute recovery and performance, it has been difficult to demonstrate clear benefits to repeated exercise performance over 7–28 days (Sherman & Wimer 1990). Theoretically, inadequate CHO intake during repeated days of exercise will lead to gradual depletion of muscle glycogen stores, and subsequent impairment of exercise endurance. This hypothesis, based on observations of reduced muscle glycogen levels following successive days of running, was represented in a schematic in an early review paper by Costill (Costill & Miller 1980). Although this figure (Figure 15.2) has become perhaps the most well-known diagram in sports nutrition, and is often used to illustrate the relationship between high CHO intake and recovery, the results for the high-CHO diet are hypothetically derived rather than experimentally determined. In fact, a number of training studies have failed to find that a high-CHO diet (8–10 g CHO/kg BM/d) clearly enhances training adaptation or performance compared with a moderate CHO intake (5–7 g/kg BM/d), despite reports of local muscular fatigue or 'staleness' in the moderate-CHO group (see reviews by Sherman & Wimer 1990; Burke et al. in press). Whether this reflects the inadequacy of study design (e.g. type II errors in the measurement of performance; confusion over 'moderate' versus 'high' CHO intakes) is hotly debated. However, until further studies are undertaken, and in view of the data which support the benefits of CHO availability and acute exercise performance, it is sensible for the current sports nutrition guidelines to promote a high-CHO diet during periods of prolonged strenuous training or competition.

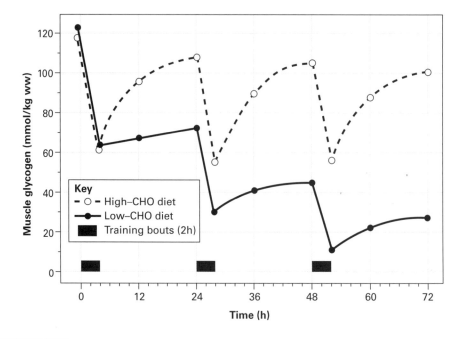

Figure 15.2 *Graph prepared by Costill and Miller (1980), depicting the effect of moderate and high CHO intakes on restoration of muscle glycogen between daily training sessions. Although this figure has become famous as support for the benefits of high-CHO training diets, some of the data in this graph are extrapolated rather than taken from actual studies. Reprinted with permission International Journal of Sports Medicine*

15.4 *ISSUES IN POST-EXERCISE REHYDRATION*

As discussed in Chapter 14, hypohydration has a deleterious effect on exercise performance, causing impairment of prolonged aerobic exercise and thermoregulation (particularly when exercise is performed in a hot environment) (see Sawka & Pandolf 1990), impairment of gastric emptying and comfort (Rehrer et al. 1991), and reduced cognitive functioning (Gopinathan et al. 1988). Performance impairments can be detected when fluid deficits are as low as 1.8% of BM (Walsh et al. 1994); however, the effects are progressive throughout all levels of hypohydration (Montain & Coyle 1992). It is, therefore, undesirable to begin an exercise session with a pre-existing fluid deficit, as a result of failure to rehydrate after previous exercise sessions, or as a result of dehydration protocols undertaken to make weight in a weight division event (see Chapter 8).

In normal healthy people, the daily replacement of fluid losses and maintenance of fluid balance are well regulated by thirst and urine losses. However, under conditions of stress (for example: exercise, environmental heat and cold, altitude) thirst may not be a sufficient stimulus for maintaining euhydration (Greenleaf 1992). Furthermore, there may be a considerable lag of four to 24 hours before body fluid levels are restored following moderate to severe hypohydration.

Studies of voluntary fluid intake patterns across a range of sports show that athletes typically replace only 30–70% of the sweat losses incurred during exercise (Noakes et al. 1988; Broad et al. 1996). As a result, most athletes can expect to finish training or competition sessions with a mild to moderate level of hypohydration. After exercise, people fail to drink sufficient volumes of fluid to restore fluid balance, even when drinks are made freely available. Therefore, the fluid deficit can remain for prolonged periods. Adolph and co-workers first described the failure to fully replace fluid losses as 'voluntary dehydration' and noted that it was exacerbated by factors that reduced the availability or palatability of fluids (Rothstein et al. 1947). However, this phenomenon has been more recently renamed 'involuntary dehydration' to recognise that the dehydrated individual has no volition to rehydrate even when fluids and opportunity are available (Nadel et al. 1990). The factors affecting self-chosen drinking patterns are multifaceted, and include behavioural issues such as social customs of drinking, as well as a genetic predisposition to be a reluctant or heavy drinker (Greenleaf 1992).

An additional challenge to post-exercise rehydration is that the athlete may continue to lose fluid during this phase, partly due to continued sweat losses, but principally due to urination. The success of post-exercise rehydration ultimately depends on the balance between fluid intake and urine losses. Ideally, an athlete should aim to fully restore fluid losses between exercise sessions so that the new event or workout can be commenced in a euhydrated state. This is difficult in situations where moderate to high levels of hypohydration have been incurred (i.e. deficits of 2–5% BM or greater) and the interval between sessions is less than six to eight hours. Optimal rehydration requires a scheduled plan of fluid intake, to overcome both physiological challenges such as inadequate thirst, as well as practical problems such as poor access to fluids. A number of factors affecting post-exercise rehydration have been identified and will now be discussed.

15.4.1 *Palatability of fluid*

Numerous studies have reported that the palatability of fluids affects *ad libitum* intake, with quality, flavour and temperature being identified as important variables (for review see Hubbard et al. 1990). Since many of these studies have investigated rehydration during exercise, it is uncertain whether the findings apply directly to post-exercise recovery (i.e. at rest). Perceptions may change with environmental conditions and with the degree of dehydration, and interestingly there is some evidence that perception of palatability or pleasure may not always correlate with total intake of a rehydration fluid. Hubbard and co-workers (1990) review that while very cold water (0°C) may be regarded as the most pleasurable, cool water (15°C) may be consumed in larger quantities.

Flavouring of drinks has also been considered to contribute to voluntary fluid intake, with studies reporting greater fluid intake during post-exercise recovery with sweetened drinks than with plain water. For example, Carter and Gisolfi (1989) investigated fluid intake during the recovery after subjects had undertaken prolonged cycling to produce a fluid deficit of 2% BM. They found that subjects consumed significantly greater amounts of fluid when presented with a glucose–electrolyte drink than when plain water was provided. Water intake resulted in replacement of 63% of sweat losses, while the sweetened drink resulted in replacement of 79% ($P < 0.05$) of fluid losses. In both cases, *ad libitum* intake of fluid failed to meet total fluid losses, and the rate of intake decreased with time despite the continued fluid deficit. Whether subjects are responding to a sweet flavour or to energy replacement has not been systematically studied. There is some evidence that extreme sweetness and high CHO concentrations reduce voluntary intake, and that initial preferences for CHO-containing beverages may decrease after several hours (see Hubbard et al. 1990).

15.4.2 *Replacement of electrolytes*

When water is ingested following exercise-induced dehydration, there is a dilution of plasma osmolality and sodium content, which results in an increased diuresis and reduced thirst. Nose and co-workers compared rehydration with water plus sodium capsules with water plus a placebo capsule in subjects who had been dehydrated by approximately 2.5% BM (Nose et al. 1988). They found that intake of sodium (equivalent to a solution of approximately 80 mmol/L⁻¹) achieved more rapid restoration of plasma volume than the water trial, due to a greater voluntary intake of fluid and lower urine output.

Maughan and Leiper (1995) dehydrated subjects by 2% BM via exercise in a hot environment, then observed them for six hours of recovery after they had consumed 150% of their fluid losses with test drinks providing varying levels of sodium. Fluid was consumed over a 30-minute period, beginning 30 minutes after the end of the exercise bout. After 90 minutes of recovery there was a significant treatment effect, with greater urine losses being observed with 2 mmol/L (no sodium) and 26 mmol/L sodium (low sodium) drinks than with the 52 mmol/L and 100 mmol/L sodium solutions (see Figure 15.3). After six hours, the difference in mean urine output between the no-sodium and 100 mmol/L sodium drinks was in the order of 800 mL. Subjects were in fluid balance by the end of the recovery period when they consumed the two higher sodium beverages, but were still in net negative fluid balance on the no-sodium and low-sodium trials, despite the intake of a volume of fluid that was 1.5 times their estimated sweat losses. Retention of the ingested fluid was related to the sodium content, however, there was no difference in net fluid balance between the 52 mmol/L⁻¹ and 100 mmol/L⁻¹ sodium trials.

There is some argument about the optimal sodium level for a post-exercise rehydration fluid. The World Health Organisation recommends a sodium level of

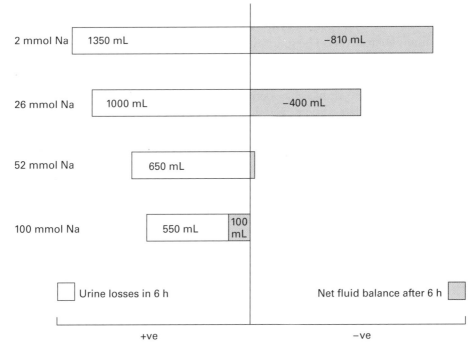

Figure 15.3 *Effect of sodium content of fluid on urine losses and restoration of fluid balance following intake of volumes of fluid representing 150% of fluid deficit incurred by exercising in the heat. Fluids contain sodium content of 2 mmol/L, 26 mmol/L, 52 mmol/L and 100 mmol/L*
*significantly different to pre-exercise
#significantly different to 2 mmol/L
! significantly different to 26 mmol/L
Data redrawn from Maughan & Leiper 1995

90 mmol/L for oral rehydration solutions used in the treatment of diarrhoea-induced dehydration (Walker-Smith 1992). However, this is based on the need to replace the sodium lost through diarrhoea as well as the need to optimise intestinal absorption of fluid and retention of ingested fluid. Sodium losses in sweat vary markedly, with typical sweat sodium levels believed to be in the range of 20–80 mmol/L[-1] (Verde et al. 1982; Armstrong et al. 1987). Therefore, a post-exercise recovery drink with sodium levels of around 50 mmol/L may well be justified. Nevertheless, to be palatable and to have commercial appeal across a wide market, sports drinks have gravitated to a more moderate sodium concentration (10–25 mmol/L).

The effectiveness of such moderate sodium levels in restoring hydration appears to be slight. Gonzalez-Alonso et al. (1992) reported that a commercial sports drink (6% CHO; 20 mmol/L sodium) was more effective than plain water in promoting restoration of fluid levels after exercise-induced dehydration. Subjects were dehydrated by approximately 2.5% BM and were studied during two hours of rehydration while consuming a volume of fluid equal to this deficit, as two equal boluses consumed at zero and 45 minutes of recovery. The sports drink trial achieved greater restoration of body weight (73% of the volume was retained) than the water trial (65% volume retained), principally due to decreased urine losses. Thus it appears from this and other studies that commercial sports drinks may confer some rehydration advantages over plain water, in terms of palatability as well as fluid retention. Nevertheless, where maximum fluid retention is desired, there may be benefits in increasing the sodium levels of rehydration fluids to levels above those provided in typical sports drinks (Maughan & Leiper 1995).

Alternatively, additional sodium may be ingested via sodium-containing foods or salt added to meals. Studies by Maughan et al. (1996) and Ray et al. (1998) have both shown that the intake of salt via everyday food choices enhances the retention of fluid consumed to rehydrate after exercise-induced dehydration. In the case of the study by Maughan and co-workers (1996), greater fluid retention (less urine production) was seen following the consumption of food plus fluid, than a drink only, potentially because of the greater electrolyte content. In this study subjects were dehydrated by 2% BM by exercising in the heat, and over 60 minutes (beginning 30 minutes into the recovery period) they consumed fluid equal to 150% of sweat losses either in the form of a sports drink (20 mmol/L sodium) or as a meal plus a low sodium drink (the water content of the meal was included to match the total fluid intake of the other trial). At the end of six hours of recovery, total urine production was lower following the meal plus drink, and subjects were in a euhydrated state. The sports drink trial resulted in a net negative fluid balance of approximately 350 mL over the same period.

The addition of potassium (25 mmol/L) to a rehydration beverage is equally as effective as sodium (60 mmol/L) in retaining fluids ingested during recovery from exercise-induced dehydration (Maughan et al. 1994). However, there is no additive effect of including both electrolytes, and the replacement of sodium would appear to be a priority since sweat losses of sodium can be significant. Nevertheless, replacement of potassium losses may be important for full restoration of intracellular fluid levels.

15.4.3 *Volume and pattern of drinking*

As sweating and obligatory urine losses continue during the rehydration phase, fluids must be consumed in volumes greater than the post-exercise fluid deficit (i.e. exercise sweat loss) to restore fluid balance. A general finding of the previously reviewed studies is that replacement of fluid in volumes equal to sweat losses results in 50–70% rehydration over 2–4 hours of recovery (based on body weight restoration). Two studies have reported on the effect of the volume of rehydration fluids on restoration of body water deficit. Mitchell and co-workers (1994) dehydrated subjects by 2.5% BM by exercising in a hot environment, then rehydrated them using a dilute electrolyte solution (15 mmol/L sodium) in volumes equivalent to 100% or 150% of their body weight deficit. Thirty per cent of the total volume was consumed as a priming dose, with the remainder of the fluid being consumed in five equal volumes at 30-minute intervals. Gastric emptying was measured, and fluid restoration was determined as body weight gain corrected for fluid remaining in the stomach. During the three-hour rehydration period, the 150% rehydration protocol resulted in greater rates and amounts of fluid emptied from the stomach, and a greater net fluid restoration (68% restoration of BM losses versus 48% restoration). The rate of gastric emptying and regain of body weight decreased over time. Interestingly, there was no further restoration of fluid balance achieved through hours two to three of recovery with either protocol, due to an increase in urine production. Even the 150% rehydration protocol only achieved restoration of 68% of loss of BM, although this figure may be lower than results calculated from other studies due to the correction for gastric contents. Thus, these authors conclude that even forced rehydration with a low-electrolyte beverage does not achieve restoration of fluid balance, and while ingestion of large volumes of fluid is more effective than an equal replacement of the lost fluid, this must be countered against the possible gastrointestinal fullness and discomfort which follow. This may be a practical consideration if a subsequent bout of exercise is scheduled within two to four hours post-recovery.

Similar conclusions were reported by Shirreffs et al. (1996) regarding the volume of fluid required to restore hydration after exercise. They studied subjects who exercised to dehydrate by 2% BM, then consumed volumes equivalent to 50%, 100%, 150% and 200% of BM loss, of solutions containing sodium concentrations of 23 mmol/L or 61 mmol/L^{-1}. Fluids were consumed in four equal volumes at 15-minute intervals, and fluid balance was monitored over six hours of recovery. They found that urine production was related to the volume of fluid consumed. In the case of the high-sodium fluids, consumption of 150% and 200% of fluid losses resulted in euhydration and hyperhydration, respectively, after six hours of recovery. All other trials resulted in residual hypohydration. These results show that a drink volume greater than the sweat loss during exercise must be ingested to restore fluid balance, but unless the sodium content of the beverage is sufficiently high this will merely result in an increased urinary output.

Finally, the consumption of a meal may be a useful adjunct to rehydration. Hubbard et al. (1990) note that food consumption may provide a social or psychological stimulus to increase voluntary fluid intake. Furthermore, the sodium content of the meal will enhance fluid retention (Maughan et al. 1996; Ray et al. 1998).

15.4.4 *Caffeine and alcohol—potential diuretics*

Diuresis may be stimulated by several factors commonly found in beverages consumed by dehydrated athletes. Gonzalez-Alonso et al. (1992) reported that consumption of a diet cola drink containing caffeine resulted in less effective regain of body fluid losses than their water or sports drink trials (see Section 15.4.3). Ingestion of diet cola in a volume equal to sweat losses resulted in restoration of 54% of BM losses; urine losses were significantly increased compared to the other trials and there was a small but significantly greater loss of fluid through continued sweating and respiratory losses (Gonzalez-Alonso et al. 1992).

Alcohol consumption has also been shown to increase urinary losses during post-exercise recovery. Subjects consuming drinks containing 4% alcohol reported greater urinary losses than when drinks containing 0, 1 or 2% alcohol were consumed (Shirreffs & Maughan 1995). Subjects exercised in the heat to dehydrate by 2% BM and rehydrated over a 60-minute period by consuming drinks equivalent to 150% of their fluid deficit of varying alcohol content. The total volume of urine produced over the six-hour recovery period was related to the alcohol content of the fluid; however, only the 4% alcohol drink trial approached significance with a net retention of 40% of ingested fluid compared to 59% in the no-alcohol trial.

15.4.5 *IV rehydration*

In the situation of severe dehydration, especially when fluid intake is compromised by gastrointestinal dysfunction and/or the collapse of the subject, rapid rehydration may be attempted via IV delivery of saline solutions. It has become fashionable in some sports for athletes to receive IV rehydration at the end of their event, to aid recovery. This is understandable in events such as the Tour de France cycling and tennis tournaments where moderate–severe fluid deficits are usual, the period between games or stages is brief, and the athlete has to juggle the time needed to allow adequate sleep as well as recovery nutrition. However, it has recently become more common across a range of sports in which athletes incur moderate fluid deficits and have no gastrointestinal impediments to oral rehydration. Many athletes and coaches believe that IV rehydration has advantages *per se* in enhancing recovery and the performance of subsequent exercise. This idea needs to be considered, and balanced against the expense and slight medical risk involved with IV procedures (especially when carried out in the field).

Armstrong and colleagues have undertaken a series of studies comparing the effects of oral and IV rehydration on restoration of fluid balance, and thermoregulation, metabolism and performance in subsequent exercise trials (Castellani et al. 1997; Riebe et al. 1997). Protocols involved exercise-induced dehydration, followed by no rehydration, or matched replacement of fluid via oral or IV delivery. After a period of recovery, subjects undertook a second bout of exercise in hot conditions. These studies have shown that fluid-replacement protocols achieved equal improvement in plasma volume and thermoregulation during subsequent exercise, compared with the no-rehydration trial (Castellani et al. 1997). However, oral rehydration was superior to IV rehydration in relation to reducing thirst and lowering the perception of effort in the second exercise trial (Riebe et al. 1997). Exercise tolerance was better following oral rehydration compared with IV fluid replacement, apparently because of the reduced perception of workload. Therefore, oral rehydration is at least as effective as IV therapy in treating moderate and uncomplicated situations of dehydration. The psychological sensation of drinking appears to provide an important component of recovery, enabling the athlete to feel better when tackling the next event or workout.

15.5 *ALCOHOL AND RECOVERY*

Although it is difficult to gain reliable data on the alcohol intake practices of people, there is at least preliminary evidence and testimonials of binge-drinking behaviour by some athletes, particularly during the post-competition period. This appears to be most prevalent in team sports where the culture may promote, or at least fail to discourage, post-game alcohol binges (see Burke & Maughan 2000). Unfortunately, post-exercise intake of alcohol is subject to many rationalisations and justifications by athletes including 'everyone is doing it', 'I only drink once a week' and 'I can run/sauna it off the next morning'.

Heavy intake of alcohol may interfere with post-exercise recovery in a number of ways. As reviewed by O'Brien (1993) and Burke and Maughan (2000), alcohol intake has a major impact on the behaviour of athletes during the post-exercise recovery period. There is some evidence that alcohol may directly affect physiological processes such as rehydration and glycogen storage (Burke & Maughan 2000). Many sporting activities are associated with muscle damage and soft-tissue injuries, either as a direct consequence of the exercise, as a result of accidents, or due to the tackling and collisions involved in contact sports. Standard medical practice is to treat soft-tissue injuries with vasoconstrictive techniques (e.g. rest, ice, compression, elevation). Since alcohol is a potent vasodilator of cutaneous blood vessels, it has been suggested that the intake of large amounts of alcohol might cause or increase undesirable swelling around damaged sites, and might impede repair processes. Although this effect has not been systematically studied, there are case histories that report these findings. However, the most important effects of excessive alcohol intake are the impairment of judgement and reduced inhibition. Intoxicated athletes are more likely to undertake high-risk behaviour and suffer an increased risk of accidents. Alcohol consumption is highly correlated with accidents of drowning, spinal injury and other problems in recreational water activities (see O'Brien 1993), and is a major factor in road accidents. Overall, the major impact of heavy alcohol intake after exercise is the failure by the athlete to follow guidelines for optimal recovery.

Alcohol is strongly linked with modern sport. The alcohol intakes and drinking patterns of athletes merit further study and a well-considered plan of education, particularly to target binge-drinking practices that are often associated with post-competition socialising. In addition to being targeted for education about sensible drinking practices, athletes might be used as spokespeople for community education messages. Athletes are admired in the community and may be effective educators in this area. Alcohol is consumed by the vast majority of adults around the world, and merits education messages about how it might be used to enhance lifestyle rather than detract from health and performance.

15.6 *SUMMARY*

Recovery after exercise poses an important challenge to the modern athlete. Important nutrition goals include restoration of liver and muscle glycogen stores, and the replacement of fluid and electrolytes lost in sweat. Rapid resynthesis of muscle glycogen stores is aided by the immediate intake of CHO (1 g/kg BM each two hours), particularly of CHO-rich foods of high GI, towards a total CHO intake over 24 hours of 7–10 g/kg BM. Rapid refuelling may be important for the athlete who has less than eight hours between lengthy exercise sessions. Provided adequate CHO is consumed, it appears that the frequency of intake, the form (liquid versus solid) and the presence of other macronutrients does not appear to affect the rate of glycogen storage. Practical considerations, such as the availability and appetite appeal of foods or drinks, and gastrointestinal comfort may determine ideal CHO choices and intake patterns. Rehydration requires a special fluid intake plan since thirst and voluntary intake will not provide for full restoration of sweat losses in the acute phase (zero to six hours) of recovery. Steps should be taken to ensure that a supply of palatable drinks is available after exercise. Sweetened drinks are generally preferred and can contribute towards achieving CHO intake goals. Replacement of sodium lost in sweat is important in maximising the retention of ingested fluids. A sodium content of 50–90 mmol/L may be necessary for optimal rehydration, however, commercial sports drinks are formulated with a more moderate sodium content (10–25 mmol/L) to allow a greater overall use and palatability. Of course, sodium replacement can occur via salt added or eaten within meals and snacks. Caffeine- and alcohol-containing beverages are not ideal rehydration fluids since they promote an increased rate of diuresis. It may be necessary to consume 150% of fluid losses to allow for complete fluid restoration. Since athletes often compete in a foreign environment, the practical issues of food availability and food preparation facilities must be considered when making recommendations for post-exercise nutrition.

15.7 *PRACTICE TIPS*

Refuelling after exercise

- Effective refuelling begins only after a substantial amount of CHO has been consumed. When there is less than eight hours between workouts or events that deplete glycogen stores, the athlete should maximise effective recovery time by consuming a high-CHO meal or snack within 30 minutes of completing each session. This will mean being organised to have suitable food and drinks available—at the exercise venue if necessary.

- The athlete should aim to consume 50–100 g CHO (1 g CHO/kg BM) immediately after exercise, and repeat after two hours or until normal meal patterns are resumed (see Table 15.5). A daily CHO intake of 7–10 g/kg BM is required to optimise muscle glycogen storage.

- When CHO needs are high, and appetite is suppressed or gastric comfort is a problem, the athlete should focus on compact forms of CHO—low-fibre choices of CHO foods, sugar-rich foods and special sports supplements such as sports bars.

- CHO-containing fluids are also low in bulk and may be appealing to athletes who are fatigued and dehydrated. These include sports drinks, soft drinks and fruit juices, commercial liquid meal supplements, milkshakes and fruit smoothies.

- Low-GI CHO foods such as lentils and legumes may be less suitable for speedy glycogen recovery and should not be the principal CHO source in recovery meals. This is generally not a problem as typical Western diets are generally based on CHO-rich foods of moderate and high GI.

- Small, frequent meals may assist the athlete to achieve high CHO intakes without the discomfort of overeating. However, the athlete should organise their routine of meals and snacks to suit individual preferences, timetable, appetite and comfort. As long as enough CHO is consumed, it doesn't appear to matter how intake is spaced throughout the day.

- When gastric comfort or total energy requirements limit total food intake, high-fat foods and excessive amounts of protein foods should not be consumed at the expense of CHO choices.

- Nutritious CHO foods and drinks may provide protein and other nutrients (vitamins and minerals) that are important in other post-exercise recovery processes. These will be important in the overall diet. Future research may show that intake early after exercise could enhance other activities of repair and rebuilding, and immune processes.

- Muscle damage interferes with glycogen storage—this may be partially offset by increasing CHO intake during the first 24 hours of recovery. CHO needs may also be increased if exercise is undertaken during the recovery period.

Rapid rehydration

- The athlete is reminded not to rely on thirst or opportunity to dictate fluid intake after exercise-induced dehydration or dehydration caused by other

Table 15.5 *CHO recovery snacks and meals*

Each of the following selections provides approximately 50 g of CHO. The athlete should eat at least one or two of these portions soon after exercise to provide 1 g CHO/kg BM, and ensure speedy recovery of glycogen stores. This strategy should be repeated after two hours or until normal eating patterns have been resumed.

- 800 mL–1000 mL of sports drink
- 800 mL of cordial
- 500 mL of fruit juice, soft drink or flavoured mineral water
- 250 mL of CHO loader drink
- 60 g packet of jelly beans or jube sweets
- 3 medium pieces of fruit
- 1 round of jam or honey sandwiches (thick-sliced bread and plenty of jam/honey)
- 3 muesli bars
- 1 large Mars bar or chocolate bar (70 g)
- 2 breakfast bars or cereal bars
- 3 rice cakes with jam or honey
- 2 crumpets or English muffins with vegemite
- 1 cup of thick vegetable soup with large bread roll
- Jaffle/toasted sandwich with banana filling (using whole banana)
- 1–2 sports bars or sports gels (check the labels)
- 100 g (1 large or 2 small) American muffin, fruit bun or scones
- 250 g (1 cup) creamed rice
- 250 g (large) baked potato with salsa filling
- 100 g pancakes (1–2 large) + 30 g syrup

50 g CHO snacks that also contain at least 10 g of protein
- 250–350 mL of liquid meal supplement
- 250–350 mL of milkshake or fruit smoothie
- Some sports bars (check labels)
- 2 × 200 g cartons of fruit-flavoured yoghurt
- Bowl of breakfast cereal with milk
- 200 g carton of fruit-flavoured yoghurt or fromage frais topped with 1 cup of breakfast cereal
- 250 g tin of baked beans or spaghetti on 2 slices of toast or in jaffle/toasted sandwich
- 1 round of sandwiches including cheese/meat/chicken in filling, plus 1 piece of fruit
- 1.5 cups of fruit salad with ½ carton of fruit-flavoured yoghurt or frozen yoghurt
- 1 carton of fruit-flavoured yoghurt and a muesli bar
- 2 crumpets or English muffins with thick spread of peanut butter
- 250 g (large) baked potato with cottage cheese or grated cheese filling
- 150 g thick crust pizza

Adapted from Hawley and Burke 1998

means. A hit-and-miss approach may be acceptable when fluid deficits are one litre or less, but when fluid losses are greater, an organised schedule is required.

- The athlete should monitor changes in BM from pre- to post-exercise to evaluate the success of drinking strategies during exercise, and the residual fluid deficit that must now be replaced. A loss of one kilogram is equivalent to one litre of fluid. Since fluid losses will continue during the recovery period via urine losses and ongoing sweating, the athlete will need to consume additional fluid to counter this. Typically, a volume equal to ~150% of the post-exercise fluid deficit should be consumed over the subsequent two to four hours to fully restore fluid balance.

- It is important to ensure that an adequate supply of palatable drinks is available. This may be difficult when the athlete is at a remote competition venue, or travelling in a country where bottled water must be consumed instead of the local water supply.

- In situations where fluid intake needs to be encouraged, the provision of flavoured drinks is a useful strategy. Since most people prefer sweet-tasting drinks, they are likely to increase their voluntary intake of such fluids. Keeping drinks at a refreshing temperature is also known to encourage greater intake. Cool drinks (10–15°C) are preferred in most situations. Very cold fluids (0–5°C) may seem ideal when the environment or the athlete is hot, however, it is often challenging to drink them quickly or in large volumes.

- CHO-containing drinks are also useful in assisting with refuelling goals and allow the athlete to tackle a number of recovery goals simultaneously.

- In the situation of moderate–large fluid deficits (e.g. > 2 L), sodium replacement will assist the retention of ingested fluids, by minimising urine losses. Options include sports drinks, commercial oral rehydration solutions (e.g. Gastrolyte), salty foods or salt added to post-exercise meals. A high-sodium beverage such as an oral hydration solution (50–90 mmol/L or 2–5 g of salt per litre), or salt added to post-exercise meals along with substantial fluid intake should guarantee that sufficient fluid and sodium have been replaced.

- Caffeine-containing fluids (e.g. cola drinks) and alcohol are not ideal rehydration beverages since they may increase urine losses. Alternative drinks should be used for early post-exercise rehydration. Later, when fluid balance has been substantially restored, the athlete may have greater freedom in making drink choices.

- Where possible, the athlete should avoid post-exercise activities that exacerbate sweat losses—for example, long exposure to hot-spas, saunas or the sun.

Alcohol intake and sport (taken from Burke & Maughan 2000)

- Alcohol is not an essential component of a diet. It is a personal choice of the athlete whether to consume alcohol at all. However, there is no evidence of impairments to health and performance when alcohol is used sensibly.

- The athlete should be guided by community guidelines, which suggest general intakes of alcohol that are safe and healthy. This varies from country to country, but in general, it is suggested that mean daily alcohol intake should be less than 40–50 g (perhaps 20–30 g/d for females), and that 'binge' drinking is discouraged. Since individual tolerance to alcohol is variable, it is difficult to set a precise definition of heavy intake or an alcohol binge. However, intakes of about 80–100 g at a single sitting are likely to constitute a heavy intake for most people.

- Alcohol is a high-energy (and nutrient-poor) food and should be restricted when the athlete is attempting to reduce body fat.

- The athlete should avoid heavy intake of alcohol on the night before competition. It appears unlikely that the intake of 1–2 standard drinks will have negative effects in most people.

- The intake of alcohol immediately before or during exercise does not enhance performance and in fact may impair performance in many people. Psychomotor performance and judgement are most affected. Therefore the athlete should not consume alcohol deliberately to aid performance, and should be wary of exercise that is conducted in conjunction with the social intake of alcohol.

- Heavy alcohol intake is likely to have a major impact on post-exercise recovery. It may have direct effects on rehydration, glycogen recovery and repair of soft-tissue damage. More importantly, the athlete is unlikely to remember or undertake strategies for optimal recovery when they are intoxicated. Therefore, the athlete should attend to these strategies before any alcohol is consumed. No alcohol should be consumed for 24 hours in the case of an athlete who has suffered a major soft-tissue injury.

- The athlete should rehydrate with appropriate fluids in volumes that are greater than their existing fluid deficit. Suitable fluid choices include sports drinks, fruit juices, soft drinks (all containing CHO) and water (when refuelling is not a major issue). However, sodium replacement via sports drinks, oral rehydration solutions or salt-containing foods is also important to encourage the retention of these rehydration fluids. Low-alcohol beers and beer–soft drink mixes may be suitable and seem to encourage large volume intakes. However, drinks containing greater than 2% alcohol are not recommended as ideal rehydration drinks.

- Before consuming any alcohol after exercise, the athlete should consume a high-CHO meal or snack to aid muscle glycogen recovery. Food intake will also help to reduce the rate of alcohol absorption and thus reduce the rate of intoxication.

- Once post-exercise recovery priorities have been addressed, the athlete who chooses to drink is encouraged to do so in moderation. Drink-driving education messages in various countries may provide a guide to sensible and well-paced drinking.

- Athletes who drink heavily after competition, or at other times, should take care to avoid driving and other hazardous activities.

- It appears likely that it will be difficult to change the attitudes and behaviours of athletes with regard to alcohol. However, coaches, managers and sports medicine staff can encourage guidelines such as these, and specifically target the fallacies and rationalisations that support binge-drinking practices. Importantly, they should reinforce these guidelines with an infrastructure that promotes sensible drinking practices. For example, alcohol might be banned from locker rooms, and fluids and foods appropriate to post-exercise recovery provided instead. In many cases, athletes drink in a peer-group situation and it may be easier to change the environment in which this occurs than the immediate attitudes of the athletes.

REFERENCES

American Dietetic Association. Position stand of the American Dietetic Association and Canadian Dietetic Association: nutrition for physical fitness and athletic performance for adults. J Am Diet Assoc 1995;93:691–6.

Armstrong LE, Costill DL, Fink WJ. Changes in body water and electrolytes during heat acclimation: effects of dietary sodium. Aviat Space Environ Med 1987;58:143–8.

Bergstrom J, Hermansen L, Hultman E, Saltin B. Diet, muscle glycogen and physical performance. Acta Physiol Scand 1967;71:140–50.

Blom CS. Post-exercise glucose uptake and glycogen synthesis in human muscle during oral or IV glucose intake. Eur J Appl Physiol 1989;58:327–33.

Blom PSC, Hostmark AT, Vaage O, Kardel KR, Maehlum S. Effect of different post-exercise sugar diets on the rate of muscle glycogen synthesis. Med Sci Sports Exerc 1987;19:491–6.

Broad EM, Burke LM, Gox GR, Heeley P, Riley M. Body weight changes and voluntary fluid intakes during training and competition sessions in team sports. Int J Sport Nutr 1996;6:307–20.

Burke LM. Nutrition for the female athlete. In: Krummel D, Kris-Etherton P, eds. Nutrition in women's health. Maryland: Aspen Publishers, 1995:263–98.

Burke LM. Nutrition for post-exercise recovery. Aust J Sci Med Sports 1996;29(1):3–10.

Burke LM, Collier GR, Beasley SK, et al. Effect of coingestion of fat and protein with CHO feedings on muscle glycogen storage. J Appl Physiol 1995;78:2187–92.

Burke LM, Collier GR, Davis PG, Fricker PA, Sanigorski AJ, Hargreaves M. Muscle glycogen storage following prolonged exercise: effect of the frequency of CHO feedings. Am J Clin Nutr 1996;64:115–19.

Burke LM, Collier GR, Hargreaves M. Muscle glycogen storage following prolonged exercise: effect of the glycaemic index of CHO feedings. J Appl Physiol 1993;75:1019–23.

Burke LM, Cox GR, Cummings N, Desbrow B. Guidelines for daily CHO intake: do athletes achieve them? Sports Med 2001;31:267–299.

Burke LM, Maughan RJ. Alcohol in sport. In: Maughan RJ, ed. IOC Encyclopaedia on Sports Nutrition. London: Blackwell, 2000:405–16.

Carter JE, Gisolfi CV. Fluid replacement during and after exercise in the heat. Med Sci Sports Exerc 1989;21:532–9.

Castellani JW, Maresh CM, Armstrong LE, et al. Intravenous versus oral rehydration: effects on subsequent exercise–heat stress. J Appl Physiol 1997;82:799–806.

Costill DL. CHOs for exercise: dietary demands for optimal performance. Int J Sports Med 1988;9:1–18.

Costill DL, Miller JM. Nutrition for endurance sport: CHO and fluid balance. Int J Sports Med 1980;1:2–14.

Costill DL, Pascoe DD, Fink WJ, Robergs RA, Barr SI, Pearson D. Impaired muscle glycogen resynthesis after eccentric exercise. J Appl Physiol 1991;69:46–50.

Costill DL, Pearson DR, Fink WJ. Impaired muscle glycogen storage after muscle biopsy. J Appl Physiol 1988;64:2245–8.

Costill DL, Sherman WM, Fink WJ, Maresh C, Witten M, Miller JM. The role of dietary CHOs in muscle glycogen resynthesis after strenuous running. Am J Clin Nutr 1981;34:1831–6.

Coyle EF. Timing and method of increased CHO intake to cope with heavy training, competition and recovery. J Sports Sci 1991;9(special issue):29–52.

Danforth W. Glycogen synthase activity in skeletal muscle. J Biol Chem 1965;240:588–93.

Doyle JA, Sherman WM, Strauss RL. Effects of eccentric and concentric exercise on muscle glycogen replenishment. J Appl Physiol 1993;74:1848–55.

Ekblom B, Williams C, eds. Final consensus statement: foods, nutrition and soccer performance. J Sports Sci 1994;12:S3.

Fallowfield JL, Williams C. CHO intake and recovery from prolonged exercise. Int J Sport Nutr 1993;3:150–64.

Foster-Powell K, Brand Miller J. International tables of glycaemic index. Am J Clin Nutr 1995;62;S817–S93.

Gonzalez-Alonso J, Heaps CL, Coyle EF. Rehydration after exercise with common beverages and water. Int J Sports Med 1992;13:399–406.

Gopinathan PM, Pichan G, Sharma VM. Role of dehydration in heat-stress induced variations in mental performance. Arch Environ Health 1988;43:15–17.

Greenleaf JE. Problem: thirst, drinking behaviour, and involuntary dehydration. Med Sci Sports Exerc 1992;24:645–56.

Hansen BF, Asp S, Kiens B, Richter E. Glycogen concentration in human skeletal muscle: effect of prolonged insulin and glucose infusion. Scand J Med Sci Sports 1999;9:209–13.

Hargreaves M. Metabolic responses to CHO ingestion: effect on exercise performance. In: Lamb DR, Murray R, eds. Perspectives in exercise science and sports medicine. Vol 12: The metabolic basis of performance in exercise and sport. Carmel, Indiana: Cooper Publishing Company, 1999:93–124.

Hawley J, Burke L. Peak performance: training and nutrition strategies for sport. Sydney: Allen & Unwin, 1998.

Hermansen L, Vaage O. Lactate disappearance and glycogen synthesis in human muscles after maximal exercise. Am J Physiol 1977;233:E422–E9.

Hubbard RW, Szlyk PC, Armstrong LE. In: Gisolfi CV, Lamb DR, eds. Influence of thirst and fluid palatability on fluid ingestion during exercise: perspectives in exercise science and sports medicine. Vol 3: Fluid homeostasis during exercise. Carmel, Indiana: Benchmark Press, 1990:39–96.

Ivy JL, Katz AL, Cutler CL, Sherman WM, Coyle EF. Muscle glycogen synthesis after exercise: effect of time of CHO ingestion. J Appl Physiol 1988b;64:1480–5.

Ivy JL, Kuo CH. Regulation of GLUT-4 protein and glycogen synthase during muscle glycogen synthesis after exercise. Acta Physiol Scand 1998;162:295–304.

Ivy JL, Lee MC, Bronzinick JT, Reed MC. Muscle glycogen storage following different amounts of CHO ingestion. J Appl Physiol 1988a;65:2018–23.

Jenkins DJA, Cuff D, Wolever TMS, et al. Digestibility of CHO foods in an ileostomate: relationship to dietary fibre, in vitro digestibility, and glycemic response. Am J Gastroenterol 1987;82:709–17.

Jenkins DJA, Jenkins AL, Wolever TMS, et al. Low glycemic index: lente CHOs and physiological effects of altered food frequency. Am J Clin Nutr 1994;59(suppl):S706–S9.

Joszi AC, Trappe TA, Starling RD, et al. The influence of starch structure on glycogen resynthesis and subsequent cycling performance. Int J Sports Med 1996;17:373–8.

Keizer HA, Kuipers H, van Kranenburg G, Guerten P. Influence of liquid and solid meals on muscle glycogen resynthesis, plasma fuel hormone response, and maximal physical work capacity. Int J Sports Med 1986;8:99–104.

Kiens B, Raben AB, Valeur AK, Richter EA. Benefit of simple CHOs on the early post-exercise muscle glycogen repletion in male athletes (abst). Med Sci Sports Exerc 1990;22(suppl4):88.

Kiens B, Richter EA. Types of carbohydrate in an ordinary diet affect insulin action and muscle substrates in humans. Am J Clin Nutr 1996;63:47–53.

Kuipers H, Keizer HA, Brouns F, Saris WHM. CHO feeding and glycogen synthesis during exercise in man. Pflugers Arch 1987;410:652–6.

McCoy M, Proietto J, Hargreaves M. Skeletal muscle GLUT-4 and postexercise muscle glycogen storage in humans. J Appl Physiol 1996;80:411–15.

Maehlum S, Hermansen L. Muscle glycogen concentration during recovery after prolonged severe exercise in fasting subjects. Scand J Clin Lab Invest 1978;38:447–60.

Maughan RJ, Horton ES, eds. Final consensus statement: current issues in nutrition in athletics. J Sports Sci 1995;13:S1.

Maughan RJ, Leiper JB. Sodium intake and post-exercise rehydration in man. European J Appl Phys 1995;71:311–19.

Maughan RJ, Leiper JB, Shirreffs SM. Restoration of fluid balance after exercise-induced dehydration: effects of food and fluid intake. Eur J Appl Physiol 1996;73:317–25.

Maughan RJ, Owen JH, Shirreffs SM, Leiper JB. Post-exercise rehydration in man: effects of electrolyte addition to ingested fluids. Eur J Appl Physiol 1994;69:209–15.

Mitchell JB, Grandjean PW, Pizza FX, Starling RD, Holtz RW. The effect of volume ingested on rehydration and gastric emptying following exercise-induced dehydration. Med Sci Sports Exerc 1994;26:1135–43.

Montain SJ, Coyle EF. Influence of graded dehydration on hyperthermia and cardiovascular drift during exercise. J Appl Physiol 1992;73:1340–50.

Nadel ER, Mack GW, Nose HN. Influence of fluid replacement beverages on body fluid homeostasis during exercise and recovery. In: Gisolf CV, Lamb DR, eds. Perspectives in exercise science and sports medicine. Vol 3: Fluid homeostasis during exercise. Carmel, Indiana: Benchmark Press, 1990:181–205.

National Health & Medical Research Council. Dietary guidelines for Australians. Canberra, Australia: Australian Government Publishing Service, 1992.

New Zealand Dietetic Association. Position paper update: nutritional considerations for physically active adults and athletes in New Zealand. J New Zealand Diet Assoc 1998;52:5–13.

Noakes TD, Adams BA, Myburgh KH, Greff C, Lotz T, Nathan M. The danger of inadequate water intake during prolonged exercise. Eur J Appl Physiol 1988;57:210–19.

Nose H, Mack GW, Shi X, Nadel ER. Role of osmolality and plasma volume during rehydration in humans. J Appl Physiol 1988;65:325–31.

O'Brien CP. Alcohol and sport: impact of social drinking on recreational and competitive sports performance. Sports Med 1993;15:71–7.

Parkin JAM, Carey MF, Martin IK, Stojanovska L, Febbraio MA. Muscle glycogen storage following prolonged exercise: effect of timing of ingestion of high glycemic index food. Med Sci Sports Exerc 1997;29:220–4.

Piehl Aulin K, Soderlund K, Hultman E. Muscle glycogen resynthesis in humans after supplementation of drinks containing CHOs with low and high molecular masses. Eur J Appl Physiol 2000;81:346–51.

Ray ML, Bryan MW, Ruden TM, Baier SM, Sharp RL, King DS. Effect of sodium in a rehydration beverage when consumed as a fluid or meal. J Appl Physiol 1998;85:1329–36.

Reed MJ, Brozinick JT, Lee MC, Ivy JL. Muscle glycogen storage postexercise: effect of mode of CHO administration. J Appl Physiol 1989;66:720–6.

Rehrer NJ, Beckers EJ, Brouns F, ten Hoor F, Saris WHM. Effects of dehydration on gastric emptying and gastrointestinal distress while running. Med Sci Sports Exerc 1991;22:790–5.

Riebe D, Maresh C, Armstrong LE, et al. Effects of oral and intravenous rehydration on ratings of perceived exertion and thirst. Med Sci Sports Exerc 1997;29:117–24.

Roberts KM, Noble EG, Hayden DB, Taylor AW. Simple and complex CHO-rich diets and muscle glycogen content of marathon runners. Eur J Appl Physiol 1988;57:70–4.

Rothstein A, Adolph EF and Wills JH. Voluntary dehydration. In: Adolph, et al. Physiology of man in the desert. Interscience: New York, 1947:254–320.

Roy BD, Tarnopolsky MA. Influence of differing macronutrient intakes on muscle glycogen resynthesis after resistance exercise. J Appl Physiol 1998;84:890–6.

Saris WHM, van Erp-Baart MA, Brouns F, Westerterp KR, ten Hoor F. Study on food intake and energy expenditure during extreme sustained exercise: the Tour de France. Int J Sports Med 1989;10(suppl1):S26–S31.

Sawka MN, Pandolf KB. Effects of body water loss on physiological function and exercise performance. In: Gisolfi CV, Lamb DR, eds. Perspectives in exercise science and sports medicine. Vol 3: Fluid homeostasis during exercise. Carmel, Indiana: Benchmark Press, 1990:3–38.

Sherman WM, Costill DL, Fink WJ, Miller JM. The effects of exercise and diet manipulation on muscle glycogen and its subsequent use during performance. Int J Sports Med 1981;2:114–18.

Sherman WM, Wimer GS. Insufficient dietary CHO during training: does it impair athletic performance? Int J Sport Nutr 1990;1:28–44.

Shirreffs SM, Maughan RJ. The effect of alcohol consumption on fluid retention following exercise-induced dehydration in man. J Physiol 1995;489:P33–P4.

Shirreffs SM, Taylor AJ, Leiper JB, Maughan RJ. Post-exercise rehydration in man: effects of volume consumed and sodium content of ingested fluids. Med Sci Sports Exerc 1996;28:1260–71.

Tarnopolsky MA, Atkinson SA, Phillips SM, MacDougall JD. CHO loading and metabolism during exercise in men and women. J Appl Physiol 1995;78:1360–8.

US Department of Agriculture and Health and Human Services. Dietary guidelines for Americans. Home and Garden Bulletin no. 232. Washington, DC: United States Department of Agriculture and Health and Human Services, 1990.

Verde T, Shepherd RJ, Corey P, Moore R. Sweat composition in exercise and in heat. J Appl Physiol 1982;53:1540–5.

Walker-Smith JA. Recommendations for composition of oral rehydration solutions for children in Europe. J Pediat Gastro 1992;14:113–15.

Walsh RM, Noakes TD, Hawley JA, Dennis SC. Impaired high-intensity cycling performance time at low levels of dehydration. Int J Sports Med 1994;15:392–8.

Widrick JJ, Costill DL, Fink WJ, Hickey MS, McConell GK, Tanaka H. CHO feedings and exercise performance: effect of initial muscle glycogen concentration. J Appl Physiol 1993;74:2998–3005.

Williams C, Brewer J, Walker M. The effect of a high-CHO diet on running performance during a 30-km treadmill time trial. Eur J Appl Physiol 1992;65:18–24.

Wolever TMS, Cohen Z, Thompson LU, et al. Ileal loss of available CHO in man: comparison of a breath hydrogen method with direct measurement using a human ileostomy model. Am J Gastroenterol 1986;81:115–22.

Zachwieja JJ, Costill DL, Pascoe DD, Robergs RA, Fink WJ. Influence of muscle glycogen depletion on the rate of resynthesis. Med Sci Sports Exerc 1991;23:44–8.

Zawadzki KM, Yaspelkis BB, Ivy JL. CHO–protein complex increases the rate of muscle glycogen storage after exercise. J Appl Physiol 1992;72:1854–9.

CHAPTER 16

Nutritional strategies to enhance fat oxidation during aerobic exercise

John Hawley

16.1 INTRODUCTION

Compared with the finite stores of carbohydrate (CHO), endogenous fat depots are large, and represent a potentially unlimited source of fuel for skeletal muscle during aerobic exercise. However, fatty acid (FA) oxidation by muscle is limited, especially during the high-power outputs and intensities sustained by athletes in training and competition. In the never-ending search for strategies to improve athletic performance there has been considerable interest in several nutritional interventions which might, theoretically, promote FA oxidation, attenuate the rate of muscle glycogen utilisation, and improve exercise performance. This chapter:

- presents an overview of the role of endogenous fat as an energy substrate for skeletal muscle during exercise;
- discusses the methods for quantifying fat oxidation during exercise;
- examines the effect of exercise intensity on the regulation of fat metabolism; and
- provides a synopsis of some of the processes that could limit FA oxidation during exercise.

Given this theoretical background, some of the nutritional procedures that may enhance fat utilisation and improve aerobic exercise performance in humans are reviewed, and practical recommendations on their use are provided for the practitioner.

16.2 *DIGESTION AND ABSORPTION OF LIPID*

The vast majority of articles examining fat metabolism during exercise have focussed exclusively on the factors that limit FA oxidation by skeletal muscle, ignoring the obvious fact that lipids first have to be digested, absorbed, and transported to their site of storage before subsequent utilisation. As most of the nutritional strategies to enhance FA oxidation during exercise detailed later in this chapter involve manipulation and/or modification of dietary fat intake, it seems relevant to give a brief overview of the digestion and absorption of fat.

Lipids provide the largest nutrient store of chemical energy that can be used to power biological work (see Figure 16.1). In the normal Western diet, the typical intake of lipids constitutes ~35% of daily energy intake (~100–150 g/d). Lipids are found in both animal and plant foodstuffs and can be classified into three basic types: simple lipids, or triacylglycerols (TG), phospholipids (or compound lipids) and cholesterol (derived lipid). Of these, TG constitute 90–95% of the total dietary fat. The majority of TG is stored in the cytoplasm of white adipose-tissue cells, although the muscle and liver contain stores of important physiological significance (see Section 16.3). The TG molecule consists of a glycerol three-carbon molecule backbone to which are attached three molecules of FA. Nearly all FA have an even number of carbon atoms. Those FA with a chain length from C14–C22 are called long-chain FA (LCFA), while those with a chain length of C8–C10 are termed medium-chain fatty acids (MCFA). Short-chain fatty acids (SCFA) are those with a chain length of C6 or less. Fatty acids that contain carbon atoms joined together by only single covalent bonds are called 'saturated' (e.g. palmitic acid) and are usually semi-solid.

Dietary sources of saturated lipids include meats, egg yolk and dairy products, while plant sources include coconut and palm oil, and hydrogenated margarine. Fatty acids that contain at least one double bond along the main carbon chain are classified as 'unsaturated' and are usually liquid at room temperature (e.g. monounsaturated such as oleic acid, and polyunsaturated such as sunflower oils). The typical breakdown of ingested lipid is 40% oleate, 25% palmitate, 15% stearate, 10% linoleate, and 5% palmitoleate, with the remainder a mixture of saturated and unsaturated FA with chain lengths of C12–C20.

Lipids are digested by gastric and pancreatic lipases. The digestion of lipid is initiated in the stomach by an acid-stable lipase, which converts TG to FA and diacylglycerols. However, the major enzyme for TG hydrolysis is the pancreatic lipase which is specific for, although not exclusive to, LCFA with more than C10. The products of TG hydrolysis are free fatty acids (FFA) and ß-monoacylglycerols, which are released at the surface of fat emulsion droplets. Both FFA and monoacylglycerols are slightly water-soluble, and molecules at the surface equilibrate with those in solution and become incorporated into bile micelles. These micelles provide the major vehicle for the transport of lipid from the intestinal lumen to the cell surface where absorption occurs. The fate of absorbed FA depends on their chain length: MCFA are able to directly pass through the cell into the portal blood and reach the liver directly. In contrast, LCFA bypass the liver and are released in the form of chylomicrons and are delivered to the circulation via the lymphatic system. As such, chylomicrons are the lipoprotein particles found in the systemic circulation and contain the highest proportion (~85%) of TG. The bypassing of the liver by LCFA may have evolved to protect the liver from a lipid overload after a large (fatty) meal.

16.3 *TRIACYLGLYCEROL AS AN ENERGY SOURCE DURING EXERCISE*

As an energy source, TG has several advantages over carbohydrate (CHO): the energy density of lipid is higher (37.5 kJ/g for stearic acid versus 16.9 kJ/g for glucose), while the relative weight as stored energy is lower. TG also provides more adenosine triphosphate (ATP) per molecule than glucose (147 versus 38 ATP), although the complete oxidation of FA requires more oxygen than the oxidation of CHO (six versus 26 mol of oxygen per mole of substrate for glucose and stearic acid oxidation, respectively). Adipose tissue TG constitutes by far the largest energy store in the body (see Figure 16.1) (sufficient to sustain skeletal muscle contraction for ~120 h at marathon running pace). On the other hand, if only CHO were utilised as a fuel, it would only deliver energy for ~90 min of running. As the men's world record for the marathon is ~125 min, this highlights the importance of the integration of fuels during prolonged exercise. The size of the adipose tissue TG pool is difficult to estimate, and obviously depends on the fat mass of each individual, but is likely to range from 5000–10 000 g in the trained athlete (see Figure 16.1). In order for this TG to be used as a substrate for oxidative metabolism, it has to be exported from adipose tissue and transported by the blood to the active tissues where it will be utilised.

Another important physiological store of TG can be found within the skeletal muscle mostly adjacent to the mitochrondria. The total active muscle mass may contain up to 350 g of intra-muscular tricylglyceride (IMTG) within the myocyte as small lipid droplets, although this amount can vary substantially due to individual differences in fibre type (type I fibres contain a greater concentration of IMTG than type II fibres), endurance training status (Kiens et al. 1993; Martin et al. 1993; Martin 1996), and diet (Starling et al. 1997). Paradoxically, although regular endurance training elicits an increase in IMTG concentration in healthy individuals, an adaptation viewed as beneficial for training and performance (Kiens et al. 1993), IMTG stores are also increased in patients with insulin-dependent diabetes mellitus (Ebeling et al. 1998). This latter condition is associated with the features of insulin resistance syndrome (Phillips et al. 1996).

Finally, FA can also be derived from circulating TG (chylomicrons) and very low-density lipoproteins (VLDL) formed from dietary fat in the postabsorptive state

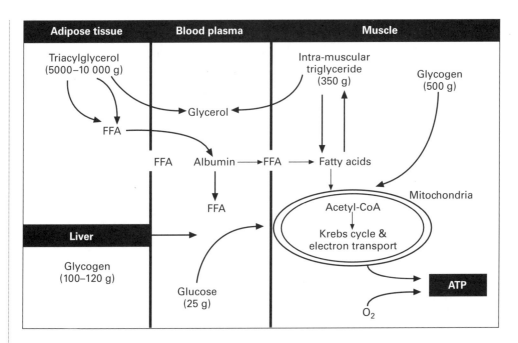

Figure 16.1 *A schema of the major endogenous storage sites of carbohydrate and fat in the trained athlete. Redrawn from Coyle (1997)*

(discussed previously). Recent evidence suggests that if all the circulating VLDL-TG were taken up and oxidised, VLDL-TG degradation could contribute up to 50% of the lipid oxidised during sub-maximal exercise (Kiens 1998).

16.4 PROCESSES THAT COULD LIMIT FATTY ACID OXIDATION DURING EXERCISE

Despite the vast stores of endogenous TG, the capacity for FA oxidation during exercise is limited. Unlike CHO oxidation, which is closely geared to the energy requirements of the working muscle, there are no mechanisms for matching the availability and utilisation of FA to the rate of energy expenditure. Indeed, there are many potential sites at which the ultimate control of FA oxidation may reside (see Figure 16.2), with the relative importance of each site depending on a large number of external factors such as the aerobic training status of the individual, habitual dietary intake, ingestion of substrates (CHO and fat) before and during exercise, gender, and the relative and absolute intensity of exercise. A comprehensive analysis of the processes that potentially limit FA oxidation during exercise is beyond the scope of this chapter, and the reader is referred to several excellent reviews of the topic (van der Vusse & Reneman 1996; Jeukendrup 1997; Wolfe 1998).

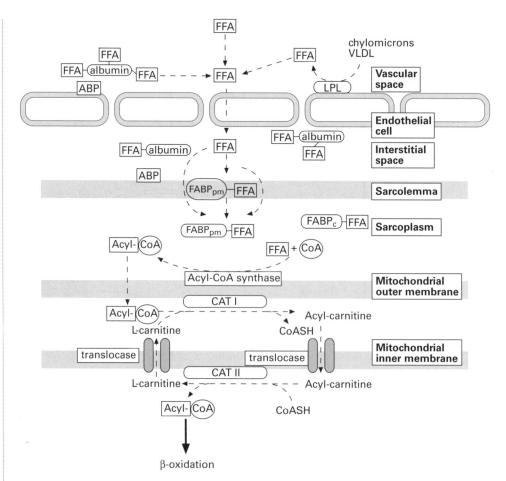

Figure 16.2 *A schema of the transport of fatty acids from the vascular space to the inner mitochondria of the skeletal muscle where ß-oxidation occurs. CAT1 = cartintinecarnitine acyl transferase I; CAT II = carnitine acyl transferase II; FABP$_c$ = fatty acid binding protein; FABP$_{pm}$ = plasma membrane bound fatty acid binding protein; FFA = free fatty acid; VLDL = very low density lipoprotein. The various processes are described in detail in the text. Reproduced from Jeukendrup (1997) with permission*

16.4.1 *Mobilisation of fatty acids from adipose triacylglycerol: Lipolysis*

Triacylglycerols cannot be oxidised by skeletal muscle directly: first they must be hydrolysed into their components, non-esterified fatty acids (NEFA) and glycerol. This process, called lipolysis, is largely dependent on the activation of the enzyme hormone sensitive TG lipase (HSL) in adipose tissue. Binding of hormone to plasma membrane receptors on adipocytes activates adenyl cyclase and initiates the lipolytic cascade (see Figure 16.2). Epinephrine and glucagon activate HSL, while high levels of plasma glucose and insulin inhibit the activity of the lipase and reduce lipolysis. FA and glycerol derived from lipolysis in adipose tissue are released into the circulation: FA are bound by serum albumin and transported to tissues for oxidation and production of ATP (discussed subsequently), while glycerol returns to the liver and can be either phosphorylated to glycerol 3-phosphate and used to form TG, or converted to dihydroxyacetone and enter the glycolytic or gluco-neogenic pathways. An isoform of the enzyme HSL is also present in skeletal muscle where it acts to break down IMTG stores.

16.4.2 *Transport of fatty acids across the sarcolemmal membrane into skeletal muscle*

The precise regulatory mechanisms of lipid uptake by skeletal muscle are not completely understood. This is somewhat surprising since muscle represents ~40% of body mass and has a highly variable metabolic rate. During transport of FA from blood to muscle, there are several potential processes that might limit eventual FA uptake. These are the membranes of the vascular endothelial cells, the interstitial space between endothelium and muscle cell, and finally the muscle cell membrane. Although FA transport across the sarcolemmal membrane into the muscle fibre was originally thought to occur exclusively by simple passive diffusion along a concentration gradient, there is now good evidence of a LCFA transport system involving FA binding proteins (FABP), FA translocases (FAT) and FA transport proteins (FATP). Of interest is the finding that FABP content is higher in type I (slow twitch) than type II (fast twitch) muscle fibres, and also increased with endurance training. This suggests a functional relationship between the FA binding capacity and the degree of oxidative metabolism in the muscle (Kiens 1998). Once FA enter the cytoplasm of muscle cell they can either be esterified and stored as IMTG or the FA can be bound to FABP for transport to the site of oxidation and activated to a fatty acyl-CoA by the enzyme acyl-CoA synthase.

16.4.3 *Oxidation of fatty acids*

Whereas most fatty acyl-CoA is formed outside the mitochondria, the oxidative machinery is inside the inner membrane, which is impermeable to CoA. To over-come this problem, there exists a specific carnitine-dependent shuttle to carry acyl groups across the membrane (see Figure 16.3).

Enzymes on both sides of the membrane transfer acyl groups between CoA and carnitine. On the outer mitochondrial membrane, the acyl group is transferred to carnitine catalysed by carnitine palmitoyltransferase I (CPTI). Acyl-carnitine then exchanges across the inner mitochondrial membrane with free carnitine by a carnitine-acylcarnitine translocase. Finally, the fatty acyl group is transferred back

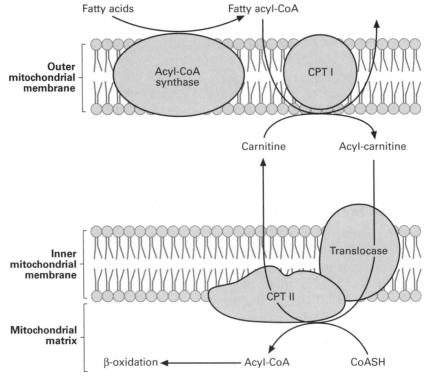

Figure 16.3 *The transport of long-chain fatty acids from the cytosol through the inner mitochondrial membrane for oxidation is dependent on the carnitine palmitoyltransferase complex (see text for further details). Reproduced from Devlin TM (editor). Textbook of biochemistry (fourth edition). Wiley-Liss: New York, 1997*

to CoA by carnitine palmitoyltransferase II (CPTII) located on the matrix side of the inner membrane. This mitochondrial transport of fatty acyl-CoA functions primarily with chain lengths of C12–C18. Medium and SCFA can freely diffuse into the mitochondrial matrix and do not require a carnitine-dependent shuttle mechanism to allow transport across the mitochondrial inner membrane. There is some evidence to suggest that carnitine-dependent transport of LCFA into the mitochondria might be a rate-limiting step for FA oxidation (see below).

The process of ß-oxidation, which occurs in the mitochondria, comprises four separate reactions in which the fatty acyl-CoA is sequentially degraded to acetyl-CoA and an acyl-CoA residue that has had 2C sequestered. The acetyl-CoA units enter the tricarboxylic acid (TCA) cycle and follow the same pathway as acetyl-CoA units from pyruvate. The rate at which FA are oxidised depends on the chain length and the degree of saturation: MCFA are oxidised more rapidly and more completely than LCFA.

16.5 METHODS TO QUANTIFY LIPID METABOLISM DURING EXERCISE

A background knowledge of some of the methods used to measure substrate metabolism during laboratory-based investigations would seem essential for the sports practitioner striving to comprehend and interpret the findings of such studies in a meaningful and practical manner to athletes and coaches. Our understanding of the regulation of fat metabolism has been advanced considerably by modern-day investigations which have used a combination of stable isotope techniques in association with conventional indirect calorimetry (Romijn et al. 1992, 1993). As the three most abundant FA are oxidised in proportion to their relative concentration in the plasma FA pool, total plasma FA kinetics can be estimated from stable isotope infusions of either oleate or palmitate. The rate of appearance (Ra) of a FA (i.e. palmitate) in the bloodstream gives an index of the release of FA into the plasma and represents the net balance between the rate of adipose tissue lipolysis and the rate of FA uptake and re-esterification. Glycerol, on the other hand, cannot be produced by the body other than from lipolysis. Furthermore, all glycerol released during lipolysis, whether from adipose tissue or skeletal muscle, appears in the plasma. Accordingly, the Ra of glycerol provides a useful indicator of the rate of whole body lipolysis. An estimation of total fuel utilisation (fat and CHO) during steady-state exercise can be obtained from the respiratory exchange ratio, the volume of carbon dioxide produced (VCO_2) divided by the oxygen consumed (VO_2).

$$\text{CHO oxidation (g/min)} = 4.585\ VCO_2 - 3.226\ VO_2$$
$$\text{Fat oxidation (g/min)} = 1.695\ VO_2 - 1.701\ VCO_2$$

Rates of substrate oxidation are usually expressed relative to an individual's body mass (or sometimes their lean muscle mass, or fat-free mass). Accordingly, the rate of CHO oxidation (μmol/kg/min) is determined by converting the g/min rate of CHO oxidation to its molar equivalent assuming 6 mol of O_2 are consumed and 6 mol of CO_2 produced for each mole (180 g) oxidised. Rates of FA oxidation (μmol/kg/min) are determined by converting the g/min rate of TG oxidation to its molar equivalent assuming the average molecular weight of TG to be 855.26 g/mol and multiplying the molar rate of TG oxidation by three, because each molecule contains 3 mmol of FA.

Given the tracer-derived rates of total lipolysis and total FA released into the plasma, it is possible to distinguish peripheral lipolysis from adipose TG and intramuscular lipolysis.

$$\text{IMTG oxidation (μmol/kg/min)} = \text{Total FA oxidation} - \text{FA uptake (FFA Rd)}$$
$$\text{(μmol/kg/min)} \qquad \text{(μmol/kg/min)}$$

For every three FA released from the IMTG pool, one glycerol molecule will be released into the plasma. Consequently, the minimum rate of release of glycerol from the IMTG pool gives an estimation of IMTG lipolysis and can be estimated from the following equation:

$$\text{IMTG lipolysis (μmol/kg/min)} = \text{IMTG oxidation (μmol/kg/min)} / (\text{μmol/FFA/μmol glycerol})$$

The rate of total glycerol release (Ra glycerol) equals the glycerol released from adipocyte TG and glycerol released from the IMTG pool. Accordingly, it is possible to calculate the rate of adipose (peripheral) TG lipolysis from the following equation:

$$\text{Adipose lipolysis (μmol/kg/min)} = \text{Total Ra glycerol} - \text{IMTG lipolysis}$$
$$\text{(μmol/kg/min)} \quad \text{(μmol/kg/min)}$$

Using a combination of these techniques, it has been possible to estimate the effect of exercise intensity and duration on fat metabolism (Romijn et al. 1993).

16.6 *THE EFFECTS OF EXERCISE INTENSITY ON LIPID METABOLISM*

In the post-absorptive state, FA oxidation provides a major portion of the energy requirements for skeletal muscle: at rest, the rate of total FA oxidation is ~4 μmol/kg/min, which represents about 50% of oxygen consumption. The rate of lipolysis at rest is usually in excess of that required to provide resting energy requirements such that at the onset of low- to moderate-intensity exercise, a significant increase in FA oxidation could occur even if there was no instant increase in lipolysis. During low-intensity exercise (25% of $VO_{2\text{ max}}$), an intensity comparable to walking, most of the energy requirements can be met from plasma FA oxidation, with a small contribution from the oxidation of plasma glucose. At exercise of low intensity the Ra of FA in plasma matches closely the rate of FA oxidation (see Table 16.1). Even when low-intensity exercise is sustained for one to two hours, the pattern of fuel utilisation does not change considerably. Presumably this is because the muscle energy requirements can be met almost exclusively from the oxidation of the FA mobilised from the large adipose TG stores, and lipolysis is not limited by blood flow.

With an increase in exercise intensity from 25% to 65% of $VO_{2\text{ max}}$ (the pace that could be sustained by a trained person for up to eight hours), total fat oxidation reaches it peak, despite a slight decline in the Ra of plasma FA (see Table 16.1). The higher rate of total FA oxidation at 65% compared to 25% of $VO_{2\text{ max}}$ reflects a substantial increase in the oxidation of IMTG. Of interest is that even when the absolute rate of FA oxidation is at a peak (i.e. 42.8 μmol/kg/min), fat only contributes about 50% to the total fuel requirements of exercise, with the remainder of the energy coming from CHO (see Figure 16.4).

During high-intensity exercise at 85% of $VO_{2\text{ max}}$ (race pace for endurance events lasting ~1 h) there is a decline in total FA oxidation (from 42.8 to 29.6 μmol/kg/min) compared to moderate-intensity exercise (see Figure 16.4). This

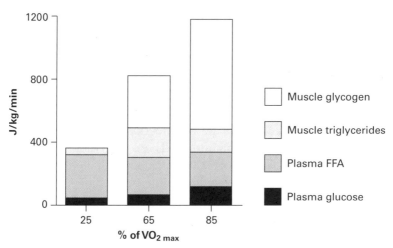

Figure 16.4 *The effect of exercise intensity on the contribution from the four major substrates to energy expenditure. Redrawn from Romijn et al. (1993). Reproduced with permission from the American Physiological Society*

Table 16.1 *The effect of exercise intensity on the rates of lipolysis and whole body fat oxidation*

Intensity (%VO$_{2\,max}$)	Ra glycerol (peripheral)	Ra glycerol (intra-muscular)	RaFFA	Fat oxidation
25	10.9 ± 1.0	0.3 ± 0.7	25.8 ± 2.4	26.8 ± 1.9
65	10.8 ± 3.1	4.5 ± 1.9	21.7 ± 2.8	47.6 ± 2.3
85	8.9 ± 2.3	4.5 ± 0.9	15.9 ± 2.7	29.6 ± 2.9

VO$_{2\,max}$ = maximal oxygen uptake; Ra = rate of appearance; FFA = free fatty acids
All values (μmol/kg/min) are mean ± SEM of 6 subjects
Data are from Romijn et al. (1992)

is largely due to a marked reduction in the Ra of plasma FA (see Table 16.1). It is likely the Ra for plasma FA decreases with increasing exercise intensity because of an insufficient blood-flow and albumin delivery to transport FA from adipose tissue into the blood stream. On the other hand, glycerol is water-soluble and so its appearance in the plasma is not blood-flow dependent: consequently the Ra for glycerol is not affected (see Table 16.1). In addition, continuous high-intensity exercise is associated with high rates of glycogenolysis (see Figure 16.4) and the concomitant production of lactic acid which accumulates in muscle and blood. This increased glycolytic flux also acts to inhibit FA oxidation by skeletal muscle (see below).

16.7 WHY CAN'T FATTY ACID OXIDATION SUSTAIN INTENSE EXERCISE?

At rest, the Ra FA (i.e. lipolysis) normally exceeds energy requirements of skeletal muscle. During low-intensity exercise, when lipolysis increases further, there is still a sufficient supply of FA to meet the muscles' energy demands. However, there is little further increase in lipolysis when exercise intensity increases to 65% of $VO_{2\,max}$: at such work rates Ra FA closely matches FA oxidation. During high-intensity exercise, lipolysis is markedly suppressed and the contribution of FA oxidation to the total energy requirements of exercise is diminished. These observations would support the notion that the reduced availability of FA (i.e. a reduction in lipolysis) may contribute to a part of the decline in FA oxidation during intense exercise.

To evaluate the extent to which decreased FA availability contributes to the lower rates of FA oxidation during intense exercise, Romijn et al. (1995) studied well-trained endurance subjects during 30 minutes of intense (85% of $VO_{2\,max}$) cycling, once during a 'control' trial when plasma FFA concentration was normal (i.e. 0.3 mmol) and again when plasma FFA concentration was elevated to ~2 mmol by an infusion of lipid (Intralipid) and heparin. Total FA oxidation was increased 27% (from 26.7 to 34.0 μmol/kg/min) with the lipid infusion compared to control. However, the elevation of plasma FFA concentration (i.e. increased availability) during intense exercise only resulted in a partial restoration of FA oxidation as the rates of total fat oxidation at 85% of $VO_{2\,max}$ were still lower than those observed in normal conditions at 65% of $VO_{2\,max}$. These findings indicate that FA oxidation is impaired during intense exercise because of a failure of lipolysis to meet the energy demands of the muscle. Therefore, in theory, TG lipolysis establishes the upper limit to FA oxidation during high-intensity exercise. However, even when lipid is infused well in excess of the muscle requirements during high-intensity exercise, less than half of the total energy requirements is met by FA oxidation. This is because the muscle is also a major site of control of the rate of FA oxidation during such exercise. Specifically, the increased rate of glycogenolysis during intense exercise appears to inhibit the entry of LCFA into the mitochondria. Sidossis et al. (1997) reported that during cycling at 80% of $VO_{2\,max}$, the accelerated glycolytic flux associated with the high work rates resulted in high rates of pyruvate and acetyl-CoA formation which inhibited CPT-I activity and, in turn, FA entry into the mitochondria. Coyle et al. (1997) also showed that CHO metabolism (i.e. glycolytic flux) regulates FA oxidation during exercise. These workers had subjects ingest CHO before exercise (in order to produce high concentrations of plasma glucose and insulin) and subsequently determined the rates of oxidation of a LCFA (palmitate) and a MCFA (octanoate). The increased glycolytic flux from pre-exercise glucose ingestion significantly reduced palmitate oxidation, but had no effect on octanoate oxidation. This is because unlike palmitate which requires CPT-I for transport into skeletal muscle mitochondria, octanoate is not limited by mitochondrial transport. Even when FA availability is maintained by an infusion of lipid, CHO ingestion still inhibits LCFA oxidation

(Sidossis et al. 1996), presumably because of the anti-lipolytic effects of elevated insulin concentrations. Taken collectively, these findings suggest that although the rate of lipolysis is important, the primary site of control of FA oxidation during moderate to intense exercise resides at the muscle tissue level (Wolfe 1998). Furthermore, increased glycolytic flux resulting from either CHO ingestion (Coyle et al. 1997; Horowitz et al. 1997, 1999) and the concomitant rise in plasma insulin, or an increase in exercise intensity (Romijn et al. 1995; Sidossis et al. 1997), directly inhibits LCFA oxidation.

16.8 *NUTRITIONAL STRATEGIES TO ENHANCE FATTY ACID OXIDATION DURING EXERCISE*

As endogenous CHO reserves are limited, and as muscle and liver glycogen depletion often coincide with fatigue during both endurance events and many team sports, there has been a recent resurgence of interest by athletes, coaches and sports practitioners· in nutritional practices which, in theory at least, could promote FA oxidation, attenuate the normal rate of CHO utilisation, and improve exercise capacity. Many of these so-called 'ergogenic aids' have received scientific investigation (for reviews see Brouns & van der Vusse 1998; Hawley 1998; Hawley et al. 1998; Coyle & Hodgkinson 1999; Hawley et al. 2000). They include ingestion of fat and caffeine before exercise, LCFA and MCFA feedings during exercise, chronic adaptation to high-fat diets, diets of purportedly ideal macronutrient ratios (e.g. the 'Zone' or 40/30/30 diet), consumption of high-fat 'sports' bars, and L-carnitine supplementation. Although intravenous infusion of lipid (Intralipid) accompanied by heparin is a potent lipolytic stimulant which increases FA oxidation and spares muscle glycogen stores during both moderate (Odland et al. 1996, 1998) and intense (Dyck et al. 1993, 1996) exercise, such a procedure is impractical in most sporting environments. Furthermore, intravenous infusions contravene the International Olympic Committee's doping regulations. As such, a critique of this area has not been included in this chapter. The reader is referred to the excellent reviews of Spriet and Dyck (1996) and Spriet (1999) for further information on this topic.

16.8.1 *Caffeine ingestion before exercise*

Caffeine, a common drug used throughout the world, is a pharmacological agent used by many athletes as an ergogenic aid to improve both short-term, high-intensity and prolonged, moderate-intensity exercise performance (for review see Spriet 1997 and Chapter 17, Section 17.6.2). Caffeine has direct effects on both the central nervous system (reducing an individual's perception of effort) (Cole et al. 1996) and on neuromuscular function (Kalmar & Caferelli 1999). However, the early studies investigating the effects of caffeine ingestion on exercise capacity focussed on changes in FFA availability and subsequent FA oxidation, the so-called 'metabolic theory' (Spriet 1997).

In a series of investigations conducted nearly twenty years ago, Costill and co-workers were the first to report that the ingestion of moderate doses of caffeine (~5 mg/kg) ~1 h before exercise stimulated lipolysis, enhanced rates of total FA oxidation (as estimated from RER measurements) and decreased the utilisation of muscle glycogen (Costill et al. 1978; Ivy et al. 1979; Essig et al. 1980). Caffeine was proposed to mobilise FA from adipose tissue and/or IMTG stores by increasing plasma epinephrine concentrations and/or directly antagonising adipocyte tissue adenosine receptors. The increased circulating FFA would then increase FA uptake and oxidation by muscle and spare endogenous CHO reserves. While the metabolic theory remains plausible, there are probably several mechanisms responsible for changes in the rates of substrate oxidation after caffeine ingestion: those mechanisms may or may not involve a direct effect of caffeine (Spriet 1997). As reviewed in Section 17.6.2 the ergogenic benefits of caffeine are complex and multifactorial, and are not limited to, or even dependent on, metabolic changes.

16.8.2 *Fat feeding before exercise*

Several studies have investigated the effects of fat feeding before exercise on the subsequent rates of substrate oxidation and exercise performance. The results from these investigations are equivocal with regard to both the effect of fat feeding on metabolism, and also performance. Costill et al. (1977) first reported that fat feeding in combination with intravenous administration of heparin stimulated lipolysis, elevated plasma FFA concentrations and decreased the rate of muscle glycogen utilisation by 40% compared to a control condition during 30 minutes of running at 70% of $VO_{2\,max}$. A recent study from the same laboratory also reported muscle glycogen sparing with fat feeding and i.v. heparin compared to control during 60 minutes of cycling at 70% of $VO_{2\,max}$ (Vukovich et al. 1993).

On the other hand, Okano et al. (1996, 1998) reported only small differences in the rates of fat and CHO oxidation in response to high-fat or high-CHO meals ingested four hours before prolonged submaximal cycling (two hours at 67% of $VO_{2\,max}$ followed by a ride to exhaustion at 78% of $VO_{2\,max}$). Furthermore, most of the differences in metabolism (i.e. a lower RER) after the fat feeding were only evident in the early stages of exercise, and did not result in an improved performance time. Whitley et al. (1998) also found that high-fat or high-CHO meals ingested four hours before exercise failed to substantially alter the pattern of fuel utilisation during 90 minutes of moderate intensity cycling, or affect a subsequent ten kilometre cycle time trial. Wee et al. (1999) fed six endurance-trained runners a random order of either a high-fat, a high-CHO or a high-fat high-CHO meal, three hours before a run to exhaustion at 71% of $VO_{2\,max}$. Despite the rate of fat oxidation being elevated after the high-fat compared to the high-CHO and high-fat high-CHO meals (19% and 14%, respectively), endurance time was 14% less after the high-fat meal. These workers concluded that CHO rather than fat availability before exercise exerts a predominant control over substrate selection during subsequent exercise.

Only one study has compared the effect of fat feeding versus CHO feeding on metabolism and performance during intense (80% of $VO_{2\,max}$) exercise. Hawley et al. (2000) reported that a high-fat feeding increased fat availability and elevated rates of FA oxidation during 20 minutes of exercise, but that the small reduction in CHO oxidation after such a regimen did not enhance a subsequent bout of intense exercise lasting ~30 minutes.

The only study to find an increase in exercise capacity with fat feeding was that of Pitsaladis et al. (1999). These workers found that cycling time to exhaustion was prolonged (from 118 to 128 minutes) when their trained subjects ingested a high-fat (90% of energy) versus a high-CHO (70% of energy) meal, four hours prior to exercise. As no differences in total CHO oxidation were reported between trials (383 versus 362 g for the CHO and fat meals respectively), it is difficult to explain the prolonged exercise time in that study.

16.8.3 *Long- and medium-chain triglyceride ingestion during exercise*

Twenty years ago Ivy et al. (1980) were the first to compare the effects of MCFA and LCFA ingestion on FA oxidation during exercise. Lipids (~30 g) were ingested by ten well-trained subjects, one hour before a bout of moderate intensity exercise lasting 60 minutes. LCFA ingestion increased serum TG concentrations but neither MCFA or LCFA had any effects on the rates of FA oxidation. These workers did report that when more than 50 g of MCFA or LCFA were ingested, severe gastrointestinal problems were experienced by the majority of subjects, and recommended a maximum amount of 30 g that could be tolerated by most athletes (Ivy et al. 1980).

Satabin et al. (1987) also compared the effect of MCFA with LCFA on rates of fat and CHO oxidation and exercise time to exhaustion at 60% of $VO_{2\,max}$. These workers used stable isotope tracers ((1-^{13}C) octanoate, (1-^{13}C) palmitate) to track the fate of ingested substrates during exercise. The most striking effect of MCFA ingestion was a rise in blood ketone bodies. On the other hand, blood ketone concentrations were unchanged with LCFA ingestion. Not surprisingly, the ingested LCFA were oxidised to a lesser extent than the MCFA (9% versus 43% of the amount ingested) although exercise times to exhaustion were similar.

In contrast to LCFA which slow the rate of gastric emptying and enter the systemic circulation as chylomicrons, MCFA are emptied very rapidly from the stomach and are absorbed into the bloodstream almost as fast as glucose (Beckers et al. 1992). As such, recent interest has focussed on the potential ergogenic effect of ingesting MCFA solutions on endurance performance (Jeukendrup et al. 1995, 1996, 1998; Goedecke et al. 1999a; Angus et al. 2000).

The first study to investigate the effects of MCT ingestion during exercise was undertaken by Massicotte et al. (1992). These researchers compared the oxidation of ingested MCFA to glucose during two hours of cycling at 65% of $VO_{2\,max}$. They found that the contribution of fat and CHO to total energy requirements during exercise was similar between the two interventions. More recently, Jeukendrup and co-workers (1995) investigated the effects of a combination of CHO and MCFA ingested during three hours of moderate-intensity (57% $VO_{2\,max}$) exercise in well-trained cyclists. When 10 g of MCFA was co-ingested with CHO each hour, ~70% of the MCFA consumed was oxidised compared to only 33% when the MCFA was ingested alone. Towards the end of exercise the rate of ingested MCFA oxidation closely matched the rate of ingestion. Even so, the contribution of ingested MCFA to total energy expenditure was only 7%. In a separate study (Jeukendrup et al. 1996), these workers examined the effects of MCFA ingestion on the rates of muscle glycogen utilisation during 180 minutes of moderate-intensity cycling. MCFA ingested at a rate of ~10 g/h had no effect on the rates of total CHO oxidation, nor the rates of muscle glycogen utilisation. Even when subjects commence exercise with low muscle glycogen content, MCT ingestion has no effect on CHO utilisation (Jeukendrup et al. 1996). Recently, Angus et al. (2000) compared the ingestion of CHO (60 g/h) plus MCFA solution (~24 g/h) on cycling time trial performance. Subjects completed a set amount of work equal to ~100 kilometres as fast as possible. Compared to a placebo (178 ± 11 minutes), the time to complete the ride was reduced after the ingestion of both CHO (166 ± 7 minutes) and CHO plus MCFA (169 ± 7 minutes). However, the addition of the MCFA did not provide any further performance improvement over CHO alone.

To date, only one study has reported a beneficial effect of MCFA ingestion on FA metabolism and performance. Van Zyl et al. (1996) reported that when large doses (~30 g/h) of MCFA were co-ingested with a 10% glucose beverage, serum FA concentrations were elevated, FA oxidation was increased, estimated muscle glycogen utilisation reduced, and 40-kilometre cycle performance (which followed two hours of sub-maximal exercise at 60% of $VO_{2\,max}$) improved by 2.5% compared to when glucose was ingested alone. However, that study is the exception. Recently, Jeukendrup et al. (1998) fed well trained subjects a similar MCFA-CHO solution to that given by van Zyl et al. (1996) and found no difference in the performance of a work bout lasting ~15 minutes which was preceded by two hours at 60% of $VO_{2\,max}$. Interestingly, both these investigations reported that when MCFA was ingested alone, performance was reduced compared to CHO. Jeukendrup et al. (1998) also found that MCFA ingestion resulted in a worse performance than when subjects ingested a water placebo. On a practical note, the ingestion of large (> 15 g/h) amounts of MCFA are likely to produce gastrointestinal problems in most athletes, which would be expected to be detrimental to performance.

16.8.4 *Adaptation to high-fat, low-carbohydrate diets*

It has long been known that modifying an individual's habitual diet can significantly alter the subsequent patterns of substrate utilisation during aerobic exercise, and impact on performance (Christensen & Hansen 1939). The consumption of a high-fat (> 60% of energy intake), low-CHO (less than 15% of energy) diet for one to three days markedly reduces resting muscle glycogen content and increases FA oxidation during sub-maximal exercise (Jansson & Kaijser 1982). Such a shift in substrate utilisation is commonly associated with impairment in exercise capacity (for review see Hawley et al. 1998). Indeed, only one study has found a positive effect on performance after short-term exposure to a high-fat diet (Muoio et al. 1994).

In contrast to the negative effects on exercise capacity that seem to result from short-term (one to three days) exposure to high-fat diets, there is some evidence to suggest that longer (five to seven day) periods of adaptation to high-fat diets may induce adaptive responses that are fundamentally different to the acute lowering of body CHO reserves. Such adaptations have been proposed to eventually induce a reversal of some of the mitochondrial adaptations that favour CHO oxidation and 'retool' the working muscle to increase its capacity for FA oxidation (Lambert et al. 1997).

The most frequently cited study to support the use of high-fat diets to improve athletic performance was that conducted by Phinney and co-workers (1983) who examined the effects of 28 days of a high-fat diet (85% of energy) versus a eucaloric diet containing 66% of energy from CHO, on sub-maximal cycle time to exhaustion. The high-fat diet reduced the average resting muscle glycogen content of their five trained subjects by 47% (143 versus 76 mmol/kg wet weight (ww)). Consequently, when cycling at ~63% of $VO_{2 \, max}$, the RER values were 0.72 (95% of energy from fat, 5% from CHO) and 0.83 (56% of energy from fat, 44% from CHO) for the high-fat and normal diets, respectively. Remarkably, the mean exercise time at this moderate work intensity was not statistically significantly different after the two dietary interventions (147 versus 151 minutes for the eucaloric versus high-fat diets, respectively). However, this performance result needs to be interpreted with caution. Firstly, it has previously been reported that trained subjects can ride for 3–4 hours at moderate intensities when fasted and fed CHO throughout exercise (Coyle et al. 1986). Secondly, the performance data are heavily skewed in favour of the fat diet largely as a result of one individual who rode ~60% longer after the high-fat compared to the normal diet. Finally, competitive endurance athletes training and racing in events lasting less than four hours rarely exercise at such low intensities (Bergman & Brooks 1999).

Lambert et al. (1994) used a random crossover design to investigate the effects of 14 days of a high-fat (67% MJ) and a high-CHO (74% MJ) diet in five trained cyclists. After dietary adaptation, subjects undertook a comprehensive battery of physical tests including a 30-second Wingate anaerobic test, a ride to exhaustion at ~90% of $VO_{2 \, max}$, and, following a 30-minute rest, a further ride to volitional fatigue at 60% of $VO_{2 \, max}$. Although the high-fat diet significantly reduced pre-exercise muscle glycogen content from (121 mmol/kg ww after the normal diet to 68 mmol/kg ww after the high-CHO diet), mean 30-second anaerobic power was similar between the two conditions (862 versus 804 W for the high-fat and CHO diet, respectively). Neither was there an effect of dietary manipulation on the time subjects could ride for at a work rate eliciting ~90% of $VO_{2\,max}$ (8.3 versus 12.5 minutes for the high-fat and CHO trials). However, although failing to attain statistical significance, a margin of 4.2 minutes at such a work rate would result in a huge difference in athletic performances (Hopkins et al. 1999). The only effect of the high-fat diet was to prolong sub-maximal endurance time during the third and final laboratory test (the ride to exhaustion at 60% of $VO_{2\,max}$) from 42 to 80 minutes, despite significantly lower starting muscle glycogen content (32 versus 73 mmol/kg ww). Such increases in endurance were associated with a marked decrease in the average rate of CHO oxidation (2.2 versus 1.4 g/min) and a significant increase in the rate of fat oxidation from 0.3 to 0.6 g/min. The results of this investigation are difficult to interpret because of the unorthodox study design, but they strongly suggest that sub-maximal exercise capacity can be preserved in spite of low pre-exercise muscle glycogen content when trained individuals are adapted to a high-fat diet.

Probably the longest exposure to a CHO-restricted diet was the recent investigation of Helge et al. (1996) who examined diet-training interactions in two groups of ten untrained subjects participating in a seven-week endurance-training program while consuming either a high-fat (62% MJ) or high-CHO (65% MJ) diet. Cycle time to exhaustion at 70% of $VO_{2\,max}$ increased by 191% after the high-CHO diet, but only by 68% in those subjects who consumed the high-fat diet. In order to determine if the impairment in endurance observed after the high-fat diet could be reversed, subjects then switched to a high-CHO diet during the eighth week of the study and the exercise task was repeated. Even after a week of ingesting CHO, the mean performance time only improved by 12 minutes, leading these workers to conclude, 'a combination of training and a fat-rich diet did not reveal an additive effect on physical performance'.

In summary, compared to a high-CHO diet, a period of adaptation to a high-fat diet will increase the relative contribution from FA oxidation by ~40% to the total energy requirements of exercise. However, adaptation to high-fat diets does not appear to alter the rate of muscle glycogen utilisation or improve prolonged, moderate-intensity exercise (for review, see Kiens & Helge 2000). Although it has been suggested that as long as 20 weeks of exposure should be allowed if humans wish to adapt to high-fat diets (Kronfeld 1973) such a time frame is impractical, and could also pose health problems for athletes (see below). Adaptation to high-fat diets are only likely to impact on endurance performance in sporting situations where CHO availability is limiting. More to the point, such nutritional strategies are only likely to be of benefit to a small group of highly trained endurance or ultra-endurance athletes (Hawley & Hopkins 1995). Even if such a dietary regimen was shown to enhance performance, high-fat diets are associated with increased risk of a number of diseases (Sternfeld 1992; Sarna & Kaprio 1994) and although regular physical activity attenuates these risks, individuals should limit their long-term exposure to high-fat diets. Short-term exposure to high-fat diets are also associated with insulin resistance in the liver (Kraegen et al. 1991) resulting in a failure to suppress hepatic glucose output, and an attenuation of liver glycogen synthesis. For these reasons, caution should always be exercised when sports practitioners recommend high-fat diets to athletes.

16.8.5 *Chronic high-fat diets followed by acute high-carbohydrate diets*

Recently it was proposed that nutritional preparation for endurance and ultra-endurance events should encompass periods of 'nutritional periodisation' (Hawley & Hopkins 1995). In such a scenario athletes might train for most of the year on a high-CHO diet, adapting to a high-fat diet for three to five days early in the week prior to a major event, then CHO-loading in the final 48 hours immediately prior to competition. Since the results of a recent study suggested that most of the adaptive responses that facilitate an increased rate of fat oxidation are complete after five days (Goedecke et al. 1999b), this nutritional periodisation would still permit endurance athletes to train hard throughout the year, and maximise their endogenous CHO stores before competition while, theoretically, allowing the working muscles to optimise their capacity for FA oxidation during a major endurance race. More to the point, a five-day period of exposure to a high-fat diet represents a more manageable period for extreme dietary change while minimising any potential health risks.

In order to test this hypothesis, Burke et al. (2000a, 2000b) determined the effects of either five days of adaptation to a high-fat diet (4.0 g/kg of fat/d, 2.4 g/kg of CHO/d) followed by one day of CHO restoration, or an isoenergetic CHO diet (9.6 g/kg of CHO/d) on exercise metabolism and endurance cycling performance. Competitive cyclists or triathletes who had a history of regular endurance training were recruited for this study; such individuals would be expected to have the muscle adaptations which favour FA oxidation (Brooks & Mercier 1994). At the end of each dietary program, which was separated by a two-week wash-out period, subjects cycled for two hours at 70% of $VO_{2\ max}$ and then completed a time trial, lasting ~30 minutes, as fast as possible. Two investigations were undertaken: during the first (Burke et al. 2000a) but not the second (Burke et al. 2000b) study, muscle biopsies and tracer-derived estimates of blood glucose oxidation were determined. The only other difference between studies was that in the first investigation (Burke et al. 2000a) subjects completed the exercise task after an overnight fast and consumed only water throughout the ride. Such a scenario would be likely to maximise rates of FA oxidation. During the second experiment (Burke et al. 2000b), subjects were given a pre-trial breakfast similar in size and composition to that they might consume before a race. In addition, they were allowed to consume CHO throughout the ride. Such nutritional practices are currently recommended by sports nutritionists (Burke 1995).

In agreement with other investigations (Phinney et al. 1983; Lambert et al. 1994), five days of the high-fat diet drastically reduced resting muscle glycogen concentration (from 451 to 255 mmol/kg dry weight (dw)). However, one day of a high-CHO diet was sufficient to restore muscle glycogen concentration to 554 mmol/kg dw (the corresponding value for the high-CHO diet was 608 mmol/kg dw). During two hours of cycling at 70% of $VO_{2\ max}$, muscle glycogen utilisation was less after fat adaptation (554 to 294 mmol/kg dw) than the high-CHO diet (608 to 248 mmol/kg dw). This glycogen 'sparing' (100 mmol/kg dw) occurred because the rates of FA oxidation were elevated by ~50% above the CHO trial. Yet despite such substantial glycogen sparing, the performance of the time trial was similar between dietary treatments.

Unfortunately, the techniques utilised in this study did not enable the determination of whether the elevated rates of FA oxidation were due to an increase in FFA release, uptake and oxidation, or an increased reliance on IMTG. However, despite the brevity of the adaptation period, the high-fat diet elicited large shifts in favour of FA oxidation. Such an adaptation is impressive in light of the already enhanced capacity for FA oxidation in such highly trained subjects. In the second study, the cycling bout was undertaken after a CHO-rich meal and with CHO intake during the ride (Burke et al. 2000b). As CHO ingestion effectively eliminates any rise in plasma FFA concentration, an effect which can persist for several hours after ingestion (Horowitz et al. 1997), it would be expected that FA oxidation would also be suppressed during exercise. Indeed, compared to the first experiment (Burke et al. 2000a), the overall rate of FA oxidation was lower. However, total FA oxidation was still higher after the high-fat compared to the high-CHO diet, indicating that there are persistent metabolic adaptations to a high-fat diet even when CHO availability during exercise is high. Although time-trial performance was similar after the two dietary regimens, the results of this study provide strong evidence that the muscle can be 'retooled' to enhance FA oxidation in as little as five days, even when CHO is ingested before and throughout exercise. Nevertheless, this strategy has not been shown to be of benefit to the performance of exercise lasting 2–3 hours. It is possible that this nutritional periodisation may still confer a positive benefit to those athletes involved in ultra-endurance sports lasting longer than five hours, when the need to conserve glycogen as long as possible is of utmost importance for performance. This theory remains to be tested.

16.8.6 *The Zone diet and high-fat sports bars*

An unusual diet, the Zone diet or 40/30/30 diet, has recently become popular due to the successful sales of books written by Dr Barry Sears (Sears 1995, 1997). This diet, if followed according to the details provided in the books, is low in total energy and restricts CHO intake to levels that could not sustain daily athletic training. For example, the Zone diet recommends that a 75 kg athlete should be consuming ~2000 kcal/d of which the contribution from CHO would be only ~800 kcal (~200 g of CHO, or less than 3 g of CHO/kg body mass/d). Such a CHO intake is well below the self-reported daily intakes of athletes (for review see Hawley et al. 1995) and far less than currently recommended by sports nutritionists (Burke 1995) and exercise physiologists (Costill & Miller 1980; Costill 1988; Sherman & Lamb 1988; Hawley & Burke 1998). The rationale for such low energy and CHO intakes, or the energy ratio of 40% CHO, 30% fat and 30% protein, in the Zone diet is the belief that such an eating pattern will promote FA oxidation. However, there is no scientific evidence to support such claims (Hawley & Burke 1998). On the contrary: the Zone diet is very similar to that utilised in two studies which have shown impaired endurance performance on CHO restricted compared to diets high in CHO (Helge et al. 1996, 1998).

In addition to the many fad diets currently being advocated to improve training capacity and enhance endurance performance, a variety of sports bars have been promoted as 'fat burners' capable of reducing CHO metabolism. Most commercially available bars contain a 40/30/30 mixture of CHO, fat and protein. To date, only one study has examined the effects of ingestion of a 40/30/30 sports bar on metabolism and ultra-endurance performance. Rauch et al. (1999) studied six highly trained endurance cyclists who rode for 5.5 hours at ~55% of $VO_{2\,max}$ before performing a time trial lasting ~25 minutes. During the 5.5 hour ride subjects ingested 1.5 sports bars and 700 mL of water every hour, or 700 mL of a 10% glucose polymer solution such that the total energy ingested during the two prolonged rides was similar. Although the rates of fat oxidation were significantly greater at the end of the sub-maximal ride when subjects ingested the bar compared to CHO (1.09 versus 0.73 g/min), two subjects were so fatigued that they failed to complete the time trial. Furthermore, the drop-off in time trial performance following ingestion of the bar was directly related to the drop in the rate of CHO oxidation, suggesting that even when FA oxidation is increased, it is insufficient to meet the demands of intense exercise (see Section 16.7).

16.8.7 *L-carnitine supplementation*

The carnitine pool in a healthy individual is about ~100 mmol, of which ~98% is found in skeletal and cardiac muscle, 1.6% in the liver and kidneys, and 0.4% in the extracellular fluid. Over half of the daily requirements of carnitine are found in a balanced diet, which includes meat, poultry, fish and some dairy products. The remainder is synthesised from methionine and lysine. Daily urine losses of carnitine are usually less than 2% of the total body carnitine store.

LCFA oxidation in all tissues is carnitine dependent (see Section 16.4.3). Therefore, hereditary and acquired conditions associated with carnitine deficiency result in TG accumulation in the skeletal muscles, insulin resistance, and an impaired utilisation of FA and reduced exercise capacity. These pathological changes can normally be reversed by carnitine supplementation. It has been hypothesised that increased availability of L-carnitine by supplementary ingestion might up-regulate the capacity to transport FA into the mitochondria and increase FA oxidation. If this were possible, then carnitine supplementation would be of significant benefit to both endurance athletes, and to individuals wishing to increase their lean body mass by reducing their levels of adipose tissue.

There have been many well-controlled studies examining the effects of carnitine supplementation on metabolism and athletic performance in both moderately trained individuals and well trained athletes (see Chapter 17, Section 17.8.2 for review). The doses administered in these studies have varied between 2–6 g/d, with the length of administration from five days up to four weeks. The results of these and many other investigations convincingly demonstrate that carnitine supplementation has no effect on patterns of fuel utilisation either at rest or during exercise. As lipid metabolism during exercise is unaltered after supplementation regimens, it is not surprising that there is no change in the rate of working muscle glycogen utilisation (Vukovich et al. 1994). Even when CHO availability has been compromised before exercise by reducing muscle glycogen stores, carnitine supplementation still fails to alter substrate utilisation (i.e. lipid metabolism) during sub-maximal exercise (Decombaz et al. 1993).

As carnitine has a physiological role in the metabolism of FA, it is not surprising that it has also been marketed as a potential fat-loss agent. In those sports in which making weight and body-fat loss are deemed important for successful performance (wrestling, rowing, gymnastics, body building), carnitine use has been vigorously promoted. However, there is no scientific evidence to suggest that carnitine enhances FA oxidation, nor helps reduce body fat or aids an athlete to make weight.

Finally, many studies have shown that there is little or no loss of carnitine from skeletal muscle during either low- or high-intensity exercise (see Heinonen 1996 for review). More to the point, in healthy athletes eating conventional diets, training does not appear to induce any physiologically substantial changes in muscle carnitine levels. Even massive doses of carnitine only increase muscle carnitine levels by only 1–2%. Therefore, there is little reason for carnitine supplementation in moderately active individuals, or athletes in hard training.

16.9 SUMMARY AND RECOMMENDATIONS FOR SPORTS PRACTITIONERS

Many nutritional strategies have been employed in an attempt to promote FA oxidation, attenuate the rate of utilisation of endogenous CHO stores, and thereby enhance athletic performance. Some of these practices have not been subjected to *any* rigorous scientific testing (e.g. the Zone diet) and should not be recommended to athletes. Others (e.g. L-carnitine supplementation) have been well investigated and clearly have no effect on the rates of FA oxidation, muscle glycogen utilisation or subsequent performance.

While the ingestion of moderate doses of caffeine (4–6 mg/kg BM) in most individuals has been shown to improve FA oxidation and enhance endurance capacity in endurance events, the ingestion of small (10 g/h) amounts of MCFA have no major effects on fat metabolism, nor do they improve exercise performance. Although the ingestion of larger (30 g/h) quantities of MCFA *may* increase fat availability and rates of FA oxidation, such amounts are likely to produce gastrointestinal problems in most athletes, which would be expected to be detrimental to performance.

With regard to the ingestion of high-fat diets, the results of several studies show that both acute (2–3 days) and more prolonged (7 days to 4 weeks) exposure to such diets reduce resting muscle glycogen levels, and increase the relative contribution from FA oxidation to the total energy requirements of sub-maximal exercise. However, such diets significantly impair subsequent endurance performance. While dietary periodisation (i.e. high-fat diets followed by acute high-carbohydrate diets) may be of benefit to a select group of ultra-endurance athletes, there is currently insufficient scientific evidence to recommend that athletes 'fat load' during training or before competition.

Finally, even those agents which have been shown to have an ergogenic effect when tested under well-controlled conditions may be ergolytic in certain individuals: there are likely to be many scientific studies which, because of a lack of a positive finding, have never been published. Accordingly, it is important for sports practitioners to recognise that there is wide inter-individual variability in the response to many fat-enhancing, performance-enhancing substances. Any nutritional strategies should be undertaken under the supervision of qualified medical personnel, and fine-tuned during daily training to suit each individual's specific needs.

REFERENCES

Angus DJ, Hargreaves M, Dancey J, Febbraio MA. Effect of carbohydrate plus medium chain triglyceride ingestion on cycling time trial performance. J Appl Physiol 2000;88:113–19.

Beckers EJ, Jeukendrup AE, Brouns F, Wagenmakers AJM, Saris WHM. Gastric emptying of carbohydrate-medium chain triglyceride suspensions at rest. Int J Sports Med 1992;13:581–4.

Bergman BC, Brooks GA. Respiratory gas-exchange ratios during graded exercise in fed and fasted trained and untrained men. J Appl Physiol 1999;86:479–87.

Brooks GA, Mercier J. Balance of carbohydrate and lipid utilization during exercise: the 'crossover' concept. J Appl Physiol 1994;76:2253–61.

Brouns F, van der Vusse. Utilization of lipids during exercise in human subjects: metabolic and dietary constraints. Br J Nutr 1998;79:117–28.

Burke LM. The complete guide to food for sports performance, 2nd edn. Sydney: Allen and Unwin, 1995.

Burke LM, Angus DJ, Clark S, et al. Metabolic adaptations following fat adaptation persist despite high-CHO availability during prolonged cycling (abst). Med Sci Sports Exerc 2000b (32:S259).

Burke LM, Angus DJ, Cox GR, et al. Effect of fat adaptation and carbohydrate restoration on metabolism and performance during prolonged cycling. J Appl Physiol 2000a;89:2413–21.

Christensen EH, Hansen O. Zur methiodik der respiratorischem quotientbestimmung in ruhe und bei arbeit. III: Arbeitsfahigkeit und ernahrung. Scand Arch Physiol 1939;81:160–71.

Cole KJ, Costill DL, Starling RD, Goodpaster BH, Trappe SW, Fink WJ. Effect of caffeine ingestion on perception of effort and subsequent work production. Int J Sport Nutr 1996;6:14–23.

Costill DL. Carbohydrates for exercise: dietary demands for optimal performance. Int J Sports Med 1988;9:1–18.

Costill DL, Coyle EF, Dalsky G, Evans W, Fink W, Hoopes D. Effects of elevated plasma FFA and insulin on muscle glycogen usage during exercise. J Appl Physiol 1977;43:695–9.

Costill DL, Dalsky GP, Fink WJ. Effects of caffeine ingestion on metabolism and exercise performance. Med Sci Sports 1978;10:155–8.

Costill DL, Miller JM. Nutrition for endurance sport: carbohydrate and fluid balance. Int J Sports Med 1980;10:155–8.

Coyle EF. Fuels for sports performance. In: Lamb DR, Murray R, eds. Perspectives in exercise science and sports medicine. Vol 10: Optimising sport performance. Carmel, Indiana: Cooper Publishing Group, 1997:95–129.

Coyle EF, Coggan AR, Hemmert MK, Ivy JL. Muscle glycogen utilization during prolonged strenuous exercise when fed carbohydrate. J Appl Physiol 1986;61:165–72.

Coyle EF, Hodgkinson BJ. Influence of dietary fat and carbohydrate on exercise metabolism and performance. In: Lamb DR, Murray R, eds. Perspective in exercise science and sports medicine. Vol 12: The metabolic basis of performance in exercise and sport. Carmel, Indiana: Cooper Publishing Group, 1999:165–98.

Coyle EF, Jeukendrup AE, Wagenmakers AJM, Saris WHM. Fatty acid oxidation is directly regulated by carbohydrate metabolism during exercise. Am J Physiol 1997;273:E268–E75.

Decombaz J, Deriaz O, Acheson K, Gmuender B, Jequier E. Effect of L-carnitine on sub-maximal exercise metabolism after depletion of muscle glycogen. Med Sci Sports Exerc 1993;25:733–40.

Dyck DJ, Peters SA, Wendling PS, Chesley A, Hultman E, Spriet LL. Regulation of muscle glycogen phosphorylase activity during intense aerobic cycling with elevated FFA. Am J Physiol 1996;265:E116–E25.

Dyck DJ, Putman CT, Heigenhauser GJF, Hultman E, Spriet LL. Regulation of fat–carbohydrate interaction in skeletal muscle during intense aerobic cycling. Am J Physiol 1993;265:E852–E9.

Ebeling P, Essen-Gustavsson B, Tuominen JA, Koivisto VA. Intramuscular triglyceride content is increased in IDDM. Diabetologica 1998;41:111–15.

Essig D, Costill DL, van Handel PJ. Effects of caffeine ingestion on utilization of muscle glycogen and lipid during ergometer cycling. Int J Sports Med 1980;1:86–90.

Goedecke JH, Christie C, Wilson C, et al. Metabolic adaptations to a high-fat diet in endurance cyclists. Metabolism 1999b;48:1509–17.

Goedecke JH, Elmer-English R, Dennis SC, Schloss I, Noakes TD, Lambert EV. Effects of medium-chain triacylglycerol ingested with carbohydrate on metabolism and exercise performance. Int J Sport Nutr 1999a;9:35–47.

Hawley JA. Fat burning during exercise: can ergogenics change the balance? Phys Sportsmed 1998;26:56–68.

Hawley JA, Brouns F, Jeukendrup AE. Strategies to enhance fat utilisation during exercise. Sports Med 1998;25;241–57.

Hawley JA, Burke LM. Peak performance: training and nutritional strategies for sport. Sydney: Allen and Unwin, 1998;372–4.

Hawley JA, Burke LM, Angus DJ, et al. Effect of altering fat availability on metabolism and performance during intense exercise. Brit J Nutr 2000;84:829–38.

Hawley JA, Dennis SC, Lindsay FH, et al. Nutritional practices of athletes: are they sub-optimal? J Sports Sci 1995;13:S75–S87.

Hawley JA, Hopkins WG. Aerobic glycolytic and aerobic lipolytic power systems: a new paradigm with implications for endurance and ultraendurance events. Sports Med 1995;19:240–50.

Hawley JA, Jeukendrup AE, Brouns F. Fat metabolism during exercise. In: Maughan RJ, ed. Nutrition in sport. Oxford: Blackwell Science, 2000:192–7.

Heinonen OJ. Carnitine supplementation and physical exercise. Sports Med 1996;22:109–32.

Helge JW, Richter EA, Kiens B. Interaction of training and diet on metabolism and endurance during exercise in man. J Physiol 1996;492:293–306.

Helge JW, Wulff B, Kiens B. Impact of a fat-rich diet on endurance in man: role of the dietary period. Med Sci Sports Exerc 1998;30:456–61.

Hopkins WG, Hawley JA, Burke LM. Design and analysis of research on sport performance. Med Sci Sports Exerc 1999;31:472–85.

Horowitz JF, Mora-Rodriguez R, Byerley LO, Coyle EF. Lipolytic suppression following carbohydrate ingestion limits fat oxidation during exercise. Am J Physiol 1997;273:E768–E75.

Horowitz JF, Mora-Rodriguez R, Byerley LO, Coyle EF. Substrate metabolism when subjects are fed carbohydrate during exercise. Am J Physiol 1999;E828–E35.

Ivy JL, Costill DL, Fink WJ. Contribution of medium and long chain triglyceride intake to energy metabolism during prolonged exercise. Int J Sports Med 1980;1:15–20.

Ivy JL, Costill DL, Fink WJ, Lower RW. Influence of caffeine and carbohydrate feedings on endurance performance. Med Sci Sports 1979;11:6–11.

Jansson E, Kaijser L. Effect of diet on the utilization of blood-borne and intramuscular substrates during exercise in man. Acta Physiol Scand 1982;115:19–30.

Jeukendrup AE. Aspects of carbohydrate and fat metabolism. Haarlem: De Vriesebosch, 1997.

Jeukendrup AE, Saris WHM, Brouns F, Halliday D, Wagenmakers AJM. Effects of carbohydrate (CHO) and fat supplementation on CHO metabolism during prolonged exercise. Metabolism 1996;45:915–21.

Jeukendrup AE, Saris WHM, Schrauwen P, Brouns F, Wagenmakers AJM. Metabolic availability of medium chain triglycerides co-ingested with carbohydrates during prolonged exercise. J Appl Physiol 1995;79:756–62.

Jeukendrup AE, Thielen JJ, Wagenmakers AJM, Brouns F, Saris WHM. Effect of MCT and carbohydrate ingestion on substrate utilization and cycling performance. Am J Clin Nutr 1998;67:397–404.

Kalmar JM, Cafarelli E. Effects of caffeine on neuromuscular function. J Appl Physiol 1999;87:801–8.

Kiens B. Training and fatty acid metabolism. In: Richter EA, Kiens B, Galbo H, Saltin B, eds. Advances in experimental medicine and biology. Vol 441: Skeletal muscle metabolism in exercise and diabetes. New York: Plenum Press, 1998:229–38.

Kiens B, Essen-Gustavsson B, Christensen NJ, Saltin B. Skeletal muscle substrate utilization during submaximal exercise in man: effect of endurance training. J Physiol 1993;469:459–78.

Kiens B, Helge J. Adaptations to a high-fat diet. In: Maughan R, ed. Nutrition in Sport. Oxford: Blackwell Science Ltd, 2000:192–202.

Kraegen EW, Clark PW, Jenkins AB, Daley EA, Chisolm DJ, Storlien LH. Development of muscle insulin resistance after liver insulin resistance in high-fat fed rats. Diabetes 1991;40:1397–403.

Kronfeld DS. Diet and the performance of racing sled dogs. J Am Vet Med Assoc 1973;162:470–3.

Lambert EV, Hawley JA, Goedecke J, Dennis SC. Nutritional strategies for promoting fat utilization and delaying the onset of fatigue during prolonged exercise. J Sports Sci 1997;15:315–24.

Lambert EV, Speechly DP, Dennis SC, Noakes TD. Enhanced endurance in trained cyclists during moderate intensity exercise following 2 weeks adaptation to a high-fat diet. Eur J Appl Physiol 1994;69:287–93.

Martin WH. Effects of acute and chronic exercise on fat metabolism. In: Holloszy JO, ed. Exercise and sport sciences reviews. Vol 24: Baltimore: Williams and Wilkins, 1996;203–31.

Martin WH, Dalsky GP, Hurley BF, et al. Effect of endurance training on plasma free fatty acid turnover and oxidation during exercise. Am J Physiol 1993;265:E708–E14.

Massicotte D, Peronnet F, Brisson GR, Hillaire-Marcel C. Oxidation of exogenous medium-chain free fatty acids during prolonged exercise–comparison with glucose. J Appl Physiol 1992;73:1334–9.

Muoio DM, Leddy JJ, Horvarth PJ, Awad AB, Pendergast DR. Effect of dietary fat on metabolic adjustments to maximal VO_2 and endurance in runners. Med Sci Sports Exerc 1994;26:81–8.

Odland LM, Heigenhauser GJF, Lopaschuk GD, Spriet LL. Human skeletal muscle malonyl-CoA at rest and during prolonged submaximal exercise. Am J Physiol 1996;270:E541–E4.

Odland LM, Heigenhauser GJF, Wong D, Hollidge-Horvat MG, Spriet LL. Effects of increased fat availability on fat–carbohydrate interaction during prolonged aerobic exercise in humans. Am J Physiol 1998;274:R894–R902.

Okano G, Sato Y, Murata Y. Effect of elevated blood FFA levels on endurance performance after a single fat meal ingestion. Med Sci Sports Exerc 1998;30:763–8.

Okano G, Sato Y, Takumi M, Sugawara M. Effect of 4-h pre-exercise high-carbohydrate and high-fat meal ingestion on endurance performance and metabolism. Int J Sports Med 1996;17:530–4.

Phillips DIW, Caddy S, Illic V, et al. Intramuscular triglyceride and muscle insulin sensitivity: evidence for a relationship in nondiabetic subjects. Metabolism 1996;45:947–50.

Phinney SD, Bistrian BR, Evans WF. The human metabolic response to chronic ketosis without caloric restriction: preservation of submaximal exercise capacity with reduced carbohydrate oxidation. Metabolism 1983;32:769–76.

Pitsiladis YP, Smith I, Maughan RJ. The effects of altered fat and carbohydrate availability on the capacity to perform prolonged cycling in trained humans. Med Sci Sports Exerc 1999;31:1570–9.

Rauch LGH, Hawley JA, Woodey M, Dennis SC, Noakes TD. Effects of ingesting a sports bar versus glucose polymer on substrate utilization and ultra-endurance performance. Int J Sports Med 1999;20:252–7.

Romijn JA, Coyle EF, Hibbert J, Wolfe RR. Comparison of indirect calorimetry and a new breath $^{13}C/^{12}C$ ratio method during strenuous exercise. Am J Physiol 1992;263:E64–E71.

Romijn JA, Coyle EF, Sidossis LS, et al. Regulation of endogenous fat and carbohydrate in relation to exercise intensity. Am J Physiol 1993;E380–E91.

Romijn JA, Coyle EF, Sidossis LS, Zhang XJ, Wolfe RR. Relationship between fatty acid delivery and fatty acid oxidation during strenuous exercise. J Appl Physiol 1995;79:1939–45.

Sarna S, Kaprio J. Life expectancy of former athletes. Sports Med 1994;17:149–51.

Satabin P, Portero P, Defer G, Bricout J, Guezennec CY. Metabolic and hormonal responses to lipid and carbohydrate diets during exercise in man. Med Sci Sports Exerc 1987;19:218–23.

Sears B. The Zone diet: a dietary road map. New York: Regan Books, 1995.

Sears B. Mastering the Zone: the next step in achieving superhealth and permanent fat loss. New York: Regan Books, 1997.

Sherman WM, Lamb DR. Nutrition and prolonged exercise. In: Lamb DR, Murray R, eds. Perspectives in exercise science and sports medicine. Vol 1: Prolonged exercise. Indianapolis: Benchmark Press, 1988;213–80.

Sidossis LS, Gastaldelli A, Klein S, Wolfe RR. Regulation of plasma fatty acid oxidation during low- and high-intensity exercise. Am J Physiol 1997;272:E1065–E70.

Sidossis LS, Stuart CA, Schulman GI, Lopaschuk GD, Wolfe RR. Glucose plus insulin regulate fat oxidation by controlling the rate of fatty acid entry into the mitochondria. J Clin Invest 1996;98:2244–50.

Spriet LL. Ergogenic aids: recent advances and retreats. In: Lamb DR, Murray R, eds. Perspectives in exercise science and sports medicine. Vol 10: Optimizing sports performance. Carmel, Indiana: Cooper Publishing Company, 1997:185–234.

Spriet LL. Biochemical regulation of carbohydrate-lipid interaction in skeletal muscle during low and moderate intensity exercise. In: Hargreaves M, Thompson M, eds. Biochemistry of exercise X. Champaign, Illinois: Human Kinetics, 1999:241–61.

Spriet LL, Dyck DJ. The glucose-fatty acid cycle in skeletal muscle at rest and during exercise. In: Maughan RJ, Shirreffs SM, eds. Biochemistry of exercise IX. Champaign, Illinois: Human Kinetics, 1996:127–55.

Starling RD, Trappe TA, Parcell AC, Kerr CG, Fink WJ, Costill DL. Effects of diet on muscle triglyceride and endurance performance. J Appl Physiol 1997;82:1185–9.

Sternfeld B. Cancer and the protective effect of physical activity: the epidemiological evidence. Med Sci Sports Exerc 1992;4:195–209.

van Vusse D, Reneman RS. Lipid metabolism in muscle. In: Rowell LB, Shepherd JT, eds. Handbook of physiology. Exercise: Regulation and integration of multiple systems. Chapter 21. New York: American Physiological Society, Oxford Press, 1996:952–94.

van Zyl CG, Lambert EV, Hawley JA, Noakes TD, Dennis SC. Effects of medium-chain triglyceride ingestion on carbohydrate metabolism and cycling performance. J Appl Physiol 1996;80:2217–25.

Vukovich MD, Costill DL, Fink WJ. Carnitine supplementation: effect on muscle carnitine and glycogen content during exercise. Med Sci Sports Exerc 1994;26:1122–9.

Vukovich MD, Costill DL, Hickey MS, Trappe SW, Cole KJ, Fink WJ. Effect of fat emulsion, infusion and fat feeding on muscle glycogen utilization during cycle exercise. J Appl Physiol 1993;75:1513–18.

Wee SL, Williams C, Garcia-Roves P. Carbohydrate availability determines endurance running capacity in fasted subjects. Med Sci Sports Exerc 1999;31:S91.

Whitley HA, Humphreys SM, Campbell IT, et al. Metabolic and performance responses during endurance exercise after high-fat and high-carbohydrate meals. J Appl Physiol 1998;85:418–24.

Wolfe RR. Fat metabolism in exercise. In: Richter EA, Kiens B, Galbo H, Saltin B, eds. Advances in experimental medicine and biology. Vol 441: Skeletal muscle metabolism in exercise and diabetes. New York: Plenum Press, 1998:147–56.

Dietary supplements and nutritional ergogenic aids in sport

Louise Burke, Ben Desbrow and Michelle Minehan

17.1 INTRODUCTION

The sports world is filled with special foods, potions, pills and powders that promise to provide the athlete with a performance edge. Advertisements and testimonials for these products claim prolonged endurance, faster recovery, increases in muscle mass and strength, losses of body fat, and resistance to fatigue, illness or infection. Such promises are attractive to athletes and coaches, especially in elite competition where very small differences separate the fame and fortune of winning from the anonymity of the rest of the field. Yet external rewards provide only part of the drive to find a 'magic bullet', because even non-elite and recreational athletes show considerable interest in using sports supplements.

In the general community, supplement use continues to increase. In 1996, consumer spending on supplements in the United States was $6.5 billion, doubling the expenditure of 1990–91. In 1997 the market increased to $12.8 billion (Camire & Kantor 1999). Traditional markets of health food shops and pharmacies have been expanded to include sports shops, multilevel marketing, mail-order and Internet sales. Supplements targeted at athletes and sports performance provide an important niche in this market. Sales figures provided for some contemporary sports supplements illustrate the rapid response of consumers to marketing and word of mouth publicity for these products. Creatine supplements, first brought to public attention after the 1992 Barcelona Olympics, now have annual sales estimated at 2.7 million kilograms (Williams et al. 1998). Hydroxy-methyl butyrate (HMB), a supplement which received its first mention in sports science literature in 1995–96, reached sales figures of $30–50 million in the United States during 1998 (Slater, in press), in the absence of clear proof of its success in increasing muscle mass and strength.

This chapter will review the supplement practices of athletes, discussing the science behind commonly used supplements. It will be seen that the evidence to support the claims of many products is absent, but that there are specific situations in which athletes may benefit from the use of nutritional supplements. To help simplify the vast array of products on offer to athletes we will continue to use a system that identifies two separate categories or applications of nutritional supplements, classifying these either as dietary supplements or nutritional ergogenic aids.

17.2 *SUPPLEMENTATION PRACTICES OF ATHLETES*

In a previous summary of the literature (Burke & Heeley 1994), we noted that few formal studies have focussed solely on the use of nutritional supplements by athletes. Most of the information about the supplementation practices of athletes is provided, in brief, from surveys of dietary intake of athletic populations. Exceptions to this include surveys of the supplementation practices of marathon runners (Nieman et al. 1989), swimmers (Baylis et al. in press) and high school athletes (Sobal & Marquart 1994; Krumbach et al. 1999). A large survey of drug use among Australian athletes (Australian Sports Medicine Federation 1983) also included a section on the use of nutritional supplements.

Table 17.1 summarises the prevalence of supplement use reported among a variety of athletic groups, and shows that more than half the athletic population are supplement users, although the prevalence ranges between sports. Of course, some of the variation in the supplement use reported by different athletic groups is due to methodological differences in collecting this information. First, there are differences between surveys with respect to the definition of 'nutritional supplements', with some surveys limiting supplements to vitamin and mineral preparations (Moffatt 1984) while others include items such as sports drinks and other sports food products (Australian Sports Medicine Federation 1983). The definition of 'regular', 'routine', 'irregular' and 'occasional' use may also differ. Finally, the method of collecting information (e.g. questionnaire/self-report versus actual record of intake) also influences the results. For example, Nieman and colleagues (1989) found a higher percentage of runners reported using vitamin or mineral supplements when responding to a frequency questionnaire (69% usage) than when recording actual use over a three-day period (48%). Methodological differences aside, the literature shows that supplement use by athletes is a popular and widespread activity, with considerable variability between and among different sports with regard to the number and type of products used. It is also apparent that supplement use moves in cycles or trends, with new supplements quickly becoming popular and others disappearing from fashion.

Table 17.1 *Prevalence of supplement use by athletes*

Reference	Population	N	% use
Adams et al. 1982	College swimmers (F)	12	33
Australian Sports Medicine Federation 1983	All athletes (M, F)	4063	47
Barr 1986	Marathon runners (F)	104	75
	Fitness class runners (F)	105	64
Barr 1987	College athletes (F)	70	76
Barr & Costill 1992	College swimmers (M)	24	17
Barry et al. 1981	Mixed elite athletes (M, F)	143	55
Baylis et al. in press	Elite swimmers (M, F)	77	99
Bazzarre et al. 1993	Recreational athletes (M, F)	91	51
Berning 1986	Elite swimmers (M, F)	NA	63
Bobb et al. 1969	College athletes (M)	28	25
Brill & Keane 1994	Body builders (M, F)	309	100
Burke et al. 1991	Elite triathletes (M)	25	44
	Elite marathon runners (M)	19	95
	Australian footballers (M)	56	46
	Olympic weightlifters (M)	19	100
Campbell & MacFadyen 1984	Swimmers (M, F)	101	61
Clark et al. 1988	Elite runners (F)	93	71
Cross 1997	Olympic swimmers (M, F)	28	89
Deuster et al. 1986	Runners (F)	57	54
Douglas & Douglas 1984	Marathon runners (M, F)	943	58
Ersoy 1991	Competitive gymnasts (F)	20	45
Faber & Spinnler-Benade 1987	Body builders (M)	76	63
Faber & Spinnler-Benade 1991	National field athletes (M)	20	35
	National field athletes (F)	10	33
Felder et al. 1998	Elite surfers (F)	10	50
Frederick & Hawkins 1992	College track athletes (F)	13	62
Grandjean 1983	Elite athletes (M, F)	69	92
Grandjean 1985	Elite athletes (M, F)	150	52

(continues)

(continued)

Reference	Population	N	% use
Grandjean et al. 1992	Elite road cyclists (F)	3	100
Houston 1980	Elite swimmers (M)	8	75
	Elite swimmers (F)	12	50
Jonnalagadda et al. 1998	Elite gymnasts (F)	33	92
Khoo et al. 1987	Ironman triathletes (M)	19	60
	Ironman triathletes (F)	10	80
Kleiner et al. 1990	Body builders (M)	8	90
	Body builders (F)	19	100
Krowchuk et al. 1989	High school athletes (M, F)	298	33
Krumbach et al. 1999	Collegiate athletes (M, F)	411	57
Lamar-Hildebrand et al. 1989	Competitive body builders (F)	6	100
	Non-competitive body builders (F)	4	50
Lawrence et al. 1975a and 1975b	Swimmers (M, F)	48	52
	Swimmers (M, F)	72	54
Loosli et al. 1986	Club gymnasts (F)	97	43
Moffatt 1984	Elite high school gymnasts (F)	13	23
Nieman et al. 1989	Non-elite runners (M)	285	86
	Non-elite runners (F)	54	70
Nowak et al. 1988	College basketball (F)	10	50
	College basketball (M)	15	6
Oppliger et al. 1993	High school wrestlers (M)	713	40
Parr et al. 1984	High school/college athletes (M)	1432	56
	High school/college athletes (F)	1547	33
Peters et al. 1986	Ultra-distance runners (M)	15	80
Sandoval et al. 1989	Body builders (M)	5	20
	Body builders (F)	6	50
Saris et al. 1989	Elite road cyclists (M)	5	100
Schulz 1988	College athletes (M, F)	127	44
Short & Short 1983	College football players (M)	40	43
	College basketballers (M)	12	42
	College wrestlers (M)	38	13
Singh et al. 1993	Ultra-marathoners (M)	10	66
	Ultra-marathoners (F)	2	100
Slavin et al. 1984	Bicycle racers (M)	76	32
	Bicycle racers (F)	32	64

Reference	Population	N	% use
Snyder et al. 1989	Elite speed skaters (M)	10	60
	Elite speed skaters (F)	7	86
Sobal & Marquart 1994	High school athletes (M, F)	742	38
Steel 1970	Olympic athletes (M, F)	80	49
Thibault et al. 1984	Marathon runners (M, F)	1123	20
Werblow et al. 1978	College athletes (F)	94	37
Worme et al. 1990	Triathletes (M, F)	71	39

Unfortunately, most studies reporting the supplementation practices of athletes fail to provide the most interesting information: the type of supplements used, the amounts taken and the rationale for their use. However, several authors have commented that at least some athletes use a large number of supplements concurrently, often resulting in nutrient intakes that are very high in comparison with normal dietary intakes (Grandjean 1993). The Australian Sports Medicine Federation Report (1983) expressed concern about the 'significant minority' of athletes who reported intakes of six to 15 supplement preparations daily. We also noted 'polypharmacy' in our survey of elite swimmers; 71% of swimmers reported the use of more than one vitamin and mineral preparation and one swimmer recorded 28 different supplement products in regular use (Baylis et al. in press).

There is little information about why athletes choose their supplement patterns. In a study of 347 marathon runners (n=347), Nieman et al. (1989) failed to find significant associations between supplement use and gender, race, marital status, education, dietary intake or training level. By contrast, Krumbach and colleagues found that male and female college athletes were motivated by different beliefs in deciding to use supplements (Krumbach et al. 1999). The Australian Sports Medicine Federation survey (1983) reported that the beliefs within a particular sport, particularly emanating from a coach, strongly influenced supplementation practices. The role of the coach as nutrition adviser has been highlighted in other studies, with 35% of coaches in one survey (Wolf et al. 1979) and 68% in another (Bentivegna et al. 1979) reporting that they had recommended their athletes to take supplements on some occasions. Despite often following supplement practices that are not generally supported by scientific evidence, elite swimmers nominated professional advice from dietitians, doctors, pharmacists and sports scientists as the most important information to consider before trying a new supplement product (Baylis et al. in press). In this survey, the advice of a coach was ranked highly as a supporting source of information, but expense was not considered to be very important (Baylis et al. in press).

Generally, there are three reasons put forward by athletes in support of their supplement use (Nieman et al. 1989):

1. to compensate for less than adequate diets or lifestyles;

2. to meet unusual nutrient demands induced by heavy exercise; and
3. to produce a direct (e.g. ergogenic) effect on performance.

Although some surveys have suggested that certain types of athletes use supplements to compensate for poor food intake, in our experience, the majority of current athletes are motivated by the direct performance or health claims made for various supplements. To better understand the variety of products marketed to athletes we have devised a simple classification system, dividing supplements into two categories.

17.3 CLASSIFICATION OF SUPPLEMENTS USED BY ATHLETES

17.3.1 *Definition of dietary supplements*

Previously we have proposed the following definitions for a 'dietary supplement' or 'sports supplement' (Burke & Read 1993):

- contains nutrients in amounts generally similar to the levels specified in the recommended dietary intakes or allowances (RDIs/RDAs), and similar to the amounts found in food;
- provides a convenient or practical means of ingesting these nutrients, particularly in the athletic setting;
- allows or aids the achievement of known physiological or nutritional requirements of an athlete;
- contains nutrient(s) in large amounts for use in treating a known nutrient deficiency;
- has been shown to meet a specific physiological or nutritional need that improves sports performance; and
- is generally acknowledged as a valuable product by sports medicine and science experts.

Sports supplements that meet the definition of the dietary supplement are summarised in Table 17.2. This table shows some of the specific applications of those products that have been demonstrated to assist in the achievement of optimal sports performance. More information on the composition and use of these products can be found in other chapters of this book, as shown in Table 17.2.

It is important for athletes to appreciate that sports supplements *per se* do not produce a performance enhancement. Rather, it is the use of a supplement to achieve sports nutrition goals or guidelines that allows the athlete to perform optimally. Nutrition education of athletes is needed to ensure that dietary supplements are used appropriately. In many cases, this information is specific to the athlete or the sports situation and may require one-on-one counselling. In most situations, the use of the supplement will be part of a larger plan of optimal sports nutrition or the clinical management of a nutritional problem. Effective education will not only ensure that dietary supplements are used for maximum benefit, but will also highlight the general importance of optimal nutrition for the athlete.

Table 17.2 Dietary supplements and their use by athletes

Supplement	Form	Composition	Sports-related use	Chapter
Sports drink	Powder	5–7% CHO	Optimum delivery of fluid + CHO during exercise	14
	Liquid	10–25 mmol/L Na	Post-exercise rehydration	15
Sports gel	Gel	60–70% CHO	Supplement high-CHO training diet	15
	30–40 g	(~25 g CHO per sachet)	Carbohydrate loading	13
	sachets or larger	Some contain MCTs or caffeine	Post-exercise CHO recovery	15
	tubes		May be used during exercise when CHO needs exceed fluid requirements	14
High-CHO supplement	Powder	10–25% CHO	Supplement high-CHO training diet	15
	Liquid	(+ some B vitamins)	Carbohydrate loading	13
			Post-exercise CHO recovery	15
			May be used during exercise when CHO needs exceed fluid requirements	14
Liquid meal supplement	Powder (mix with water or milk) or liquid	1–1.5 kcal/mL 15–20% protein 50–70% CHO Low to moderate fat Vitamins/minerals: 500–1000 mL supplies RDIs/RDAs	Supplement high-energy/CHO nutrient diet (especially during heavy training/competition or weight gain) Low-bulk meal replacement (especially pre-event meal) Post-exercise recovery Portable nutrition for travelling athlete	5, 15 13 15 24
Sports bar	Bar (50–60 g)	40–50 g CHO 5–10 g protein Usually low in fat Vitamins/minerals: 50–100% of RDIs/RDAs	CHO source during exercise Post-exercise recovery Supplement high-energy/CHO/nutrient diet Portable nutrition (travelling)	14 15 15 24
Vitamin/mineral supplement	Capsule/tablet	Broad range 1–4 × RDIs/RDAs of vitamins and minerals	Micronutrient support for low-energy or weight-loss diet Micronutrient support for restricted variety diets (e.g. vegetarian diet) Micronutrient support for unreliable food supply (e.g. travelling athlete)	7, 12 9, 12, 21 24
Iron supplement	Capsule/tablet	Ferrous sulfate/gluconate/fumarate	Supervised management of iron deficiency	11
Calcium supplement	Tablet	Calcium carbonate/ phosphate/lactate	Calcium supplementation in low-energy or low dairy food diet? Treatment/prevention of osteopenia	10

Since the dietary guidelines for exercise are well documented, and their application can provide a substantial enhancement of performance, it should be relatively simple to demonstrate beneficial uses of common sports supplements. In fact, many products such as sports drinks, carbohydrate (CHO) gels and liquid meal supplements have been specially manufactured in response to needs identified by applied sport science research. Pharmaceutical and food companies that produce and market dietary supplements provide much of the financial support for this research. In this way, a beneficial relationship between the company, the sports science or medicine professional and the athlete is nurtured.

17.3.2 *Definition of nutritional ergogenic aids*

The second broad category of sports supplements might be termed nutritional ergogenic aids, described by the following characteristics (Burke & Read 1993):

- contain nutrients or other food components in amounts greater than nutrient RDI levels, or the amounts typically provided by food;
- propose a direct ergogenic (work-enhancing) effect on sports performance, often through a pharmacological rather than a physiological effect;
- often rely on theoretical or anecdotal support rather than on documented support from scientific trials; and
- are generally not supported by sports nutrition experts, except where scientific trials have documented a significant ergogenic effect.

It is the use of these supplements that continue to escalate, and to cycle in and out of fashion. It is difficult for scientists and practitioners to stay abreast of the number of new products that emerge onto the market each year. In this chapter, we review the use and scientific support for a number of nutritional ergogenic aids that are of current interest. However, before this summary is presented, it is useful to understand the processes of government regulation of sports supplements, and the processes needed to provide suitable proof of performance enhancements resulting from the use of a product.

17.4 THE SPORTS SUPPLEMENT INDUSTRY

In Australia, the production and sale of sports supplements falls under the jurisdiction of two government bodies: the Australian and New Zealand Food Authority (ANZFA), which controls food products, and Therapeutic Goods Administration (TGA), which controls pills and other formulations marketed as therapeutic goods (Baylis et al. in press). Sports foods such as sports drinks, sports bars, sports gels and liquid meal supplements generally fall within Standards R9 and R10 of the ANZFA Foods Standards Code. These standards make provision for a range of acceptable formulations and permitted additives, as well as a list of permitted or compulsory education messages for presentation on product packaging. It is the responsibility of individual states and territories to adopt these standards within their Food Laws, and to check and regulate that these laws are upheld. In reality, there are some sports foods, available on the Australian market, that do not meet these Standards, either by containing ingredients that are in contravention to the Code, or by carrying illegal claims. This is not the case for the larger number of mainstream products such as commercial sports drinks and bars. However, there are some sports foods, usually produced by smaller manufacturers targeting a niche market of athletes, which fail to comply. As ANZFA codes move towards the goal of developing a largely self-regulated industry of food manufacture and marketing, there is a greater likelihood that sports foods will contain non-permitted substances and/or incomplete or inaccurate labelling information.

According to our recent review (Baylis et al. in press), the availability and marketing of dietary supplements fitting the description of pills, powders or other non-food forms, fall within the jurisdiction of the TGA, under the Australian Therapeutic Goods Act 1989. This Act distinguishes two classes of products: drugs and therapeutic devices. Although dietary supplements may be packaged in a way suggesting medical or scientific rigour, as therapeutic devices they are regulated at an entirely different level to prescription pharmaceutical products. Therapeutic devices are further classified into categories of 'registrable' and 'listable' products, with almost all dietary supplements falling within the 'listable' or less regulated category. Although they need to comply with relevant statutory standards, for example to exclude ingredients banned by Australian Customs laws, they are considered low-risk self-medications and are not subjected to a comprehensive review of quality, safety and efficacy. They are expected to comply with Good Manufacturing Practice, and to advertising regulations, making limited therapeutic claims. In practice, these products receive little investigation of quality and advertising claims, unless they are the subject of serious complaints regarding health and safety issues (Baylis et al. in press).

Since supplements that are imported via mail order, Internet sales or personal importation are not subject to any scrutiny in the country of destiny, it is important for athletes to have a global understanding of the regulation of supplements. In other countries, including the United States, there is less regulation of the production and marketing of supplements than under the Australian system. In the US, all supplements (food and non-food forms) fall under the jurisdiction of the Food and Drug Administration. The Dietary Supplement Health and Education Act, passed in 1994, reduced the regulation of dietary supplements and broadened the category to include new ingredients such as herbal and botanical products, and constituents or metabolites of other dietary supplements. This Act shifted responsibility from the manufacturer to the FDA to enforce safety and claim guidelines. Since then manufacturers have not been required to comply with Good Manufacturing Practice.

In the absence or minimisation of rigorous government evaluation, quality control of supplement manufacturing is trusted to supplement companies. Large companies that produce conventional supplements such as vitamins and minerals, particularly to manufacturing standards used in the preparation of pharmaceutical products, are likely to achieve good quality control. This includes precision with ingredient levels and labelling, and avoidance of undeclared ingredients or contaminants. However, this does not appear to be true for all supplement types or manufacturers. Independent testing of 16 commercial dehydroepiandrosterone (DHEA) products revealed that only half the products contained the amount of DHEA stated on the product label, with actual levels varying between 0–150% of the stated content (Parasrampuria et al. 1998). Melatonin supplements have been found to fail to meet quality claims or delivery profiles stated on their labels (Hahm et al. 1999). Investigation of supplements containing Ephedra Sinica (Ma Huang) showed variability in alkaloid content between various brands of supplements, failure to report the Ephedra content on product labels, and batch-to-batch variability within the same product of nearly 140% (Gurley et al. 1998).

Although manufacturers are guided not to make unsupported claims about health or performance benefits from the use of supplements, product advertisements and testimonials show ample evidence that this aspect of supplement marketing is unregulated and exploited. For example, a survey of five issues of body building magazines found 800 individual performance claims for 624 different products within advertisements (Grunewald & Bailey 1993). Similarly large numbers of claims were found in another survey of health and body building magazines (Philen et al. 1992). The enthusiasm and emotive nature of these claims provide a false sense of confidence about the products. Most consumers are unaware that such advertising is not regulated. Therefore, they are likely to believe that claims about supplements are medically and scientifically supported, simply because they believe that untrue claims would not be allowed to exist. The undeserved credibility of supplement products derived from such claims not only continues to promote sales, but lures athletes into a false sense of security about aspects of quality and safety of products.

Later in this chapter, we will examine the process of undertaking rigorous scientific research, and appreciate that it is costly in time, money and resources. In the case of pharmaceutical products, which need to meet stringent regulations for therapeutic use and for safety, a company can expect to spend two to ten years and two million dollars in testing to gain approval for a new drug (Bucci 1998). Few of even the largest supplement manufacturers have the resources to comprehensively study the existing range of ergogenic aids and their combinations of use. Of course, it may not always be in the interests of a company to test some of their supplements in case they find negative results. In any case, a company might consider it wasteful to spend money on research, which they are not forced to do and which the market does not appear to demand.

17.5 *WHAT IS PROOF?*

The process of substantiating the performance benefits or outcomes from supplementation is difficult. In exploring the concept of 'proof', it will be seen that there are different levels of support that appeal to different audiences.

17.5.1 *Scientific theories*

A hypothesis is a line of enquiry that attempts to uncover or explain important relationships between factors. Historically, the dietary practices of athletes have evolved from hypotheses based on the contemporary understanding of exercise metabolism. Centuries ago, athletes were guided to eat the flesh of 'athletic' animals on the superstition that they might gain whatever factors underpinned the animal's prowess. Later on, high-protein diets were recommended, based on the belief that exercise was fuelled by protein, the key component of muscle. As our understanding of exercise metabolism has become more sophisticated, it has produced a huge number of new theories about factors that might play an important role in various reactions.

The current focus of the sports supplement industry is on compounds and nutrients that act as cofactors, intermediary metabolites or stimulants of key reactions in exercise metabolism. The rationale behind supplementation is simple and attractive: when the system is 'supercharged' with additional amounts of these compounds, metabolic processes will proceed faster or longer, thus enhancing sports performance. The marketing of most contemporary supplements is accompanied by sophisticated descriptions of metabolic pathways and biochemical reactions whose enhancement will lead to athletic success. To the scientist, a theory that links an increased level of a compound with performance enhancement may be a hypothesis that is worthy of testing, but it does not constitute proof or support for the idea. However, to the public, a hypothesis can be made to sound like a *fait accompli*, and athletes can be induced to buy products on the strength of a 'scientific breakthrough' which exists only on paper. In an era when sports scientists feel challenged by the apparent sophistication of the scientific theories presented by supplement companies, it is unlikely that athletes will possess sufficient scientific knowledge to be critical of these proposals.

While a 'supercharging' hypothesis may appear plausible at first glance, there are many reasons why it may not occur. Other issues to be considered include:

1. Will oral ingestion of the compound increase concentrations at the sites that are critical?
2. Does the present level of compound fall below the critical level for optimal metabolism?
3. Is this reaction the rate limiting step in metabolism or are other reactions setting the pace?

A scientific theory or hypothesis should be developed and fine-tuned before setting up a supplementation study. Since studies are expensive in time, money and resources, it is important that ideas that make it to trial are based on sound logic. But while a scientific theory should be developed in preparation for a study (or to explain the data collected in a study), it cannot be touted or accepted as evidence or practice until verified by actual research.

17.5.2 *Anecdotal support*

Testimonials provide a powerful force in the advertising and marketing of sports supplements, particularly products that target the body building or resistance training industry. This is also true of supplements sold through multilevel marketing schemes. Advertisements highlight the successful health or performance outcomes that people have achieved, allegedly as a result of their use of a supplement product. Often famous athletes or media stars supply these testimonials, but sometimes they also feature the exploits of 'everyday' people. Although cynics may note that people receive payment for these endorsements, testimonials, nevertheless, provide an emotive argument in favour of the supplement involved. Some athletes, including elite sportspeople, have financial interests in the supplement industry. For example, the body building guru, Joe Weider, not only publishes the magazine *Muscle and Fitness*, which has a world-wide circulation of over seven million readers, but also owns a number of supplement lines such as the Weider and Victory ranges. Other athletes may have a smaller role, by acting as distributors for supplement ranges that are sold through multilevel marketing.

However, not all testimonials are paid for. Since the sports world lends itself to the swapping of ideas, it is not surprising for an athlete to become interested in a supplement on the direct recommendation or hearsay from another supplement user. Successful athletes and teams are perpetually asked to nominate the secrets of their success in the media. In the following reviews of well-known ergogenic aids, we will see that public interest in a product can often be traced back to the recommendation or testimonial of a winning sportsperson.

It is hard for athletes to understand that success in sport results from a complicated and multifactorial recipe, and that even the most successful athletes may not fully appreciate the factors behind their prowess. In many cases, it is likely that the athlete has succeeded without the effects of the supplements they are taking—and in some cases perhaps, in spite of them! Unsupported beliefs and superstition are key reasons behind many decisions to use supplements. The idea that 'everyone is doing it' provides a powerful motivation to the athlete contemplating a new product. Sometimes, this manifests as a fear that 'others may have a winning edge that I don't have'. The *ad hoc* and undiscriminating patterns of supplement use reported by some athletes are testament to the power of 'word of mouth'.

Of course, the anecdotal experiences of athletes may be useful when considering the scientific investigation of a supplement. These experiences may support the case for expending resources on a study, or help in deciding on protocols for using the supplement or for measuring the outcomes. However, by themselves they provide very weak support for the benefits of a supplement. Many of the benefits perceived by athletes who try a new supplement result from the psychological boost, which accompanies a new experience or special treatment.

17.5.2.1 *Placebo and other effects*

People who participate in a study experience various psychological responses. One response, known as the 'Hawthorne effect', occurs as a result of the 'special treatment' or monitoring received by subjects who know they are participating in a study. This was first identified during a series of management studies undertaken in the 1920s at the Hawthorne works of an electric company in the United States. The studies monitored the work output of a group of individuals under varying conditions of light. First, the lighting was increased in intensity and work output was found to increase—even in conditions exceeding the levels that were typically tolerated. However, when the light was then progressively reduced to very low levels, the work output of the subjects also improved. The researchers concluded that subjects improved their performance simply as a result of being involved in the experiment, or more likely, having their output closely monitored.

The Hawthorne effect predicts that athletes will improve their training or competition performances if they receive extra interest or monitoring. This is a common scenario for athletes who 'test' a new supplement, especially when this is done under the scrutiny of the coach, the manufacturer or other athletes in the group. These athletes might undergo some new testing or monitoring processes which they tackle more enthusiastically because they are under scrutiny and being encouraged. While the improvement in performance is a welcome outcome for the athlete, it is not necessarily the result of the supplement. The effect of the supplement can only be isolated by comparing the outcome with changes that occur in a 'control' group of athletes, who are similarly encouraged and monitored without receiving a new treatment.

The 'placebo' effect describes a favourable outcome arising simply from the belief that you have received a beneficial treatment. In a clinical environment, a placebo is often given in the form of a harmless but inactive substance or treatment that satisfies the patient's symbolic need to receive a 'therapy'. Despite our belief that the placebo effect is real and potentially substantial, only a few studies have tried to document the size or characteristics of the effect. Beecher (1959) reported that an injection of saline solution was 70% as effective as morphine in reducing pain for hospital patients. In another study, weightlifters who received injections described as anabolic steroids increased their gains in lean body mass despite receiving an inert (water) treatment (Arial 1972). A recent investigation where athletes were given either a sports drink or a sweetened placebo during a one-hour cycling time trial found that performance was affected by the information provided to the subjects (Clark et al. in press). The placebo effect caused by thinking they were receiving a CHO drink allowed the subjects to achieve a small but worthwhile increase in performance of 4%. Being unsure of which treatment was being received increased the variability of performance, illustrating that the greatest benefits from supplement use occur when athletes are confident they are receiving a useful product (Clark et al. in press). Further work is needed to better describe the potential size and duration of this effect, and whether it applies equally to all athletes and all types of performance testing.

In the meantime, we can be satisfied that the placebo effect exists and may explain, at least partially, why athletes have a positive experience when trying a new supplement or dietary treatment. However, while the experience of other athletes provides a powerful incentive (or fear) to promote the use of nutritional ergogenic aids, it does not provide sufficient proof of beneficial effects.

17.5.3 *The scientific trial*

The scientific trial remains the 'gold standard' for investigating the effects of dietary supplements and nutritional ergogenic aids on sports performance. Scientists undertaking scientific trials should test the effects of the supplement in a context that simulates sports performance as closely as possible. Additional studies might be needed to elucidate the mechanisms by which these effects occur, but overall, sports science research must be able to deliver answers to questions related to real-life sport.

There are many variables that interfere with the outcomes of research. A researcher must design a protocol that eliminates extraneous or confounding variables and monitors a set of carefully chosen independent and dependent variables. Factors to consider include:

1. subject variables (characteristics including age, gender, level of training, experience with test protocols, psychological effects, nutritional status);
2. measurement variables (taking into account the validity and reproducibility of techniques, costs, availability of equipment, subjective versus objective measures, and the application to the hypothesis being tested);
3. study design (acute versus chronic supplementation protocols, laboratory versus field settings, blinding of subjects and researchers, crossover versus parallel group design, placebo control);
4. supplementation protocols (timing and quantity of doses, duration of supplementation period); and
5. statistical procedures (how best to examine the data generated by the studies).

At times, a series of studies might need to be undertaken to systematically address the range of questions that must be answered. It is beyond the scope of this chapter to fully explore the characteristics of good research design. However, the following ideas are useful in designing trials to test the effects of supplements on sports performance.

1. Recruit well trained athletes as subjects, unless the aim of the study is to test the effects of supplementation at different levels of training. The level of training may alter the effect of the supplement. Most importantly, it will affect the precision of measurements of performance. A homogenous group of well-trained athletes will generally show less intra- and inter- subject variability in performance, thus increasing the statistical power of the study.

2. Incorporate the use of a placebo treatment to overcome the psychological effect of supplementation. If practical, add a control (no treatment) trial so that the magnitude of the placebo effect can be determined.

3. Where possible, use repeated measures or 'crossover' design, in which each subject acts as their own control by undertaking both the treatment and placebo trials. This offers the benefit of increasing statistical power (reduced variability between treatments) and/or decreasing the number of subjects required. Take care to allow a suitable wash-out period so that the effects of the supplement are removed before the group which received the experimental treatment first begins the placebo trial.

4. Randomly assign subjects to treatment and placebo groups, and counter-balance the order of treatment, to remove the effect of time or training on study outcomes.

5. Employ a double-blind allocation of treatments to remove the subjective bias of both researcher and subjects. Blinding of the researchers will help to control the occurrence of the 'halo effect' where an observer, who believes an effect is likely, 'marks up' or encourages the performance of subjects.

6. Standardise the pre-trial training and dietary status of subjects.

7. Design the experimental conditions to mimic real-life practices of athletes. For example, allow athletes to consume a pre-event meal or to consume fluid and CHO during the performance according to usual or recommended practices.

8. Choose measurement variables that are sufficiently reliable to allow changes due to the supplement to be detected, and that are applicable to the hypothesis being tested.

9. Choose a performance test that is highly reliable and applicable to the real-life performances of athletes.

10. Choose a supplementation protocol that maximises the likelihood of a positive outcome. If a positive effect is found, doses can be manipulated in further trials to refine the optimal supplementation protocol.

11. Interpret results in light of what is important to sports performance.

17.5.3.1 *Are we testing the athlete's definition of performance enhancement?*

Although some of the features of a well designed scientific study have been outlined above, we must also consider whether the conditions and issues that satisfy a scientist are shared by the athlete. There are a number of ways in which scientific testing fails to provide answers to the questions that are asked by athletes.

When traditional scientific testing is applied to sports science, performance enhancement is tested according to the statistician's viewpoint. In human studies which involve a large number of experimental variables, typical outcome measurements of performance are highly variable. When variability between and within subjects is considerable, a large change or difference in performance (effect size) will be required to meet the 0.05 level of probability that is considered statistically significant. Therefore, most traditional intervention studies are biased towards detecting treatments that cause large changes, and ignoring treatments that produce only small changes.

Dwyer and Brotherhood (1981) first drew attention to this issue in sport, calculating relationships between sample sizes and critical levels of performance change, modelled from existing experimental-placebo trials of vitamin supplementation. Accepting the typical variability in performance measurements seen in these studies, they estimated that a subject sample of ~5000 would be needed to allow a 1–2% change in performance to become statistically significant (e.g. two to four seconds in a four-minute event such as the 1500 m run or 400 m swim). Conversely, a 12.5% improvement (e.g. 30 seconds) would be needed in a sample size of 20 before significance would be achieved. Of course, the critical change would be substantially smaller if within- and between-subject variation was reduced in such trials, and the use of repeated-measures design would reduce subject numbers. However, the point is clearly made that athletes might still be interested in improving their performance by margins that are smaller than considered 'significant' in most scientific studies.

So what is a substantial or worthwhile improvement for an elite athlete? In a sophisticated review, Hopkins and colleagues (1999) used simulations and the results of recent elite competitions to define the magnitude of the smallest enhancement that might be of interest to an elite athlete. Although the tight finishes that are typical of elite sports suggest that a tiny improvement in performance would make a difference, in fact, the situation is complicated by two important factors. These are the variation in an athlete's performance between events (also known as within-athlete variation), and the variation in performance between athletes in the same event (also known as between-athlete variation). Modelling suggests that an improvement equal to 0.4–0.7 times the typical within-athlete co-efficient of variation (CV) of performance will be worthwhile in changing the outcome of an event. For example, a 0.6 CV improvement would lift the athlete who is a true 4th place getter into winning 19% of races instead of 9% of races. The true top performer, who statistically wins 38% of races, will win 48% of races after a 0.3 CV enhancement. Analysis of competition shows that the typical CV of elite sports events ranges from 1–4%, although the top athletes are likely to be the most reliable performers (Hopkins et al. 1999).

According to Hopkins and colleagues, researchers would need a sample of 16–65 athletes in crossover studies, and 65–260 in a controlled experimental-placebo study to delimit performance enhancements of this size. Since most studies are undertaken in laboratories, and enhancements in laboratory tests and real-life events may differ, they point out the need for validity studies that combine reliability data for laboratory performances and actual competition. At the very least, studies should be conducted using performance tests of known and high reliability. This review concludes by recommending features of study design that reinforce the guidelines provided in this chapter. The authors argue against using the traditional measures of statistical significance to interpret the results of intervention studies. Instead, they encourage researchers to report their performance outcomes expressed as a percentage change, with confidence limits to define the true outcome in a similar population (Hopkins et al. 1999). Researchers should then consider whether such changes are meaningful to the outcome of an elite sports event, or calculate sample sizes necessary to delimit the size and direction of worthwhile changes.

By incorporating our recommended features into research design (see Section 17.5.3), sports scientists should be able to detect performance changes of 2–5% and greater. Dietary interventions which produce performance enhancements of this order include providing fluid or CHO in events of one hour or greater (Below & Coyle 1995; Jeukendrup et al. 1997) or CHO loading before endurance events (Hawley et al. 1997). However, without performance tests of greater reliability and sample sizes that are larger than are currently typical of sports science research, scientists will be unable to rule out the merits of interventions that produce smaller enhancements. It is likely that some supplements may produce changes in this 'grey' area. A final but important issue is that the results of studies should only be applied to populations that are similar to the test group.

17.5.3.2 *Individual responses*

Notwithstanding the general variability in performance, there is evidence that some treatments cause a range of different responses in individual athletes. In some cases, the same intervention can produce favourable responses in some individuals, neutral responses in others, and sometimes, detrimental outcomes to another group. For example, research has identified that some athletes are 'non-responders' to caffeine or creatine supplementation (Graham & Spriet 1991; Greenhaff et al. 1994). It is useful to have metabolic or other mechanistic data to substantiate real differences in response, and to differentiate these from the general variability of performance. For example, it has been shown that subjects whose muscle creatine levels did not increase by at least 20% as a result of creatine supplementation did not show the functional changes and performance enhancements seen by the rest of the experimental group (Greenhaff et al. 1994).

Studies employing simple group analysis and small sample sizes are hampered by situations where there is true variability in the size and direction of the response to an intervention. Such studies will fail to detect a difference in performance, even though this is a real outcome for some subjects in the group. Ideally, studies employing large sample sizes and co-variate analysis should be used; this approach will allow real changes to be detected and may also identify the characteristics of individuals which predict 'response' and 'non-response'. At present, such studies are rare.

17.6 NUTRITIONAL ERGOGENIC AIDS WITH CLEAR SCIENTIFIC SUPPORT

Well-conducted scientific trials have produced evidence that some ergogenic aids **can** enhance sporting performance. In this section, we review several products which enjoy such support. It should be noted that each work within a specific and narrow set of exercise situations, and should not be considered a universal sports supplement. Athletes need to be educated on appropriate situations of use, and appropriate supplementation protocols. Even so, studies show that some athletes are 'non-responders' to these protocols and some may actually experience side-effects or negative outcomes. Ideally, athletes should experiment with supplements before using them during important competitions, and will benefit from the assistance and monitoring provided by sports scientists.

17.6.1 *Creatine*

At the 1992 Barcelona Olympic Games, testimonials and gold-medal performances by British sprinters propelled a new supplement, creatine, into the limelight. Scientists were intrigued by the timely publication of a study which showed increases in muscle creatine stores following the oral intake of large doses of creatine (Harris et al. 1992). Since then, creatine has become the fastest selling and best-researched ergogenic aid. It is not often that scientists and athletes are excited by the same product. The coincidental rise of the Internet has assisted the rapid spread of scientific and testimonial information.

Although some lay publications and manufacturers have labelled creatine as a 'legal steroid', this is an incorrect and unfair comparison. In fact, creatine is a muscle fuel, and the ability of creatine supplementation to increase muscle creatine stores makes it similar to CHO loading. Creatine (methylguanidine-acetic acid) is a compound derived from amino acids which is stored primarily in skeletal muscle at typical concentrations of 100–150 mmol/kg/dry weight (dw) of muscle. About 60–65% of this creatine is phosphorylated. Creatine phosphate (CrP) provides a rapid but brief source of phosphate for the resynthesis of ATP during maximal exercise, and is therefore an important fuel source in maximal sprints of 5–10 seconds. Other functions of creatine phosphate metabolism are the buffering of hydrogen ions produced during anaerobic glycolysis and the transport of ATP, generated by aerobic metabolism, from the muscle cell mitochondria to the cytoplasm where it can be utilised for muscle contraction. Creatine metabolism is covered in more detail in Chapter 2 and in the following reviews of creatine metabolism and supplementation: Spriet 1997; Williams et al. 1998; Juhn & Tarnopolsky 1998a, 1998b; Kraemer & Volek 1999; Demant & Rhodes 1999; Greenhaff 2000.

The daily turnover of creatine, eliminated as creatinine, is approximately 1–2 g/d. This can be partially replaced from dietary creatine intake, found in animal muscle products such as meat and eggs, and typically consumed in amounts of ~1–2 g/d in an omnivorous diet. Additional creatine needs are endogenously synthesised from arginine, glycine and methionine, principally in the liver, and transported to the muscle for uptake. Creatine is transported into the muscle against a high concentration gradient, via saturable transport processes that are stimulated by insulin (Green et al. 1996a, 1996b). High dietary intakes temporarily suppress endogenous creatine production. Vegetarians who do not consume a dietary source of creatine are believed to have a reduced body creatine store, suggesting that they do not totally compensate for the lack of dietary intake (Green et al. 1997). The reason for the variability of muscle creatine concentrations between individuals is uncertain. There are some suggestions that females typically have higher muscle creatine concentrations (Fosberg et al. 1991), and it appears that creatine stores decline with ageing. The effect of training on creatine concentrations also requires further study.

In 1992, Harris and colleagues published the watershed study that showed that muscle creatine levels were increased as a result of supplementation with repeated doses of creatine, large enough to sustain plasma creatine levels above the threshold for maximal creatine transport into the muscle cell (Harris et al. 1992). They used a protocol providing four to six doses of 5 g creatine (monohydrate) for five days to increase total muscle creatine concentrations by 20%, and reach an apparent muscle threshold of ~150–160 mmol/kg dw. About 20% of the increased muscle creatine content was stored as CrP and saturation occurred after two to three days. Increases in muscle creatine stores were greatest in those who had the lowest pre-supplementation concentrations and when coupled with intensive daily exercise (Harris et al. 1992).

Although this discovery appears to be recent, in fact, studies showing that oral creatine doses are largely retained in the body were available over 70 years ago (Chanutin 1926). However, it is only now that muscle biopsy procedures and imaging techniques are available to enable scientists to monitor muscle stores of creatine and investigate the success of creatine-loading protocols. Over the past decade a number of studies have refined our knowledge of supplementation protocols. Rapid loading is achieved by consuming a daily creatine dose of 20–25 g, in split doses, for five days. Alternatively, a daily dose of 3 g/d will achieve a slow loading over 28 days (Hultman et al. 1996). Elevated muscle creatine stores are maintained by continued daily supplementation of 2–3 g (Hultman et al. 1996). Across studies there is evidence that the creatine-loading response varies between individuals, with ~30% of individuals being 'non-responders' or failing to significantly increase muscle creatine stores

(Spriet 1997; Greenhaff 2000). Co-ingestion of substantial amounts of CHO (75–100 g) with creatine doses has been shown to enhance creatine accumulation (Green et al. 1996a, 1996b) and to assist individuals to reach the muscle creatine threshold of 160 mmol/kg dw. Creatine appears to be trapped in the muscle: in the absence of continued supplementation, it takes ~4–5 weeks to return to resting creatine concentrations (Hultman et al. 1996). Many studies have reported an acute gain in body mass (BM) of ~1 kg during rapid creatine loading. This is likely to be primarily a gain in body water, and is mirrored by a reduction in urine output during the loading days (Hultman et al. 1996).

Many studies have investigated the effect of creatine supplementation on muscle function exercise and performance. Studies vary according to the characteristics of subjects (gender, age, training status), the mode of exercise, and whether supplementation involved an acute loading intervention, or a chronic effect on training adaptations. In the Appendix to this chapter we have summarised the results of studies fully published in peer-reviewed journals in Tables 17.5 (acute supplementation) and 17.6 (chronic supplementation). All studies were undertaken using an experimental-placebo design unless otherwise indicated. This is the most suitable design for such studies since the wash-out period is of a lengthy duration. We offer the following summary of this literature, and of recent reviews (Spriet 1997; Juhn & Tarnopolsky 1998a, 1998b; Williams et al. 1998; Demant & Rhodes 1999; Kraemer & Volek 1999; American College of Sports Medicine 2000; Greenhaff 2000).

1. The major benefit of creatine supplementation appears to be an increase in the rate of creatine phosphate resynthesis during the recovery between bouts of high-intensity exercise, producing higher creatine phosphate levels at the start of the subsequent exercise bout. Creatine supplementation can enhance the performance of repeated 6–30 sec bouts of maximal exercise, interspersed with short recovery intervals (20 sec–5 min), where it can attenuate the normal decrease in force or power production that occurs over the course of the session.

2. Oral creatine supplementation cannot be considered ergogenic for single-bout or first-bout sprints because the likely benefit is too small to be consistently detected.

3. The exercise situations that have been most consistently demonstrated to benefit from creatine supplementation are laboratory protocols involving isolated muscular efforts or weight-supported activities such as cycling.

4. Evidence that creatine supplementation is of benefit to endurance exercise or weight-bearing activities (e.g. running and swimming) is absent or inconsistent.

5. Performance responses to creatine supplementation vary considerably between subjects in a study, and between studies.

6. In theory, acute creatine supplementation might be beneficial for a single event in sports involving repeated high-intensity intervals with brief recovery periods. This description includes team games and racquet sports. Similarly, chronic creatine supplementation may enhance training performance and long-term

adaptation to exercise programs based on repeated high-intensity exercise. These benefits may apply to the across-season performance of athletes in team and racquet sports, as well as the preparation of athletes who undertake interval training and resistance training (e.g. swimmers and sprinters).

7. These benefits remain theoretical since few studies have been undertaken with elite athletes or as 'field studies'. Performance enhancements will only occur in weight-bearing and weight-sensitive sports (e.g. light-weight rowing and rock climbing) if gains in muscular output compensate for increases in body mass. Performance enhancements may not always occur in complex games and sports; even if changes in strength or speed are achieved by creatine-assisted training, these may not translate into improvements in game outcomes (i.e. goals scored).

8. Whether the long-term gains in muscle mass reported in studies of resistance training are caused by direct stimulation of increased myofibrillar protein synthesis by creatine, enhanced ability to undertake resistance training, or a combination of both factors, remains to be determined.

Whether there are side-effects from long-term use of creatine, particularly with the large doses associated with rapid loading, remains to be determined. To date, there are anecdotal reports of nausea, gastrointestinal upset, headaches and muscle cramping/strains linked to some creatine supplementation protocols. Some of these adverse effects are plausible, particularly in light of increased water retention within skeletal muscle (and perhaps brain) cells. At this time, however, studies have not found evidence of an increased prevalence or risk of these problems among creatine users. Some concern is directed to long-term creatine users, particularly those who self-medicate with doses far in excess of the recommended creatine usage protocols in this chapter. Since creatine may affect fluid balance or fluid distribution within various body compartments, athletes are warned to pay additional attention to fluid needs in hot weather. It may also be prudent to avoid rapid loading regimens in situations where there is a high risk of dehydration. Similarly, rapid creatine loading is unwise for athletes who need to meet weight (body mass) targets. Although it is commonly suggested that creatine supplementation may cause renal impairments, the only case report of such a problem occurred in a patient with pre-existing renal dysfunction (Prichard & Kalra 1998). Poortmans and Francaux (1999) found creatine intake had no detrimental effects on renal responses. Nevertheless, until long-term and large population studies can be undertaken, bodies such as the American College of Sports Medicine (2000) have taken a cautious view on the benefits and side-effects of creatine supplementation.

17.6.2 *Caffeine*

Caffeine is the best known member of the methyl xanthines: a family of naturally occurring stimulants found in the leaves, nuts and seeds of a number of plants. Major dietary sources of caffeine, such as tea, coffee, chocolate and cola drinks, typically provide 30–100 mg of caffeine per serve, while some non-prescriptive medications contain 100–200 mg of caffeine per tablet.

The physiological actions of caffeine are well documented and include stimulation of the central nervous system, cardiac muscle, diuresis, and epinephrine release and activity. Caffeine has several effects on skeletal muscle involving calcium handling, sodium-potassium pump activity, elevation of cyclic-AMP and direct action on enzymes such as glycogen phosphorylase. Increased catecholamine action, and the direct effect of caffeine on cyclic-AMP, may both act to increase lipolysis in adipose and muscle tissue, causing an increase in plasma-free fatty acid concentrations, and increased availability of intra-muscular triglyceride. It has been proposed that an increased potential for fat oxidation during moderate-intensity exercise promotes glycogen sparing. Caffeine may also influence athletic performance via central nervous system effects, such as a reduced perception of effort or an enhanced recruitment of motor units. Breakdown products of caffeine such as paraxanthine and theophylline may also have actions within the body. Caffeine supplementation is a fascinating and complex issue to investigate due to the difficulty in isolating individual effects of caffeine, and the potential for variability between subjects. Further information on the effects of caffeine can be found in the following reviews: Graham et al. 1994; Tarnopolsky 1994; Graham 1997.

Interest in the effect of caffeine on exercise performance dates back almost a century, but it is only the last forty years that controlled studies have been conducted and extensively reviewed. Early research in the 1970s focussed on the effects of caffeine on metabolism and performance during endurance events. A resurgence of interest in caffeine supplementation during the 1990s expanded the focus of studies to include exercise performances such as sprints (< 90 secs), and short (~5 min) and long (~20 min) events involving high intensity effort. Studies of caffeine supplementation and performance have been summarised in Tables 17.7 and 17.8 in the Appendix to this chapter, with divisions into categories based on the type of exercise protocol and the timing of caffeine intake.

In 1984, caffeine was added back to the International Olympic Committee (IOC) list of banned substances, as a restricted substance. Caffeine usage is monitored via a single urine sample taken post-event, and concentrations of caffeine, representing the 1–5% of an ingested caffeine dose that is excreted unchanged, are measured. Athletes whose urinary concentrations of caffeine exceed 12 µg/mL are considered to have 'doped'. It has been noted that there is a wide intra- and inter-individual variability in urinary caffeine concentrations (Birket & Miners 1991). However, few people exceed these levels as a result of normal coffee drinking and dietary practices (Delbeke & Debackere 1984). Studies document that at caffeine doses of 5–6 mg/kg, which produce ergogenic benefits in a number of exercise protocols, positive drug test outcomes are unlikely (Pasman et al. 1995). Furthermore, increased doses of 9 mg/kg at which a substantial percentage of subjects begin to show 'illegal' urinary caffeine concentrations do not produce an additional performance advantage. Therefore, athletes may be able to explore ergogenic benefits from caffeine supplementation while keeping well within the doping laws of elite sport.

We offer the following summary of our present knowledge about caffeine supplementation and exercise performance based on Tables 17.7 and 17.8 and reviews of caffeine (Graham et al. 1994; Tarnopolsky 1994; Graham 1997; Spriet 1997).

1. Caffeine supplementation causes various effects on a range of body tissues, at a range of doses. Overall, beneficial effects begin to be detectable at intakes of 3 mg/kg. The optimal dose for a variety of effects appears to be ~5–6 mg/kg. Above this intake no further benefits are seen, and there is an increased risk of side-effects or a 'positive' urinary caffeine level (> 12 μg/mL).

2. There appears to be a range of exercise activities that may benefit from caffeine supplementation. Further research is needed to clarify the applied situations in which benefits are seen and to fine-tune supplementation protocols.

3. Most studies of caffeine supplementation have used the protocol of ingesting caffeine one hour pre-event. Recently, benefits have been seen when caffeine was fed in association with CHO at modest doses throughout the exercise bout (Kovacs et al. 1998). Further research is needed to explore the timing of doses, particularly in events of 60 min or greater.

4. At present there is no clear mechanism to explain beneficial effects of caffeine supplementation. If glycogen sparing occurs during submaximal exercise events, it appears to be limited to the first 15–20 mins of exercise. Epinephrine changes also do not appear to be critical for performance changes.

5. The effects of caffeine supplementation differ between individuals. Some people are non-responders and some people experience negative side-effects such as tremors, increased heart rate and headaches.

6. Factors that may explain differences between performance outcomes in various studies include:
   • mode of exercise (cycling studies seem to be more likely to show benefits than running studies);
   • training status of subjects (exercise performances of well-trained subjects are more reliable and may allow smaller changes to be detected);
   • habitual caffeine intake of subjects;
     nutritional status of subjects (fasting versus pre-event CHO feeding, CHO intake during exercise versus water); and
   • gender.
     At present the role of each of these factors is not clear.

7. Individuals who want to try caffeine supplementation during their competition performances should experiment in training situations or less important competitions to determine whether there is a safe, legal and efficacious protocol for their event.

17.6.3 *Bicarbonate*

As far back as the 1930s, exercise scientists discovered that the intake of acid salts by runners decreased blood pH and impaired performance of high intensity exercise, while the addition of alkalotic therapies improved running time (Denig et al. 1931; Dill et al. 1932). Anaerobic glycolysis provides the primary fuel source for exercise of near maximal intensity lasting longer than approximately 20–30 sec. The total capacity of this system is limited. A progressive increase in the acidity of the intracellular environment, caused by the accumulation of lactate and hydrogen ions, results in muscular fatigue and an inability to maintain the exercise intensity. Although the precise mechanism is not fully clear, it is believed that the intracellular accumulation of hydrogen ions directly inhibits muscle contraction by impairing the role of calcium in this process. It may also reduce the activity of glycolytic enzymes such as phosphofructokinase (see Chapter 2, Figure 2.1). When intracellular buffering capacity is exceeded, lactate and hydrogen ions diffuse into the extracellular space, perhaps aided by a positive pH gradient. Bicarbonate represents one of the most important extracellular buffers.

In theory, an increase in blood bicarbonate levels should delay the onset of muscular fatigue during prolonged anaerobic metabolism, by increasing extracellular buffering capacity and the muscle's ability to dispose of excess H^+ ions. 'Soda loading' or 'bicarbonate loading', the ingestion of sodium bicarbonate to increase blood bicarbonate levels, has been trialled by athletes and studied by scientists for over 70 years. Sodium citrate has also been used as a buffering agent. The science and practice of ingesting buffering salts have been conflicting and inconsistent.

The general protocol for bicarbonate loading is to ingest 0.3 g of sodium bicarbonate per kilogram BM, one to two hours prior to the exercise task. Sodium bicarbonate is available as the household product 'bicarb soda' or as pharmaceutical urinary alkaliners such as 'Ural'; the typical athlete requires a dose of approximately 4–5 teaspoons. Bicarbonate loading is not considered to pose any major health risk, although some individuals suffer gastrointestinal distress such as cramping or diarrhoea. Consuming the sodium bicarbonate with plenty of water (e.g. a litre or more) may help to prevent hyperosmotic diarrhoea. Sodium citrate is also usually ingested in doses of 0.3–0.5 g/kg BM.

Theoretically, bicarbonate loading might enhance the performance of athletic events that are otherwise limited by excess hydrogen ion accumulation. These include events conducted at near maximum intensity for the duration of 1–7 min—for example 400–1500 m running, 100–400 m swimming, kayaking, rowing and canoeing events. Sports that are dependent on repeated anaerobic bursts may also benefit from bicarbonate loading. Neither the IOC, nor the governing bodies of sport, bans bicarbonate and citrate loading. However, it might be argued that it contravenes the spirit of anti-doping rules, which ban the use of 'any physiological substances taken in an attempt to artificially enhance performance'. Alternatively, one could argue that bicarbonate loading is similar to CHO loading or creatine loading, and that it represents an extension of dietary practice. In any case, it is difficult to detect the use of bicarbonate- or citrate-loading strategies by athletes, since urinary pH varies according to dietary practices such as vegetarianism and high CHO intake (Heigenhauser & Jones 1991).

There have been at least 40 studies of the effects of bicarbonate loading on athletic or exercise performance in humans (for reviews see Heigenhauser & Jones 1991; Linderman & Fahey 1991; Maughan & Greenhaff 1991; McNaughton 2000). It is beyond the scope of this chapter to review all of these studies. An alternative approach to summarise a large but narrowly defined group of studies is to undertake a meta-analysis. This statistical treatment is able to integrate and quantify results to uncover trends or relationships that might not be evident in individual studies, or from the subjective bias of a narrative review. This is a particularly useful way to review the bicarbonate-loading literature since it compacts the large number of individual studies, overcomes the limitations of small sample sizes, and helps to overview the problem of inconsistent and contradictory findings. Such a meta-analysis was published in 1993, and included 29 randomised double-blind crossover trials, published in English, with a primary purpose of investigating the effect of bicarbonate loading on physical performance (Matson & Tran 1993).

Since several studies compared multiple doses or modes of exercise, a total of 35 effect sizes were available for study (Matson & Tran 1993). A total of 285 subjects were represented, with the vast majority being healthy male, college-aged students. There was some variation in the protocol of bicarbonate loading, with different doses and times of ingestion being employed. While cycling was the most frequently used mode of exercise, performance was measured in a variety of ways. Performance times varied from 30 sec to 5–7 min of near maximal intensity, and included repeated intervals of one minute with short rest times between. Performance outcomes included changes in power over a given time period, total work performed in a specified time, or time to exhaustion at a specific exercise intensity. Only five studies included in this meta-analysis measured performance in an outcome that would mimic real-life sport, using trained subjects. These studies are summarised in Table 17.9 (see Appendix 17) along with more recent studies which feature a sports-specific design. It is worth noting some recent studies featured in Table 17.9 that showed that bicarbonate loading enhanced cycling performance of approximately one hour duration (Potteiger et al. 1996; McNaughton et al. 1999).

The 1993 meta-analysis of bicarbonate literature concluded that the ingestion of sodium bicarbonate has a positive effect on exercise performance. The weighted effect size was 0.44, meaning that the mean performance of the bicarbonate trial was, on average, 0.44 standard deviations better than the placebo trial. In statistical terms, this is considered a moderate effect size. Factors that were associated with a larger effect size included mode of exercise (exercise producing a larger anaerobic component, measuring time to exhaustion, or involving repeated work intervals) and large doses of sodium bicarbonate. In trials that measured time to exhaustion there was a mean increase in duration of 27% ± 20%. It was noted that strategies that reduced the variability in performance, such as using a homogenous subject pool, particularly of well-trained athletes, would significantly improve the strength of the statistical analysis.

There was only a weak relationship reported between the alkalinity (increase in pH and bicarbonate) attained in the bicarbonate trial and the performance outcome. However, the greater the level of metabolic acidosis achieved during the exercise, the greater the ergogenic effect. Thus, it was concluded that a key factor associated with an ergogenic effect is the attainment of a threshold pH gradient across the cell membrane, resulting from the accumulation of intracellular H^+ as well as the extracellular alkalosis. Significant variability within studies suggests that bicarbonate ingestion has an individual effect on different subjects, and that the effect on performance is more complicated than the simple mechanisms suggested above. It has been suggested that an anaerobically trained athlete would have better intrinsic buffering capacity, and would be less likely to show a positive effect from bicarbonate loading. However, the meta-analysis provided no clarification of this theory. In concluding their findings, Matson and Tran (1993) recommended that further research be undertaken, particularly with subjects matched in VO_{max} anaerobic capacity, fibre type and performance times, and with exercise protocols that are specific to the subjects' training as well as actual athletic performance.

It is worth considering that an improvement in actual athletic performance (as studied by the trials summarised in Table 17.9) might only be achieved if the athlete is able to pace their performance to exploit the increased buffering capacity. Studies that fail to show an enhancement effect may result from exercise modes that are too short or insufficient in intensity to produce a critical H^+ load, or from the failure of the athlete to judge a challenging pace. Sports performance that might benefit from bicarbonate loading may therefore be very specific to the type of event, the individual athlete, and their ability to challenge their buffering system. Until further research can clarify the range of exercise activities that are potentially capable of performance enhancement, the individual athlete is advised to experiment in training to judge their own case. Experimentation in a competition-simulated environment should be considered crucial; the athlete needs to discover not only the potential for performance improvement, but also the likelihood of unwanted side-effects.

17.7 NUTRITIONAL ERGOGENIC AIDS WITH MIXED SCIENTIFIC SUPPORT

17.7.1 Antioxidant supplements

Exercise has been linked with an increased production of free oxygen radical species capable of causing cellular damage. A sudden increase in training stress (such as an increase in volume or intensity) or a stressful environment (training in hot conditions or at altitude) is believed to increase the production of these free oxygen radicals, leading to an increase in markers of cellular damage. Supplementation with antioxidant vitamins such as vitamin C or vitamin E is postulated to increase antioxidant status and provide protection against this damage (see Chapter 12, Section 12.6.2).

The literature on the effects of antioxidant supplementation on antioxidant status, cellular damage and performance is complex and confusing. Some, but not all, studies of acute supplementation during periods of increased stress may provide bridging protection until adaptation processes can increase the host antioxidant status (for review see Dekkers et al. 1996; Packer 1997). It is possible that benefits may occur at a subtle and cellular level that are too small to translate into detectable performance benefits. Whether ongoing supplementation is necessary for optimal training adaptations and competition performance of athletes is similarly unknown, and any benefits may be too small to detect.

17.7.2 *Protein and amino acids*

Protein metabolism and protein requirements for training and competition are summarised in Chapter 5. This chapter concluded that protein supplements are expensive and are unnecessary for achieving an increase in muscle mass or strength. However, mixed-macronutrient products, such as liquid meal supplements, could be useful in situations where a compact source of CHO and protein was desirable. Such scenarios might include:

1. meeting the high-energy needs of an athlete undertaking heavy training, a growth spurt or an increase in muscle mass; and
2. a post-exercise recovery meal promoting enhanced protein status and glycogen restoration simultaneously.

In both situations, a liquid meal supplement might provide a practical alternative or adjunct to everyday foods. The cost of such supplements is usually considerably less than high-protein or all-protein products, but is typically greater than normal foods. Nevertheless, this expense may be justified when convenience is an important issue in achieving nutrient intake goals.

Several individual amino acids, or amino acid groups, have been singled out for special attention in sports nutrition. During the 1980s, preparations of individual amino acids were the most successfully marketed 'designer' supplement, despite a lack of evidence that 'free-form' preparations of amino acids were superior in digestion/absorption than amino acids found in intact proteins (i.e. in everyday foods). In the 1990s, special forms of 'ion-exchanged whey protein powder' received a similar but unsubstantiated hype. Contemporary products include tablets or powders containing individual amino acids as the sole ingredients, as well as general sports supplements (sports drinks, liquid meal powders, bars) fortified with additional amino acids. Many of these specialised amino acid products are expensive and provide amino acid intakes that can easily be consumed from everyday foods at more reasonable cost. We will now explore the evidence that particular amino acids have a special role in athletic performance and recovery from exercise.

17.7.2.1 *Branched-chain amino acids (BCAAs)*

Interest in the branched-chain amino acids (leucine, isoleucine and valine) is based on their important role in protein metabolism and on their hypothesised role in the development of central fatigue. BCAAs in the muscle are able to transaminate pyruvate to form alanine, which is recycled to glucose in the liver via the Cori cycle (see Chapter 5, Section 5.2.2). There is significant oxidation of these amino acids during exercise, and tracer studies that follow leucine kinetics are often used as an estimation of protein turnover. Supplements containing BCAAs are claimed to enhance recovery after exercise, although there is no proof that BCAAs are unique in promoting an enhanced reversal of protein catabolism. Instead, intake of CHO and protein, as provided by everyday foods and supplements such as liquid meal preparations, is the recommended dietary strategy for post-exercise recovery (see Chapter 15).

Supplementation with BCAAs during exercise has been claimed to reduce or delay the onset of 'central fatigue', described as fatigue emanating from the central nervous system rather than the muscle. Over the last decade, theories about the role of neurotransmitters in the psychological sensations of mood, drive, pain, weariness and fatigue have become popular. It has been suggested that neurochemicals such as serotonin, dopamine and norepinephrine play a role in the determination of exercise performance. Since it is difficult to undertake a direct examination of brain function during exercise in humans, we are reliant on monitoring indirect markers such as plasma levels of neurotransmitter precursors, or monitoring the effects of drugs that are known agonists or antagonists of neurotransmitter function.

Briefly, it has been hypothesised that central fatigue occurs due to increased brain levels of serotonin, which result from greater amounts of free (unbound) tryptophan being able to cross the blood–brain barrier (for review see Davis 1995). A key factor in this increased uptake is an increase in the plasma ratio of free tryptophan to BCAAs (tryptophan:BCAA), which compete for the same transporters into the brain. The ratio changes during exercise as BCAAs are oxidised by the muscle. However, it also changes because the rise in free fatty acids (FFAs), which occurs during exercise, displaces tryptophan from its binding site on the albumin molecule and increases the plasma concentration of free tryptophan. It has been theorised that supplementation of BCAAs during exercise might prevent the drop in plasma BCAAs, attenuate the rise in free tryptophan:BCAA, and reduce the likelihood of fatigue arising from increased brain serotonin concentrations.

Studies that have investigated the effect of BCAA supplementation immediately before or during endurance exercise are summarised in Table 17.10 (see Appendix 17). At first glance it seems that this might be a successful strategy to enhance sports performance. However, several of the studies summarised in this table can be criticised on methodological grounds. For example, the running studies by Blomstrand and colleagues (1991) only found a performance enhancement by undertaking an artificial statistical procedure whereby 'randomly selected' groups of subjects were subdivided according to an arbitrary finishing time. There is no rationale to justify this classification and no proof that the random allocation of subjects would not have produced slight mismatches in the calibre of each group, independent of the intervention received. The application of the cognitive test to sports performance has also been questioned. Finally, in these studies the researchers failed to control factors such as fluid and CHO intake during exercise (Davis 1995). Other studies have failed to confirm an enhancement in the performance of prolonged exercise following BCAA supplementation.

There are several arguments against an endorsement of BCAA supplementation during exercise. The first issue is that many studies have only compared BCAA supplementation with a water placebo. Interestingly, the ingestion of CHO during exercise minimises the unfavourable change in plasma free tryptophan:BCAA. Carbohydrate ingestion during exercise suppresses the rise in FFA concentrations, thus attenuating the increase in free tryptophan concentrations (Davis et al. 1992). Thus, CHO intake during endurance exercise provides an effective strategy against both peripheral and central mechanisms of fatigue. Studies comparing the co-ingestion of CHO and BCAAs with the intake of CHO alone are needed to settle the issue of BCAA supplementation. To date, convincing evidence of this type is lacking. Furthermore, the rise in plasma ammonia concentrations that accompanies the intake of substantial amounts of BCAAs must be considered. Ammonia is known to be toxic to the brain and muscle and may produce its own effect on exercise capacity and performance. At present, despite an intriguing theory of potential performance benefits, there is no substantial proof that BCAA supplementation enhances exercise performance.

17.7.2.2 *Arginine, ornithine and lysine*

Arginine, ornithine and lysine have been claimed individually, and in combinations, to promote the release of growth hormone, leading to an increase in muscle mass and a decrease in body fat. Arginine and ornithine have also been purported to stimulate insulin release when consumed in combination with CHO, enhancing anabolic activities including glycogen storage. These amino acids have been marketed as 'legal anabolic compounds', recovery agents and stimulators of muscle growth. Two studies by Elam and associates (1988, 1989) are often cited in support of gains in muscle size and strength in subjects undertaking body building training while supplementing with arginine and ornithine (2 g/d). However, these studies are flawed in design, and lacking an appropriate measure of pre- and post-measures in the 'control' group. Therefore, it is not possible to demonstrate whether any purported changes in this study are due to the amino acid supplementation.

Data supporting the stimulation of growth hormone following oral intake of amino acids are sketchy and inconsistent. Lemon (1991) found only modest changes in growth hormone release following ingestion of large amounts of arginine and ornithine (up to 20 g/d). Furthermore, he reported that growth hormone release was greater following heavy resistance training, and was not further stimulated by the addition of these amino acids. Studies at the Australian Institute of Sport also failed to find improvements in growth hormone release following intake of 3–4 g/d of these amino acids (Fricker et al. 1988, 1991). In a series of studies investigating the interaction of training, food and supplements on acute or late-night release of growth hormone, researchers found that exercising in a fasted state produced the greatest growth hormone stimulus (Fricker et al. 1988, 1991). Finally, inconsistent effects on growth hormone release were observed over three hours following the intake of ~2 g of arginine/lysine and ornithine/tyrosine amino acid combinations by body builders (Lambert et al. 1993).

Effects of amino acid intake on insulin responses are equally unconvincing. Studies of ornithine supplementation (170 mg/kg) and post-exercise arginine supplementation (80 mg/kg/h) in combination with CHO feedings have failed to find an enhanced insulin response (Bucci et al. 1992; Yaspelkis & Ivy 1999). Chronic intake of arginine/lysine supplements (132 mg/kg LBM) for ten weeks failed to change oral glucose tolerance test parameters in inactive subjects or subjects undertaking resistance training (Gater et al. 1992a). It also failed to alter body composition or strength changes (Gater et al. 1992b).

Overall, it appears that the oral intake of amino acids fails to achieve the hormonal stimulation seen when amino acids are intravenously administered in clinical situations. Furthermore, very high intakes of some amino acids are associated with cramping and diarrhoea (Yaspelkis & Ivy 1999). To date there is no convincing evidence to prove that amino acids supplements promote an enhanced hormonal response and/or an increased response to resistance training. Furthermore, the 2–3 g doses recommended by many amino acid manufacturers can easily be obtained by eating common foods such as milk, yoghurt and eggs.

17.7.2.3 *Glutamine*

Glutamine is the most abundant amino acid in muscle and plasma. It is considered important or essential for many activities of the immune system such as lymphocyte-activated natural killer cell activity, lymphocyte proliferation and macrophage phagocytosis. Glutamine is used at a high rate by these cells as an oxidative fuel and as a source of purine intermediates. Plasma glutamine concentrations are maintained by the balance between glutamine utilisation and release. Plasma glutamine concentrations fall during prolonged exercise and other catabolic states such as trauma or surgery, possibly as a result of increased liver uptake for gluconeogenesis. Glutamine concentrations may remain lowered for a period during the recovery phase, depending on the intensity and duration of the exercise (for review see Walsh et al. 1998).

It has been suggested that the acute effects of several bouts of exercise may be cumulative, since some researchers have found that over-trained athletes have lower plasma glutamine values than healthy athletes (Rowbottom et al. 1996). Indeed, it has been theorised that a chronic glutamine debt may be responsible for the immunosuppression suffered by some athletes, and that glutamine supplementation may overcome the problems of over-training, or the impaired immunity suffered by athletes undertaking repeated bouts of heavy training. However, the data showing a link between lowered glutamine levels and susceptibility to illness in athletes are not consistent (Mackinnon et al. 1996; Kingsbury et al. 1998). One study has reported that glutamine supplementation after a heavy exercise session decreased the incidence of infection suffered during the following week (Castell et al. 1996). However, the interpretation of these results should be carried out with caution since there are flaws in the methodology, such as the failure to monitor plasma glutamine concentrations and the reliance on self-reports of illness. At present the data suggest that glutamine supplementation is only of benefit for athletes who show a true glutamine deficiency, and that this problem is less common than originally proposed. Therefore, glutamine supplementation does not provide a general cure or prevention for immune problems suffered by athletes.

17.7.3 *Glycerol*

Glycerol, a three-carbon alcohol, provides the backbone to triglyceride molecules and is released during lipolysis (see Chapter 16, Sections 16.2 and 16.5). Within the body it is evenly distributed throughout fluid compartments and exerts an osmotic pressure. When consumed orally, it is rapidly absorbed and slowly metabolised via the liver and kidneys. When consumed in combination with a substantial fluid intake, the osmotic pressure will enhance the retention of this fluid and expansion of the various body fluid spaces. Effective protocols for glycerol hyperhydration are 1–1.5 g/kg glycerol with an intake of 25–35 mL/kg of fluid. Typically, this allows a fluid expansion or retention of ~600 mL above a fluid bolus alone, by reducing urinary volume. A thorough review of glycerol and its role as a hyperhydrating agent is provided by Robergs (1998).

Glycerol can be consumed by using commercially available glycerine solutions, or more recently, special hyperhydration supplements targeted at athletes. Glycerol hyperhydration may be useful as a preparation strategy for events that are likely to challenge fluid status and thermoregulation (see Chapter 14). This includes exercise of high intensity and/or hot and humid environments, where sweat losses are high and opportunities to replace fluid are substantially less than the rates of fluid loss. It may also be useful as a rehydration agent for situations requiring the quick recovery from a moderate to large fluid deficit. This includes situations where there is a short recovery period between events or important training sessions and the athlete has a significant fluid loss from the first session. Athletes who dehydrate to make weight might also benefit by enhancing their fluid retention during the recovery period between the weigh-in and competition (see Chapter 8).

Although glycerol may provide a logical aid for the rapid reversal of dehydration in the situations described above, such protocols have not been studied. Therefore, we can not be certain of any benefits or side-effects, or ways in which protocols might be fine-tuned. Research is needed to examine this idea. However, glycerol hyperhydration strategies have received a small amount of attention from sports scientists, and studies investigating the effects on sports performance are summarised in the Appendix (Table 17.11). At present, there is insufficient evidence to make a decision about the value of glycerol hyperhydration on performance. The literature appears inconsistent, at least partly because of differences in study methodologies. For example, some studies have investigated the effect of glycerol in assisting the body to retain larger amounts of a fluid bolus consumed in the hours before exercise, while others have used protocols in which glycerol is consumed with only a modest fluid intake. Other protocols have added glycerol to fluids consumed during exercise. At present, the most promising scenario involves the use of glycerol to maximise the retention of fluid bolus just prior to an event in which a substantial fluid deficit cannot be prevented. In some, but not all, studies of this type, glycerol hyperhydration has been associated with performance benefits. However, the mechanism for this effect is not clear, since the theoretical advantages of increased sweat losses and greater capacity for heat dissipation, and attenuation of cardiac and thermoregulatory challenges, are not consistently seen. Further investigation is needed to replicate and explain performance benefits.

Finally, protocols need to be fine-tuned, and perhaps individualised for specific situations. As explained in Chapter 11, the benefits of hyperhydrating with additional fluid must be measured against the energy cost of the increase in body mass. Hyperhydration techniques which increase BM by ~0.6 kg may not present a problem to weight-supported sports such as cycling on flat courses or on a laboratory ergometer. However, this may not be the case in weight-sensitive sports such as running or uphill cycling. Finally, side-effects from the use of glycerol include nausea, gastrointestinal distress, and headaches resulting from increased intracranial pressure. These problems have been reported among some but not all subjects in the current studies. Fine-tuning of protocols may reduce the risk of these problems, however, some individuals may remain at a greater risk than others. At the present time, glycerol hyperhydration should remain an activity that is supervised and monitored by appropriate sports science/medicine professionals, and only used in competition situations after adequate experimentation and fine-tuning has occurred.

17.8 NUTRITIONAL ERGOGENIC AIDS LACKING SUBSTANTIAL SCIENTIFIC SUPPORT

17.8.1 Ginseng and related herbal products

Ginseng has enjoyed popularity as a health supplement for many centuries. The chemical composition of commercial supplement products is highly variable due to differences in the genetic nature of the plant source, variation in active ingredients with cultivation and season, and differences in the methods of drying and curing. Several species of ginseng are known to exist: American, Siberian, Korean and Japanese (Bahrke & Morgan 1994). Most of these belong to the Panax species and are related. However, Russian or Siberian ginseng is extracted from a different plant (Eleutherococcus senticoccus). The root of these plants is considered the most valuable part.

A number of chemically similar steroid glycosides or saponin chemicals, known as ginsenosides, have been identified as active ingredients in ginsengs. Unfortunately for the process of scientific study, the variability of active ingredients within and between species is great, and the processes involved in the preparation of supplement products exaggerates these differences. The bioavailability of supplements varies according to the method of administration (chewing gum, pill, capsule, tablet or liquid). Some ginseng preparations also provide additional agents such as vitamins, minerals or other herbal compounds.

Ginseng has been used widely in herbal medicines of oriental cultures to cure fatigue, relieve pain and headaches, and improve mental function and vigour. It is also claimed to increase non-specific resistance to various stressors, described by Russian and Eastern European scientists as an adaptogenic response. An adaptogen is a substance purported to normalise physiology after exposure to a variety of stresses. It exhibits a lack of specificity in its actions and can both reduce or increase a response that has been altered by a stressor. This theory represents a philosophy of physiology or medicine different from the traditional Western understanding.

Despite the history of use in Eastern or traditional medicine, ginseng has only recently emerged as a purported ergogenic aid for exercise performance. In athletes, ginseng is claimed to reduce fatigue, and improve aerobic conditioning, strength, mental alertness and recovery. Table 17.12 in the Appendix summarises the few controlled studies that have investigated the effect of ginseng and related products on exercise or sports performance. Other studies presented in reviews or discussions of ginseng supplementation (Bahrke & Morgan 1994; Dowling et al. 1996) have not been included due to flaws in research design (failure to include a control or placebo group) and lack of availability of details due to publication in a foreign language journal. Conference presentations, which have not been published in a peer-reviewed forum, have also been omitted. We included a study on a supplement containing ciwujia since the active ingredients are extracted from the leaves of the plant whose roots provide Siberian ginseng.

In view of the paucity of literature and failure to utilise trained subjects in most studies, it is fair to say that the effect of ginseng supplementation and athletic performance has not been thoroughly researched. However, the variability of the content of commercial ginseng supplements creates a difficulty in undertaking well-controlled research, as well as advising athletes about any favourable results. Chong and Oberholzer (1998) assayed 50 commercial ginseng preparations and noted that 44 products ranged in ginsenoside concentration from 1.9–9.0%, and six preparations failed to produce a detectable level of ginsenosides. Thus, even if scientific evidence showed that ginseng could enhance exercise performance, athletes could not be certain of receiving the appropriate dose and type of active ingredients from all preparations in the commercially available range. Furthermore, one product that was assayed by Chong and Oberholzer (1988) contained large amounts of ephedrine, confirming expert opinion that herbal preparations present an unknown risk of causing an inadvertent doping outcome for elite athletes (Baylis et al. in press). At the current time there is no substantial evidence to support testimonial claims that ginseng is of benefit to performance or recovery.

17.8.2 *Carnitine*

Carnitine is a non-essential nutrient, first described early in the 1900s. It was first considered to be an essential vitamin until the discovery that it could be manufactured in the liver and kidney from amino acid precursors (lysine and methionine). Dietary sources of carnitine include most animal foods, but due to losses in cooking and preparation of foods there are few data on the total content of the diet. Carnitine ingested or synthesised by humans is in the L-isoform, and is carried via the blood for storage, predominantly in heart and skeletal muscle.

One of the chief roles of carnitine is, as a component of the enzymes carnitine-palmityltransferase I, carnitine-palmityltransferase II and carnitine-acylcarnitine translocase, to transport long chain fatty acids (LCFAs) across the mitochondrial membrane to the site of their oxidation (see Chapter 16). Because of this function, it has been suggested that carnitine supplementation might enhance fatty acid transport and oxidation, potentially decreasing body fat levels. This claim has been widely embraced by body builders and other groups conscious of body-fat levels, where carnitine supplements are consumed for 'cutting up' or 'getting ripped'. Carnitine is an ingredient in many purported weight-loss products. Endurance athletes might also benefit from carnitine supplementation, if it can enhance fatty acid oxidation during submaximal exercise. Theoretically, a reduced reliance on glycogen stores and blood glucose oxidation could enhance endurance in events where CHO stores are otherwise limiting.

Another role of carnitine is to act as a 'sink' for acetyl-CoA units produced during high intensity exercise. By converting this to acetyl-carnitine and CoA, carnitine could help to maintain CoA availability and to decrease the ratio of acetyl-CoA:CoA. If supplementation could increase this function it might enhance flux through the citric acid cycle. Furthermore, it could enhance the activity of the enzyme pyruvate dehydrogenase (PDH), which is otherwise inhibited by high levels of acetyl-CoA, thus increasing oxidative metabolism of glucose. If this results in lower lactate production, it might enhance exercise performance in situations that might otherwise be limited by excess lactate and hydrogen ion accumulation (see Chapter 2). Extensive reviews of carnitine function are available (Cerretelli & Marconi 1990; Wagenmakers 1991; Clarkson 1992; Heinonen 1996).

There are several inborn errors of metabolism leading to inadequate muscle carnitine activity. Individuals with such conditions experience lipid abnormalities and reduced exercise capacity, which can be attenuated by carnitine supplementation. Such uses of carnitine supplementation are established medical therapy. However, whether additional carnitine intake in healthy individuals enhances metabolism and exercise performance is another matter. Several issues must be considered if this is a possibility:

1. Does heavy training lead to a decrease and sub-optimal level of muscle carnitine?
2. Does carnitine supplementation lead to an increase in muscle carnitine concentrations?
3. Is carnitine the limiting factor in the transport of long-chain fatty acids (LCFAs) into the mitochondria?
4. Can enhanced carnitine levels enhance activities of PDH or citric-acid cycle flux?

Reviews by Wagenmakers (1991) and Heinonen (1996) cast doubt on the theoretical benefits of carnitine supplementation in healthy athletes. They summarise that there is no proof that fatty acid transport is the rate limiting step in fat oxidation, and that muscle levels of carnitine appear to be adequate for maximal function of carnitine palmityltransferase. Furthermore, PDH is believed to be fully active within seconds of high-intensity exercise, and additional carnitine is unlikely to further stimulate this activity. The issue of optimal muscle carnitine content for athletes is probably the most important issue to clarify. It is known that exercise results in increased carnitine excretion, and it is possible that muscle carnitine content may decrease during intense training. However, Clarkson (1992) maintains that a serious deficiency would not occur since carnitine and its amino acid precursors are easily obtained in the diet. Cerretelli and Marconi (1990) have summarised a series of studies of carnitine supplementation in human subjects. Although most studies show an increase in plasma carnitine levels following carnitine supplementation of 1–6 g/d, the effects on muscle carnitine content are less clear. Nevertheless, the consensus of most reviewers is that there is no compelling evidence that muscle carnitine levels are enhanced as a result of supplementation (Wagenmakers 1991; Heinonen 1996).

Studies that have investigated the effects of carnitine supplementation on exercise metabolism and/or performance are summarised in Table 17.13

(Appendix). Overall, there is little evidence that carnitine supplementation causes any change in metabolism during submaximal or high-intensity exercise. The few studies that report favourable metabolic outcomes, or an increase in exercise performance, are hard to explain. For example, it is hard to understand how a supplement taken 90 min before exercise has sufficient time to be absorbed through the gut into the bloodstream and taken up by the muscle (Siliprandi et al. 1990). However, on balance there is little evidence of increased performance resulting from carnitine supplementation. The effect of carnitine supplementation on body-fat levels, although widely publicised in supplement advertising, has not been studied.

Although studies of acute and long-term carnitine supplementation report that carnitine appears to be safe, it should be noted that this applies to L-carnitine preparations. D-carnitine, however, has been shown to cause depletion of L-carnitine in tissues, therefore creating a carnitine deficiency (Clarkson 1992). Athletes are advised to avoid commercial carnitine preparations that do not clearly specify that contents are > 99% L-carnitine.

17.8.3 *Coenzyme Q10*

Coenzyme Q10, also known as ubiquinone, is a non-essential lipid-soluble nutrient found predominantly in animal foods and in low levels in plant foods. In the body it is located primarily in the mitochondria, especially in skeletal and cardiac muscle. One of its well-known functions is as a link in the electron transport chain within the mitochondria, thus providing a part in the final production of ATP. It is also believed to have an antioxidant function, mopping up free oxygen radicals in the mitochondrial antioxidant defence system and preventing damage to DNA and cell membranes. It has been suggested that some cardiac and neuromuscular dysfunction is due to coenzyme Q10 deficiency; indeed, patients with ischaemic heart disease are shown to have lower plasma Q10 concentrations. Some studies have shown that these patients respond to coenzyme Q10 supplementation with increased exercise capacity. Coenzyme Q10 supplements have recently emerged as new products marketed in the general community to promote vigour. For athletes they are claimed to enhance energy production through the electron transport chain, and to reduce the oxidative damage of exercise.

Table 17.14 (see Appendix 17) summarises the studies, which have examined the effects of coenzyme Q10 supplementation on exercise metabolism, oxidative damage caused by exercise, and performance. Studies that have been reported only in the form of conference abstracts have not been presented. There are few data that support an ergogenic benefit of coenzyme Q10 on exercise performance. In fact, there are substantial data that show that coenzyme Q10 has an ergolytic effect on high-intensity performance and training adaptations. A series of studies undertaken at the Karolinska Institute in Sweden has produced consistent evidence that Q10 supplementation increases the oxidative damage produced by high-intensity exercise (Malm et al. 1996; Malm et al. 1997; Svennson et al. 1999). Twenty-two days of supplementation, undertaken in conjunction with high-intensity training, was shown to increase oxidative damage, as indicated by higher plasma CK levels and increased malondialdehyde levels in response to exercise (Malm et al. 1996; Malm et al. 1997). In these circumstances, Q10 was believed to act as a pro-oxidant rather than an antioxidant. Training adaptations were impaired in healthy subjects who undertook high-intensity training while taking Q10 supplements, with the placebo group out-performing the Q10 group at the end of the supplementation phase (Malm et al. 1997).

Clearly, further work is required to investigate the effects of coenzyme Q10 supplementation on exercise performance and training. However, at present there is little to recommend Q10 supplementation to athletes undertaking high-intensity training, and we are reminded that some scientific theories are not as straightforward as they seem. The issue of antioxidant supplementation is complex and as yet unsolved.

17.8.4 *Inosine*

Inosine is a nucleic acid derivative, considered to be a non-essential nutrient. Major dietary sources include yeast and organ meats. Inosine is a precursor of the nucleotide inosine monophosphate (IMP), and may also lead to the production of ATP. In-vitro tests suggest that inosine may enhance the levels of 2,3-diphosphoglycerate (2,3-DPG) in red blood cells. Potential mechanisms by which inosine supplementation might enhance exercise performance include an increased ATP supply, and increased release of oxygen from erythrocytes to the muscle, via a shift in the oxyhaemoglobin curve mediated by increased 2,3-DPG concentrations. Inosine is believed to have vasodilatory effects and antioxidant properties, and may lead to the formation of fumarate, a citric acid cycle substrate. Further information on the functions of inosine is provided by Williams et al. (1990) and Starling et al. (1996). However, these are only hypothetical situations that have not been supported by research.

The major support for inosine supplementation comes from testimonials from successful athletes, with reports that it is a favourite supplement of Russian and Eastern European athletes. In 1988, *Muscle and Fitness*, a popular magazine, carried an article describing a six-week study of inosine supplementation on four trained athletes (Colgan 1988). The report claimed the study was undertaken using a double-blind crossover design, and found strength gains as a result of the supplementation. No data or statistical analyses were presented. This study has not appeared in a peer-reviewed publication or in adequate detail to judge the validity of these claims. Interestingly, the athletes were reported to suffer irritability and fatigue while on inosine treatment.

Only three well-controlled crossover designed studies of inosine supplementation have been published in the scientific literature (see Table 17.15 in Appendix 17).

It should also be noted that inosine was an ingredient in a multicompound ergogenic aid (CAPS) that failed to enhance performance of triathletes in a study by Snider and colleagues (1992); this study has been reviewed in the section on coenzyme Q10 above. The three studies of isolated inosine supplementation used well-trained athletes as subjects and all failed to find performance benefits following inosine supplementation (Williams et al. 1990; Starling et al. 1996; McNaughton et al. 1999).

Metabolic data from these studies failed to show any favourable enhancements that could improve sports performance, or support the theoretical actions of supplemental inosine. For example, 2,3-DPG levels were not increased following inosine supplementation and there was no evidence from blood metabolites or respiratory exchange data of enhancement of CHO metabolism. Although muscle substrates were not directly measured, purported changes to ATP concentrations are unlikely to enhance exercise performance, since ATP is not depleted by exercise, even at the point of fatigue (see Chapter 2). Interestingly, two of the studies reported that subjects performed the high-intensity tasks better on the placebo treatment than following inosine supplementation (Williams et al. 1990; Starling et al. 1996). This suggests that inosine might actually **impair** the performance of high-intensity exercise. Potential mechanisms for exercise impairment include an increased formation of inosine monophosphate (IMP) in the muscle, either at rest or during exercise. High IMP concentrations have been found at the point of fatigue in many exercise studies; furthermore, IMP has been shown to inhibit ATPase activity (Sahlin 1992). It is possible that increased resting muscle IMP concentrations could reduce the duration of high intensity exercise before critically high levels were reached, causing premature fatigue. Such a theory can only be investigated by direct measurements of muscle nucleosides.

Ultimately, inosine is degraded to uric acid for excretion. It is possible that inosine supplementation could lead to elevated uric acid levels, providing an alternative mechanism of performance impairment as well as an increased risk of gout. In the present studies, two days of inosine supplementation did not change uric acid levels; however, five days and ten days of intake doubled blood concentrations to levels above the normal range (Williams et al. 1990; Starling et al. 1996; McNaughton et al. 1999). Thus, chronic inosine supplementation may pose a health risk. In summary, since there is a lack of evidence of performance benefits, and the possibility of performance decrements and side-effects, there is little to recommend the use of inosine supplements by athletes.

17.8.5 *Chromium picolinate*

Chromium is an essential element, required in trace amounts. An Australian RDI for chromium has not been set, however, the US Food and Nutrition Board established an Estimated Safe and Adequate Daily Dietary Allowance (ESADDA) within the range of 50–200 µg/d (National Research Council 1989). Dietary sources of chromium include yeast, nuts and legumes, some fruit and vegetables, chocolate, wine and beer. Dietary surveys often report the estimated chromium intake of many populations to be below this recommended range. However, in light of criticism that ESADDA ranges for chromium have been set artificially high, and the lack of reliable food composition data for chromium, it is difficult to assess the likelihood of an inadequate chromium intake (for review see Clarkson 1997). There is some evidence that daily training may increase urinary chromium losses, increasing chromium requirements and the risk of sub-optimal chromium intakes. However, adaptations may also occur to improve absorption or retention of chromium in compensation (see Clarkson 1997). As is the case for many micronutrients, athletes with restricted energy intakes are most at risk of low chromium intakes.

One of the best known roles of chromium in the body is to potentiate insulin action. This action enhances glucose uptake, as well as lipid and amino acid metabolism (for review see Stoecker 1996). Chromium may also have a role in immune function. Subjects with chromium deficiencies often show improvements in growth or glucose tolerance in response to chromium supplementation (Stoecker 1996). In the case of the athletic population, individuals with inadequate dietary intake of chromium may respond positively to supplemental chromium intake. However, the major market is focussed on claims that chromium supplements will enhance handling of glucose, amino acids and fatty acids, allowing dramatic gains in muscle mass and strength, while reducing body fat.

Chromium supplements are available in the form of chromium nicotinate, chloride and picolinate. Chromium picolinate is claimed to be the most biologically active form, and the claims for the efficacy of chromium picolinate have caused an interesting public debate between the patent holders (Evans and colleagues) and other trace element/mineral experts such as Levafi, and Lukaski. Examples of this discussion include a review on chromium supplementation (Levafi et al. 1992) followed by a series of letters published in *International Journal of Sport Nutrition* (Evans 1993; Levafi et al. 1993). One concern about chromium supplementation is that chromium potentially competes with trivalent iron for binding to transferrin, thus predisposing those with chronically high intakes of chromium to iron deficiency (Lukaski et al. 1996). Some (Lukaski et al. 1996), but not all (Campbell et al. 1997), studies have reported a reduction in iron status as a result of chromium picolinate supplementation.

Table 17.16 (Appendix 17) summarises studies of chromium piconate supplementation and effect on body composition and exercise performance. Not included in this table are the studies responsible for motivating the original interest in chromium picolinate. These studies claimed significant increases in lean body mass in subjects undertaking aerobic exercise classes (Evans 1993) and weight training (Evans 1989) while supplementing with chromium picolinate. However, Levafi has provided a thorough criticism of these studies (Levafi et al. 1992; Levafi

1993), identifying methodological flaws. He pointed out that the earlier study (Evans 1989) failed to control for training experience of subjects or their compliance with the study protocol. Furthermore, positive anabolic results were estimated through the use of anthropometric techniques that carry significant measurement and prediction error. With regard to the 1993 study claiming gains of 2 kg of lean body mass (Evans 1993), Lefavi suggests this is an unlikely outcome for subjects undertaking aerobics classes over 12 weeks. Most importantly, this study did not include a control group to verify that changes were simply the result of the chromium picolinate supplementation.

The studies summarised in Table 17.16 do not provide evidence of gains in strength and lean body mass or loss of body fat, other than what can be achieved through training alone. There is certainly no support for the dramatic claims made in some advertisements that position chromium picolinate as a 'legal anabolic' agent. The only situation in which chromium supplementation is likely to be useful is in treating individuals whose dietary intakes are inadequate.

17.8.6 *Medium chain triglycerides*

Medium chain triglycerides (MCTs) are fats composed of medium-chain fatty acids (MCFA) with a chain length of six to ten carbon molecules. As outlined in Chapter 16, Section 16.2, they differ from fats composed of LCFA in terms of digestion, absorption and uptake into the muscle mitochondria. Specifically, MCTs can be digested within the intestinal lumen with less need for bile and pancreatic juices than long-chain triglycerides, with MCFAs being absorbed via the portal circulation. MCFAs can be taken up into the mitochondria without the need for carnitine-assisted transport. In clinical nutrition, MCTs derived from palm kernel and coconut oil are used to supply energy to patients who have various digestive or lipid metabolism disorders. In the sports world, MCTs have been positioned as an easily absorbed and oxidised fuel source, and have been marketed to body builders as a fat source that is less likely to deposit as body fat. However the role of MCTs in the general diet of athletes has not been studied.

A more interesting role of MCTs in sport is as an additional fuel source during prolonged exercise (see Chapter 16, Section 16.3). If MCTs ingested during prolonged endurance and ultra-endurance events could spare glycogen, they might provide a performance advantage by prolonging the availability of important CHO stores. Although earlier studies of MCT ingestion immediately prior to or during exercise did not show much promise (Section 16.8.3), recent tracer techniques using stable isotopes have enabled a more sophisticated study of MCT metabolism during exercise. Jeukendrup and colleagues (1995) studied the ingestion of 29 g of MCT during three hours of cycling at 55% VO_2 max, alone, or with the addition of moderate and large amounts of CHO. The presence of CHO increased the rate of MCT oxidation, possibly by increasing its rate of absorption. The maximum rate of MCT oxidation was achieved in all trials between 120–180 min, at values of

~0.12 g/min. Although this suggests that MCT can supply a useful energy source, the researchers pointed out that the maximum amount of MCT that can be tolerated within the gastrointestinal tract is ~30 g in total. Therefore, they suggest that the contribution of MCTs is likely to be limited to a maximum of ~3–7% of the total energy expenditure during typical ultra-endurance events (Jeukendrup et al. 1995). In a separate study, this intake of MCTs was not shown to influence CHO utilisation or glycogen sparing (Jeukendrup et al. 1996).

Studies that have examined the effect of the co-ingestion of MCT and CHO on ultra-endurance performance are summarised in Table 17.17 (Appendix 17). These studies show inconsistent effects of MCT on fuel utilisation. In circumstances where the intake of large amounts of MCT raises plasma FFA concentrations and allows glycogen sparing, it may benefit the performance of exercise at the end of a prolonged bout (van Zyl et al. 1996). However, these metabolic (and performance) benefits may be over-ridden when exercise is commenced with higher insulin levels, as is the case following a CHO-rich pre-exercise meal (Goedecke et al. 1999; Angus et al. 2000). Critical to the whole issue is the ability of subjects to tolerate the substantial amount of MCT oils required to have a metabolic impact. Symptoms range in severity from insignificant (van Zyl et al. 1996) to performance-limiting (Jeukendrup et al. 1998). Differences in gastrointestinal tolerance between studies may reflect differences in the mean chain length of MCTs found in the supplements, or increased tolerance in some athletes due to constant exposure to MCTs. The intensity and mode of exercise may also affect gastrointestinal symptoms. For further reading on the ingestion of MCTs during exercise, see Chapter 16, Section 16.8.3.

In summary, although CHO gel supplements are marketed with the addition of MCTs, there are little data to support a beneficial use of these special products. Furthermore, the theoretical use is limited to the small population of athletes who undertake ultra-endurance sports. Further research may clarify whether MCTs can be a useful supplement for ultra-endurance sports, but significant investigation of gastrointestinal concerns is needed before any recommendations can be made.

17.9 NEW SUPPLEMENTS LACKING SUBSTANTIAL SCIENTIFIC SUPPORT

Many new ergogenic aids hit the sports world with considerable hype, testimonials, and clever marketing. The Internet has only served to exaggerate publicity about such products and accelerate the spread of unsupported information. It takes time for scientists to undertake well-controlled trials to investigate the claims made for these products, or substantiate the experiences claimed by satisfied customers. The process of peer-review and publication also adds to the time lag between the claims and the presentation of evidence. In this section we will review some of the newest and 'hottest' ergogenic aids in the sports world. By necessity we will need to present information from conference presentations and manuscripts that are still in review.

Therefore, we will be cautious in our judgement of any data that have not been fully reviewed by appropriate experts. However promising the claims and early evidence for these supplements might seem, we will need to consider that substantial scientific support is still lacking.

17.9.1 *Androstenedione, DHEA and pro-hormone supplements*

Anabolic steroids are controlled as pharmaceutical products and are listed as proscribed agents by the IOC. However, new supplements have recently appeared on the athletic market containing pro-hormones that can be converted in the body to testosterone (Blue & Lombardo 1999). These include androstenedione, dehydroepiandrosterone (DHEA), 19-norandrostenedione and other metabolites found in the steroid pathways. Theoretically, each has some androgen activity as well as being part of the pathway to testosterone production. Some herbal compounds such as Saw palmetto and Tribulus terrestris are also claimed to have anabolic activity.

Since these products are manufactured as dietary supplements rather than drugs, they enjoy a loose regulation of quality control and claims. We have already commented that independent analysis of some products has shown a variable content of the stated ingredients (Parasrampuria 1998). They are heavily promoted in the body building world where they are claimed to promote fat loss, gains in muscle mass and strength, increased libido, reversal of ageing and enhanced immunity. Some have shot to instant fame by being associated with successful performances or well-known athletes. For example, androstenedione received publicity as an ergogenic aid used by baseball player Mark McGwire during the 1998 season in which he broke the home-run record.

Pro-hormones are banned by the IOC, either directly by name, or indirectly under the umbrella of being a 'related substance' of anabolic-androgenic steroids. However, individual sporting organisations may not include these products within their own list of banned agents. There is some confusion about whether the use of these agents will cause a positive drug test. However, if they cause a large change in testosterone : epitestosterone ratio, or cause an increased excretion of banned substances such as metabolites of the anabolic steroid nandrolone, an athlete will record a positive doping outcome. To date, excretion studies have produced conflicting results with some, but not all, subjects who ingested common over-the-counter supplements experiencing differential changes in urinary testosterone and epitestosterone concentrations which increased the ratio above the legal cut-off of 6:1 (Bosy et al. 1998; Uralets & Gillette 1999). However, high concentrations of metabolites of nandrolone have been found in urine for seven to ten days following the ingestion of a single dose of 19-norandrostenedione (Uralets & Gillette 1999).

In the event that an athlete is not subject to doping restrictions, and has purchased a supplement that delivers the claimed dose of pro-hormones, they should then consider the evidence that such products can influence metabolism or performance. To date, this information is scarce. In fact the rationale for the supplements is based on limited historical studies, for example, investigations in two female subjects (Mahesh et al. 1962).

A series of studies of androstenedione, DHEA and herbal 'anabolic' supplements has been undertaken by King and colleagues from the Iowa State University. In the first study, reported in *Journal of the American Medical Association*, they investigated the effects of acute (100 mg) and chronic (300 mg for eight weeks) supplementation with androstenedione in healthy males (King et al. 1999). Androstenedione is the immediate precursor of testosterone, and possesses its own weak androgenic properties. The composition of the androstenedione supplement used in the study, derived from wild yams, was verified by independent analyses and the amounts fed to subjects exceeded the maximum doses recommended by the manufacturers. The acute feeding trial found that serum androstenedione concentrations were elevated for six hours after the intake of the supplement, however, there was no change in either free or total serum testosterone concentrations. Similarly, serum androstenedione concentrations rose during the chronic supplementation trial and remained elevated above those of the placebo group after eight weeks. Again, there were no changes in free or total testosterone concentrations in the group receiving androstenedione over the eight-week period, and no differences between the treatment and placebo groups at any time.

Interestingly, serum oestradiol and oestrone concentrations increased in the treatment group, suggesting that the exogenous androstenedione was aromatised in peripheral tissues to oestrogens rather than converted to testosterone. Furthermore, serum concentrations of HDL cholesterol were significantly reduced within two weeks of androstenedione supplementation and remained below that of the placebo group throughout the trial. Supervised resistance training was undertaken during the eight-week study, and produced significant increases in lean body mass and muscle strength, and reductions in body-fat mass in both treatment and placebo groups. There were no differences in the gains made between groups, nor changes in the histology of muscle fibres collected by the muscle biopsy technique. The authors concluded that androstenedione supplementation is not useful to subjects with normal testosterone levels, and may only increase testosterone concentrations in hypotestosterogenic populations such as women and older men. They found that the supplement was of no benefit to healthy males in enhancing the benefits gained from a resistance training program. Furthermore, there were indications of negative health outcomes such as unfavourable lipid and oestrogen profiles, which might be associated with health problems such as cardiac disease and increased risk of prostate cancers.

A separate study by this group investigated the effects of acute and chronic supplementation with DHEA (Brown et al. 1999). DHEA is the steroid hormone of greatest natural abundance in the blood, and decreases with ageing. It can be converted to androstenedione, which in turn can be converted to testosterone. In the study, young men took either a single 50 mg dose of DHEA, or an eight-week cyclical course providing 150 mg/d (two weeks on, one week off) while undertaking a supervised resistance training program. As in the androstenedione study, an independent analysis confirmed the purity of the supplements, and the chronic supplementation protocol exceeded the daily dose recommended by DHEA manufacturers. The acute intake of DHEA was found to raise serum androstenedione concentrations, peaking at 60 min and remaining elevated at six hours post-ingestion. There were no changes in serum concentrations of testosterone or other hormones, compared with the intake of a placebo. The chronic DHEA supplementation protocol resulted in increased serum androstenedione concentrations compared with baseline or placebo concentrations, at weeks two and five. However, by week eight these concentrations were not different to baseline values. There were no differences in serum testosterone or oestrogens as a result of training or supplementation with DHEA. The resistance training program increased strength and lean body mass significantly and similarly in DHEA and placebo groups. Therefore, the DHEA supplement did not enhance testosterone concentrations or adaptations associated with resistance training in young men.

The final study undertaken by the group (Brown et al. 2000) investigated the effect of a combined supplement containing androstenedione (300 mg/d), DHEA (150 mg/d) and herbal ingredients (Tribulus terristris, Saw Palmetto, Chrysin and Indole-3-carbinol). The addition of the herbal extracts is claimed to promote testosterone production by reducing the aromatisation of androgens to form oestrogens. The supplement was taken in a cyclical protocol (two weeks on, one week off) during eight weeks of supervised resistance training. Again, the supplement was found to increase serum androstenedione concentrations but to have no effect on testosterone values. A rise in serum oestrogens and decrease in HDL-cholesterol was seen, replicating the results of the previous androstenedione supplementation study (King et al. 1999). The researchers concluded that the addition of the herbal extracts, at least in the dosages found in a common body-building supplement, are insufficient to reduce the aromatisation pathways for androgen disposal. Increases in strength and lean body mass achieved by the resistance training program were not enhanced by the supplement and the potential for negative health outcomes remains a concern.

The studies undertaken by this laboratory have received considerable scientific and lay comment. The editorial accompanying the publication of the first study in JAMA advised some caution in reviewing the results (Yesalis 1999). It pointed out that although the doses used in the study were in excess of the protocols recommended by the manufacturers, they are conservative in comparison to the doses recommended and used by some athletes. It also noted that the strength gains made by previously untrained men might be sufficiently large and variable as to mask any effects from androstenedione. Nevertheless, it called for the (US) federal government to remove androstenedione and other pro-hormones from sale. Other critics have suggested that only well trained athletes who have reached a plateau in the results of their resistance training could be expected to benefit from androstenedione supplementation. Researchers were reminded that the first scientific position papers regarding anabolic steroids concluded that they were ineffective in enhancing strength or performance in sport, as a result of the failure of scientists to investigate the real practices undertaken by athletes.

However, other laboratories have begun to confirm the results reported by King and colleagues. Wallace et al. (1999) investigated the effects of 12-week supplementation with androstenedione (100 mg/d), DHEA (100 mg/d) or a placebo in middle-aged resistance-trained men. They found that the supplements failed to increase lean body mass, strength or testosterone concentrations above that seen in the placebo group. However, they saw no adverse side-effects in terms of liver function tests, lipid levels or prostate function.

Ten experienced male resistance trainers received 200 mg of androstenedione supplements or a placebo for two days in a crossover designed study undertaken by Ballantyne and colleagues (2000). Hormone levels were investigated at baseline, after the supplement and following a bout of resistance training on the second day of supplementation. Androstenedione supplementation was found to elevate plasma androstenedione concentrations, without any alteration in testosterone values. Exercise elevated testosterone equally in both supplement and placebo trials. Exercise in the supplement trial caused a significant elevation in plasma oestradiol. The researchers concluded that androstenedione supplementation is unlikely to provide male athletes with any anabolic benefit.

Finally, another group has employed tracer techniques to study muscle protein kinetics in six healthy men, before and after the intake of 100 mg/d andro-stenedione (Rasmussen et al. 2000). Muscle protein turnover was investigated before and after the supplementation, and was also compared to that of a control group. The results showed that androstenedione supplementation did not affect muscle protein anabolism. There was a trend towards increased muscle protein turnover (increased synthesis matched by increased breakdown) in the treatment group compared with control subjects. However, differences were small and did not lead to a net protein increase. Monitoring of blood hormone concentrations replicated the finding that androstenedione supplementation does not lead to increased plasma testosterone concentrations, but is associated with an increase in oestradiol concentrations (Rasmussen et al. 2000).

To date, there are no published reports of the effects of 19-norandrostenedione or related compounds on serum hormone concentrations, changes in body composition or exercise performance. In summary, although supplements containing pro-hormones and herbal 'steroids' are marketed emotively to athletes, there is no evidence to prove that they can enhance sports performance or adaptations to training. More importantly, there is evidence that these supplements may cause negative health outcomes as a result of unfavourable changes in blood lipid profiles and oestrogen hormones. For elite athletes, these products are considered to be proscribed agents and may result in a positive doping result.

17.9.2 *Hydroxy-methyl butyrate (HMB)*

B-hydroxy B-methylbutyrate (HMB) is a metabolite of the amino acid leucine. As one of the latest fast-selling dietary supplements, it is claimed to enhance gains in strength and body mass associated with resistance training, enhance loss of body fat and to enhance recovery from exercise. It is claimed to act as an anti-catabolic agent, minimising protein breakdown and the cellular damage that occurs with high intensity exercise. Leucine administration is known to influence protein metabolism, specifically to reduce protein degradation during periods of stress or trauma that are associated with elevated protein catabolism. It has been proposed that it is the increase in leucine metabolites such as ketoisocaproate (KIC) or HMB that mediates this effect. In animals, some but not all studies have found that HMB supplementation increases gains in carcass weight or feed efficiency, defined as weight gain per unit feed, during growth (for review see Slater, in press). To date, only two studies of HMB supplementation in humans have appeared in the peer-reviewed literature.

In 1996, Nissen and colleagues reported on two studies of HMB supplementation in men (Nissen et al. 1996). The first study involved healthy but untrained males who were randomised into groups receiving 0, 1.5 or 3 mg of HMB per day for three weeks, while consuming a normal (117 g/d) or supplemented (175 g/d) protein intake and undertaking resistance training. HMB supplementation was found to reduce urinary 3-methyl histidine excretion (a marker of muscle protein degradation) and plasma creatine kinase concentrations (a crude indicator of cellular damage). HMB supplementation was associated with a dose-responsive increase in weight lifted during training (particularly in lower body strength), and there was a trend for increased gain in lean body mass with the increase in HMB dose. The second study investigated seven weeks of HMB supplementation (3 mg/d) and resistance training in previously trained subjects. No dietary control was imposed during this study. The results showed that all subjects increased body mass during the study period, but there were trends for greater increases in fat-free mass (assessed by total body electrical conductivity) in the HMB group. The increases in muscle strength measurements were greater for some (upper body) but not all (lower body) lifts in the HMB-supplemented group.

Although these results are supportive of benefits from HMB supplementation, there are several methodological concerns with these investigations. Firstly, dietary intake was not controlled in the second study and HMB was provided to subjects in a protein–CHO supplement that was not matched in the placebo group. This allows the possibility that dietary differences, or additional protein and nutrients provided in this supplement, were responsible for the small differences in responses to the resistance training program between groups. Second, it is hard to explain differences in strength gains in various body parts in terms of differential effects of HMB supplementation. Examination of these data show that the groups were not equally matched for baseline values of upper body strength, despite random allocation of subjects to the treatment groups. The HMB group had lower upper body strength at the beginning of the study than the placebo group, and with a significant increase in strength over the seven-week study, still only reached the baseline values of the placebo group. Therefore, it is possible to explain the increased gains in the HMB group as the outcome of lower initial levels and a greater potential for change. Lower body strength, which was better matched at baseline, did not change over time between groups, thus providing additional support for this theory.

The other fully reported study compared changes in body composition, strength and marker of muscle damage in experienced resistance-trained males who consumed a daily supplement providing 0, 3 and 6 mg/d of HMB for 28 days (Kreider et al. 1999). All subjects throughout the study period were given individualised training programs. Changes in total body weight and body composition were not different between groups. There were no significant interactions between groups for gains in strength for bench press or leg press. There was a trend for lower plasma CK concentrations for subjects receiving the higher HMB dose compared with the placebo group. Otherwise, there were no differences in markers of muscle catabolism or damage between groups. The researchers concluded that HMB supplementation provides no ergogenic value to experienced resistance-trained athletes (Kreider et al. 1999).

There are several conference abstracts that report gains in strength and lean body mass when HMB is combined with resistance training in previously untrained men. Other studies have found variable effects on body composition and strength when HMB supplements were taken alone or in combination with creatine by college football players during pre-season training (for review see Slater, in press). However, it is difficult to fully interpret such data in the absence of details of the research design. Therefore, until further studies of HMB supplementation are conducted and reported in full, it is impossible to make a decision on the potential of this supplement.

17.9.3 *Colostrum*

Colostrum is a protein-rich substance secreted in breast milk in the first few days after a mother has given birth. It is high in immunoglobulins and insulin-like growth factors (IGFs). Unlike the adult gut, the gut of a baby has 'leaky' junctions which allows it to absorb whole proteins including immunoglobulins, thus developing the immuno-competence needed to survive outside the uterus. Recently, companies have developed supplements rich in the colostrum of cows for use by humans. In 1997, a paper published in the *Journal of Applied Physiology* reported that colostrum supplements (Bioenervie™) increased plasma IGF-1 levels in sprinters and jumpers who undertook strength and speed training sessions during the supplementation period (Mero et al. 1997). Supplementation failed to change vertical jump performance in these athletes. This study raised several controversial issues. First, it appeared to show that humans could absorb intact proteins from a supplement, and second, it appeared to provide a dietary source of IGFs, an anabolic hormone whose intentional intake is banned by the IOC. Discussion of this paper suggested that if colostrum did provide a direct source of IGF it would contravene the doping laws of sport. However, more recently it has been suggested that the data showing increased IGF concentrations are spurious and the result of inaccurate techniques for measuring these growth factors.

To date, the only other studies of colostrum and athletic performance exist only as conference papers in abstract form. In a study presented in 1998, Buckley and colleagues reported on the effects of eight weeks of running training (3 × 45 min/week) in combination with 60 g/d of a colostrum powder (Intact™) or a whey placebo in two groups of previously untrained men (Buckley et al. 1998). The test set, consisting of two incremental treadmill runs to exhaustion, with a 20 min recovery interval, was undertaken at zero, four and eight weeks. They reported that after eight weeks the treatment group completed more work and ran further in the second of two treadmill runs than subjects in the placebo group (Buckley et al. 1998). No differences were seen at four weeks, and no measurements were taken to explain the performance improvements seen in the second run at eight weeks.

In 1999 Buckley and colleagues presented the results of a one-week supplementation program with 60 g/d of colostrum or whey protein placebo on the performance of well-trained rowers undertaking a supervised training program. At weeks zero and nine, the rowers undertook two four-step rowing ergometer tests separated by a 15 min recovery period. They reported that the colostrum supplementation resulted in a greater amount of work and distance achieved in the last stage of both incremental rowing ergometer tests (Buckley et al. 1999). Criticisms of this study include small subject numbers (three in the treatment group and five in the placebo group) and failure to measure any parameters to explain their findings.

It should be noted that the studies undertaken by Buckley and colleagues (1998, 1999) were funded by the manufacturers of the colostrum supplement and both have received considerable promotion and hype. The results of the studies have been interpreted aggressively by both the researcher and the manufacturer to include claims of enhanced recovery, superior muscle buffering capacity, and increased growth of muscle contractile proteins. The benefits have been transferred to other groups including manual workers and chronic fatigue sufferers. At the present time, we believe that the data from these studies cannot be commented on until it appears in press following the appropriate peer-review process. Furthermore, we note that the studies are limited by small subject numbers (rowing study) and the failure to investigate mechanisms to support and explain the observed performance benefits (both studies). It is a concern that there does not appear to be a plausible explanation to underpin the effects of colostrum supplements on adults.

Therefore, although colostrum is a 'hot' supplement in the athletic world and merits further research, there is insufficient evidence at present to support any performance benefits. At the recommended price of $70 per week, and the suggestion that it may take at least four weeks to show benefits, athletes are reminded that colostrum supplementation involves a considerable expense.

17.10 *BALANCING ADVANTAGES AND DISADVANTAGES OF SUPPLEMENT USE*

Athletes should consider several factors before deciding to use a supplement. The likely benefits should be considered carefully, and weighed against the cost of a supplement program and the risk of negative outcomes. In the previous section of this chapter, we discussed supplements and the conditions of use that can lead to true performance benefits. We also acknowledged that placebo or psychologically mediated effects can achieve a worthwhile improvement in training or competition performance, at least in the short term. Supplement use, even when it provides a performance advantage, is an expense that the athlete must acknowledge and prioritise appropriately within their total budget. At times, it may be deemed money well spent, particularly when the supplement provides the most practical and palatable way to achieve a nutrition goal, or when ergogenic benefits have been well documented. On other occasions the athlete may choose to limit the use of expensive supplements to the most important events or training periods. The downside of supplement use includes the potential for side-effects, an inadvertent doping outcome and failure to consider other real performance-enhancing strategies. These problems are often forgotten.

17.10.1 *Doping safety*

In most sports, competition between elite athletes is conducted within a code of conduct, issued by the Governing Body of the sport or the Medical Commission of the IOC, that includes a ban against doping. Doping has been defined by the IOC as 'the administration or the use by a competing athlete of any substance foreign to the body or of any physiological substance taken in abnormal quantity or taken by an abnormal route of entry into the body, with the sole intention of increasing in an artificial or unfair manner his performance in competition'. The substances and methods that are banned by most sporting organisations are based on the list prescribed by the IOC (see Table 17.3).

Most countries have an anti-doping agency or program that provides education to athletes to distinguish between common pharmaceutical products that are permitted and those that contain substances that are banned, either totally or for competition use. Athletes, coaches and sports medicine/science professionals are responsible for applying this information to their own practice. Inadvertent doping may occur, where an athlete records a positive drug test after unintentionally taking a banned substance as an unrecognised ingredient of a product they have consumed. However, most organisations now place full liability with the athlete who tests positive, regardless of circumstance, and full penalties can be expected.

Table 17.3 List of substances or methods banned by the International Olympic Committee (IOC) 1999

Category	Examples
A. Stimulants	Pseudo-ephedrine (e.g. Sudafed) Ephedrine Amphetamines High doses of caffeine—producing a urinary caffeine level ≥ 12 μg/mL
B. Anabolic agents Anabolic and androgenic steroids Non-steroidal anabolic agents	Nandrolone DHEA Androstenedione Other agents with similar properties (e.g. 19-norandrostenedione and other pro-steroid hormones) Beta 2 agonists (except for inhalants of salbutamol and terbutaline)
C. Diuretics	Frusemide (Lasix) Spironolactone (Aldactone)
D. Narcotic analgesics	
E. Peptide and glycoprotein hormones and analogues	Human growth hormone (HGH) Human chorionic gonadotrophin Corticotrophin· Erythropoetin (EPO)
F. Blood doping	
G. Pharmacological, chemical and physical manipulations	Catheterisation (drawing urine from bladder) Masking agents Swapping urine

Although pharmaceutical products, both prescription-regulated and over-the-counter products, are the most likely source of inadvertent doping problems, supplements must also be considered. Although there are no data recording the prevalence of inadvertent doping through drug use, there are isolated reports such as the case of a Dutch professional cyclist who recorded a doping positive after using a liquid herbal supplement that declared ephedra among 15 ingredients (Ros et al. 1999). Supplements containing herbal forms of ephedrine or caffeine, and pro-hormones such as DHEA or androstenedione are either directly banned or may lead to a positive drug test (see Section 17.9.1). In fact, there has been speculation that dietary supplements, such as those containing 19-norandrostenedione, may be responsible for the recent spate of positive tests for the anabolic steroid Nandrolone among a wide range of athletes (Christie 1999).

An inadvertent doping outcome could arise from supplement use in a number of ways (Baylis et al. in press):

1. The supplement contains a banned substance as a stated ingredient but the athlete is not aware that the substance is banned or that it acts to cause a positive doping test.
2. The supplement contains a banned substance within stated ingredients but the athlete is unaware of the relationship between the products (for example, athletes may not recognise that guarana has a high caffeine level, or that Ma Huang herbal products contain ephedrine).
3. The supplement contains banned substances that are not declared as a stated ingredient. These ingredients may be added deliberately but not declared, or added inadvertently as by-products of other ingredients or contaminants of the production process. Examples include herbal preparations that inadvertently contain ephedra or other herbal alkaloid stimulants found in a common plant source, or multi-ingredient 'anabolic supplements' which have an undisclosed content of pro-hormones that convert into banned substances.

Despite the lack of data to report the actual prevalence of the problem, there is a small but real risk of inadvertent doping through supplement use (Baylis et al. in press). Admittedly, the problem exists for a minor percentage of people who undertake sport or exercise activities. However, the outcome for these athletes can be a substantial loss of success, reputation and earnings. In the case of pharmaceutical products, it is relatively easy and successful to prepare lists of proprietary products categorised into banned and permitted classifications. However, in view of the unknown and variable composition of at least some supplement formulations, such a system could not be applied to sports supplements. Understandably, laboratories are generally unwilling to test supplements because of the considerable liability involved with providing a false clearance. We have recently suggested a more suitable classification system would include four categories: low risk, unknown risk, restricted and banned. Examples of general classes of supplements that would fit these categories in Australia are summarised in Table 17.4. It would be useful to have an accredited program to test individual supplement products and perhaps place individual products within the classification system. However, any such program would need to be underpinned by the acceptance of liability by supplement manufacturers and the education of athletes about supplement use. The use of dietary supplements and some sports foods is never risk-free, and each athlete must make their own decision about whether or not to accept the risk (Baylis et al. in press).

Table 17.4 Suggested categorisation of general groups of supplements and sports foods in Australia according to 'Sports safety'

Low risk	Unknown risk	Restricted	Banned
The supplements in this category include only ingredients that are permitted in sport. These supplements are least likely to result in an athlete testing positive to a banned substance	The supplements in this category contain ingredients about which there is insufficient information and, hence, cause for concern. With these supplements there is an athlete testing positive to a banned substance	The supplements in this category contain ingredients that are banned when consumed in amounts that produce a urinary caffeine level of 12 µg/mL or greater	The supplements in this category are known to contain banned substances Examples include supplements containing:
Examples: • Most sports foods (sports drinks, bars, gels, liquid meal supplements) • Vitamin and mineral supplements from pharmaceutical companies or established manufacturers	Examples: • Supplements obtained via Internet, mail-order, personal import from overseas	Examples: • Supplements containing caffeine and guarana	• Ephedra and related compounds • Strychnine • DHEA • Androstenedione • 19-norandrostenedione, 19-norandrostenediol and other pro-hormones

The responsibility for the risk associated with the use of any supplements lies with the athlete
Baylis et al. In press

17.10.2 *Toxicity and side-effects*

Most supplements fall under the banner of foods or 'listable' therapeutic goods and are considered to be relatively safe. As such, there may be no official or mandatory accounting processes to document adverse side-effects arising from the use of these products. Nevertheless, some information about toxicological problems arising from the use of supplements and herbal medicines can be found in various medical registers. Reviews from around the world summarise that while the overall risk to public health from the use of supplements, herbal and traditional remedies is low, cases of toxicity and side-effects include allergic reactions to some products (such as royal jelly), overexposure as a result of self-medication, and poisoning due to contaminants (Perharic et al. 1994; Kozyrskyj 1997; Shaw et al. 1997). These reports call for better regulation and surveillance of supplements and herbal products, and increased awareness of potential hazards.

The problems that occurred with tryptophan supplements provide a good warning of the potential problems associated with poor regulation and heavy marketing of supplements. During 1989–90, regulatory bodies in most countries recalled the sale of supplements containing synthetic forms of the amino acid tryptophan. This occurred after a large number of cases of eosinophilia-myalgia syndrome were reported over the previous five years, leading to several deaths and chronic illness (Roufs 1992). The problem was linked to the use of certain tryptophan supplements produced by microbial fermentation processes (Roufs 1992). Whether these adverse effects were due to the amino acid *per se*, a contaminant in products, or a combination of these factors has not been resolved. However, according to the FDA (1998), impurities were recently found in some supplements containing 5-hydroxy-L-tryptophan, adding weight to the continuing caution regarding tryptophan supplements.

In summary, athletes should not regard supplements and herbal remedies as harmless substances. Although some of the solutions to problems lie with better regulation of manufacturing and marketing processes, the athlete must also bear some responsibility to promote safer use of products. Practices should include avoidance of unknown or 'backyard' brands in favour of products made by larger companies known to implement good manufacturing practice, and careful adherence to recommended doses.

17.10.3 *Misplaced priorities and use of resources*

The claims made for many supplements are emotive and tempting. The promise of instant and dramatic results is alluring to all athletes, regardless of their true talent. It is understandable that athletes want to use these supplements, especially when they hear reports that their opponents or other successful competitors are using them. In our experience, many athletes do not understand that the claims made for many supplements result from lack of regulation rather than the results of rigorous research. As a result, athletes can be drawn to products that are insubstantial and faddish rather than strategies that provide a worthwhile and lasting contribution to sports performance.

Successful sports performance is the product of genetics, long-term training, optimal nutrition, state-of-the-art equipment, and a committed attitude. These factors cannot be replaced by the use of supplements. However, if these are all in place, then an athlete may 'fine-tune' their performance capacity through the use of certain well supported supplements. Since all athletes have limited resources of time and money, it is possible that they will be tempted to see supplements as a short cut to success. Unfortunately, the supplements that receive the most attention and publicity are those with little or no documented benefits for exercise performance. At best, the use of these supplements may be a waste of money. At worst, they may distract the athlete from the use of important training strategies and tools. As nutrition practitioners we commonly see evidence of athletes who do not eat well, and who shun scientifically supported supplements, such as the intake of sports drinks during prolonged training sessions, yet are fascinated by the latest new pill or potion on the sports scene. Equally we are concerned by coaches and parents who want to introduce supplements, including products with credible uses such as creatine, to young and adolescent athletes. We feel that young athletes can make important gains in sports performance through training and adoption of good eating habits. The use of such specialised supplement products should be left until a later stage of a sporting career when goals are to fine-tune rather than lay the foundation.

17.11 SUMMARY

Athletes and coaches are convinced that a performance edge can be found through the use of sports supplements. In our experience, in order to retain a 'real world' credibility, sports scientists need to accept this belief and work within such a framework. This does not mean abandoning critical thinking or downplaying the role of nutrition in optimal performance. Rather, the sports scientist should work with the athlete and coach to allow them to make informed choices about their use of supplements. Ideally, this will mean choosing supplements which have been shown to assist in achieving their specific training and competition goals, and incorporating the appropriate use of these supplements as part of their total nutritional program. In this chapter, we divided supplements into two categories: dietary supplements and nutritional ergogenic aids. We showed that dietary supplements, such as sports drinks, liquid meal supplements, and sports bars, have a variety of well supported roles in helping the athlete to achieve their nutritional goals for optimal performance. While research may continue to refine the composition of these supplements and, perhaps, add to the family of products, the greatest need is for education of athletes to ensure the appropriate use of these dietary supplements. In many cases the information is specific to the individual athlete or sports situation and will require one-to-one counselling. In most situations, the use of the dietary supplement will simply be part of a large plan of optimal sports nutrition or the clinical management of a nutritional disorder. Effective education will not only ensure that the dietary supplement is used correctly, but will highlight the importance of optimal eating strategies.

By contrast, the role of most of the commonly sold nutritional ergogenic aids remains unsupported. There is good evidence that caffeine, bicarbonate and creatine offer the potential of performance benefits for specific athletes in specific situations. Well-conducted research is helping to produce better guidelines for the appropriate use of such supplements. Further research is needed to clarify the potential for glycerol and antioxidant vitamins. However, the majority of nutritional ergogenic aids sold to athletes seem unlikely to produce benefits, other than a placebo effect for the athletes that believe in their promises. The supplement industry is an extremely profitable business, relying mainly on testimonials and scientific theories to market the majority of the nutritional ergogenic aids. The production and marketing of such supplements is poorly regulated with respect to quality control and the scientific support for claims. Athletes appear to be unaware of these issues and are vulnerable to problems such as wasting money and overlooking superior performance-enhancing activities. The risk of side-effects and inadvertent doping arising from the use of many supplements is small but real.

A mutual benefit for all parties (athletes, supplement manufacturers and sports scientists) will only be achieved through co-operation and pooling of resources to undertake further well-designed research and to support appropriate education programs. However, such research needs to be carefully planned and executed so that it can answer questions that are relevant to athletes and real-life sports competition.

Even where the benefits of supplements to athletic performance can be proven, it is important to put their role into perspective. The effects of training and other factors (e.g. inherited talent, equipment, mental preparation and motivation) will provide a greater influence on sports performance than the effects of a dietary supplement or nutritional ergogenic aid. But when these issues are already optimised, as in the case of the well-prepared elite athlete, the effects of supplements might provide another small but significant improvement in performance. The nutrients that can be provided by supplements to greatest effect are fluid and CHO. Other supplements are unlikely to ever provide a substitute for the factors that are basic to sports performance.

17.12 *PRACTICE TIPS*

Glenn Cardwell

• Each month it seems there is a new supplement or ergogenic aid produced, which is widely and frantically marketed, before taking a back seat to the next product. This constant activity makes it difficult to keep up-to-date with what is available to athletes. It is wise to make regular visits to health stores, use the

Internet, read the latest sports magazines and ask athletes about their supplements in order to keep up-to-date with what is on the market. Many supplements will clearly be of little value, while a small proportion may have enough plausibility and merit to warrant further enquiries.

- It is vital to keep up-to-date with the latest research on products. Strategies include:
  — doing frequent searches for articles on new supplements through the Internet;
  — undertaking Medline searches for scientific references;
  — checking information from manufacturers and distributors of products, some of which list references which may be of assistance;
  — searching websites for universities and professional bodies such as sports dietitians Australia and other health professionals for their comments; and
  — looking at the National Institute of Health (USA) website on dietary supplements (http://www.odp.od.nih.gov/ods/databases/ibids.html).

- Dietitians are often stereotyped as being 'anti-supplements'. It is important to check that you have no such biases, or project this view to athletes and coaches. There are some sports supplements and sports foods that have a proven worth in sports performance. These products include sports drinks, creatine, and meal-replacement drinks. Although some useful products are more expensive than the supermarket equivalent, their superior taste and convenience might be an attraction to the athlete. Athletes should be aware that various products can be beneficial to their training and competition performance, but that the value of these products is specific to the conditions of use. It is important to remain up-to-date with research that illustrates the specific uses of these products. The sports dietitian can provide a valuable service to athletes by being the interface between the science and practice of this area of sports nutrition. It is good to have fact sheets and other educational tools on various supplements that can provide information to athletes about the conditions under which they might be used. Be prepared to be make your advice practical and specific to individual sports or individual athletes.

- Companies who make useful sports supplements and sports foods may also fund research, education resources or conferences and seminars. They may also employ sports dietitians or sports science teams who should not be overlooked as valuable contacts for nutrition information. Check for websites, education resources and other items that can keep you up-to-date, or provide information for your athletes.

- Athletes will frequently ask for your advice about a new supplement that has taken their interest. Ask them to bring in supplement packaging or information. Discuss what the label says, any performance-enhancing claims and each of the ingredients. Make every effort to find out if there is any scientific validity for the product using the strategies outlined previously. Write to the company for scientific support for their product. If they don't answer, then tell the athlete that the manufacturer is unable to furnish any supporting evidence for their product. If they provide references, check their relevance and quality. If they provide only testimonials or non-peer-reviewed articles, then it is likely they have no quality research to back their claims.

- Provide copies of good research or quality reviews that discuss the merits or drawbacks of each product. Point out that many products are claimed to have almost drug-like properties, yet have not undergone the rigorous testing that is required for pharmaceutical products. Some products have been used in studies run over six weeks. Explain that this does not indicate the long-term effects of the product.

- Many products are sold through a multilevel marketing (MLM) process. Product distributors are recruited by friends and colleagues with the promise of an 'exciting business opportunity' that can make you 'financially independent'. Testimonials from the top salespeople suggest that MLM is a quick and efficient way of becoming rich, making it attractive to many people wanting extra income. It is very rare to find anyone with tertiary nutrition qualifications involved in MLM sales. Most MLM products specifically marketed to athletes are sold on their performance-enhancing properties, usually backed by testimonials from athletes who have received free product and sponsorship. Their sporting prowess is claimed to be due to the nutrition product, with little reference to their genetic background, the hours of training and the power of psychology. Distributors are generally encouraged to make verbal health or performance claims, claims that are often illegal to make in company brochures.

- Be careful when accepting supplement products from distributors, and particularly from MLM salespeople, as acceptance of the product can imply your endorsement. Distributors may use the line 'many sports dietitians are trying our product' when the dietitian has, in fact, only been given a free sample. It may be safer to get your product samples through other means, such as simply purchasing it from a store or as an anonymous sale. If you are comfortable with the benefits of the product and the ethics of the company, then you may choose to recommend the product to athletes.

- Frequently, sports supplements provide similar nutrient value to common supermarket items or other cheaper supplements. The glamour of sport is used as a hook to increase the price. Check the ingredients of products to see if they can be duplicated by a cheaper product. For example, sports bars may be replaced by breakfast bars or muesli bars, powdered weight-gain products may be similar to pharmaceutical liquid meal products or even skim milk powder, and amino acid supplements may provide the same dose of amino acids as a carton of yoghurt. While sometimes the packaging or form of the sports supplement makes it particularly practical for use by an athlete, on many occasions a cheaper food product or alternative supplement can be found.

- Part of the marketing of products is to state that the product meets all of the health regulations of the country of sale. Sometimes this is given a twist in terminology, for example to state that the product is 'endorsed' by TGA or ANZFA. Although the product may meet the guidelines or codes of these agencies, it generally doesn't follow that the product has any therapeutic or performance-enhancing properties. These agencies are concerned mainly with issues of safety rather than efficacy.

- There are some groups of athletes that should be particularly careful before using sports supplements. Strongly dissuade children, growing teenagers, pregnant or breast-feeding women, and women attempting conception from taking new products. It is extremely unlikely that products have been tested on such groups, and we are unaware of their effect on the growth and development of the foetus, infants and children.

- There is a small but real risk that the use of some sports supplements will lead to a positive doping test. Elite athletes should never take any supplement without first consulting their physician or sports dietitian, as it may contain ingredients that have been banned by their sporting authority. Not all of the ingredients may be listed on a label.

- Since sports supplements are a challenging and often frustrating area of sports nutrition, it is important to be realistic about your goals. The role of a sports dietitian is to provide a balanced, rational and dispassionate evaluation of each product so that the athlete can make an informed choice. This information will need to be regularly updated. The athlete will make the final choice. Do not expect to change the views of every athlete. They have various reasons for wanting to try products. For example:
  — They are curious after hearing about the product.
  — 'Everyone else is using the product, so it must work.'
  — Everyone else is using the product, so they must take it to remain on level terms with the opposition.
  — It adds a little variety and interest to their sports preparation.
  — Your views may not change them. Whether or not they continue to use a product will be based on the perceived benefits to their sports performance.

- A supplement will always be an adjunct to, not replace, a well-chosen diet. It is unlikely that any supplement in the near future will be able to redress the harm of poor quality eating, or failure to address well-supported nutritional strategies for sport, such as achieving adequate fuel intake or fluid levels. As many athletes can't get the basics right, it is the duty of the sports dietitian to stress the value of good nutrition, before an athlete considers taking a supplement.

REFERENCES

Adams MM, Porcello LP, Vivian VM. Effect of a supplement on dietary intake of female collegiate swimmers. Phys Sportsmed 1982;10:122–34.

Allen JD, McLung J, Nelson AG, Welsch M. Ginseng supplementation does not enhance healthy young adults' peak aerobic exercise performance. J Am Coll Nutr 1999;17:462–6.

American College of Sports Medicine. Position Statement: the physiological and health consequences of oral Cr supplementation. Med Sci Sports Exerc 2000;32:706–17.

Anderson MJ, Cotter JD, Garnham AP, Casley DJ, Febbraio MA. Effect of glycerol–induced hyperhydration on thermoregulation and metabolism during exercise in the heat. Int J Sport Nutr Exerc Metab 2001;11:315–33.

Angus DJ, Hargreaves M, Dancey J, Febbraio MA. Effect of carbohydrate or carbohydrate plus medium chain triglyceride ingestion on cycling time trial performance. J Appl Physiol 2000;88:113–19.

Anselme F, Collomp K, Mercier B, Ahmaïdi S, Prefaut C. Caffeine increases maximal anaerobic power and blood lactate concentration. Eur J Appl Physiol 1992;65:188–91.

Ariel G, Saville W. Anabolic steroids: the physiological effects of placebo. Med Sci Sports 1972;4:124–6.

Australian Sports Medicine Federation. Survey of drug use in Australian sport. Melbourne: Australian Sports Medicine Federation, 1983.

Bahrke MS, Morgan WP. Evaluation of the ergogenic properties of ginseng. Sports Med 1994;18:229–48.

Ballantyne CS, Phillips SM, MacDonald JR, Tarnopolsky M, MacDougall JD. The acute effects of androstenedione supplementation in healthy young males. Can J Appl Physiol 2000;25:68–78.

Balsom PD, Harridge SDR, Soderland K, Sjodin B, Ekblom B. Creatine supplementation per se does not enhance endurance exercise performance. Acta Physiol Scand 1993;149:521–3.

Balsom PD, Soderland K, Sjodin B, Ekblom B. Skeletal muscle metabolism during short duration high-intensity exercise: influence of creatine supplementation. Acta Physiol Scand 1995;154:303–10.

Barnett C, Costill DL, Vukovich MD, et al. Effect of L-carnitine supplementation on muscle and blood carnitine content and lactate accumulation during high-intensity sprint cycling. Int J Sport Nutr 1994;4:280–8.

Barnett C, Hinds H, Jenkins DG. Effects of oral creatine supplementation on multiple sprint cycle performance. Aust J Sci Med Sport 1996;28:35–9.

Barr SI. Nutrition knowledge and selected nutritional practices of female recreational athletes. J Nutr Ed 1986;18:167–74.

Barr SI. Nutrition knowledge of female varsity athletes and university students. J Am Diet Assoc 1987;87:1660–4.

Barr SI, Costill DL. Effect of increased training volume on nutrient intake of male collegiate swimmers. Int J Sports Med 1992;13:47–51.

Barry AT, Cantwell F, Doherty JC, et al. A nutritional study of Irish athletes. Brit J Sports Med 1981;15:99–109.

Baylis A, Cameron-Smith D, Burke LM. Inadvertent doping through supplement use by athletes: assessment and management of the risk. In press.

Bazzarre TL, Scarpino A, Sigmon R, Marquart LF, Wu SL, Izurieta M. Vitamin–mineral supplement use and nutritional status of athletes. J Am Coll Nutr 1993;12:162–9.

Beecher HK. Measurement of subjective responses: quantitative effects of drugs. New York: Oxford University Press, 1959.

Bell DG, Jacobs I, Zamecnik J. Effects of caffeine, ephedrine, and their combination on time to exhaustion during high-intensity exercise. Eur J Appl Physiol 1998;77:427–33.

Below PR, Mora-Rodiguez R, Gonzalez-Alonso J, Coyle EF. Fluid and carbohydrate ingestion independently improve performance during 1 h of intense exercise. Med Sci Sports Exerc 1995;27:200–10.

Bentivenga A, Kelly E, Kalenak A. Diet, fitness and athletic performance. Phys Sportsmed 1979;7:100–5.

Berglund B, Hemmingsson P. Effects of caffeine ingestion on exercise performance at low and high altitudes in cross-country skiers. Int J Sports Med 1982;3:234–6.

Berning J. Swimmers nutrition knowledge and practice. Sports Nutrition News. 4, 1986.

Birch R, Noble D, Greenhaff PL. The influence of dietary creatine supplementation on performance during repeated bouts of maximal isokinetic cycling in man. Eur J Appl Physiol 1994;69:268–70.

Birkett DJ, Miners JO. Caffeine renal clearance and urine caffeine concentrations during steady-state dosing: implications for monitoring caffeine intake during sports events. Br J Clin Pharmacol 1991;31:405–8.

Blomstrand E, Hassmen P, Ekblom B, Newsholme EA. Administration of branched-chain amino acids during sustained exercise—effects on performance and on plasma concentration of some amino acids. Eur J Appl Physiol 1991;63:83–8.

Blomstrand E, Hassmen P, Ek S, Ekblom B, Newsholme EA. Influence of ingesting a solution of branched-chain amino acids on perceived exertion during exercise. Acta Physiol Scand 1997;159:41–99.

Blomstrand E, Hassmen P, Newsholme EA. Effect of branched-chain amino acid supplementation on mental performance. Acta Physiol Scand 1991;143:225–6.

Blue JG, Lombardo JA. Steroids and steroid-like compounds. Clin Sports Med 1999;18:667–89.

Bobb A, Pringle D, Ryan AJ. A brief study of the diet of athletes. J Sports Med. 1969;9:255–62.

Bond V, Adams R, Balkissoon B, et al. Effects of caffeine on cardiorespiratory function and glucose metabolism during rest and graded exercise. J Sports Med 1987;27:47–52.

Bond V, Gresham K, McRae J, Tearney RJ. Caffeine ingestion and isokinetic strength. Brit J Sports Med 1986;20:135–7.

Bosco C, Tihanyi J, Pucspk J, et al. Effect of oral creatine supplementation on jumping and running performance. Int J Sports Med 1997;18:369–72.

Bosy TZ, Moore KA, Polkis A. The effect of oral dehydroepiandrosterone (DHEA) on the urine testosterone/epitestosterone (T/E) ratio in human male volunteers. J Anal Toxicol 1998;22:455–9.

Braun B, Clarkson PM, Freedson PS, Kohl RL. Effects of coenzyme Q10 supplementation on exercise performance, VO_2 max, and lipid peroxidation in trained cyclists. Int J Sport Nutr 1991;1:353–65.

Brill JB, Keane MW. Supplementation patterns of competitive male and female body builders. Int J Sport Nutr 1994;4:398–412.

Brown GA, Vukovich MD, Reifenrath TA, et al. Effects of anabolic precursors on serum testosterone adaptations to resistance training in young men. Int J Sports Nutr Exerc Metab 2000;10:340–359.

Brown GA, Vukovich MD, Sharp RL, Reifenrath TA, Parsons KA, King DS. Effect of oral DHAE on serum testosterone and adaptations to resistance training in young men. J Appl Physiol 1999;87:2274–83.

Bucci LR. Dietary supplements as ergogenic aids. In: Wolinsky I, ed. Nutrition in exercise and sport, 3rd edn. Boca Raton: CRC Press, 1998:315–68.

Bucci LR, Hickson JF, Wolinksy I, Pivarnik JM. Ornithine supplementation and insulin release in body builders. Int J Sports Nutr 1992;2:287–91.

Buckley J, Abbott M, Martin S, Brinkworth G, Whyte P. Effect of an oral bovine colostrum supplement (intact™) on running performance (abst). Adelaide: Proc Aust Conf Sci Med Sport, 1998:79.

Buckley JD, Brinkworth GD, Bourdon PC, et al. Oral supplementation with bovine colostrum (intact™) improves performance in elite female rowers (abst). Sydney: Proc 5th IOC World Congress, 1999:246.

Burke LM, Gollan RA, Read RSD. Dietary intakes and food use of groups of elite Australian male athletes. Int J Sport Nutr 1991;1:378–94.

Burke LM, Heeley P. Dietary supplements and nutritional ergogenic aids in sport. In: Burke L, Deakin V, eds. Clinical Sports Nutrition. Sydney, Australia: McGraw Hill, 1994:227–84.

Burke LM, Pyne DB, Telford RD. Effect of creatine supplementation on single-effort sprint performance in elite swimmers. Int J Sport Nutr 1996;6:222–33.

Burke LM, Read RSD. Dietary supplements in sport. Sports Med 1993;15(1):43–56.

Camire ME, Kantor MA. Dietary supplements: nutritional and legal considerations. Food Tech 1999;53:87–96.

Campbell ML, MacFadyen KL. Nutrition knowledge, beliefs and dietary practices of competitive swimmers. Can Home Econ J 1984;34:47–51.

Campbell WW, Beard JL, Joseph LJ, Davey SL, Evans WJ. Chromium picolinate supplementation and resistive training by older men: effects on iron-status and hematologic indexes. Am J Clin Nutr 1997;66:644–9.

Casey A, Constantini-Teodosiu, Howell S, Hultman E, Greenhaff P. Creatine ingestion favorably affects performance and muscle metabolism during maximal exercise in humans. Am J Physiol 1996;271:E31–E7.

Castell LM, Poortmans JR, Newsholme EA. Does glutamine have a role in reducing infections in athletes? Eur J Appl Physiol 1996;73:488–90.

Cerretelli P, Marconi C. L-carnitine supplementation in humans: the effects on physical performance. Int J Sports Med 1990;11:1–14.

Chanutin A. The fate of creatine when administered to man. J Biol Chem 1926;67:29–37.

Cheuvront SN, Moffatt RJ, Biggerstaff KD, Bearden S, McDonough P. Effect of ENDUROX™ on metabolic responses to submaximal exercise. Int J Sport Nutr 1999;9:434–42.

Chong SKF, Oberholzer VG. Ginseng—is there a clinical use in medicine? Postgrad Med J 1988;65:841–6.

Christie J. U.S. stars assail drug detection system. Mail and Globe, Sports Section, August 26 1999, 34.

Clancy S, Clarkson PM, De Cheke M, et al. Effects of chromium picolinate supplementation on body composition, strength, and urinary chromium loss in football players. Int J Sport Nutr 1994;4:142–53.

Clark GR, Hawley JA, Burke LM, Hopkins WG. Placebo effect of carbohydrate feedings during a 40 km cycling time trial. Med Sci Sports Exerc 2000;32:1642–7.

Clark N, Nelson M, Evans W. Nutrition education for the elite female runners. The Phys Sportsmed 1988;16(2):124–36.

Clarkson PM. Nutritional ergogenic aids: carnitine. Int J Sport Nutr 1992;92:185–90.

Clarkson PM. Effects of exercise on chromium levels: is supplementation necessary? Sports Med 1997;23:341–9.

Cohen BS, Nelson AG, Prevost MC, Thompson GD, Marx BD, Morris GS. Effects of caffeine ingestion on endurance racing in heat and humidity. Eur J Appl Physiol 1996;73:358–63.

Cole KJ, Costill DL, Starling RD, Goodpaster BH, Trappe SW, Fink WJ. Effect of caffeine ingestion on perception of effort and subsequent work production. Int J Sports Nutr 1996;6:14–23.

Colgan M. Inosine—the latest Weider-sponsored research. Muscle & Fitness 1988;49(1):94–6.

Collomp K, Ahmaidi S, Audran M, Chanal J-L, Préfaut C. Effects of caffeine ingestion on performance and anaerobic metabolism during the windgate test. Int J Sports Med 1991;12:439–43.

Collomp K, Ahmaidi S, Chatard JC, Audran M, Préfaut C. Benefits of caffeine ingestion on sprint performance in trained and untrained swimmers. Eur J Appl Physiol 1992;64:377–80.

Colombani P, Wenk C, Kunz I, et al. Effects of L-carnitine supplementation on physical performance and energy metabolism of endurance-trained athletes: a double-blind crossover field study. Eur J Appl Physiol 1996;73:434–9.

Cooke WH, Barnes WS. The influence of recovery duration on high-intensity exercise performance after oral creatine supplementation. Can J Appl Physiol 1997;22(5):454–67.

Cooke WH, Grandjean PW, Barnes WS. Effect of oral creatine supplementation on power output and fatigue during bicycle ergometry. J Appl Physiol 1995;78(2):670–3.

Costill DL, Dalsky GP, Fink WJ. Effects of caffeine ingestion on metabolism and exercise performance. Med Sci Sports 1978;10:155–8.

Cross N. Nutrition and the elite athlete: implications for the management of coaching practices. Swimming Times 1997:25–6.

Davis JM. Carbohydrates, branched-chain amino acids and endurance: the central fatigue hypothesis. Int J Sport Nutr 1995;5(suppl):S29–S38.

Davis JM, Bailey SP, Woods JA, Galiano FJ, Hamilton M, Bartoli WP. Effects of carbohydrate feedings on plasma free tryptophan and branched-chain amino acids during prolonged cycling. Eur J Appl Physiol 1992;65:513–19.

Dawson B, Cutler M, Moody A, Lawrence S, Goodman C, Randall N. Effects of oral creatine loading on single and repeated maximal short sprints. Aust J Sci Med Sport 1995;27(3):56–61.

Decombaz J, Deriaz O, Acheson K, Gmuender B, Jequier E. Effect of L-carnitine on submaximal exercise metabolism after depletion of muscle glycogen. Med Sci Sports Exerc 1993;25:733–40.

Dekkers JC, van Dooren LJ, Kemper HC. The role of antioxidants and enzymes in the prevention of exercise muscle damage. Sports Med 1996;21:213–38.

Delbeke FT, Debackere M. Caffeine: use and abuse in sports. Int J Sports Med 1984;5:179–82.

Demant TW, Rhodes EC. Effects of creatine supplementation on exercise performance. Sports Med 1999;28:49–60.

Denadai BS, Denadai MLDR. Effects of caffeine on time to exhaustion in exercise performed below and above the anaerobic threshold. Braz J Med Biol Res 1998;31:581–5.

Dennig H, Talbot JH, Edwards HT, Dill B. Effects of acidosis and alkalosis upon the capacity for work. J Clin Invest 1931;9:601–13.

Deuster PA, Kyle SB, Moser PB, Vigersky RA, Singh A, Schoomaker EB. Nutritional survey of highly trained women runners. Am J Clin Nutr 1986;45:954–62.

Dill DB, Edwards HT, Talbot JH. Alkalosis and the capacity for work. J Biol Chem 1932;97:58–9.

Dodd SL, Brooks E, Powers SK, Tulley R. The effects of caffeine on graded exercise performance in caffeine naïve versus habituated subjects. Eur J Appl Physiol 1991;2:424–9.

Doherty M. The effect of caffeine on the maximal accumulated oxygen deficit and short term running performance. Int J Sport Nutr 1998;8:95–104.

Douglas PD, Douglas JD. Nutritional knowledge and food practices of high school athletes. J Am Diet Assoc 1984;84:1198–202.

Dowling EA, Redondo DR, Branch JD, Jones S, McNabb G, Williams MH. Effect of eleutherococcus senticosus on submaximal and maximal exercise performance. Med Sci Sports Exerc 1996;28:482–9.

Dwyer T, Brotherhood J. Long-term dietary considerations in physical training. Proc Nutr Soc Aust 1981;6:31–40.

Earnest CP, Almada AL, Mitchell TL. Effects of creatine monohydrate ingestion on intermediate duration anaerobic treadmill running to exhaustion. J Strength Cond Res 1997;11(4):234–8.

Earnest CP, Snell PG, Rodriguez R, Almada AL. The effect of creatine monohydrate ingestion on anaerobic power indices, muscular strength and body composition. Acta Physiol Scand 1995;153:207–9.

Elam RP. Morphological change in adult male from resistance training and amino acid supplementation. J Sports Med Phys Fitness 1988;28:35–9.

Elam RP, Hardin DH, Sutton RAL, Hagen L. Effects of arginine and ornithine on strength, lean body mass, and urinary hydroxyproline in adult males. J Sports Med Phys Fitness 1989;29:52–6.

Engelhardt M, Neumann G, Berbalk A, Reuter I. Creatine supplementation in endurance sports. Med Sci Sports Exerc 1998;30:1123–9.

Engels HJ, Wirth JC. No ergogenic effects of ginseng (Panax ginseng C.A. Meyer) during graded maximal aerobic exercise. J Am Diet Assoc 1997;97:1110–15.

Ersoy G. Dietary status and anthropometric assessment of child gymnasts. J Sports Med Phys Fitness 1991;31:577–80.

Evans GW. The effect of chromium picolinate on insulin controlled parameters in humans. Int J Biosocial Med Res 1989;11:163–80.

Evans GW. Chromium picolinate is an effective and efficacious and safe supplement (letter to the editor). Int J Sport Nutr 1993;3:117–19.

Faber M, Spinnler-Benade AJ. Nutrient intake and dietary supplementation in body builders. S Afr Med J 1987;72:831–4.

Faber M, Spinnler-Benade AJ. Mineral and vitamin intake in field athletes (discus-, hammer-, javelin-throwers and shotputters). Int J Sports Med 1991;12:324–7.

Falk B, Burstein R, Ashkenazi I, et al. The effect of caffeine ingestion on physical performance after prolonged exercise. Eur J Appl Physiol 1989;59:168–73.

Febbraio MA, Flanagan TR, Snow RJ, Zhao S, Carey MF. Effect of creatine supplementation on intramuscular TCr, metabolism and performance during intermittent, supramaximal exercise in humans. Acta Physiol Scand 1995;155:387–95.

Felder JM, Burke LM, Lowdon BJ, Cameron-Smith D, Collier GR. Nutritional practices of elite female surfers during training and competition. Int J Sport Nutr 1998;8:36–48.

Ferrauti A, Weber K, Strüder HK. Metabolic and ergogenic effects of carbohydrate and caffeine beverage in tennis. J Sports Med Phys Fitness 1997;37:258–66.

Flinn S, Gregory J, McNaughton LR, Davies P. Caffeine ingestion prior to incremental cycling to exhaustion in recreational cyclists. Int J Sports Med 1990;11:188–93.

Food and Drug Administration (online). Impurities confirmed in dietary supplement 5-hydroxy-L-tryptophan. FDA Talk Paper T98–T48 Aug 31. http://www.fda.gov/bbs/topics/ANSWERS/ANS00953.html, 1998.

Forsberg AM, Nilsson E, Werneman J, Bergstrom J, Hultman E. Muscle composition in relation to age and sex. Clin Sci 1991;81:249–56.

Frederick L, Hawkins ST. A comparison of nutrition knowledge and attitudes, dieting practices and bone densities of post-menopausal women, female college athletes, and nonathletic women. J Am Diet Assoc 1992;92:299–305.

French C, McNaughton L, Pavies P, Tristram S. Caffeine ingestion during exercise to exhaustion in elite distance runners. J Sports Med Phys Fitness 1991;31:425–32.

Fricker PA, Beasley SK, Copeland IW. Physiological growth hormone responses of throwers to amino acids, eating and exercise. Aust J Sci Med Sport 1988;20:21–3.

Fricker PA, Beasley SK, Copeland IW. A preliminary study on the effects of amino acids, fasting and exercise on nocturnal growth hormone release in weightlifters. Excel 1991;79(2):2–5.

Fulco CS, Rock PB, Trad LA, et al. Effect of caffeine on submaximal exercise performance at altitude. Aviat Space Environ Med 1994;65:539–45.

Gaesser GA, Rich RG. Influence of caffeine on blood lactate response during incremental exercise. Int J Sports Med 1985;6:207–11.

Gao J, Costill DL, Horswill CA, Park SH. Sodium bicarbonate ingestion improves performance in interval swimming. Eur J Appl Physiol 1988;58:171–4.

Gater DR, Gater DA, Uribe JM, Bunt JC. Effects of arginine/lysine supplementation and resistance training on glucose tolerance. J Appl Physiol 1992a;72:1279–84.

Gater DR, Gater DA, Uribe JM, Bunt JC. Impact of nutritional supplements and resistance training on body composition, strength and insulin-like growth factor-1. J Appl Sport Sci Res 1992b;6:66–76.

Goedecke JH, Elmer-English R, Dennis SC, Schloss I, Noakes TD, Lambert EV. Effects of medium-chain triacylglycerol ingested with carbohydrate on metabolism and exercise performance. Int J Sport Nutr 1999;9:35–47.

Goldfinch J, McNaughton L, Davies P. Induced metabolic alkalosis and its effects on 400m racing time. Eur J Appl Physiol 1988;57:45–8.

Gorostiaga EM, Maurer CA, Eclache JP. Decrease in respiratory quotient during exercise following L-carnitine supplementation. Int J Sports Med 1989;10:169–74.

Graham TE, Hibbert E, Sathasivam P. Metabolic and exercise endurance effects of coffee and caffeine ingestion. J Appl Physiol 1998;85:883–9.

Graham TE, McLean C. In: Tarnopolsky M, ed. Gender differences in the metabolic responses to caffeine. Boca Raton: CRC Press, 1999:301–27.

Graham TE, Rush JWE, van Soeren MH. Caffeine and exercise: metabolism and performance. Can J Appl Physiol 1994;19(1):111–38.

Graham TE, Sathasivam P, MacNaughton KW. Influence of cold, exercise and caffeine on catecholamines and metabolism in men. J Appl Physiol 1991;70:2052–8.

Graham TE, Spriet LL. Performance and metabolic responses to a high caffeine dose during prolonged exercise. J Appl Physiol 1991;71:2292–8.

Graham TE, Spriet LL. Metabolic, catecholamine and exercise performance responses to various doses of caffeine. J Appl Physiol 1995;78:867–74.

Grandjean AC. Vitamins, diet, and the athlete. Clin Sports Med 1983;2:105–14.

Grandjean AC. Profile of nutritional beliefs and practices of elite athletes. In: Butts NK, Gushiiken T, Zarins B, eds. The elite athlete. New York: Spectrum, 1985:239–47.

Grandjean AC, Lolkus LJ, Lind R, Schaefer AE. Dietary intake of female cyclists during repeated days of racing. Cycling Science 1992;4:21–5.

Grant KE, Chandler RM, Castle AL, Ivy JL. Chromium and exercise training: effect on obese women. Med Sci Sport Exerc 1997;29:992–8.

Green AL, Hultman E, Macdonald IA, Sewell DA, Greenhaff PL. Carbohydrate ingestion augments skeletal muscle creatine accumulation during supplementation in man. Am J Physiol 1996a;271:E812–E26.

Green AL, Macdonald IA, Greenhaff PL. The effects of creatine and carbohydrate on whole body creatine retention in vegetarians. Proc Nutr Soc 1997;56:81A.

Green AL, Simpson EJ, Littlewood JJ, Macdonald IA, Greenhaff PL. Carbohydrate ingestion augments creatine retention during creatine feeding in man. Acta Physiol Scand 1996b;158:195–202.

Greenhaff PL, Bodin K, Soderlund K, Hultman E. Effect of oral creatine supplementation on skeletal phosphocreatine resynthesis. Am J Physiol 1994;266:E725–E30.

Greenhaff PL, Casey A, Short AH, Harris R, Soderland K, Hultman E. Influence of oral creatine supplementation of muscle torque during repeated bouts of maximal voluntary exercise in man. Clin Sci 1993;84:565–71.

Greer F, Mclean C, Graham TE. Caffeine, performance, and metabolism during repeated windgate exercise tests. J Appl Physiol 1998;85:1502–8.

Greig C, Finch KM, Jones DA, Cooper M, Sargeant AJ, Forte CA. The effect of oral supplementation with L-carnitine on maximum and submaximum exercise capacity. Eur J Appl Physiol 1987;56:457–60.

Grindstaff PD, Kreider R, Bishop R, et al. Effects of creatine supplementation on repetitive sprint performance and body composition in competitive swimmers. Int J Sport Nutr 1997;7:330–46.

Grunewald KK, Bailey RS. Commercially marketed supplements for body building athletes. Sports Med 1993;15:90–103.

Gurley BJ, Wang P, Gardner SF. Ephedrine-type alkaloid content of nutritional supplements containing Ephedra Sinica (Ma Huang) as determined by high performance liquid chromatography. J Pharm Sci 1988;87:1547–53.

Hahm H, Kujawa J, Ausberger L. Comparison of melatonin products against USP's nutritional supplements standards and other criteria. J Am Pharm Assoc 1999;39:27–31.

Hallmark MA, Reynolds TH, DeSouza CA, Dotson CO, Anderson RA, Rogers MA. Effects of chromium and resistive training on muscle strength and body composition. Med Sci Sports Exerc 1996;28:139–44.

Harris RC, Soderlund K, Hultman E. Elevation of creatine in resting and exercise muscle of normal subjects by creatine supplementation. Clin Sci 1992;83:367–74.

Hasten DL, Rome EP, Franks BD, Hegsted M. Effects of chromium picolinate on beginning weight training students. Int J Sport Nutr 1992;2:343–50.

Hawley JA, Schabort EJ, Noakes TD, Dennis SC. Carbohydrate-loading and exercise performance: an update. Sports Med 1997;24:73–81.

Heigenhauser GFJ, Jones NJ. Bicarbonate loading. In: Lamb DR, Williams MH, eds. Perspectives in exercise science and sports medicine. Vol 4: Ergogenics. Carmel, Indiana: Cooper Publishing Group, 1991:183–212.

Heinonen OJ. Carnitine and physical exercise. Sports Med 1996;22:109–32.

Hitchins S, Martin DT, Burke LM, et al. Glycerol hyperhydration improves cycle time trial performance in hot humid conditions. Eur J Appl Physiol 1999;80:494–501.

Hopkins WG, Hawley A, Burke LM. Design and analysis of research on sport performance enhancement. Med Sci Sports Exerc 1999;31:472–85.

Houston ME. Diet, training and sleep: a survey study of elite Canadian swimmers. Can J Appl Sports Sci 1980;5:161–3.

Hultman E, Soderlund K, Timmons JA, Cederblad G, Greenhaff PL. Muscle creatine loading in men. J Appl Physiol 1996;81:232–7.

Inder, WJ, Swanney MP, Donald RA, Prickett TCR, Hellemans J. The effect of glycerol and desmopressin on exercise performance and hydration in triathletes. Med Sci Sports Exerc 1998;30:1263–9.

International Olympic Committee. Doping: an IOC White paper. Lausanne, Switzerland: IOC, 1999.

Ivy JL, Costill DL, Fink WJ, Lower RW. Influence of caffeine and carbohydrate feedings on endurance performance. Med Sci Sports 1979;11:6–11.

Jackman M, Wendling P, Friars D, Graham TE. Metabolic, catecholamine, and endurance responses to caffeine during intense exercise. J Appl Physiol 1996;81:1658–63.

Jacobs I, Bleue S, Goodman J. Creatine ingestion increases anaerobic capacity and maximum accumulated oxygen deficit. Can J Appl Physiol 1997;22(3):231–43.

Jeukendrup AE, Saris WHM, Schrauwen P, Brouns F, Wagenmakers AJM. Metabolic availability of medium-chain triglycerides coingested with carbohydrates during prolonged exercise. J Appl Physiol 1995;79:756–62.

Jeukendrup AE, Saris WHM, Brouns F, Halliday D, Wagenmakers AJM. Effects of carbohydrate and fat supplementation on carbohydrate metabolism during prolonged exercise. Metabolism 1996;46:915–21.

Jeukendrup AE, Thielen JJHC, Wagenmakers AJM, Brouns F, Saris WHM. Effects of MCT and carbohydrate ingestion during exercise on substrate utilisation and subsequent performance. Am J Clin Nutr 1998;67:397–404.

Jonnalagadda SS, Benardot D, Nelson M. Energy and nutrient intakes of the United States national women's artistic gymnastics team. Int J Sport Nutr 1998;8:331–44.

Juhn MS, Tarnopolsky M. Oral creatine supplementation and athletic performance: a critical review. Clin J Sport Med 1998;8:286–97.

Juhn MS, Tarnopolsky M. Potential side-effects of oral creatine supplementation: a critical review. Clin J Sport Med 1998;8:298–304.

Kaikkonen J, Kosonen L, Nyyssonen K, et al. Effect of combined coenzyme Q10 and d-a-tocopheryl acetate supplementation on exercise-induced lipid peroxidation and muscular damage: a placebo-controlled double-blind study in marathon runners. Free Radical Res 1998;29:85–92.

Kelly VG, Jenkins DG. Effect of oral creatine supplementation on near-maximal strength and repeated sets of high-intensity bench press exercise. J Strength Cond Res 1998;12(2):109–15.

Khoo CS, Rawson NE, Robinson ML, Stevenson RJ. Nutrient intake and eating habits of triathletes. Ann Sports Med 1987;3:144–50.

Kindermann W, Keul J, Huber G. Physical exercise after induced alkalosis (bicarbonate or tris-buffer). Eur J Appl Physiol 1977;37:197–204.

King DS, Sharp RL, Vukovich MD. Effect of oral androstenedione on serum testosterone and adaptations to resistance training in young men. JAMA 1999;281:2020–2028.

Kingsbury KJ, Kay L, Hjelm M. Contrasting plasma free fatty amino acid patterns in elite athletes: association with fatigue and infection. Br J Sports Med 1998;32:25–32.

Kleiner SM, Bazzarre TL, Litchford MD. Metabolic profiles, diet, and health practices of championship male and female body builders. J Am Diet Assoc 1990;90:962–7.

Kovacs EM, Stegen JHCH, Brouns F. Effect of caffeinated drinks on substrate metabolism, caffeine excretion, and performance. J Appl Physiol 1998;85:709–15.

Kozyrskyj, A. Herbal products in Canada: how safe are they? Can Fam Phys 1997;43:697–702.

Kraemer W, Volek JS. Creatine supplementation: its role in human performance. Clin Sports Med 1999;18:651–66.

Kreider RB, Ferreira M, Wilson M, et al. Effects of creatine supplementation on body composition, strength, and sprint performance. Med Sci Sports Exerc 1998;30:73–82.

Kreider RB, Ferreira M, Wilson M, Almada AL. Effects of calcium B-hydroxy B-methyl butyrate supplementation during resistance training on markers of catabolism, body composition and strength. Int J Sports Med 1999;20:503–9.

Krowchuk DP, Anglin TM, Goodfellow DB, et al. High school athletes and the use of ergogenic aids. Am J Dis Child 1989;143:486–9.

Krumbach CJ, Ellis DR, Driskell JA. A report of the vitamin and mineral supplement use among university athletes in a Division 1 institution. Int J Sport Nutr 1999;9:416–25.

Laaksonen R, Fogelholm M, Himberg JJ, Laaksoc J, Salorinne Y. Ubiquinone supplementation and exercise capacity in trained young and older men. Eur J Appl Physiol 1995;72:95–100.

Lamar-Hildebrand N, Saldanha L, Endres J. Dietary and exercise practices of college-aged female body builders. J Am Diet Assoc 1989;89:1308–10.

Lawrence JD, Bower RC, Riehl WP, Smith JL. Effects of a-tocopherol acetate on the swimming endurance of trained swimmers. Am J Clin Nutr 1975a;28:205–8.

Lawrence JD, Smith JL, Bower RC, Riehl WP. The effect of alpha-tocopherol (vitamin E) and pyridoxine HCI (vitamin B6) on the swimming endurance of trained swimmers. J Am Coll Health Assoc 1975b;23:219–22.

LeBlanc J, Jobin M, Côté J, Samson P, Labrie A. Enhanced metabolic response to caffeine in exercise-trained human subjects. J Appl Physiol 1985;59:832–7.

Leenders N, Sherman WM, Lamb DR, Nelson TE. Creatine supplementation and swimming performance. Int J Sport Nutr 1999;9:251–62.

Lefavi RG. Response to Evans—Chromium picolinate. Int J Sport Nutr 1993;3:120–2.

Lefavi RG, Richard AA, Keith RE, Wilson GD, McMillan JL, Stone MH. Efficacy of chromium supplementation in athletes: emphasis on anabolism. Int J Sport Nutr 1992;2:111–22.

Lemon PWR, Effects of carbohydrate feedings on plasma free tryptophan and branched-chain amino acids during prolonged cycling. Int J Sport Nutr 1991;1:127–45.

Linderman J, Fahey TD. Sodium bicarbonate ingestion and exercise performance. Sports Med 1991;11:71–7.

Loosli AR, Benson DM, Gillien DM, Bourdet K. Nutrition habits and knowledge in competitive adolescent female gymnasts. Phys Sportsmed 1986;14:118–30.

Lukaski HC, Bolonchik WW, Siders WA, Milne DB. Chromium supplementation and resistance training: effects on body composition, strength, and trace element status of men. Am J Clin Nutr 1996;63:954–65.

Lyons TP, Riedesel ML, Meuli LE, Chick TW. Effects of glycerol-induced hyperhydration prior to exercise in the heat on sweating and core temperature. Med Sci Sports Exerc 1990;22:477–83.

MacIntosh BR, Wright BM. Caffeine ingestion and performance of a 1500 metre swim. Can J Appl Physiol 1995;20(2):168–77.

MacKinnon LT, Hooper S. Plasma glutamine and upper respiratory tract infection during intensified training in swimmers. Med Sci Sports Exerc 1996;28:285–90.

McNaughton LR. Bicarbonate and citrate. In: Maughan RJ, ed. IOC Encyclopedia of Sports Nutrition. London: Blackwell, 2000:393–404.

McNaughton L, Cedaro R. The effect of sodium bicarbonate on rowing ergometer performance in elite rowers. Aust J Sci Med Sport 1991;23:66–9.

McNaughton L, Dalton B, Palmer G. Sodium bicarbonate can be used as an ergogenic aid in high intensity, competitive cycling ergometry of 1 hour duration. Eur J Appl Physiol 1999;80:64–9.

McNaughton LR, Dalton B, Tarr J. The effects of creatine supplementation on high-intensity exercise performance in elite performers. Eur J Appl Physiol 1998;78:236–40.

McNaughton LR, Dalton B, Tarr J. Inosine has no effect on aerobic or anaerobic cycling performance. Int J Sport Nutr 1999;9:333–44.

McNaughton L, Egan G, Caelli G. A comparison of Chinese and Russian ginseng as ergogenic aids to improve various facets of physical fitness. Int Clin Nutr Rev 1989;9:32–5.

Madsen K, MacLean DA, Kiens B, Christensen D. Effects of glucose, glucose plus branched-chain amino acids, or placebo on bike performance over 100 km. J Appl Physiol 1996;81:2644–50.

Maganaris CN, Maughan RJ. Creatine supplementation enhances maximum voluntary isometric force and endurance capacity in resistance trained men. Acta Physiol Scand 1998;163:279–87.

Mahesh VB, Greenblatt RB. The in vivo conversion of dehydroepiandosterone and androstenedione to testosterone in the human. Acta Endocrinol 1962;41:400–6.

Malm C, Svensson M, Ekblom B, Sjodin B. Effects of ubiquinone-10 supplementation and high intensity training on physical performance in humans. Acta Physiol Scan 1997;161:379–84.

Malm C, Svensson M, Sjoberg B, Ekblom B. Supplementation with ubiquinone-10 causes cellular damage during intense exercise. Acta Physiol Scand 1996;157:511–2.

Marconi C, Sassi G, Carpinelli A, Cerretelli P. Effects of L-carnitine loading on the aerobic and anaerobic performance of endurance athletes. Eur J Appl Physiol 1985;54:131–5.

Massad SJ, Shier NW, Koceja DM, Ellis NT. High school athletes and nutritional supplements: a study of knowledge and use. Int J Sport Nutr 1995;5:232–45.

Matson LG, Tran ZT. Effects of sodium bicarbonate ingestion on anaerobic performance: a meta-analytic review. Int J Sports Nutr 1993;3:2–28.

Maughan R, Greenhaff P. High intensity exercise performance and acid-base balance: the effect of diet and induced alkalosis. In: Brouns F, ed. Advance in nutrition and top sport. Med Sports Sci 32: Basel: Karger 1991:147–65.

Mero A, Mikkulainen H, Riski J, Pakkanen R, Aalto J, Takala T. Effects of bovine colostrum supplement on serum IGF-1, IgG, hormone and saliva IgA during training. J Appl Physiol 1997;83:1144–51.

Mittleman KD, Ricci MR, Bailey SP. Branched-chain amino acids prolong exercise during heat stress in men and women. Med Sci Sports Exerc 1999;30:83–91.

Moffatt RJ. Dietary status of elite female high school gymnasts: inadequacy of vitamin and mineral intake. J Am Diet Assoc 1984;84:1361–3.

Mohr T, Van Soeren M, Graham TE, Kjær M. Caffeine ingestion and metabolic responses of tetraplegic humans during electrical cycling. J Appl Physiol 1998;85:979–85.

Montner P, Stark DM, Riedesel ML, et al. Pre-exercise glycerol hydration improves cycling endurance time. Int J Sports Med 1996;17:27–33.

Morris AC, Jacobs I, McLellan TM, Klugerman A, Wang LCH, Zamecnik J. No ergogenic effects of ginseng ingestion. Int J Sport Nutr 1996;6:263–71.

Mujika I, Chatard J, Lacoste L, Barale F, Geyssant A. Creatine supplementation does not improve sprint performance in competitive swimmers. Med Sci Sports Exerc 1996;28:1435–41.

Murray R, Eddy DE, Paul GL, Seifert JG, Halaby GA. Physiological responses to glycerol ingestion during exercise. J Appl Physiol 1991;71:144–9.

National Research Council. Recommended Dietary Allowances. Washington, DC: National Academy Press, 1989.

Nielsen AN, Mizuno M, Ratkevicius A, et al. No effect of antioxidant supplementation in triathletes on maximal oxygen uptake, 31P-NMRS detected muscle energy metabolism and muscle fatigue. Int J Sports Med 1999;20:154–8.

Nieman DC, Gates JR, Butler JV, Pollet LM, Dietrich SJ, Lutz RD. Supplementation patterns in marathon runners. J Am Diet Assoc 1989;89:1615–19.

Nissen S, Sharp R, Ray M, et al. Effect of leucine metabolite B-hydroxy-B-methyl butyrate on muscle metabolism during resistance-exercise training. J Appl Physiol 1996;81:2095–104.

Noonan D, Berg K, Latin RW, Wagner JC, Reimers K. Effects of varying dosages of oral creatine relative to fat free body mass on strength and body composition. J Strength Cond Res 1998;12(2):104–8.

Nowak RK, Knudsen KS, Schultz LO. Body composition and nutrient intakes of college men and women basketball players. J Am Diet Assoc 1988;88:575–8.

Odland LM, MacDougall JD, Tarnopolsky MA, Elorriaga A, Borgmann A. Effect of oral creatine supplementation on muscle [PCr] and short-term maximum power output. Med Sci Sports Exerc 1997;29:216–19.

Oppliger RA, Landry GL, Foster SW, Lambracht AC. Bulimic behaviours among interscholastic wrestlers: a statewide survey. Pediatrics 1993;91:826–31.

Oyono-Enguelle S, Freund H, Ott C, et al. Prolonged submaximal exercise and L-carnitine in humans. Eur J Appl Physiol 1988;58:53–61.

Packer L. Oxidants, antioxidant nutrients and the athlete. J Sports Sci 1997;15:353–63.

Parasrampuria J, Schwartz K, Petesch R. Quality control of dehydroepiandrosterone dietary supplement products. JAMA 1998;280:1565.

Parr RB, Bachman LA, Moss RA. Iron deficiency in female athletes. Phys Sportsmed 1984;12:81–6.

Pasman WJ, van Baak MA, Jeukendrup AE, de Haan A. The effect of different dosages of caffeine on endurance performance time. Int J Sports Med 1995;16:225–30.

Perharic L, Shaw D, Collbridge M, House I, Leon C, Murray V. Toxicological problems resulting from exposure to traditional remedies and food supplements. Drug Safety 1994;11:284–94.

Peters AJ, Dressendorfer RH, Rimar J, Keen CL. Diets of endurance runners competing in a 20-day road race. Phys Sportsmed 1986;14:63–70.

Peyrebrune MC, Nevill ME, Donaldson FJ, Cosford DJ. The effects of oral creatine supplementation on performance in single and repeated sprint swimming. J Sports Sci 1998;16:271–9.

Philen RM, Ortiz DI, Auerbach SB, Falk H. Survey of advertising for nutritional supplements in health and body building magazines. JAMA 1992;268:1008–11.

Pieralisi G, Ripari P, Vecchiet L. Effects of standardised ginseng extract combined with dimethylaminoethanol bitartrate, vitamins, minerals and trace elements on physical performance during exercise. Clin Therapeut 1991;12:373–82.

Poortmans JR, Francaux M. Long-term oral creatine supplementation does not impair renal function in healthy athletes. Med Sci Sports Exerc 1999;31:1108–10.

Potteiger JA, Nickel GL, Webster MJ, Haub MD, Palmer RJ. Sodium citrate ingestion enhances 30km cycling performance. Int J Sports Med 1996;17:7–11.

Powers SK, Byrd RJ, Tully R, Callender T. Effects of caffeine ingestion on metabolism and performance during graded exercise. Eur J Appl Physiol 1983;50:301–7.

Prevost MC, Nelson AG, Morris GS. Creatine supplementation enhances intermittent work performance. Res Q Exerc Sport 1997;68:233–40.

Rasmussin BB, Volpi E, Gore DC, Wolfe RR. Androstenedione does not stimulate muscle protein anabolism in young healthy men. J Clin Endocrinol Metab 2000;85:55–9.

Redondo DR, Dowling EA, Graham BL, Almada AL, Williams MH. The effect of oral creatine monohydrate supplementation on running velocity. Int J Sport Nutr 1996;6:213–21.

Robergs RA, Griffin SE. Glycerol: biochemistry, pharmacokinetics and clinical and practical applications. Sports Med 1998;26:145–67.

Ros JJ, Pelders MG, de Smet PA. A case of positive doping associated with a botanical food supplement. Pharm World Sci 1999;21:44–6.

Rossiter HB, Cannell ER, Jakeman PM. The effect of oral creatine supplementation on the 1000 m performance of competitive rowers. J Sports Sci 1996;14:175–9.

Roufs JB. Review of L-tryptophan and eosinophilia-myalgia syndrome. J Am Diet Assoc 1992;92:844–50.

Rowbottom DG, Keast D, Goodman C, et al. The hematological, biochemical and immunological profile of athletes suffering from the over-training syndrome. Eur J Appl Physiol 1995;70:502–7.

Sahlin K. Metabolic aspects of fatigue in human skeletal muscle. In: Marconnet P, Komi PV, Saltin B, Sejersted OM, eds. Muscle fatigue mechanisms in exercise and training. Vol 34. Basel: Karger, 1992:54–68.

Sandoval WM, Heyward VH, Lyons TM. Comparison of body composition, exercise and nutritional profiles of female and male body builders at competition. J Sports Med Phys Fitness 1989;29:63–70.

Saris WHM, Van Erp-Baart MA, Brouns F, Westerterp KR, Ten Hoor F. Study on food intake and energy expenditure during extreme sustained exercise: the Tour de France. Int J Sports Med 1989;10:S26–S31.

Sasaki H, Meada J, Usui S, Ishiko T. Effect of sucrose and caffeine on performance of prolonged strenuous running. Int J Sports Med 1987;8:261–5.

Schneider DA, McDonough PJ, Fadel PJ, Berwick JP. Creatine supplementation and the total work performed during 15-s and 1-min bouts of maximal cycling. Aust J Sci Med Sport 1997;29:65–8.

Schulz LO. Factors influencing the use of nutritional supplements by college students with varying levels of physical activity. Nutr Res 1988;8:459–66.

Shaw D, Leon C, Kolev S, Murray V. Traditional remedies and food supplements: a 5-year toxicological study (1991–1995). Drug Safety 1997;17:342–56.

Short SH, Short WR. Four year study of university athletes' dietary intake. J Am Diet Assoc 1983;82:632–45.

Siliprandi N, Di Lisa F, Pieralisi G. Metabolic changes induced by maximal exercise in human subjects following L-carnitine administration. Biochimica et Biophysica Acta 1990;1034:17–21.

Singh A, Evans P, Gallagher KL, Deuster PA. Dietary intakes and biochemical profiles of nutritional status of ultramarathoners. Med Sci Sports Exerc 1993;25:28–34.

Slater, G. HMB supplementation and the promotion of muscle growth and strength. Sports Med 2000;30:105–16.

Slavin J, McNamara EA, Lutter J. Nutritional practices of women cyclists, including recreational riders and elite races. In: Katch F, ed. Sport Health and Nutrition: The 1984 Olympic Scientific Congress Proceedings. Vol 2. Champaign, Illinois: Human Kinetics, 1984.

Smith JC, Stephens DP, Hall EL, Jackson AW, Earnest CP. Effect of creatine ingestion on parameters of the work rate-time relationship and time to exhaustion in high-intensity cycling. Eur J Appl Physiol 1998;77:360–5.

Smith SA, Montain SJ, Matott RP, Zientara GP, Jolesz FA, Fielding RA. Creatine supplementation and age influence muscle metabolism during exercise. J Appl Physiol 1998;85:1349–56.

Smith SA, Montain SC, Matott RP, Zientara GP, Jolesz FA, Fielding RA. Effects of creatine supplementation on the energy cost of muscle contraction: a ^{31}P-MRS study. J Appl Physiol 1999;87:116–23.

Snider I, Bazzarre TL, Murdoch SD, Goldfarb A. Effects of coenzyme athletic performance system as an ergogenic aid on endurance performance to exhaustion. Int J Sport Nutr 1992;2:272–86.

Snow RJ, McKenna MJ, Selig SE, et al. Effect of creatine supplementation on sprint exercise performance and muscle metabolism. J Appl Physiol 1998;84:1667–73.

Snyder AC, Schulz LO, Foster C. Voluntary consumption of a carbohydrate supplement by elite speed skaters. J Am Diet Assoc 1989;89:1125–7.

Sobal J, Marquart LF. Vitamin/mineral supplement use among high school athletes. Adolescence 1994;29:835–43.

Soop M, Bjorkman O, Cederblad G, Hagenfeldt L, Wahren J. Influence of carnitine supplementation on muscle substrate and carnitine metabolism during exercise. J Appl Physiol 1998;64:2394–9.

Spriet LL. Ergogenic aids: recent advances and retreats. In: Lamb DR, Murray R, eds. Perspectives in exercise science and sports medicine. Vol 10: Optimizing Sports Performance. Carmel, Indiana: Cooper Publishing Company, 1997:185–238.

Spriet LL, MacLean DA, Dyck DJ, Hultman E, Cederblad G, Graham TE. Caffeine ingestion and muscle metabolism during prolonged exercise in humans. Am J Physiol 1992;262(Endocrinol. Metab. 25):E891–E8.

Starling RD, Trappe TA, Short KR, et al. Effect of inosine supplementation on aerobic and anaerobic cycling performance. Med Sci Sports Exerc 1996;28:1193–8.

Steel JE. A nutritional study of Australian Olympic athletes. Med J Aust 1970;2:119–23.

Stoecker BJ. Chromium. In: Ziegler EE, Filer LJ, eds. Present knowledge in nutrition, 7th edn. Washington: ILSI press, 1996:344–52.

Stone MH, Sanborn K, Smith LL, et al. Effects of in-season (5 weeks) creatine and pyruvate supplementation on anaerobic performance and body composition in American football players. Int J Sport Nutr 1999;9:146–65.

Svennson M, Malm C, Tonkonogi M, Ekblom B, Sjodin B, Sahlin K, Effect of Q10 supplementation on tissue Q10 levels and adenine nucleotide catabolism during high-intensity exercise. Int J Sport Nutr 1999;9:166–80.

Tarnopolsky MA. Caffeine and endurance performance. Sports Med 1994;18:109–25.

Tarnopolsky MA, Atkinson SA, Macdougall JD, Sale DG, Sutton JR. Physiological responses to caffeine during endurance running in habitual caffeine users. Med Sci Sports Exerc 1989;21:418–24.

Telford RD, Catchpole EA, Deakin V, Hahn AG, Plank AW. The effect of 7 to 8 months of vitamin/mineral supplementation on athletic performance. Int J Sport Nutr 1992;2:135–53.

Terrillion KA, Kolkhorst FW, Dolgener FA, Joslyn SJ. The effect of creatine supplementation on two 700-m maximal running bouts. Int J Sport Nutr 1997;7:138–43.

Theodorou AS, Cooke CB, King RFGJ, et al. The effect of longer-term creatine supplementation on elite swimming performance after an acute creatine loading. J Sports Sci 1999;17:853–9.

Thibault G, Lambert J, Rivard M, Brodeur JM, St Jacques B. Utilization of ergogenic aids and the attitude toward safety in marathon runners. In: Katch F, ed. Sport, health and nutrition: the 1984 Olympic Scientific Congress Proceedings. Vol 2. Champaign, Illinois: Human Kinetics, 1984.

Thompson CH, Kemp GJ, Sanderson AL, et al. Effect of creatine on aerobic and anaerobic metabolism in skeletal muscle in swimmers. Br J Sports Med 1996;30:222–5.

Tiryaki GR, Atterbom HA. The effects of sodium bicarbonate and sodium citrate on 600m running time of trained females. J Sports Med Phys Fitness 1995;35:194–8.

Trappe SW, Costill DL, Goodpaster MD, Fink WJ. The effects of L-carnitine supplementation on performance during interval swimming. Int J Sports Med 1994;15:181–5.

Trent LK, Thieding-Cancel D. Effects of chromium picolinate on body composition. J Sports Med Phys Fitness 1995;35:273–80.

Trice I, Haymes EM. Effects of caffeine ingestion on exercise induced changes during high intensity, intermittent exercise. Int J Sports Nut 1995;5:37–44.

Uralets VP, Gillette PA. Over-the-counter anabolic steroids 4-androsten-3,17-dione;4-androsten-3beta,17beta-diol; and 19-nor-4-androsten-3,17-dione: excretion studies in men. J Anal Toxicol 1999;23:357–66.

Urbanski RL, Loy SF, Vincent WJ, Yaspelkis III BB. Creatine supplementation differentially affects maximal isometric strength and time to fatigue in large and small muscle groups. Int J Sport Nutr 1999;9:136–45.

Vandenberghe K, Gillis N, van Leemputte M, van Hecke P, Vanstapel F, Hespel P. Caffeine counteracts the ergogenic action of muscle creatine loading. J Appl Physiol 1996;80:452–7.

Vandenberghe K, Goris M, Van Hecke P, et al. Long-term creatine intake is beneficial to muscle performance during resistance training. J Appl Physiol 1997;83:2055–63.

Vandenbuerie F, Vanden Eynde B, Vandenberghe K, Hespel P. Effect of creatine loading on endurance capacity and sprint power in cyclists. Int J Sports Med 1998;19:490–5.

Van Leemputte M, Vandenberghe K, Hespel P. Shortening of muscle relaxation time after creatine loading. J Appl Physiol 1999;86:840–4.

Van Soeren MH, Graham TE. Effect of caffeine on metabolism, exercise endurance, and catecholamine responses after withdrawal. J Appl Physiol 1998;85:1493–501.

Van Soeren MH, Sathasivam P, Spriet LL, Graham TE. Caffeine metabolism and epinephrine responses during exercise in users and nonusers. J Appl Physiol 1993;75:805–12.

Van Zyl CG, Lambert EV, Hawley JA, Noakes TD, Dennis SC. Effects of medium-chain triglyceride ingestion on fuel metabolism and cycling performance. J Appl Physiol 1996;80:2217–25.

Vecchiet L, Di Lisa F, Pieralisi G. Influence of L-carnitine administration on maximal physical exercise. Eur J Appl Physiol 1990;61:486–90.

Volek JS, Kraemer WJ, Bush JA, et al. Creatine supplementation enhances muscular performance during high-intensity resistance exercise. J Am Diet Assoc 1997;97:765–70.

Volek JS, Duncan ND, Mazzetti SA, et al. Performance and muscle fiber adaptations to creatine supplementation and heavy resistance training. Med Sci Sports Exerc 1999;31:1147–56.

Vukovich MD, Costill DL, Fink WJ. Carnitine supplementation: effect on muscle carnitine and glycogen content during exercise. Med Sci Sports Exerc 1994;26:1122–9.

Wagenmakers AJM. L-carnitine supplementation and performance in man. In: Brouns F, ed. Advances in nutrition and top sport: medicine and sport science. Basel: Karger, 1991:110–27.

Walker LS, Bemben MG, Bemben DA, Knehans AW. Chromium picolinate effects on body composition and muscular performance in wrestlers. Med Sci Sports Exerc 1998;30:1730–7.

Wallace MB, Lim J, Cutler A, Bucci L. Effects of dehydroepiandrosterone vs androstenedione supplementation in men. Med Sci Sports Exerc 1999;31:1788–92.

Walsh NP, Blannin AK, Robson PJ, et al. Glutamine, exercise and immune function: links and possible mechanisms. Sports Med 1998;26:177–91.

Wemple RD, Lamb DR, McKeever KH. Caffeine vs caffeine-free sports drinks: effects on urine production at rest and during prolonged exercise. Int J Sports Med 1997;18:40–6.

Werblow JA, Fox HM, Henneman A. Nutritional knowledge, attitudes, and food patterns of women athletes. J Am Diet Assoc 1978;73:242–5.

Weston SB, Zhou S, Weatherby RP, Robson J. Does exogenous coenzyme Q10 affect aerobic capacity in endurance athletes? Int J Sport Nutr 1997;7:197–206.

Wiles JD, Bird SR, Hopkins J, Riley M. Effect of caffeinated coffee on running speed, respiratory factors, blood lactate and perceived exertion during 1500-m treadmill running. Br J Sports Med 1992;26(2):116–20.

Wilkes D, Gledhill N, Smyth R. Effect of acute induced metabolic acidosis on 800 m racing time. Med Sci Sports Exerc 1983;15:277–80.

Williams MH, Kreider R, Branch JD. Creatine. Champaign, Illinois: Human Kinetics, 1998:10.

Williams MH, Kreider R, Hunter DW, et al. Effect of inosine supplementation on 3-mile treadmill run performance and VO_2 peak. Med Sci Sport Exerc 1990;22:517–22.

Williams JH, Signorile JF, Barnes WS, Henrich TW. Caffeine, maximal power output and fatigue. Brit J Sports Med 1988;22(4):132–4.

Wolf E, Wirth J, Lohman T. Nutritional practices of coaches in the Big Ten. Phys Sportsmed 1979;7(2):113–24.

Worme JD, Doubt TJ, Singh A, Ryan CJ, Moses FM, Deuster PA. Dietary patterns, gastrointestinal complaints, and nutritional knowledge of recreational triathletes. Am J Clin Nutr 1990;51:690–7.

Yaspelkis BB, Ivy JL. The effect of a carbohydrate-arginine supplement on postexercise carbohydrate metabolism. Int J Sport Nutr 1999;9:241–50.

Yesalsis CE. Medical, legal, and societal implications of androstenedione. JAMA 1999;281:2043–4.

Ylikoski T, Piirainen J, Hanninen O, Penttinen J. The effect of coenzyme Q10 on the exercise performance of cross-country skiers. Molec Aspects Med 1997;18:S283–S90.

Ziemba AW, Chmura J, Kaciuba-Uscilko H, Nazar K, Wisnik P, Gawronski W. Ginseng treatment improves psychomotor performance at rest and during graded exercise. Int J Sport Nutr 1999;9:371–7.

APPENDIX: **Summary of the research literature on common sports supplements**

Table 17.5 *Studies of acute creatine loading on performance (< 10 d)*

Study	Event	Subjects	Creatine dose	Enhanced performance	Comments
Smith et al. 1998	Cycling 4 maximal bouts on ergometer	15 untrained M & F	20 g/d for 5 d	Yes	Improved time to exhaustion at shorter, higher-intensity exercise bouts
Vandebuerie et al. 1998	Cycling Progressive cycle to exhaustion (~2 h 30 min) + 5 × 10 sec maximal sprints	12 well trained amateur cyclists M	25 g/d for 4 d with or without 5 g at 0, 60 and 120 min of exercise	Yes	Improved power output for the 5 × 10 sec maximal sprints Creatine during exercise counteracted improvements caused by creatine loading
Snow et al. 1998	Cycling 20 sec maximal sprint	8 untrained M	30 g/d for 5 d	No	No change to any measurements of power ~1 kg ↑ BM
Engelhardt et al. 1998	Cycling 60 min submaximal exercise + 15 sec maximal sprints	12 regional class triathletes	6 g/d for 5 d	Yes	Endurance performance not affected. Interval power performance increased by 18%
Cooke & Barnes 1997	Cycling 2 sprints separated by either 30, 60, 90 or 120 sec of recovery	80 M	20 g/d for 5 d	No	No effect on maximum power, ability to maintain peak power (PP) output or restoration of PP after 30, 60, 90 or 120 sec ~1 kg ↑ BM
Jacobs et al. 1997	Cycling Cycle to exhaustion at 125% VO₂ max Maximal Accumulated Oxygen Deficit (MAOD) calculated	26 M & F of varying training status	20 g/d for 5 d	Yes	Increased MAOD and time to exhaustion. Large individual variation 0.7 kg ↑ BM
Schneider et al. 1997	Cycling (A) 5 × 15 sec maximal sprints (B) 5 × 1 min cycling bouts	9 untrained M	(A) 25 g/d for 7 d (B) 25 g/d for 9 d	Yes	(A) Improved work during each 15 sec bout of maximal cycling (B) No effect on work completed
Odland et al. 1997	Cycling 30 sec Wingate test	9 active but untrained M	20 g/d for 3 d	No	No effect on any recorded exercise measures
Casey et al. 1996	Cycling 2 × 30 sec sprints with 4 min recovery	9 healthy M (chosen for good reliability) Pre- and post-trial	20 g/d for 5 d	Yes	4% increase in total work done in both bouts
Barnett et al. 1996	Cycling 7 × 10 sec sprints	17 recreationally active M	280 mg/kg for 4 d	No	No effect on multiple sprint cycle performance

(continues)

(continued)

Study	Event	Subjects	Creatine dose	Enhanced performance	Comments
Cooke et al. 1995	Cycling 2 × 15 sec maximal sprints	12 untrained M	20 g/d for 5 d	No	No effect on power output or fatigue
Balsom et al. 1995	Cycling 5 × 6 sec sprints + 1 × 10 sec sprint Counter-movement jump + squat jump	7 untrained M	20 g/d for 6 d	Yes	No difference in jump performance Subjects better able to maintain power output during 10 sec exercise period
Dawson et al. 1995	Cycling (A) 1 × 10 sec sprints (B) 6 × 6 sec sprints	(A) 18 active M (B) 22 active M	20 g/d for 5 d	Yes	(A) No effect on 1 × 10 sec sprint performance (B) Improved total work, work completed in sprint 1 and peak power
Febbraio et al. 1995	Cycling 4 × 1 min cycling bouts at 115–125% VO_2 max + fifth bout to fatigue	6 active but untrained M	20 g/d for 5 d Crossover design	No	No difference in exercise duration in the fifth work bout
Birch et al. 1994	Cycling 3 × 30 sec sprints	14 untrained M	20 g/d for 5 d	Yes	Work output increased during exercise bouts 1 and 2 but not 3
Theodorou et al. 1999	Swimming Interval set (5–10 repeats on 1 or 2 min, according to the event/distance of swimmer)	22 elite swimmers (M & F) Pre- and post-test in all swimmers (order effect)	25 g/d for 4 d	Yes	Improvement of 1.5% in mean swim time in interval set. ↑ BM. Order effect dismissed by failure to improve further with longer-term study
Peyrebrune et al. 1998	Swimming 1 × 50 yd maximal swim 8 × 50 yd maximal swims	14 elite M swimmers	9 g/d for 5 d	Yes	Reduced total sprint time for 8 × 50 yd swims. Percentage decline in performance times reduced
Grindstaff et al. 1997	Swimming 3 × 100 m freestyle sprints + 3 × 20 sec arm ergometer maximal sprints	18 M & F junior competitive swimmers	21 g/d for 9 d	Yes	Improved swim time in heats 1 and 2
Mujika et al. 1996	Swimming 25 m, 50 m, 100 m swim	20 national and international level swimmers (M & F)	20 g/d for 5 d	No	No significant performance changes Significant ↑ BM
Burke et al. 1996	Swimming 25 m, 50 m, 100 m swim, 10 sec maximal leg ergometry test	32 national and international swimmers (M & F)	20 g/d for 5 d	No	No significant differences between group means for sprint swim times or 10 sec leg ergometry performance

Study	Event	Subjects	Creatine dose	Enhanced performance	Comments
Rossiter et al. 1996	Rowing 1000 m rowing ergometer time trial	38 competitive, club standard rowers (M & F)	0.25 g/kg for 5 d	No	Improved 100 m rowing performance by ~1% (P = 0.088)
Terrillion et al. 1997	Running 2 × maximal 700 m run on outdoor track	12 well-trained, competitive M runners	20 g/d for 5 d	No	No significant difference between placebo or supplemented groups
Redondo et al. 1996	Running 3 × 60 m sprints	18 trained team-sport athletes and sprinters (M & F)	25 g/d for 7 d	No	No significant difference
Balsom et al. 1993	Running Treadmill run at ~120% VO$_2$ max to exhaustion 6 km terrain run	14 habitually active to well-trained M	20 g/d for 6 d	No	No effect on treadmill run performance. Impaired terrain run due to ↑ BM
Harris et al. 1993	Running 4 × 300 m with 4 min rest plus 4 × 1000 with 3 min rest	10 trained M middle-distance runners	30 g/d for 6 d	Yes	Reduction in running time in the final 300 and 1000 m runs
Bosco et al. 1997	Jumping and Running 5 sec and 45 sec continuous jumping exercises Treadmill running at 20 km/hr to exhaustion	8 sprinters + 6 jumpers M	20 g/d for 5 d	Yes	Improved jumping performance in the first and second 15 sec period of the jumping test Improved intensive running time to exhaustion
McNaughton et al. 1998	Kayaking 90 sec, 150 sec, 300 sec kayak ergometer tests	16 elite surf-ski/ white-water kayak paddlers (M)	20 g/d for 5 d	Yes	Subjects completed significantly more work in all tests. ↑ BM
Volek et al. 1997	Resistance exercise Bench presses + jump squat to exhaustion	14 active M	25 g for 6 d	Yes	Significant increase in reps to exhaustion and peak power for squats ↑ BM
Van Leemputte et al. 1999	12 maximal isometric elbow flexions on isokinetic dynamometer	16 untrained M	20 g/d for 5 d	Yes	Relaxation time reduced following creatine
Urbanski et al. 1999	Maximal and submaximal isometric knee extension and handgrip exercise	10 active but untrained M	20 g/d for 5 d	Yes	Increased maximal knee-extension torque and time to fatigue during submaximal knee extension and submaximal handgrip. No significant ↑ BM

(continues)

(continued)

Study	Event	Subjects	Creatine dose	Enhanced performance	Comments
Smith et al. 1999	Single leg knee extension exercise to exhaustion	9 active but untrained M & F	0.3 g/kg per d for 5 d	No	Muscle ATP cost of contraction not affected
Manganaris & Maughan 1998	Maximal knee extension + knee extension to exhaustion	10 weight-trained males	10 g/d for 5 d	Yes	Maximal voluntary contraction and endurance capacity increased ↑ BM
Smith et al. 1998	Single leg knee extension exercise to exhaustion	$4 \times > 50$yr $+ 5 \times < 40$yr M & F	0.3 g/kg for 5 d	Yes	Time to exhaustion increased in both groups combined
Vandenberghe et al. 1996	Single leg knee extension exercise	9 active but untrained M	0.5 g/kg/d for 6 d	Yes	Dynamic torque production increased. No ↑ BM
Greenhaff et al. 1993	Maximal knee extension exercise	12 M	20 g/d for 5 d	Yes	Increased muscle peak torque production

M = male, F = female

Table 17.6 Studies of chronic creatine supplementation on performance in athletes (> 10 d)

Study	Event	Subjects	Creatine dose	Enhanced performance	Comments
Theodorou et al. 1999	Swimming Interval session according to usual stroke/event	22 elite swimmers (M & F)	5 g/d for 8 w (following loading dose)	No	No difference between groups or across time in mean interval swim times
Leenders et al. 1999	Swimming 6 × 50 m swims 10 × 25 yd swims	32 college swimmers (M & F)	20 g/d for 6 d + 10 g/d for 8 d	Yes (M only)	Mean overall swimming velocity improved in the 6 × 50 m intervals for M. (P = 0.02) Body composition not changed
Thompson et al. 1996	Swimming Resistance calf exercise to fatigue + 100 m and 400 m swim	10 university swimmers (F)	2 g/d for 6 w	No	No effect on calf-exercise duration or swim time No ↑ in LBM
Prevost et al. 1997	Cycling 4 × protocols on different days @ 150% peak work-load to exhaustion A = continuous, B = 30 sec: 60 sec recovery, C = 20 sec: 40 sec, D = 10 sec: 20 sec	18 active M & F	19 g/d for 5 d + 2 g for 6 d	Yes	Increase in time to exhaustion and work output in all protocols, with protocol D showing greatest increase and protocol A showing smallest improvement
Earnest et al. 1997	Running 2 × treadmill runs to exhaustion (~90 sec)	11 interval- and strength-trained M	20 g/d for 4 d + 10 g/d for 6 d	Yes	Mean time to exhaustion improved Running times improved more during second run trial than first No ↑ in BM
Stone et al. 1999	Resistance exercise 1-RM parallel squat and bench press + counter-movement vertical jump and static vertical jump + 15 × 5 sec cycle ergometer sprints	42 collegiate American football players (M)	0.22 g/kg for 7 w	Yes	Increased squat and bench press, static vertical jump power output ↑ BM and LBM

(continues)

(continued)

Study	Event	Subjects	Creatine dose	Enhanced performance	Comments
Volek et al. 1999	Resistance exercise 1-RM bench press + squat strength, power production during jump squat, muscular endurance during bench press	19 resistance-trained M	25 g/d for 1 w + 5 g/d for 11 w	Yes	Improved bench press and squat. Greater increases in Type I, IIA and IIAB muscle fibre cross-sectional areas ↑ BM and FFM.
Kelly & Jenkins 1998	Resistance exercise 3-RM bench press, 85% of 1-RM bench press	18 M power lifters	20 g/d for 5 d + 5 g/d for 21 d	Yes	Improved 3-RM strength ↑ BM and LBM
Kreider et al. 1998	Resistance exercise Progressive resistance training + 12 x 6 sec maximal cycle ergometer sprints	25 NCAA division 1A American football players (M)	15.75 g/d for 4 w	Yes	Increased work during sprints 1–5. Increased bench press lifting volume and total lifting volume Total ↑ BM = 2.4 ±1.4 kg
Noonan et al. 1998	Resistance exercise 1-RM bench press, 40 yd dash time, vertical jump height	30 M college athletes	20 g/d for 5 d + 100 mg/kg FFM or 300 mg/kg FFM for 51 d	Yes	Improved bench press Improvement greatest in 300 mg/kg FFM group Improved 40 yd dash time in 100 mg/kg FFM group No significant differences in body composition
Vandenberghe et al. 1997	Resistance exercise Resistance training + intermittent right arm exercise test on isokinetic dynamometer	19 sedentary F	20 g/d for 4 d + 5 g/d for 10 w	Yes	No change in arm-flexion torque or body composition after high dose creatine. Improved leg press, leg extension, squat performance, and arm-flexion torque with long term creatine ↑ FFM
Earnest et al. 1995	Resistance exercise 3 x 30 sec Wingate cycle tests + 1-RM bench press + 70% x 1-RM bench press to fatigue	8 weight-trained M	28 d (dosage n.a.)	Yes	Improved anaerobic work for Wingate tests and bench press performance ↑ BM

M = male, F = female   n.a. not available

Table 17.7 Studies of caffeine intake and endurance performance (> 60mins)

Reference	Event	Subjects	Caffeine dose	Performance benefits	Summary
			Caffeine taken 1 h pre-exercise		
Van Soeren & Graham 1998	Cycling 80–85% $VO_{2\,max}$ to exhaustion	6 M (habitual caffeine users)	6 mg/kg (after 0, 2 & 4 days' withdrawal)	Yes	Increased time to exhaustion in all caffeine trials regardless of period of withdrawal
Trice & Haymes 1995	Cycling Bouts of 30 min alternating 1 min exercise: 1 min rest to exhaustion	8 untrained M (caffeine naive)	5 mg/kg (taken in decaf coffee)	Yes	Time to exhaustion increased 29% with caffeine. Increased FFA and trend for decreasing RPE with caffeine
Spriet et al. 1992	Cycling 80% $VO_{2\,max}$ to exhaustion	8 recreational cyclists (M & F)	9 mg/kg	Yes	Increased time to exhaustion. Glycogen sparing by 55% in the first 15 min of exercise
Costill et al. 1978	Cycling 80% $VO_{2\,max}$ to exhaustion	9 recreational cyclists (M & F)	330 mg (in decaf coffee) (= 4.4 mg/kg for M, 5.8 mg/kg for F)	Yes	Increased time to exhaustion. Evidence of increased lipolysis. Reduced RPE
Cohen et al. 1996	Running Half-marathon in hot conditions	7 trained runners (M & F)	5 and 9 mg/kg	No	No effects on RPE or performance at either dose
French et al. 1991	Running 75%$VO_{2\,max}$ for 45 min then + incremental to exhaustion	6 M recreational runners	10 mg/kg (immediately before exercise)	Yes	Caffeine increased total distance run. Elevated glucose and lactate values only seen at exhaustion. No RER data collected
Berglund & Hemmingsson 1982	Cross country skiing Field study 23 km (high altitude) & 20 km (low altitude) races	High: 13 well-trained skiers (M & F) Low: 14 well-trained skiers (M & F)	6 mg/kg	High: Yes Low: No	Trend to improved performance in low-altitude study. No metabolic data collected. Difficult to standardise environmental conditions

(continues)

(continued)

Reference	Event	Subjects	Caffeine dose Caffeine taken 1 h pre-exercise and during event	Performance benefits	Summary
Wemple et al. 1997	Cycling 3 h (60% $VO_{2\,max}$) + time trial	6 active subjects (M & F)	1 h before + every 20 min until 160 min of ride. Total caffeine = 8.7 mg/kg	No	CHO intake during exercise. No difference in performance, RPE or urine losses with caffeine
Ivy et al. 1979	Cycling 2 h isokinetic cycling @ 80 rpm	9 active cyclists (M & F)	Total caffeine = 500 mg. 250 mg at 1 h then 7 x doses during exercise	Yes	Increase in total work. Increased mobilisation and utilisation of fat. RPE same despite increased work
Falk et al. 1989	Marching 8 h at 45–50% $VO_{2\,max}$. Followed by 90% $VO_{2\,max}$ cycle to fatigue	23 untrained M (caffeine naive) Experimental-placebo design	Total caffeine = 10 mg/kg (5 mg/kg prior, then 2.5 mg/kg at 3 & 5 h)	No	No elevation in FFA with caffeine. RPE differences between groups were marginal (P = 0.05)
Ferrauti et al. 1997	Tennis (240 min of competition singles followed by hitting accuracy & tennis sprint test)	16 division II tennis players (M & F)	Total caffeine = 364 mg (M) & 260 mg (F) ~4–4.5 mg/kg	Yes (F only)	Caffeine suggested to improve metabolic transition from rest to play, but is unlikely to induce metabolic effects during event

M = male, F = female

Table 17.8 *Effects of caffeine supplementation on non-endurance performance (60 min or less)*

Reference	Event	Subjects	Dose	Performance benefits	Summary
			30–60 min event **Caffeine taken 1 h pre-event**		
Denadai & Denadai 1998	Cycling Cycling to exhaustion @ 10% below anaerobic threshold	8 healthy M	5 mg/kg	Yes	Increased time to exhaustion (46 vs 32 min) and reduced RPE
Cole et al. 1996	Cycling 30 min: 3 x 10 min @ RPE of 9, 12 & 15	10 healthy M	6 mg/kg	Yes	Average of 12.6% increase in work produced for same perception of effort No differences seen in RER despite higher intensity
Pasman et al. 1995	Cycling 80%W_{max} to exhaustion	9 well trained cyclists	0, 5, 9 & 13 mg/kg	Yes	Time to exhaustion was 27% longer in caffeine trials No greater gains with increasing caffeine doses Large individual variation in urinary caffeine response
Graham et al. 1998	Running 85% $VO_{2\,max}$ to exhaustion	9 well trained M	4.5 mg/kg Caffeine, decaf coffee and coffee	Yes	Increase in time to exhaustion with caffeine Other components of coffee antagonise the responses of caffeine
Graham & Spriet 1995	Running 85% $VO_{2\,max}$ to exhaustion	8 trained M runners	3, 6, 9 mg/kg	Yes (3 & 6 mg/kg only)	Highest dose of caffeine had the greatest effect on epinephrine and metabolites, yet had the least effect on performance
Graham & Spriet 1991	Running ~85% $VO_{2\,max}$ to exhaustion Cycling ~85% $VO_{2\,max}$ to exhaustion	7 well trained M runners	9 mg/kg	Yes (both running and cycling)	3 of 13 caffeine trials above IOC limit No metabolic explanation for performance improvement Non-responder noted

(continues)

(continued)

Reference	Event	Subjects	Dose	Performance benefits	Summary
			30–60 min event Caffeine intake before and during event		
Kovacs et al. 1998	Cycling ~60 min time trial	14 well trained M	Total caffeine = 2.1, 3.2 & 4.5 mg/kg (equal doses at 75 min pre-exercise and at 20 and 40 min during time trial)	Yes (3.2 & 4.5 mg/kg < 2.1 mg/kg < Placebo)	Addition of caffeine to CHO/electrolyte drinks improved 60 min time trial performance Performance threshold at 3.2 mg/kg Dose well within legal limits
Saski et al. 1987	Running 80% $VO_{2\,max}$ for 45 min rest—then to fatigue	5 well trained males	Total caf. = 420 mg (mean ~7.25 mg/kg)	Yes	Caffeine + sucrose not significantly different from caffeine or sucrose alone, despite changes in substrate metabolism
			~20 min events		
Denadai & Denadai 1998	Cycling Cycling to exhaustion @ 10% above anaerobic threshold	8 healthy M	5 mg/kg	No	No difference in time to exhaustion (18.5 vs 19.2 min) or RPE
Mohr et al. 1998	Cycling Electronic stimulation of limbs	7 Tetraplegic (C_{5-7}) & 2 Paraplegic (T_4) males	6 mg/kg	Yes	Time to exhaustion 6% longer in caffeine trials Supports caffeine having a direct ergogenic effect on skeletal muscle
Bell et al. 1998	Cycling 85% VO_2 peak to fatigue	8 untrained M	5 mg/kg (90 min prior)	No	Caffeine elevated epinephrine, FFA, glycerol and glucose yet had no effect on performance
Fulco et al. 1994	Cycling 80% $VO_{2\,max}$ at sea level and altitude	8 untrained M	4 mg/kg	Yes	Caffeine increased time to exhaustion during acute altitude exposure only Influence of caffeine seemed to decrease with exposure to altitude

Reference	Event	Subjects	Dose	Performance benefits	Summary
Dodd et al. 1991	Cycling Incremental test to exhaustion	17 untrained M (8 caffeine naive & 9 habitual users)	3 & 5 mg/kg	No	Time to exhaustion unaffected by caffeine dose or intake history Caffeine-naive subjects showed heightened resting V_E, VO_2, HR & exercising FFA
Flinn et al. 1990	Cycling Incremental test to exhaustion	9 untrained M	10 mg/kg (3 h prior)	Yes	Increase in time to exhaustion & work completed Suggested taking caffeine 3 h prior to exercise to allow plasma FFA to peak
Bond et al. 1987	Cycling Incremental test to exhaustion	6 healthy M	5 mg/kg	No	Time to exhaustion unaffected by caffeine Caffeine failed to alter any respiratory or blood parameter other than slightly increasing blood glucose
Gaesser & Rich 1985	Cycling Incremental test to exhaustion	8 healthy M	5 mg/kg	No	Max values for work, VO_2, V_E, HR, RER and lactate along with lactate threshold were unaffected by caffeine
Powers et al. 1983	Cycling Incremental test to exhaustion	7 M recreational cyclists (2 w caffeine withdrawal)	5 mg/kg	No	Values for TTF, VO_2, HR, RER, FFA & lactate were all unaffected by caffeine. Plasma glycerol levels increased
MacIntosh & Wright 1995	Swimming 1500 m freestyle	11 well-trained M & F swimmers	6 mg/kg	Yes	23 sec improvement in swimming times Caffeine affected substrate and electrolyte balance
		~5 min events Caffeine 1 h pre-exercise			
Jackman et al. 1996	Cycling 100% $VO_{2\,max}$: 2 × 2 min, then to exhaustion	14 untrained (M & F) subjects	6 mg/kg	Yes	Increase in time to exhaustion for 10 subjects No glycogen sparing

(continues)

(continued)

Reference	Event	Subjects	Dose	Performance benefits	Summary
Doherty et al. 1998	Running Time to exhaustion (3–4 min) MAOD	9 trained M	5 mg/kg	Yes	10–14% improvement in time to exhaustion Increased MAOD Mechanism unclear
Wiles et al. 1992	Running 1500 m time trial	18 trained M	3 g caffeinated coffee (~150–200 mg caffeine)	Yes	Av 4.2 sec faster over 1500 m
	1100 m constant speed + 1 min max: 'final burst' at self-selected pace	10 well trained athletes	As above	Yes	Caffeine improved speed of final 1 min 'burst', reduced RER and increased VO_2
	1500 m @ 0.5 km/h below max 1500 m pace	6 well trained M athletes	As above	Not measured	Caffeine increased VO_2 However RER, lactate and RPE unaffected by caffeine
Sprint events					
Greer et al. 1998	Cycling 4 x 30 sec Wingate tests	9 untrained M	6 mg/kg	No	No effects on peak power, average power or rate of power loss Hence no indication for use of caf in sports requiring repeated supramaximal bouts of activity
Anselme et al. 1992	Cycling Repeated 6 sec sprints: force/velocity exercise test	14 untrained M & F subjects	250 mg (30 min prior to exercise av.~ 4 mg/kg)	Yes	Caffeine increased pedalling frequency and hence W_{max}. caffeine elevated lactate and lactate/W
Collomp et al. 1991	Cycling 1 x 30 sec Wingate test	6 untrained M & F subjects	5 mg/kg	No	No support for untrained individuals to take caffeine to enhance supramaximal exercise performance
Williams et al. 1988	Cycling 1 x 15 sec maximum power test	9 M (caffeine naive)	7 mg/kg	No	Caffeine failed to increase max power output or alter rate or magnitude of fatigue
Collomp et al. 1992	Swimming 2 x 100 m sprints	14 trained (M & F) and 7 recreational (M & F) swimmers	250 mg (~4 mg/kg)	Yes (in trained subjects)	Suggested that specific training is required for caffeine to produce improvements in anaerobic capacity

M = male, F = female

Table 17.9   *Studies of bicarbonate or citrate loading on sports specific performance: crossover designed studies*

Reference	Event	Subjects	Dose	Enhanced performance	Summary
McNaughton et al. 1999	Cycling 60 min time trial	10 well trained M cyclists	300 mg/kg sodium bicarbonate	Yes	14% more work completed with bicarbonate
Potteiger et al. 1996	Cycling 30 km time trial	8 M	500 mg/kg sodium citrate	Yes	Reduction in time trial time (57 min 36 sec vs 59 min 22 sec Sodium citrate raised pH values from 10 km onwards and improved power output in the initial 25 min
Tiryaki et al. 1995	Running 600 m	11 collegiate F runners + 4 untrained controls	300 mg/kg sodium citrate or sodium bicarbonate	No	No performance effect despite significant changes to acid/base status
Goldfinch et al. 1988	Running 400 m	6 trained M	400 mg/kg sodium bicarbonate	Yes	Improved running time [56.94 sec vs 58.63 sec (placebo) and 58.46 sec (control)] Elevated post-exercise values for pH and base excess
Wilkes et al. 1983	Running 800 m	6 varsity track M athletes	300 mg/kg sodium bicarbonate	Yes	Improved running time [2 min 2.9 sec vs 2 min 5.1 sec (placebo) and 2 min 5.8 sec (control)] Elevated post-exercise values for pH, lactate and blood bicarbonate
Kindermann et al. 1977	Running 400 m	10 healthy M	200 mg/kg infusion of bicarbonate	No	Questions the importance of pH as a limiting factor in performance of high intensity exercise
Gao et al. 1988	Swimming 5 × 100 yd swim: 2 min rest	10 US collegiate swimmers	250 mg/kg sodium bicarbonate	Yes	Faster times in 4th and 5th swim
McNaughton & Cedaro 1991	Rowing 6 min maximal effort on ergometer	5 elite M rowers	300 mg/kg sodium bicarbonate	Yes	Increased work and distance rowed (1861 m vs 1813 m) Increased lactate levels

M = male, F = female

Table 17.10 *Table of studies of BCAA supplementation and performance*

Study	Event	Subjects	BCAA dose	Enhanced performance	Comments
Mittleman et al. 1998	Cycling in the heat (34°C) Time to exhaustion at 40% $VO_{2\ max}$	13 moderately trained M & F Crossover design	9.4 g F or 15.8 g M	Yes	Increased time to exhaustion (153 vs 137 min) with BCAA trial Increase in plasma BCAA and decrease in plasma tryptophan: BCAA Trend to higher plasma ammonia No difference between sexes
Blomstrand et al. 1997	Cycling 60 min @ 70% $VO_{2\ max}$ + 20 min time trial Stroop Colour Word Test given after ride	7 trained M cyclists Crossover design	90 mg/kg (~6.5 g)	No	No differences in work done in time trial, however, RPE lower during BCAA trial during steady-state phase Index of cognitive function (Stroop Colour Word Test) improved after exercise on BCAA trial
Madsen et al. 1996	Cycling 100 km time trial	9 well trained M cyclists Crossover design	3.5 L @ 5% glucose or 5% glucose + 18 g BCAA	No	No performance differences between trials Plasma BCAA and ammonia levels higher with BCAA trial
Davis et al. 1999	Running Intermittent shuttle run to exhaustion	8 active M & F Crossover design	CHO + 7 g BCAA or CHO or placebo consumed before/during/after trial	No	CHO or CHO + BCAA increased time to fatigue compared with placebo No further enhancement with addition of BCAA
Blomstrand et al. 1991	Running Marathon or 30 km cross-country race Run time, plus Stroop Colour Word Test (CWT) given after cross-country run	25 M cross-country runners, 193 M marathon runners Experimental-placebo design	16 g (marathon) or 7.5 g (cross-country)	Yes	CWT performance improved in BCAA trial after cross-country run 'Slower runners' ran faster in BCAA group Note that the methodology of dividing group into slower and faster runners according to arbitrary timepoint has been criticised on statistical grounds
Blomstrand et al. 1991	Soccer Soccer match: Stroop Colour Word Test given after match	6 F national soccer players Crossover design	6% CHO + 7.5 g BCAA or CHO alone	Yes	Improvement in CWT test after game with CHO + BCAA

M = male, F = female

Table 17.11 Studies of glycerol hyperhydration and performance

Study	Event	Subjects	Glycerol dose	Enhanced performance	Comments
Anderson et al. 2001	Cycling 90 min @ 98% lactate threshold + 15 min time trial Hot environment (35°C)	6 well trained M cyclists Crossover design	1 g/kg with 20 mL/kg low-joule cordial (compared with low-joule cordial overload)	Yes	Glycerol allowed retention of additional 400 mL of fluid above hyperhydration with cordial alone 5% improvement in work done in 15 min time trial No change in muscle metabolism Reduced rectal temperature at 90 min with glycerol trial
Hitchins et al. 1999	Cycling 30 min @ fixed power + 30 min time trial Hot environment (32°C)	8 well trained M cyclists Crossover design	1 g/kg with 22 mL/kg dilute sports drink, 2.5 h pre-exercise (compared with sports drink overload)	Yes	Glycerol treatment expanded body water by 600 mL and increased (5%) work achieved in time trial This was achieved largely by preventing the drop in power seen at the start of placebo time trial No difference in power profile at end of time trials No difference in cardiovascular, thermoregulatory, RPE between trials despite differences in power output
Inder et al. 1998	Cycling 60 min @ 70% VO_2 max + incremental ride to exhaustion	8 highly trained M triathletes Crossover design	1 g/kg with 500 mL water, 4 h pre-exercise (compared with 500 mL water)	No	Glycerol was consumed with a modest fluid load No increase in pre-exercise hydration status, sweat losses or urine production during exercise No difference in time to exhaustion or workload reached 3 subjects experienced GI problems with glycerol
Montner et al. 1996	Cycling Cycling @ 60% W_{max} until exhaustion	11 active M & F 7 active M & F Crossover designs	1.2 g/kg with 26 mL/kg water, 1 h pre-exercise same pre-treatment + sports drink during exercise	Yes	Reduced HR and increased time to exhaustion with pre-exercise glycerol treatment by ~20%

(continues)

(continued)

Study	Event	Subjects	Glycerol dose	Enhanced performance	Comments
Murray et al. 1991	Cycling 90 min cycling @ 50% $VO_{2\,max}$	9 active M & F Crossover design	0.9 g/kg (10%) glycerol solution or 4% glycerol + sports drink consumed during exercise. Total fluid load = 12 mL/kg (compared with sports drink or water of equal volumes)	Not measured No benefits to thermo-regulation seen	No differences in hydration status, urine production, HR, sweat loss or body temperature No benefits seen to suggest superior thermoregulatory or performance outcomes
Latzka et al. 1998	Running Treadmill running at 55% $VO_{2\,max}$ until exhaustion or high rectal temperature Hot environment (35°C) without further fluid intake	8 heat-acclimatised men Crossover design	1.2 g/kg LBM + 29 mL/kg water, 1 h pre-exercise (compared with water hyperhydration or control)	Yes (better than control, but equal to water hyper-hydration)	Both hyperhydration trials increased body fluid by ~1400 mL No advantages in either trial regarding sweat losses, cardiac output or temperature control; however, time to exhaustion longer in both trials compared with control Some GI and headache symptoms with glycerol
Lyons et al. 1990	Running 90 min treadmill run @ 60% $VO_{2\,max}$	6 M & F	1 g/kg with 25 mL/kg fluid, 2.5 h pre-exercise + 0.1 g/kg/h during exercise (compared with water hyperhydration and low fluid intake)	Not measured Benefits to thermo-regulation seen	Glycerol increased fluid retention by ~500 mL over water alone Increased sweat rate and decreased rectal temperature in glycerol trial suggest thermoregulatory benefits

M = male, F = female

Table 17.12 Studies of ginseng supplementation and metabolism or performance

Study	Event	Subjects	Ginseng dose	Enhanced performance	Comments
Ziemba et al. 1999	Cycling Incremental test to exhaustion Reaction time measured at each stage	15 M soccer players Experimental-placebo design	350 mg/d for 6 w	No (but enhanced reaction time)	No change in lactate threshold or $VO_{2\,max}$ however, enhanced reaction time at submaximal workloads
Allen et al. 1998	Cycling Incremental test to exhaustion	28 healthy subjects (M & F) Experimental-placebo design	200 mg/d for 3 w	No	No enhancement of total workload, RPE and lactate at submaximal loads or $VO_{2\,max}$
Engels & Wirth 1997	Cycling Submaximal and maximal cycling test	37 healthy M Experimental-placebo design	200 mg/d or 400 mg/d for 8 w	Not measured but no metabolic changes	No change in RPE, HR or RER at submaximal or maximal workloads
Morris et al. 1996	Cycling Time to exhaustion @ 75% $VO_{2\,max}$	8 active subjects (M & F) Crossover design	8 mg/kg/d or 16 mg/kg/d for 1 w standard ginseng preparation used	No	No change in time to exhaustion or metabolic parameters No change in RPE
Dowling et al. 1996	Running 10 min treadmill test at 10 km race pace, maximal treadmill test	20 highly trained runners (M & F) Experimental-placebo design	60 drops/d (maximum recommended dose) of Russian ginseng for 6 w	No	No change in metabolic characteristics at race pace, treadmill max, RPE Low statistical power may prevent small changes from being detected
Pieralisi et al. 1991	Running Incremental treadmill test to exhaustion	49 active subjects (M) Crossover design	2 capsules/d for 6 w Ginsana 115 (ginseng + vitamins, bitartrate + minerals)	Yes	Increased $VO_{2\,max}$ and reduced O_2 consumption at submaximal workloads
McNaughton et al. 1989	Physical testing $VO_{2\,max}$, grip, pectoral and quadriceps strength	30 active subjects (M & F) Crossover design	1 g/d × 6 w of Chinese ginseng or Russian ginseng	Yes	Significantly greater increase in $VO_{2\,max}$ and pectoral and grip strength with Chinese ginseng Trends for enhancement with Russian ginseng

M = male, F = female

Table 17.13 Studies of carnitine supplementation and metabolism or performance

Study	Event	Subjects	Carnitine dose	Enhanced performance	Comments
Barnett et al. 1994	Cycling 4 min ride at 90% $VO_{2\ max}$ + 5 x 1 min rides at 115% $VO_{2\ max}$	8 untrained M Crossover design– order effect	4 g/d for 14 d	Not measured No metabolic enhance- ments	Supplementation failed to increase muscle carnitine content No change in lactate accumulation during submaximal and supramaximal performance
Vukovich et al. 1994	Cycling 60 min at 70% $VO_{2\ max}$ High-fat pre-trial diet to promote lipid availability	8 untrained M Crossover design	6 g/d for 7 and 14 d	Not measured No metabolic enhance- ments	No change in muscle carnitine content after supplementation No effect on VO_2, RER, HR or substrate utilisation Without glycogen sparing there is no mechanism to expect performance enhancements
Decombaz et al. 1993	Cycling CHO depletion regime + 20 min at 60% $VO_{2\ max}$	9 untrained M Crossover design	3 g/d for 7 d	Not measured No metabolic enhance- ments	Substrate metabolism not affected during submaximal exercise even after glycogen depletion and situation of high lipid flux
Siliprandi et al. 1990	Cycling Cycle to exhaustion	10 moderately trained M Crossover design	2 g @ 1 h before exercise (acute administration)	Yes	Increased time to exhaustion. Carnitine reduced the increase in plasma lactate and pyruvate after maximal progressive work, however, dose and timeframe for uptake into muscle seems unrealistic
Vecchiet et al. 1990	Cycling Incremental cycling to exhaustion	10 moderately trained M Crossover design	2 g @ 1 h before exercise (acute administration)	Yes	Increase in time (and work) until exhaustion Decrease in lactate production and oxygen consumption at same workload As for Siliprandi study, others have criticised the dose and timing of supplement
Gorostiaga et al. 1989	Cycling 45 min at 66% $VO_{2\ max}$ + 60 min seated recovery	10 endurance trained M & F Crossover design	2 g/d for 28 d	Not measured Metabolic enhance- ments	Reduced RER during exercise ($P < 0.05$). Non-significant trend for higher O_2 uptake, HR, blood glycerol and resting plasma FFA. Provides mechanism by which enhancement of endurance exercise might be seen

Study	Event	Subjects	Carnitine dose	Enhanced performance	Comments
Soop et al. 1988	Cycling 120 min at 50% $VO_{2\,max}$	7 moderately trained M Crossover design, with order effect	5 g/d for 5 d	Not measured No metabolic enhancements	No effect on muscle substrate utilisation during exercise or at rest
Oyono-Enguelle et al. 1988	Cycling 60 min at 50% $VO_{2\,max}$ + 120 min recovery	10 untrained males Crossover design with 2 control trials and 1 experimental trial. Order effect	2 g/d for 4 w	Not measured No metabolic enhancements	No change in in physiological parameters and blood metabolites. The increased demand for FA oxidation during exercise is adequately supported by endogenous carnitine
Greig et al. 1987	Cycling Progressive test to exhaustion	(A) 9 untrained M & F (B) 10 untrained M & F Crossover design	2 g/d for 2 w 2 g for 4 w	No	No significant physiological changes. Changes in performance were small and inconsistent
Trappe et al. 1994	Swimming 5 x 91.4 m swims	20 highly trained collegiate swimmers (M) Experimental-placebo design	4 g/d for 7 d	No	No difference in performance times between trials or between groups
Colombani et al. 1996	Running Marathon run + submaximal performance test day after marathon	7 endurance trained athletes (M) Crossover design	2 g @ 2 h before run and at 20 km mark	No	No change in exercise metabolism or marathon running time. No change in recovery and submaximal test performance on following day
Marconi et al. 1985	Running Supramaximal work (jumps) + treadmill $VO_{2\,max}$ + submaximal run	6 national class walkers Crossover design	4 g/d for 2 w	Yes	Increase in $VO_{2\,max}$ by 6%, but no effects on oxygen utilisation and RER at submaximal loads, or change in lactate accumulation with jumps. Results appear inconsistent

M = male, F = female

Table 17.14 Studies of coenzyme Q10 supplementation and performance

Study	Event	Subjects	Carnitine dose	Enhanced performance	Comments
Nielsen et al. 1999	Cycling Incremental VO$_{2\,max}$ test to exhaustion Energy status of the muscle measured by NMRS during contractions	7 well trained M triathletes	100 mg/d for 6 w (+ Vit E + Vit C)	No	No effect on maximal oxygen uptake or muscle energy metabolism
Svensson et al. 1999	Cycling 30 sec max cycle + 10 × 10 sec max cycles	17 well trained M Experimental-placebo design	110 mg/d for 20 d	Not measured No evidence of improved lipid peroxidation	Supplementation increased plasma but not muscle Q10 Q10 did not affect purine catabolism or plasma malondialdehyde (indication of lipid peroxidation) Combined with previous data from group, suggests that Q10 may reduce training adaptations*
Malm et al. 1997	Cycling Anaerobic training sessions + anaerobic + submaximal cycling tests undertaken throughout 2 d of supplementation	18 M Experimental-placebo design	120 mg/d for 22 d	No*	Q10 produced negative effect on anaerobic cycling performance— failure to achieve a training effect Increased CK levels with Q10 No effect on submaximal performance
Weston et al. 1997	Cycling Normal training undertaken during 28 d supplementation Incremental test to exhaustion undertaken pre- and post-exercise	18 trained cyclists and triathletes (M) Experimental-placebo design	1 mg/kg/d for 28 d	No	Q10 did not enhance any performance parameters
Malm et al. 1996	Cycling Anaerobic training sessions + anaerobic + submaximal cycling tests undertaken throughout 22 d of supplementation	15 healthy M Experimental-placebo design	120 mg/d for 22 d	No*	Q10 produced ergolytic effect on anaerobic cycling performance— failure to achieve a training effect No effect on submaximal performance

Study	Event	Subjects	Carnitine dose	Enhanced performance	Comments
Laaksonen et al. 1995	Cycling Prolonged endurance test to exhaustion	11 young and 8 older trained M Crossover design	120 mg/d for 6 w	No*	No change in muscle Q10 concentrations or plasma malondialdehyde as a result of Q10 supplementation Negative effect on time to exhaustion (placebo had greater endurance)
Snider et al. 1992	Cycling and running 90 min on treadmill @ 70% $VO_{2\,max}$ + cycling @ 70% $VO_{2\,max}$ to exhaustion	11 highly trained triathletes Crossover design	100 mg/d for 4 w (+ vitamin E, inosine, cytochrome C)	No	No difference in time to exhaustion between trials No differences in blood metabolites or RPE
Braun et al. 1991	Cycling Incremental test to exhaustion performance pre- and post-supplementation period Training continued during period	10 M cyclists Experimental-placebo design	100 mg/d for 8 w	No	Performance increased equally in both groups after training period Q10 had no effect on cycling performance or any measured parameters Malondialdehyde concentrations reduced in both groups after training
Kaikkonen et al. 1998	Running Marathon (field test)	37 moderately trained M runners Experimental-placebo design	90 mg/d for 3 w (+ vit E)	Not measured No change in muscle damage	No change in indices of oxidative or muscle damage following marathon run
Ylikoski et al. 1997	Cross-country skiing Treadmill pole-walking to exhaustion	25 national level cross-country skiers Experimental-placebo design	90 mg/d for 6 w	Yes	Improved $VO_{2\,max}$ with Q10 supplementation Increase in aerobic and anaerobic thresholds No control of exercise during supplementation periods

* Decrease in performance, M = male, F = female

Table 17.15 *Studies of inosine supplementation and performance*

Study	Event	Subjects	Inosine dose	Enhanced performance	Comments
McNaughton et al. 1999	Cycling 5 x 6 sec, 30 sec and 20 min time trial	7 well-trained M Crossover design	10 000 mg for 5 and 10 d	No	No improvements in sprint times or time trial performance Increase in plasma uric acid concentrations
Starling et al. 1996	Cycling Wingate bike test, 30 min self-paced cycle, supramaximal sprint to fatigue	10 competitive M cyclists Crossover design	5000 mg/d for 5 d	No*	No difference in Wingate performance or 30 min cycle Negative effect on time to fatigue Increase in plasma uric acid concentration
Williams et al. 1990	Running Submaximal warm-up run, competitive 3-mile treadmill run, maximal treadmill run	9 highly trained M & F endurance runners Crossover design	6000 mg/d for 2 d (maximum recommended dose)	No*	No effect on 3-mile run time, $VO_{2\ peak}$ or other variables Negative effect on maximal run

* *Decrease in performance, M = male, F = female*

Table 17.16 *Studies of chromium picolinate and changes in body composition*

Study	Event	Subjects	Chromium Picolinate dose	Enhanced performance	Comments
Walker et al. 1998	14 w resistance and conditioning training program and endurance testing Pre- and post-testing of strength, peak power, body composition, Wingate test, VO$_{2\,max}$ on run treadmill	20 M collegiate wrestlers Experimental-placebo design	200 µg/d for 14 w	No	Did not enhance body composition or performance variables beyond improvements seen with training alone
Grant et al. 1997	9 w supplementation with or without resistance training program Testing = BM, composition	43 obese F Experimental-placebo design	400 µg/d chromium picolinate or nicotinate for 9 w	No (↑ BM with chromium picolinate)	↑ BM in chromium picolinate group ↓ BM and insulin response with training and chromium nicotinate
Lukaski et al. 1996	8 w resistance training program Pre- and post-testing of strength, body composition and iron status	36 untrained M Experimental-placebo design	3.4 µmol/d (~200 µg/d) chromium picolinate or or chloride for 8 w	No	No beneficial effects on LBM, body fat or strength above training effect No difference between chromium preparations Trend for ↓ iron status (↓ transferrin status) with chromium picolinate
Hallmark et al. 1996	12 w resistance training program Pre- and post-testing of strength and body composition	16 untrained M Experimental-placebo design	200 µg/d for 12 w	No	No differences in body composition with training or supplement Strength increases independent of supplement

(continues)

(continued)

Study	Event	Subjects	Chromium Picolinate dose	Enhanced performance	Comments
Trent & Thieding-Cancel 1995	16 w physical conditioning program Pre- and post-testing of body composition	95 active-duty Navy personnel (M & F) Experimental-placebo design	400 µg/d for 16 w	No	No differences in BM and fat changes between groups (note body composition measured by anthropometry)
Clancy et al. 1994	9 w pre-season resistance and conditioning training Pre-, mid- and post-testing of body composition, strength	36 M collegiate football (gridiron) players Experimental-placebo design	200 µg/d for 9 w	No	No enhancement of BM, body composition or strength above placebo group
Hasten et al. 1992	12 w resistance training program Pre- and post-testing of body composition and strength	59 M & F college students Experimental-placebo design	200 µg/d for 12 w	No (but ↑ BM in F)	No differences in strength changes due to chromium picolinate Greater ↑ in BM in F with chromium but no difference with M No difference with loss of body fat

M = male, F = female

Table 17.17 *Studies of MCT + CHO supplementation and ultra-endurance performance: crossover design*

Study	Event	Subjects	MCT dose	Enhanced performance	Comments
Angus et al. 2000	Cycling 100 km time trial (~3 h)	8 endurance trained M cyclists/triathletes	1 L per h of 6% CHO + 4% MCT (vs 6% CHO or placebo) (total intake of MCT = 42 g per or ~120 g)	No	CHO-enhanced performance over placebo, but addition of MCT does not provide further benefits 4 subjects experienced GI problems with MCT No differences in fat oxidation, plasma FFA between MCT and CHO + MCT Suppression of fat oxidation due to high exercise intensity or pre-trial CHO meal causing high insulin concentrations
Goedecke et al. 1999	Cycling 2 h @ 63% VO$_{2\ max}$ + 40 km time trial (~70 min)	9 endurance trained M cyclists	1.6 L of 10% CHO or 10% CHO + 1.7% MCT or 10% CHO + 3.4% MCT (total intake of MCT = 27 or 52 g)	No	No differences in time trial performance 2 subjects experience GI distress with higher MCT intake Higher FFA with MCT but no change in CHO oxidation
Jeukendrup et al. 1998	Cycling 2 h @ 60% VO$_{2\ max}$ + time trial (~15 min)	9 endurance trained M cyclists/triathletes	20 mL/kg of 10% CHO or 10% CHO + 5% MCT or 5% MCT or placebo (total intake of MCT = 86 g)	No	No difference between CHO, CHO + MCT or placebo (~14 min) but MCT alone impaired performance (17.3 min) MCT + CHO showed slightly higher fat oxidation than CHO alone No glycogen sparing seen
Van Zyl et al. 1996	Cycling 2 h @ 60% VO$_{2\ max}$ + 40 km time trial (~70 min)	6 endurance trained cyclists	2 L of 4.3% MCT or 10% CHO or 10% CHO+ 4.3% MCT (total intake of MCT = 86 g)	Yes	MCT + CHO-enhanced time trial performance times (65.1 min) compared with CHO (66.8 min) and MCT (72.1 min) Increase in FFA and glycogen sparing with MCT + CHO

M = male, F = female, GI = gastrointestinal

CHAPTER 18

Nutrition for special populations: children and young athletes

Shona Bass and Karen Inge

18.1 INTRODUCTION

Physical activity during childhood and adolescence is widely recommended for short- and long-term physiological, sociological and psychological benefits. There are concerns, however, regarding the possible negative effects of intense training on growth and maturation, and in particular, the combination of intense training with sub-optimal energy and nutrient intakes.

Section 18.2 describes the different temporal patterns of skeletal growth and maturation, how maturation is clinically assessed, and how diet and intense exercise may affect skeletal growth and maturation. Section 18.3 considers the nutritional requirements of children and adolescents participating in sport at an elite level, and concludes with lifestyle issues, food habits and counselling strategies for sports dietitians who are working with this special population.

18.2 SKELETAL GROWTH AND MATURATION IN YOUNG ELITE ATHLETES

Growth and maturation refer to two distinct biological processes. Growth refers to an increase in the total body size, and/or the size attained by specific parts of the body. Maturation refers to the tempo and timing of progress towards the mature biological state. Growth focuses on size, and maturation focuses on the progress of attaining size (Malina & Bouchard 1991). Understanding skeletal development—growth in size and bone mass accrual—becomes clinically important when exposure to risk and protective factors (e.g. disease, poor nutrition, exercise) affect the attainment of final stature and peak bone mass.

18.2.1 *Skeletal growth*

The skeletal growth process can be viewed as two distinct but interrelated processes: an increase in bone length and an increase in bone mass (bone mass accrual). There are different temporal patterns of growth in bone length and bone mass accrual (Bass et al. 1999). These different patterns are characterised by the stage of maturation, the gender and the skeletal region (axial or appendicular). The clinical importance of understanding this heterogeneity in skeletal development lies in the site-specific (e.g. hip or spine) surfeits or deficits that may occur due to exposure to risk or protective factors at different stages of development.

18.2.1.1 *Growth in bone length*

Growth in bone length is categorised by unique biological phases that are linked to hormonal regulation. The entire growth process is divided into three additive and partly superimposed components: infancy, childhood and puberty (Karlberg 1989a, 1989b, 1990). Growth during infancy is thought to be a continuation of postnatal 'foetal growth' and is predominantly regulated by insulin and insulin-like growth factors I and II (IGF-I and IGF-II) (Gluckman 1989, 1996; Wollmann & Ranke 1996). It is independent of growth hormone (GH) and probably thyroid function. Growth hormone and IGF-I are responsible for growth during childhood, provided thyroid function is normal, while growth during puberty is related to GH and sex steroids (Karlberg 1989a, 1989b; Wollmann & Ranke 1996). The three phases of growth are also distinguished by the different temporal patterns of growth in stature. There is rapid foetal growth with a peak intra-uterine growth velocity at four months gestational age. From this point there is a marked deceleration of linear growth that continues after birth until 6 to 12 months. Childhood growth is characterised by a growth spurt occurring early, and then gradually decelerating velocity through childhood. Puberty is characterised by acceleration of growth velocity (growth spurt).

During infancy

Body size at birth is primarily dependent on intra-uterine conditions (nutrition and oxygen). After birth, most infants make growth adjustments (increased or decreased velocity) in their first two years to reach their genetically determined growth potential (Karlberg 1989b; Rogol 1995). Infants are known to 'shift centiles' during the first 12–18 months of life. The second year of life seems to be an important period of growth of bone length because environment and/or diseases may delay the onset of the GH-dependent growth spurt (Karlberg 1989b). Further, the position on the growth curve at two years of age is generally tracked for the remaining growth period (Smith et al. 1976; Karlberg 1989b; Cooper et al. 1995). Growth is more stable during the third year of life, when the infancy component of growth has virtually disappeared and growth is predominated by the childhood component.

Growth from six months to approximately four years of age is the sum of the infancy and childhood components. The influence of the infancy component finishes by about four years of age, after which growth is regulated solely by the childhood component until puberty.

During childhood

The onset of the GH-dependent childhood component is characterised by a growth spurt between the ages of 6–12 months. There is an obvious and abrupt increase in growth rate, which results in a slowing of the rapid deceleration in growth velocity. The peak velocity during this growth spurt is approximately 17 cm/yr (Karlberg 1989a, 1989b, 1990; Wollmann & Ranke 1996). Of particular interest is that this growth spurt is characterised by an acceleration of growth of the legs; growth velocity of the trunk remains constant.

The childhood component, often referred to as pre-pubertal growth, is nearly identical in girls and boys, as shown in Figure 18.1. During this phase there is an initial rapid decrease in velocity, and then a slow consistent decline in velocity to reach a minimal pre-pubertal height velocity of about 5 cm/yr in both sexes

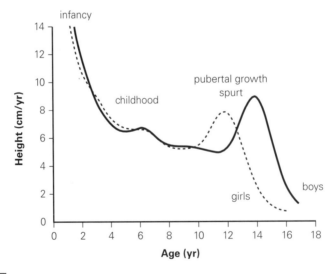

Figure 18.1 *Skeletal growth velocity*
The childhood component, often referred to as pre-pubertal growth, is nearly identical in girls and boys. During this phase there is an initial rapid decrease in velocity, and then a slow consistent decline in velocity. The pubertal component is characterised by a growth spurt. Girls generally start their growth spurt and attain their peak height velocity approximately two years earlier than boys

Adapted from Preece and Ratcliffe 1992

(Karlberg 1989a, 1989b; Prader 1992). A mid-childhood growth spurt at seven to eight years has been observed in two-thirds of healthy children. This transient acceleration in height is thought to be due to adrenal androgens, involves growth in all dimensions, and is similar for both genders. The subsequent decline in growth immediately before puberty often highlights this mid-childhood spurt (Karlberg 1989a, 1989b; Prader 1992).

The childhood patterns of long-bone growth are very stable and orderly compared to infancy and puberty. Changes in percentile levels with increasing age are minimal (Maresh 1955; Karlberg 1989b). Growth in the childhood component is dominated by growth of the legs (approximately 43.7 and 48.6 cm in girls and boys respectively) compared to trunk growth (approximately 34.7 and 36.7 cm in girls and boys respectively) (Karlberg 1989b). At 12 years of age, the gain in height for both sexes due to childhood growth is about equal (Karlberg 1989b).

During puberty

Growth during puberty is more complex than in the childhood years (when the growth rate is relatively constant). Similar to the infancy phase of growth, there is also a growth spurt during puberty. In contrast to the infancy component, however, the growth spurt during puberty is dominated by an acceleration in trunk length; growth of the legs proceeds with constant velocity. Approximately 97% of final stature has been attained by the time menarche has occurred; about 15% of the final stature is achieved during the pubertal growth spurt (Faulkner et al. 1993; Bass et al. 1999). Pubertal growth is often considered to be a growth-promoting event and the final height-limiting process. This is because height velocity is markedly increased, however, the rate of skeletal maturation is also increased, which eventually leads to fusion of the epiphyseal cartilage (Bourguignon 1988). This pubertal growth spurt is directly related to the physical and hormonal changes that accompany sexual development, and is characterised by three phases (Cara 1993):

- minimal height velocity just before the spurt (pre-pubertal growth lag);
- maximal growth—peak height velocity (PHV); and
- decreasing height velocity (epiphyses fuse and final height is achieved).

Girls generally start their growth spurt and attain their PHV two years earlier than boys (see Figure 18.1). Early in puberty, girls tend to be taller than boys because they begin their spurt earlier, and grow faster in the early phases of the growth spurt (Preece 1982; Buckler 1990; Preece & Ratcliffe 1992). Upper- and lower-body comparisons between males and females show that nearly 60% of the gender difference in total stature is due to longer leg length in males. The majority of this extra leg length in boys is attained before the pubertal growth spurt, while a greater proportion of the gender differences in sitting height is attained during the pubertal growth spurt.

18.2.1.2 *Bone mass accrual*

During skeletal growth there is an increase in bone length and a corresponding increase in bone size and bone mass. There are numerous data that describe the heterogeneity in growth of bone length between the axial and appendicular skeleton at different stages of maturation (Maresh 1955; Tanner 1962; Preece 1982; Buckler 1990; Preece & Ratcliffe 1992). In contrast, there are little data that provide the same description of the heterogeneity of bone mass accrual.

At birth, the newborn skeleton contains approximately 30 g of calcium, and in the next 20 years of life there is approximately 1500 g of calcium accrued in the skeleton. This increase is more than three times the calcium that is lost during 40 years of ageing. During childhood, bone mass is being accrued at a constant rate, similar to the pattern of longitudinal bone growth; and there are minimal differences in bone size or mass at most skeletal sites between pre-pubertal girls and boys (Faulkner et al. 1993). The pubertal growth spurt contributes proportionally more to peak bone mass than to final stature (Bass et al. 1999). Approximately 80–85% of peak bone mass has been accrued by the time menarche has occurred. About half of this is achieved during pre-pubertal growth (approximately ten to 12 years) and is non–sex-hormone dependent. The other half is achieved very rapidly during two to four years of pubertal growth (Faulkner et al. 1993; Bass et al. 1999).

There are limited data available about the gender differences in bone mass accrual during puberty; however, it has been reported that a greater proportion of peak bone mass may be accrued during puberty in females than males (Gordon et al. 1991). Females accrue up to 55% of adult lumbar spine bone mass during puberty, while males may accrue only 21% (Gordon et al. 1991). It appears that males tend to accrue bone mass at the spine slowly and gradually throughout the age range. In contrast, females tend to accrue bone mass rapidly during puberty. This sex-specific pattern in bone mass accrual is similar to the pattern of increase in body weight (Gordon et al. 1991). These results highlight the important contribution of bone mass accrual during puberty to the attainment of peak bone mass in young women (Bachrach et al. 1991).

The pubertal growth spurt is also characterised by different temporal patterns of growth in bone length and bone mass accrual (see Figure 18.2) (Bass et al. 1999). There is up to a one-year difference between the age for PHV and accrual of peak bone mass (Katzman et al. 1991; Fournier et al. 1997; Bass et al. 1999). It is thought that bone fragility increases at this time because there is a rapid increase in bone length, without a corresponding increase in bone mass. Interestingly, this time of temporal dissociation between length and mass corresponds to the time when there is an increase in the number of childhood fractures. Increased physical activity or an increase in the number of falls does not account for this increased number of fractures (Bailey et al. 1989; Blimkie et al. 1993).

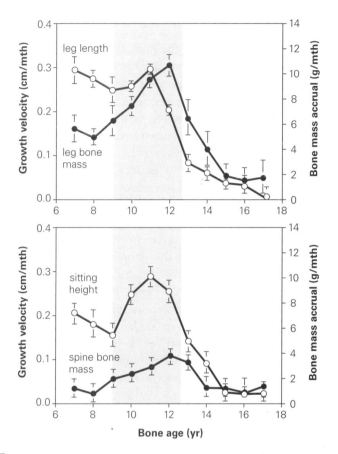

Figure 18.2   *Growth velocity and mineral accrual during childhood and adolescence*
The pubertal growth spurt is characterised by different temporal patterns of growth in bone length (cm/month) and bone mass (g/month accrual). There is up to a one-year lag between the time for PHV and peak bone mass accrual. The shaded region represents the pubertal years (Tanner stage to menarche)

Adapted from Bass et al. 1999

18.2.2   *Maturation*

Maturation refers to progress (timing and tempo) toward the biological mature state. Timing refers to when specific maturational events occur, and tempo refers to the rate at which maturation progresses. Individuals vary in the timing and tempo of maturation, this may affect the ability of some children to train and compete against other children who are the same chronological age but at a different stage of maturation. Techniques for estimating maturity vary depending on the biological system being assessed. Commonly used systems include skeletal maturation, sexual maturation, and somatic (physical) maturation. Dental maturation also can be used as a maturity indicator.

18.2.2.1 *Skeletal age*

The skeleton develops from cartilage in the prenatal period to fully developed bone in early adulthood. Skeletal age (or bone age) is based on the maturation of the skeleton—it reflects the development of calcified or ossified areas of bone and the external contour changes that result from bone growth and ossification (Malina & Bouchard 1991). As the epiphyseal growth plate matures, its shape and width change in a predictable fashion, with eventual fusion of the epiphysis and elimination of the radiological visible 'gap' between the epiphysis and its corresponding metaphysis (Gertner 1999). Therefore, a mature skeleton will have more bone development and less cartilage compared to a less mature skeleton.

X-rays are used to determine the amount of bone development and how close the shape and contours of the bones are to adult status. The left hand (wrist area) is the site most often used, as there are many bones in the area to assess, it is reasonably typical of the skeleton as a whole, and the gonads are not exposed to radiation. Bone age is assigned by averaging the developmental stage of the bones in the wrist (Tanner et al. 1975; Grimston et al. 1990). Figure 18.3 shows the different stages of skeletal maturation in the wrist bones of two individuals.

Bone age gives a better assessment of skeletal and biological maturity than chronological age (years since birth). Further, skeletal maturation is thought to be the best method for assessing biological age or maturity status, and it is the only method that spans the entire growth period—from birth to adulthood (Malina & Bouchard 1991). Three methods used to evaluate skeletal development are the Greulich-Pyle, Tanner-Whitehouse and Fels methods (Greulich & Pyle 1959; Tanner et al. 1975, 1983; Roche et al. 1988). The systems are complex and require extensive experience to be used accurately and reliably.

18.2.2.2 *Sexual maturation*

The principle physical events of puberty include the growth spurt, and the development of reproductive organs and secondary sexual characteristics. Changes also occur in body composition and in the cardiorespiratory system. While skeletal age is the only maturational indicator that can be applied over the entire growth period, it is not a good predictor of pubertal events. Assessing sexual maturation is useful because sexual maturation is highly related to the overall process of physiological maturation (Tanner 1962).

Assessing sexual maturation is based on the stage of development of secondary sex characteristics, including breast development and age of menarche in girls, genital development in boys, and pubic hair development in both sexes. Tanner (1962) devised categories based on specific secondary sex characteristics consisting of five stages of maturation from Stage 1 (pre-pubertal children) to Stage 5 (full maturation). Other maturity indicators include the development of axillary (armpit) hair in boys and girls, and facial hair and voice changes in boys.

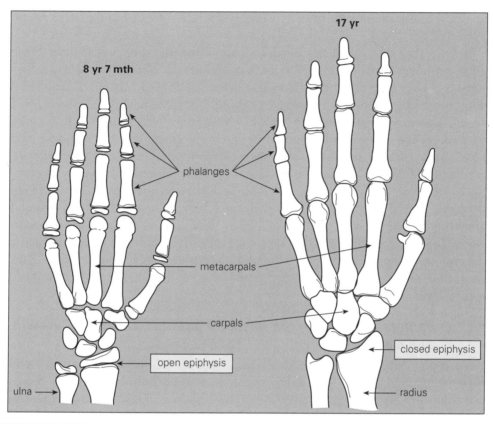

Figure 18.3 *The different stages of skeletal maturation in the wrist bones of two individuals*

The assessment of skeletal age reflects the development of calcified or ossified areas of bone and changes in shape that result from bone growth and ossification. The epiphyses are open in the younger child and closed in the adolescent

Gender differences in maturation are most apparent during puberty. While the overall sequence of maturation is similar, there are considerable differences in the timing of onset of pubertal events. In girls at approximately ten years of age, there is an increase in oestrogen secretion which signals the onset of puberty (Tanner Stage 2 for breast development); pubic hair development generally starts about six months later. Peak height velocity occurs relatively early in puberty (Tanner Stage 3 for breast development, at around 12 years), usually before the occurrence of menarche (Prader 1992; Preece & Ratcliffe 1992). Menarche signals that growth is coming to an end. Adult height is attained about 2.8 years after menarche (Prader 1992). The age of menarche influences the amount of height that is subsequently gained. For instance, on average, if menses occurs at 10 years of age, there is a further 10 cm gained in height after menarche. If, however, menses occurs at 14 years of age, the subsequent gain in height is only 5 cm (Roche & Davila 1972; Roche 1989; Buckler 1990).

In boys, the onset of puberty usually occurs 12 months after girls (Tanner Stage 2 for genitalia development, ~11 years) (Tanner 1962). The growth spurt in boys starts relatively later in puberty than girls (genitalia, Stage 3, ~12 years), and PHV also occurs later (between Tanner Stage 4 and 5 for genitalia development, ~14 years). The growth spurt of boys tends to be two years after that of girls, because boys enter puberty one year later and the relative placement of the growth spurt and PHV in male puberty is also one year later (compared with female puberty) (Preece & Ratcliffe 1992). Males are on average 12–13 cm taller than females at adulthood—they are generally 10 cm taller when they begin their growth spurt (5 cm from one year extra pre-pubertal growth, and 5 cm due to one year of pubertal growth before the growth spurt). The higher PHV in boys accounts for the additional 2–3 cm (Marshall 1978). The time between the start and the end of the pubertal development of the male genitalia is very short, only about 2.5 years. This short time reflects the powerful effect of testosterone on development of the male genitalia (Prader 1992).

18.2.3 *Factors influencing the temporal patterns of skeletal growth and maturation*

Regular physical activity in a healthy well nourished child is important for normal skeletal and muscle growth, and the development of cardiovascular fitness, neuromuscular coordination, and cognitive function (Malina 1994). The rapid increase in sex steroids and growth factors during puberty is thought to accelerate the development of these physiological characteristics, leading to increased trainability for athletic potential (Rowland 1997). In contrast, however, intense training during childhood and adolescence, particularly when combined with poor nutrition, can have negative effects on skeletal growth and maturation.

18.2.3.1 *How is reduced growth and delayed maturation detected?*

Compromised skeletal growth is characterised by:

- a slowing of pre-pubertal growth to a velocity close to zero; and
- reduced or no PHV.

Whereas delayed maturation is characterised by:

- bone age being more than two years younger than chronological age; and
- failure to have the first menstrual cycle (menarche) by the age of 16 years.

Assessing the effect of physical activity on growth and maturation is complex because it is difficult to discern what contribution was due to familial associations (genetic factors) and what was causally related to environmental conditions (training and/or nutrition).

18.2.3.2 *Reduced growth and delayed maturation in elite athletes: inherited or environmental factors?*

Genetic factors can explain many of the characteristics of reduced growth and delayed maturation reported in some athletes. For example, the age of menarche of mothers of athletes tended to be later than mothers of non-athletes, and sisters of athletes also tend to attain a later menarche than average (Malina et al. 1994). The number of siblings in the family has also been reported to influence age of menarche; girls from larger families tend to attain menarche later than those from small families (Malina et al. 1994). After accounting for these maternal influences, the next predictor for age of menarche in athletes is lean body mass (Brookes-Gunn & Warren 1988; Rees 1990, 1993). Further, familial short stature (e.g. short parents) is often used as a selection criteria in elite gymnastic programs. Retrospective data showed that elite gymnasts had short stature (−1 standard deviation from the population distribution) at two years of age, long before they commenced training for gymnastics (Peltenburg et al. 1984). Furthermore, familial short stature in healthy non-athletic children is often associated with delayed maturation (Niewoehner 1998).

While familial short stature is used as a selection criterion for many elite gymnastic programs, there is evidence that some young female gymnasts may also have attenuated skeletal growth. Several research groups have documented growth and maturation in elite gymnasts from two years (Theintz et al. 1993; Bass et al. 2000) to five years (Lindholm et al. 1994; Zonderland et al. 1997). Findings of these studies indicated that gymnasts grew more slowly than controls, their growth spurt was either absent or delayed, and the delay in skeletal maturation increased with longer duration of training. Theintz et al. (1993) observed that 22 gymnasts (aged 12.3 ± 0.2 years), followed for two years, passed through pubertal development with almost no acceleration in growth. Similar findings were reported in 28 gymnasts (aged 11–14 years) over five years (Lindholm et al. 1994). Bass et al. (2000) reported that 21 gymnasts (aged 11.0 ± 0.4 years) had short stature, and the deficit in stature became greater with longer duration of training due to a shift to the right and blunting of the growth velocity curve.

Theintz et al. (1993) and Lindholm et al. (1994) predicted gymnasts final adult height from either mid-parental equations or estimates from the relative closure of the epiphyses. Theintz et al. (1993) reported that the predicted final adult height of the gymnasts decreased over the two years of training, while Lindholm et al. (1994) reported that the final adult height in six gymnasts of the 22 gymnasts was 3.5–7.5 cm shorter than predicted heights at the end of a five-year study.

There is also evidence that intense exercise may also be associated with delayed maturation. Theintz et al. (1993) reported that skeletal maturation of the gymnasts was moderately delayed (about 1.0 year) and did not worsen during the course of the study. In contrast, Bass et al. (2000) reported that skeletal maturation in 21 gymnasts (aged 11.0 ± 0.4 years) was delayed by 1.8 ± 0.2 years and became more delayed by an additional 0.5 ± 0.1 years after two years of training. Similar findings have been reported in rhythmic gymnasts aged 11–23 years (Georgopoulos et al. 1999). Their skeletal maturation was delayed by 1.3 years, and their mean age of menarche was older than their mothers' and sisters'. In this study the delay in skeletal maturation and the age of menarche was positively correlated to the intensity of training, and negatively correlated to body fat. Furthermore, the prevalence of delayed menarche in ballet dancers varies from 5–40%, with an average delay of around two years (Warren & Brooks-Gunn 1989). Some dancers do not menstruate until their early 20s (Warren 1980, 1983; Warren & Stiehl 1999). Slowing of skeletal growth and delayed maturation associated with intense training has also been reported in case studies of young female and male athletes (Laron & Klinger 1989), monozygotic twins (Constantini et al. 1997) and triplets (Tveit-Milligan et al. 1993).

Not all elite athletes are at risk of reduced growth and delayed maturation

Large differences in growth and maturation have been observed between individual gymnasts involved in similar training regimens. In the study by Bass et al. (2000), some gymnasts had delayed skeletal maturation by up to 3.2 years and yet others of a similar age and training schedule were not delayed. Further, over the course of the study the delay in skeletal maturation improved in some but became more delayed in others. Only 13 of the 22 gymnasts followed by Lindholm et al. (1994) showed an attenuated growth curve. While in the study by Theintz et al. (1993) the height standard deviation scores in some gymnasts were positive and remained positive over the course of the study, in others the height standard deviation scores were reduced and worsened over the course of the study. These data support the notion that not all gymnasts involved in elite training programs are at risk of reduced growth and delayed maturation. Therefore, it is important to identify gymnasts who may be at risk of attenuated growth and delayed maturation (see Section 18.2.6).

18.2.3.3 *Do attenuated skeletal growth patterns occur uniformly in all bones?*

Short stature in elite young athletes may be the result of attenuated growth at one skeletal site but not others (Bass et al. 2000). For instance, Theintz et al. (1993) reported that the reduced growth of 22 gymnasts was related to a slower growth velocity of the legs, not the trunk. However, sampling bias may have affected these results, as the controls were swimmers who were taller than average, with greater than average growth velocities. In contrast, Bass et al. (2000) reported that reduced leg length in the gymnasts was present at baseline but did not worsen with increasing duration of gymnastic training; the deficit in trunk length was only detectable after two years of training and worsened with increasing years of training. Therefore, Bass et al. (2000) proposed that the reduced leg length of gymnasts may be due to selection bias, and the acquired component of the deficit in stature was the result of a progressive deficit in trunk length. Site-specific deficits in longitudinal growth have also been reported in ballet dancers—their trunk length was shorter relative to leg length as demonstrated by the decreased upper- to lower-body ratio compared to other female family members (Warren 1980).

18.2.3.4 *Other factors that may influence skeletal growth and maturation*

Slowing of skeletal growth and delayed maturation are often reported in athletes from sports where there is emphasis on leanness (10%–20% below desired weight) or in aesthetic sports where there is a focus on a petite build or small body mass (e.g. gymnastics, long distance running, skiing, figure skating and ballet) (Warren 1980; Frisch et al. 1981; Warren 1983; Neinstein 1985; Brooks-Gunn et al. 1987; Warren & Stiehl 1999). The mechanism for the attenuated growth and delayed maturation reported in athletes is unclear, but nutritional insufficiency may be a major contributing factor (see Chapter 10). Growth failure and impaired maturation have been reported in healthy non-athletic children who regularly restricted kilojoules (Pugliese et al. 1983). Similar eating behaviour is not uncommon in young athletes striving for a lean body mass. For many young athletes, energy and nutrient intakes may be insufficient to support the nutritional needs for normal growth and maturation as well as intense exercise (Caine et al. 2000, unpublished). Puberty, the period of accelerated growth, may be particularly influenced by poor nutrition (Largo 1993), and young athletes may be at increased risk if their dietary regime is designed to maintain a reduced body weight for performance. Often diets designed for elite gymnasts are nutrient dense and well balanced but may be too low in energy (Lindholm et al. 1995; Bass et al. 2000). In most instances, however, young athletes who are following very low energy diets are unsupervised—hence, their diets are unbalanced and likely to be both low in energy and sub-optimal in nutrient density.

Unfortunately, little is known about the energy requirements of gymnastic training (Van Erp-Baart et al. 1985; Davies et al. 1997; Caine et al. 2000), so determining daily energy expenditures and energy balance in gymnastics is not possible. If young athletes are in negative energy balance, chronic mild under-nutrition may result, leading to compromised skeletal growth and delayed maturation (Malina 1994). Negative energy balance is known to reduce the levels of IGF-I, and the relationship between IGF-I and growth is well known (Smith et al. 1995). Low IGF-I values have been reported in young female gymnasts (Jahreis 1991; Bass et al. 1998). In a study of 21 gymnasts, energy intake was an independent predictor of growth velocity and correlated with the delay in skeletal maturation (Bass et al. 2000).

18.2.3.5 *Environmental influences on growth and maturation*

Other factors that may interact with intense exercise and negative energy balance to alter growth potential include:

- the psychological and emotional stress associated with maintaining body weight when the natural course is to gain;

- year-long training (including training programs with little time-out);
- frequent competitions;
- altered social relationships with peers; and
- demanding parents and/or coaches (Malina 1994).

In addition, reduced skeletal growth may be due to repetitive stress and physical trauma damaging the epiphyses. Immature bones with open epiphyses are susceptible to stress injuries such as little-leaguer elbow, Osgood-Schlatter disease, and iliac crest apophysitis. Stress changes, stress fractures and abnormal bone growth in the epiphysis of the radius have also been reported in gymnasts (Micheli 1983; Caine et al. 1989, 1992; Mandelbaum et al. 1989; Meeussen & Borms 1992). However, there has been little investigation into the effects of repetitive loading on an open epiphysis (Borms 1986; Maffulli & King 1992). Interestingly, there are limited animal data that show that repetitive load may inhibit the long bone growth, and that non–weight-bearing exercise (swimming) may facilitate long bone growth (Swissa-Sivan et al. 1989; Maffulli & King 1992).

18.2.4 *Catch-up growth: can impaired growth and delayed maturation be reversed?*

The notion that negative energy balance is strongly associated with reduced growth and delayed maturation is supported by 'catch-up growth' that is observed when training is reduced or ceases (Lindholm et al. 1994; Theintz 1994; Bass et al. 2000). Catch-up growth is generally associated in a clinical sense when a temporary cause of growth retardation has been removed, and the child returns to their normal growth channel. This occurs after any type of temporary growth disturbance (e.g. after malnutrition, corticoid therapy, renal acidosis, and after initiation of substitution in growth hormone deficiency or hypothyroidism) (Boersma et al. 1995). Catch-up growth is characterised by accelerated and/or protracted skeletal growth. In some cases, prolonged catch-up growth continues until early adulthood, and in other cases, growth velocity can be as high as four times the 'usual' rate (Largo 1993; Boersma et al. 1995).

Catch-up growth may be complete or incomplete; completely or partially restoring stature to normal (Mosier 1989; Largo 1993). Usually when growth in length is retarded, so is bone maturation, but not always to the same extent. Theoretically, any imbalance could result in incomplete catch-up growth. However, catch-up of bone age may be slower than that of bone length; thus, in most cases the equilibrium of both parameters is re-established (Mosier 1986; Van den Brande 1986; Prader 1992). The timing and magnitude of the negative energy balance may also influence the ability of the child to achieve complete catch-up growth. Generally, the more severe the delay in skeletal maturation, the higher the risk of incomplete catch-up growth. In healthy, non-athletic children, normal skeletal maturation is defined as bone age being within one year of chronological age (e.g. ± 1 year). In late-maturing children, bone age is delayed between one to two years, and delayed maturation is defined as bone age being delayed by more than two years (Blethen et al. 1984; Mosier 1986; Van den Brande 1986; Prader 1992; Borer 1995; Malina 2000).

18.2.4.1 *Examples of catch-up growth in athletes*

Bass et al. (2000) monitored the growth and maturation in 13 elite gymnasts 12 months before and 12 months after retirement. Figure 18.4 shows that the gymnasts who were more than ten years of age exhibited the well-documented pattern of catch-up growth characterised by an increase and maintenance of growth velocity well above that expected for their chronological age. This catch-up growth occurred and varied according to the age at retirement from the sport. Tonz et al. (1990) also reported a slowing of growth in gymnasts during the peri-pubertal years (relative to controls) and catch-up growth later in puberty. Lindholm et al. (1994) reported that catch-up growth was evident in gymnasts during times of reduced training schedules. It has also been reported that ballet dancers progressed very rapidly through pubertal development during periods of reduced training. While normal girls progress from Tanner Breast Stage 2 to 4 over an average of 2.0 ± 1.0 years, dancers have been shown to make the same progression in as little as four months (Warren 1980). Case studies of young female and male athletes (Laron & Klinger 1989), monozygotic twins (Constantini et al. 1997) and triplets (Tveit-Milligan et al. 1993) also support the notion that catch-up growth occurs in young elite athletes when training schedules have been reduced due to vacation, injury or retirement.

18.2.4.2 *Is catch-up growth always complete?*

It is difficult to determine whether catch-up growth was complete in the aforementioned cases. In the study by Bass et al. (2000), gymnasts who had been retired for eight years did not have short stature. While these group results suggest that final height may not have been compromised, the large variation in severity of the attenuated growth patterns suggests that some individuals within the group may have had incomplete catch-up growth.

18.2.5 *Consequences of delayed skeletal growth and maturation*

Reduced final height may or may not be a problem for an athlete. Ultimately, what is important is a positive body image. Athletes and their parents should be aware that elite training, in conjunction with a diet that is in negative energy balance, might compromise the attainment of final height (Mansfield & Emans 1993). Another issue to be considered in girls is that delayed menarche is a risk factor for menstrual dysfunction (secondary amenorrhoea), and that in some athletes menstrual dysfunction results in low peak bone density (see Chapter 10). Athletes who are involved in high-volume, low-impact sports and have low body weight are at risk of menstrual dysfunction and low bone density that may be irreversible (Keen & Drinkwater 1997; Micklesfield et al. 1998). In contrast, it has been reported that athletes who are involved in high-impact sports, particularly during growth, have high bone density despite menstrual dysfunction (Lindholm et al. 1995; Robinson et al. 1995; Bass et al. 1998).

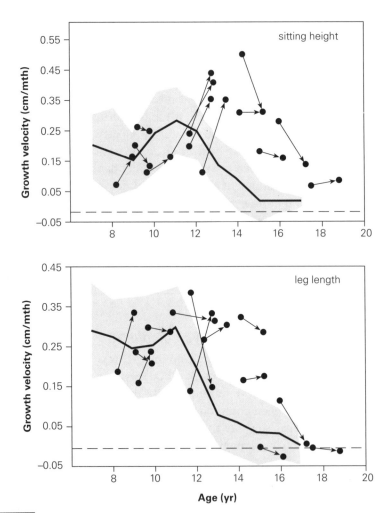

Figure 18.4 *Catch up growth in elite gymnasts.*
Growth velocity of 13 elite gymnasts, 12 months before (tail of the arrow), and 12 months after retirement (head of the arrow) from gymnastic training. Catchup growth was evident in sitting height in the gymnasts who were more than ten years of age. There was no evidence of catchup growth in leg length at any age. The shaded area represents the growth velocity of young healthy non-athletic controls (mean ± 1 SD).

Adapted from Bass et al. 2000

18.2.6 *Summary of growth and maturational issues in young athletes*

Growth and maturation are complex processes and the effect of intense exercise and diet on these processes can not easily be discerned. While some young athletes who are involved in intense training and consume low energy diets may have intrinsically short stature and familial delayed growth, the prospect of attenuated growth and delayed maturation should not be dismissed. If growth rate is reduced and maturation is delayed, catch-up growth may occur (if training intensity is reduced and energy intake is increased). Total catch-up growth may be compromised if the delay in maturation is severe. Some individuals may be more at risk of attenuated growth patterns than others; therefore the growth and maturation of young athletes should be monitored to identify those individuals who are at risk (particularly those with severe and prolonged energy-restricted diets, and who are participating in long-term intense training programs). The following annual assessments are recommended: anthropometric measures, pubertal stage, bone age, nutritional status, symptoms of eating disorders and measures of body image. These parameters should be monitored regularly in young athletes committed to long-term training programs (e.g. ballet dancers and gymnasts). Finally, it is important that these athletes and their parents are in a position to make informed choices about their participation in elite sports. Athletes, parents, coaches and dietitians need to be informed and recognise the benefits and potential risks and outcomes associated with the participation of young athletes in intense physical activity, especially when combined with low-energy diets.

18.3 *NUTRITIONAL NEEDS FOR YOUNG ELITE ATHLETES*

Often the enjoyment and appreciation of sport begins at an early age. Therefore, it is important that children and adolescents are encouraged to adopt healthy dietary practices so that adequate nutritional requirements for growth, maturation and sporting performance are attained. Unfortunately, there is little information specifically relating to the dietary needs of young elite athletes; the majority of research has focussed on adult athletes. Professor Oded Bar-Or, at McMaster University in Canada, suggests that, as there is little child-specific information regarding nutrition requirements for sport, we tend to base recommendations on the requirements of healthy non-athletic children and adult-athletes (Bar-Or 1999, personal communication). It is not known whether the population nutrient recommendation—Recommended Dietary Intakes/Recommended Dietary Allowances (RDIs/RDAs)—for healthy non-athletic children and adolescents are appropriate for young athletes. Furthermore, little research has been conducted on the use of ergogenic aids in young athletes. For the purpose of this section of the chapter, 'children' refers to those aged 5–12 years, and adolescents are those aged 13–18 years (National Health & Medical Research Council 1995).

18.3.1 *Nutrients, including energy*

18.3.1.1 *Energy*

Adequate energy intake during childhood and adolescence is vital to support normal growth as well as providing for the extra energy needs of training (American Dietetic Association 1996c, 1996d). A negative energy balance may be desirable for weight loss in some situations, however, severe and prolonged energy-restricted diets are not recommended for young athletes. Chronic negative energy balance during growth can result in short stature and delayed puberty, menstrual irregularities, poor bone health (see Section 18.2.3.2), increased incidence of injuries, and risk of developing eating disorders (Thompson 1998).

Estimates of energy requirements are derived from the summation of various components of expenditure, that is, basal metabolic rate, growth, metabolisable energy and physical activity (World Health Organisation 1985) (see Chapter 6). Very little is known, however, about the energy requirements of young athletes (Thompson 1998). Table 18.1 shows the population recommendations for energy and protein from different countries for children and adolescents (Cobiac et al. 1997). These figures, which show slight variation, are for light to moderate activity levels and should be considered the minimum for young athletes involved in intensive training programs.

Unfortunately, few studies have directly measured the energy expenditure of children and adolescents performing various sports. Estimates are often extrapolated from adult data, however, there are inherent errors associated with this approach. Children tend to be less metabolically efficient than adults (MacDoughall et al. 1979; Girandola et al. 1981), and are mechanically more inefficient with motor activities. This means that energy expenditure values extrapolated from adults for use in children are underestimated. For instance, girls have a higher energy cost for walking and running compared with women (Haymes et al. 1974), and children aged six to eight years require 20–30% more oxygen per unit body weight than adults when running at similar speeds (Astrand 1952; Daniels 1978). This indicates that children and adolescent athletes have higher energy needs than adults for similar activities. As shown in Table 18.2, there is a large variation in the energy intakes of young athletes that is age-, sport- and gender-specific. More recently, the mean energy intake of 21 female gymnasts (aged 11 years) was reported to be only 6106 kJ per day (Bass et al. 2000). This is lower than the intakes reported for other gymnasts in Table 18.2. Despite the under-reporting of energy intakes in dietary survey techniques, these apparently low energy intakes are of concern if consistently lower than energy expenditures.

18.3.1.2 *Protein*

Children and adolescents have higher protein needs than adults because of the extra protein required for growth. The population recommendations for protein of normally active children and adolescents are reported in Table 18.1. The RDIs for

Table 18.1 Recommended dietary intakes (RDIs) for energy and protein for children and adolescents

		Australia		United Kingdom		United States		Canada		WHO/ FAO/UNU
	Age (years)	RDI	Age (years)	DRV	Age (years)	RDA	Age (years)	RNI	Age (years)	
Energy (MJ/d)										
Males	4–7	6.7–7.5	4–6	7.2	4–6	7.5	4–6	7.5	4–6	7.6
	8–11	8.9	7–10	8.2	7–10	8.4	7–9	9.2	7–9	9.2
	12–15	10.5	11–14	9.3	11–14	10.5	10–12	10.5	10–12	10.9
	16–18	12.6	15–18	11.5	15–18	12.6	13–15	11.7	12–15	12.1
							16–18	13.4	15–18	12.8
Females	4–7	6.7–7.5	4–6	6.5	4–6	7.5	4–6	7.5	4–6	7.6
	8–11	7.9	7–10	7.3	7–10	8.4	7–9	8.0	7–9	9.2
	12–15	8.9	11–14	7.9	11–14	9.2	10–12	9.2	10–12	9.8
	16–18	9.4	15–18	8.8	15–18	9.2	13–15	9.2	12–15	10.4
							16–18	8.8	15–18	9.7
Protein (g/d)										
Males	4–7	18–24	4–6	19.7	4–6	24	4–6	19	4–6	20
	8–11	27–38	7–10	28.3	7–10	28	7–9	26	7–9	25
	12–15	42–60	11–14	42.1	11–14	45	10–12	34	10–12	30
	16–18	64–70	15–18	55.2	15–18	59	13–15	49	12–15	37
							16–18	58	15–18	38
Females	4–7	18–24	4–6	19.7	4–6	24	4–6	19	4–6	20
	8–11	27–39	7–10	28.3	7–10	28	7–9	26	7–9	25
	12–15	44–55	11–14	41.2	11–14	46	10–12	36	10–12	29
	16–18	57	15–18	45.0	15–18	44	13–15	46	12–15	31
							16–18	47	15–18	30

RDI = Recommended Dietary Intake
DRV = Dietary Reference Value
RDA = Recommended Dietary Allowance
RNI = Recommended Nutrient Intake
Adapted from Cobiac et al. 1997

Table 18.2 Self-reported energy intakes of young athletes

Sport	Number of subjects	Age (yr)	Height (cm)	Weight (kg)	(kJ/d)	Energy intake (kJ/kg)	(kcal/day)	(kcal/kg)
Females								
Gymnastics	29	7–10	134.9	30.6	6 908	226	1 651	53.9
	240	11–14	146.7	36.8	7 502	203	1 793	48.3
	56	15–18	160.6	51.0	7 485	149	1 789	35.6
Swimming	100	11–14	156.5	47.22	8 657	189	2 069	45.1
	22	15–18	—[a]	58.2	14 949	257	3 573	61.4
Volleyball	26	13–17	—[a]	—[a]	7 527	—[a]	1 799	—[a]
Dance	92	12–17	160.2	46.8	7 908	171	1 890	40.8
Males								
Swimming	9	11–14	—[a]	56.4	12 853	230	3 072	55.0
	42	15–18	182.0	75.1	18 983	252	4 537	60.2
Running	4	7–10	—[a]	—[a]	8 167	272	1 952	65.0
	14	11–14	—[a]	—[a]	10 632	276	2 541	66.0
	4	15–18	—[a]	—[a]	11 447	209	2 736	50.0
Wrestling	4	7–10	—[a]	—[a]	7 916	272	1 892	64.0
	50	11–14	—[a]	—[a]	10 288	222	2 459	53.0
	20	15–18	—[a]	—[a]	11 309	184	2 703	44.0
Football	46	11–14	—[a]	60.9	10 556	173	2 523	41.4
	88	15–18	—[a]	75.9	14 079	185	3 365	44.3

a = value not reported
Adapted from Thompson 1998

protein in Australian adults is 0.75 g/kg of body weight per day. The protein recommendation is higher in exercising adults to account for gains in lean body mass (during strength training), to compensate for protein used as a fuel source during physical activity and in muscle regeneration. The recommended protein intake for strength and endurance athletes is 1.6–1.7 and 1.2–1.4 g/kg body weight per day respectively (Lemon 1998). There are insufficient data to determine protein recommendations for children and adolescent strength and endurance athletes. However, it may be appropriate to suggest that young athletes have higher protein needs than population recommendations to help meet the increased demands of their sport. The latest National Nutrition Survey conducted in Australia reported the protein intakes of normally active children and adolescents (Table 18.3). Comparing these figures with those in Table 18.1, it is clear that normally active Australian children and adolescents have little difficulty in meeting their protein requirements. In fact according to the NNS, protein intakes in young people are two to three times higher than the RDI.

Table 18.3 *Protein intakes of Australian children and adolescents from the 1995 National Nutrition Survey in Australia*

Group	Age (yr)	Protein intake (g/d)	Protein intake (% of energy)
Males	4–7	64	14
	8–11	82	14.5
	12–15	101	15
	16–18	120	15.5
Females	4–7	57	14
	8–11	69	14
	12–15	74	15
	16–18	80	16

Adapted from McLennan and Podger 1998

Due to limited data on the protein needs of young athletes it is difficult to make precise recommendations (Thompson 1998; Tarnopolsky 1999). However, Lemon (1998) suggests that if total energy intake meets energy expenditure, protein needs of between 1.2–2 g/kg body weight per day should be met. Even in sports where the athletes are often on low-energy diets, the protein intakes appear to meet these levels. For instance, the protein intakes reported in gymnasts and ballet dancers range between 1.5 and 2.0 g/kg body weight per day (15–17% of energy) (Benson et al. 1985, 1990; Loosli et al. 1986; Benardot et al. 1989). Young athletes who may be at increased risk of low protein intakes include strict vegetarians and athletes striving to meet high carbohydrate (CHO) needs.

18.3.1.3 *CHO*

The benefits of high-CHO diets for enhancing athletic performance are well documented (see Chapters 13, 14 and 15); however, there is a paucity of data on the CHO requirements of young athletes. Preliminary findings in 12 adolescent boys (10–14 years (SD ± 1.11) showed that endogenous CHO from glycogenolysis or gluconeogenesis increases exercise performance and contributes more to the total energy provision than reported in adults (up to 20% more) (Riddell 1999, personal communication). There are no data in this area pertaining to girls.

The recommended CHO intake for adult athletes ranges from 55–70% of total energy intake and is dependent on the type of sporting activity (Costill 1988). Burke (1998) recommends that absolute CHO intakes are adjusted for body mass (i.e. g CHO/kg of body weight) (see Chapter 15). There are no published recommendations for CHO intakes for young athletes. Riddell (1999, personal communication) believes that substrate utilisation and CHO requirements may differ between children and adults. Until further research is undertaken, however, CHO recommendations for young athletes will be based on adult athlete recommendations; that is, a diet providing 55% of total energy intake may be the most appropriate guideline for children and adolescent athletes.

There are no known data published regarding the practice, benefits or detrimental effects of CHO loading in children and adolescents, nor is there any data on glycogen resynthesis rates in young athletes. Research on maximum glycogen storage capacity in children and adolescents would enable the determination of recommendations for CHO intake. Until such research is conducted, if at all feasible, Bar-Or and colleagues (1997) suggest that nutrition advice provided to young athletes is based on each individual's response and tolerance.

CHO intakes and dental caries

While a high-CHO diet may be beneficial for training and performance, there are concerns about the effect of some types of CHO on dental health. Dental caries or tooth decay is the result of repeated acid attacks by bacteria in dental plaque. Fermentable CHOs present in foods and beverages provide the necessary substrates for enhancing acid production (Sank 1999). Eating or drinking sugary foods and beverages between meals, without regular cleaning of teeth, promotes dental caries.

The rate of cariogenicity of a food is associated with: the amount of fermentable CHO consumed, the physical form of the CHO, the concentration of sugars in the foods consumed, the length of time the teeth are exposed to acid, the frequency of meals and snacks, and the proximity of eating before bedtime (Sank 1999). Foods likely to exacerbate dental erosion include consumption of citrus fruits and juices, carbonated and uncarbonated sugary drinks, acidic herbal teas, vinegar and vinegar products, confectionery and acidic medications (e.g. vitamin C tablets and syrups) (Sank 1999). Although there has been little research on the relationship between athletes' eating and drinking habits and their dental health (Murray & Drummond

1996), anecdotal information on athletes and population research suggest that preventive advice is warranted. Emphasis needs to be placed on reducing the cariogenicity of the fermentable CHO-containing foods or fluids by water rinsing, eating casein-containing food (preferably low-fat), or chewing gum (preferably sugar free) immediately after consumption of these substances (National Health & Medical Research Council 1995; Sank 1999). The erosive potential of foods can also be reduced by minimising contact time with the teeth by consuming fluids quickly, through a straw or from squeeze bottles directly into the mouth (Murray & Drummond 1996; Milesovic 1997). Chilling drinks is also recommended because the erosive potential (acid dissociation constant) of the acidic fluids is temperature dependent.

Saliva can also offer protection from dental caries and erosion by acting as a buffer. The buffering effect of the saliva may be reduced if the athlete is severely dehydrated (> 8%) or has a dry mouth due to excessive mouth breathing (Murray & Drummond 1996). Proper dental hygiene should be encouraged, and for adolescents wearing braces, dental hygiene should be a priority. Collaboration between dietetic and dental professionals is recommended for oral health promotion, and disease prevention and intervention (American Dietetic Association 1996a).

18.3.1.4 *Fat*

The National Health & Medical Research Council (NHMRC) (1995) recommended a mean contribution of fat to total energy of 36–38% in children aged 10–15 years. These intakes are higher than those recommended for adults. In children and adolescent athletes, fat intakes range from 30–39% of total energy (O'Connor 1994). While children and adolescent athletes are not usually concerned about the negative associations between fat intake and health, they need to recognise that high-fat diets, particularly diets high in saturated fat, are not conducive to optimal training performance and recovery, and may cause problems later in life. Another concern for endurance athletes is that a high-fat diet makes it difficult to meet high CHO requirements.

Young athletes may have a greater capacity than adults to utilise fats as a fuel source during exercise. A greater fat utilisation is demonstrated by a higher free glycerol level in the blood, increased fatty acid uptake and lower respiratory exchange ratios during exercise, indicating a greater fat utilisation (Macek & Vavra 1981; Delamarche et al. 1992; Martinez & Haymes 1992). This increased capacity does not necessarily translate to an increase in the dietary fat requirement in young athletes (Bar-Or & Unnithan 1994).

Until further research has been conducted it is prudent to encourage children and adolescent athletes to consume fat intakes that meet population dietary goals and targets, that is, less than 30% of total energy from fat for adolescents, and less than 35% for children aged 5–14 years, with no more than 10% of energy from saturated fat (National Health & Medical Research Council 1995).

18.3.1.5 *Vitamins*

If energy intakes meet energy expenditures then it is likely that vitamin needs will also be met. It has been reported that young athletes met most of their daily allowances for B vitamins (Benardot et al. 1989; Rankinen et al. 1995; Kopp-Woodroffe et al. 1999), although in some instances intakes of vitamin B6 and folate were below recommended (Loosli et al. 1986; Guilland et al. 1989; Benson et al. 1990). Vitamin intakes were also inadequate in young athletes who restricted their energy intake (Benson et al. 1985). Adolescent ballet dancers, female gymnasts and college wrestlers are all groups at risk of not meeting vitamin recommendations (Moffatt 1984; Benson et al. 1985; Loosli et al. 1986; Steen & McKinney 1986). For instance, 59% of 12–17-year-old ballet dancers (n = 92) reported consuming two-thirds of the RDA for folate (Benson et al. 1985), and 50% of gymnasts (n = 97) aged 11–17 years, failed to consume two-thirds of the RDA for vitamin E (Loosli et al. 1986). Adolescent female athletes (n = 26) on low-energy diets reported consuming marginal intakes of vitamin A, although their vitamin C intakes were well above the RDA. Other vitamins were not measured (Perron & Endres 1985). Thus, low-energy diets may place young athletes at risk of inadequacies of some but not all vitamins.

It is important to note that RDIs/RDAs are not actual requirements, but are the estimated levels of intake of essential nutrients that are judged to be adequate to meet the known needs of the majority of healthy persons (Sirota 1994). It is unknown if these RDIs/RDAs are appropriate for children and adolescent athletes who are training at an elite level. However, these recommendations are still used for comparative assessment of vitamin adequacy in groups of athletes.

Vitamin status is difficult to determine because of the difficulties in collecting reliable data on usual dietary intakes over a long period. Biochemical indices are useful indices of vitamin status, but are often invasive and may not be available for some vitamins (Haymes 1991) (see Chapter 3 and Chapter 12).

18.3.1.6 *Minerals*

Calcium and iron intakes are commonly reported below daily allowances (RDIs/RDAs) in dietary surveys of children and adolescents, particularly in girls (see Chapter 10 and Chapter 11). Adequate zinc intakes are also of concern in young athletes (Bar-Or et al. 1997), not only for zinc's role in energy processes but because of its role in growth, development and immunity.

Calcium

Calcium requirements are highest during childhood and adolescence, with the exception of pregnancy and lactation (see Chapter 10). The NNS of 1995 in Australia reported that 77% of girls and 64% of boys surveyed, aged 12–15 years, did not meet the RDI for calcium. Further, girls of all ages (4–18 years) were not consuming adequate calcium (McLennan & Podger 1997).

Young female athletes who restrict energy intake tend to restrict dairy products and thus are at an increased risk of low calcium intakes (Benson et al. 1985, 1990; Perron & Endres 1985; Benardot et al. 1989; Moen et al. 1992; Bass et al. 2000). Dairy products are the predominant source of calcium in the diets of young healthy non-athletic children and adolescents (National Health & Medical Research Council 1995), so restricting or limiting these foods usually accounts for the low calcium intakes.

Iron

Adolescent females are regarded to be at the highest risk of iron deficiency because of a combination of factors including: high iron requirements because of rapid pubertal growth, increased iron losses through menstrual bleeding, inadequate iron intakes as a consequence of low energy diets and the adoption of vegetarianism (Bergstrom et al. 1995). Weight-bearing exercise also increases the risk of iron deficiency from losses induced by haemolysis, from the GI tract, and excessive sweating (Rowland et al. 1987; Nickerson et al. 1989; Rowland 1990) (see Chapter 11). Iron depletion and deficiency in young athletes, particularly female athletes, is common, with up to 40–50% of adolescent female athletes demonstrating some degree of iron depletion (based on serum ferritin levels) (Benson et al. 1985, 1990; Perron & Endres 1985; Loosli et al. 1986; Benardot et al. 1989; Rowland 1990).

Diagnosis of true iron depletion, using serum ferritin as a biochemical marker, is difficult in children and adolescents, as the increased plasma volume associated with any growth spurt can present falsely low values (see Chapter 11). Strategies for detection and treatment of iron depletion in children and adolescents are similar to those suggested for adult athletes (see Chapter 11).

Zinc

Optimal zinc status is essential for children and adolescents because of the role it plays in growth and development. Classical symptoms of zinc deficiency are reduced linear growth velocity and delayed development of secondary sexual characteristics (Prasad et al. 1963; Sandstead 1985). In the NNS in Australia, female adolescents ($\geq$ 12 years) did not meet the RDI for zinc (McLennan & Podger 1997). Young female athletes also appear to be consuming zinc intakes below daily allowances (Benson et al. 1985; Loosli et al. 1986; Rankinen et al. 1995; Wiita & Stomabaugh 1996; Kopp-Woodroffe et al. 1999). As the best dietary sources of bioavailable zinc are from animal products, vegetarian athletes are at even greater risk of low zinc intakes.

18.3.1.7 *Vitamin and mineral supplements*

Young athletes take vitamin and mineral supplements for numerous reasons. In a survey of 742 high-school athletes (from nine schools), 38% reported taking such supplements; this is more than non-athletic adolescents (25–30%) (Sobal &

Marquart 1994). The most common supplements taken by these athletes were vitamin C (25%), multivitamins (19%), iron (11%), calcium (9%), vitamin A (9%), B vitamins (8%) and zinc (3%). Wrestlers and gymnasts were the highest users (59% and 40% respectively). While boys took more vitamin A supplements than girls, girls took more iron (Sobal & Marquart 1994).

Healthy growth was the most common reason given for taking supplements in this study, followed by treating illness and improving sports performance. Only 62% of those taking supplements believed vitamin and mineral supplements improved athletic performance (Sobal & Marquart 1994). Similar results were reported in another study of 509 high-school athletes aged 14–18 years (Massad et al. 1995). In this study, the main reason the athletes took vitamin A supplements was for the health of their skin. Around one-third of those taking vitamin A supplements did not know that it could be harmful in high doses.

The American Dietetic Association (1996) advocated that the best strategy to obtain adequate bioavailable nutrients is from a wide variety of food rather than from supplements. Vitamin and mineral supplements should, therefore, not be necessary for children and adolescent athletes, except in situations where they are monitored by a qualified health professional. Vulnerable groups of young athletes who may benefit from taking vitamin and/or mineral supplements include: vegetarians, amenorrheic athletes, iron deficient athletes and those on restricted-energy diets. Some vitamins and minerals, if misused, have adverse side-effects that may not be reversible (see Chapter 12, Section 12.7). Prescribed doses of multivitamin and multimineral supplements taken as directed, although they may not be necessary, are generally considered safe for use.

18.3.1.8 *Ergogenic aids*

Ergogenic aids (performance enhancers) have become extremely popular. Ergogenic aids are touted by manufacturers to increase muscle mass, to provide a performance boost and/or to provide increased strength (see Chapter 17). There is little scientific evidence to support the efficacy of most of these products. Young athletes are vulnerable to peer pressure and anecdotal stories, often from well-respected and famous sporting heroes, who may support the use of these products and are encouraged to use them. Young athletes should be aware that performance improvement is reliant on many factors—such as growth, physiological and sexual maturation, skill acquisition, and years of training and good nutrition—and that supplements of any kind will not give them a 'quick fix' to performance problems (Eichner et al. 1999).

Ergogenic aids frequently used by young male athletes are muscle-building supplements. These include protein powders, creatine, dehydroepiandrosterone (DHEA) and hydroxy-methyl butyrate (HMB). As the short- and long-term effects of these substances on the immature athlete are not known, caution should be used before recommending these products to young athletes (Eichner et al. 1999).

Some ingredients in these products may also be banned and could result in a positive drug test (especially DHEA and androstenedione, which may have steroid-like anabolic properties). To date, creatine seems relatively safe (see Chapter 17), however, as water is transported into the muscles with creatine, large doses may be a hazard in the heat—especially if young athletes take up to 86 g/d of creatine (Eichner et al. 1999). Product purity and quality is also a concern because, in most countries, quality control tests are not necessarily conducted. It is unknown if HMB is effective in adults, and possible adverse effects are unknown. Guidelines on HMB for children and adolescents cannot be made until further research has been conducted. It would be prudent not to recommend these types of ergogenic aids to young athletes until we understand fully their mechanisms of action.

Other popular ergogenic aids, including caffeine, bicarbonate and colostrum, cannot be recommended for young athletes until further research confirms a level of associated risk and possible side-effects. In fact, it has been suggested that athletes younger than 18 years should not consume any ergogenic aid until further scientific evidence emerges as to their safety (Eichner et al. 1999). The consensus of the American College of Sports Medicine Round Table is that athletes under the age of 18 years should not consume creatine (Eichner et al. 1999). Further, the popular belief among young athletes that all supplements available at health food stores have been scientifically tested and are safe needs to be addressed (particularly since some supplements have been shown to have harmful effects) (Cowart 1992; Friedl et al. 1992). Close to one-half of the young United States athletes (48%) (n = 509) believed this to be the case (Massad et al. 1995). Information regarding ergogenic aids should be provided by a knowledgeable sports physician or sports dietitian, and not from the health-food store, magazine advertisements, the Internet or the gym (Eichner et al. 1999).

18.4 *HYDRATION AND THERMOREGULATION*

Much is known about the fluid and electrolyte requirements of adults involved in physical activity, however, there is less research about these requirements in children and adolescents. Children have less developed and, therefore, less efficient thermoregulatory mechanisms than adults (Bar-Or et al. 1980). Risks of hypothermia in cold environments and hypohydration and hyperthermia in hot environments in young athletes are higher than in adults. Thermogenesis per kilogram of body weight is greater in children than in adolescents and adults, but their ability to transfer heat from the centre of the body to the skin by blood is less effective.

18.4.1 *Hyperthermia*

The smaller the child, the greater is the excess in heat production (Bar-Or 1989). Children also have a greater surface area to body volume ratio. Thus, they are exposed to a faster influx of heat when environmental temperature exceeds skin temperature (Bar-Or et al. 1980). These factors make it more difficult to regulate body temperature.

Dissipation of heat from the body occurs through the skin by either, or a combination of, conduction, convection, radiation or evaporation. Heat is also dissipated through the lungs (Bar-Or 1989). When heat production is high in response to physical activity, the cooling effect of evaporation of sweat from the skin (an endothermic reaction) is the body's physiological mechanism for cooling (Bar-Or 1989). Unfortunately, the sweat response is less efficient in children compared with adults. Children have a lower sweat rate than adults (~2.5 times less), not due to fewer sweat glands, but due to each gland producing less sweat. Pre-pubescents rarely produce more than 400–500 mL of sweat per m^2/h, whereas adults under the same conditions can produce more than 700–800 mL of sweat per m^2/h (Bar-Or 1989). Further, the sweating threshold (the core temperature when sweating starts) appears to be higher in children than adults (Falk 1998). The sweat rate approaches adult levels early in puberty (Falk et al. 1992). Compared to adults, children dissipate less heat through evaporative sweating and more through convection (the loss of heat through the skin) plus radiation (Bar-Or 1989). This is achieved by greater vasodilation.

Children and adolescents exercising in the heat should be monitored closely for signs of heat stress. Those with high levels of body fat and heavy builds are more susceptible to heat stress because they are less efficient in dissipating body heat. It is important that children have adequate fluid consumption and that sunscreens, light-weight clothing and hats are worn when possible.

18.4.2 *Hypothermia*

It is also important for children exercising in the cold to be monitored for signs of hypothermia. Young athletes appear to be at greater risk of hypothermia than adult athletes, because in the cold children have lower skin temperatures (due to greater vasoconstriction) and a higher rate of heat loss (due to their greater surface area to mass ratio) (Smolander et al. 1992; Falk 1998). However, children have a higher metabolic rate in the cold, compared with adults, which is advantageous for heat production (Smolander et al. 1992; Falk 1998).

18.4.3 *Hypohydration*

Hypohydration refers to a reduction in body water as the body progresses from a normally hydrated (euhydrated) to a dehydrated state. Athletes who begin exercise in a hypohydrated state are likely to experience adverse effects on cardiovascular function, temperature regulation and exercise performance (Lamb & Shehata 1999). When adults undertake prolonged exercise they rarely drink enough to replenish fluid losses, even when fluid is offered to them *ad libitum* (Bar-Or & Wilk 1996). This is especially evident in hot and humid conditions. A similar pattern has been noted in young athletes (Bar-Or et al. 1980). Like adults, young athletes dehydrate progressively when left to drink *ad libitum*. However, in young adults dehydration is accompanied by a faster rise in core temperature than in adults (Bar-Or et al. 1980; Bar-Or & Wilk 1996; Thompson 1998). The reasons for this are unclear, but may be due to lower cardiac output and lower evaporative cooling capacity in children (Bar-Or 1989).

18.4.3.1 *Fluid replacement*

Maintaining adequate hydration is crucial for the prevention of heat stress. Thirst is a late indicator of low hydration status; in fact, when thirst is apparent, dehydration has already begun and may be well advanced. Sports Medicine Australia (1997) have made recommendations for fluid intake for active children and adolescents (see Table 18.4).

Table 18.4 *Sports Medicine Australia guidelines for fluid replacement (water) for children and adolescents* (Sports Medicine Australia 1997)*

Age (yr)	Time (min)	Volume* (mL)
Approx 15	45 (before exercise)	300–400
	20 (during exercise)	150–200
	As soon as possible after exercise	Liberal until urination
Approx 10	45 (before exercise)	150–200
	20 (during exercise)	75–100
	As soon as possible after exercise	Liberal until urination

* In hot environments, fluid intake may need to be more frequent

The guidelines in Table 18.4 may need to be reviewed to reflect the popular use of (or change in attitude towards) CHO–electrolyte fluids (i.e. sports drinks). Sports Dietitians Australia (1998) has issued a consensus statement for fluid replacement. Although it is tailored for adult athletes, the principles of type of beverage, frequency of intake and timing (including drinking pre-exercise, during exercise, and post-exercise for recovery) can be applied to young athletes (see Chapter 14, Section 14.8, and Chapters 13 and 15).

While water is often described as the best choice of fluid, there are situations when drinks containing CHO are more appropriate. Studies on voluntary drinking habits and flavour preferences in children and adolescents suggest that greater consumption occurs when flavoured drinks or sports drinks are offered instead of water (Meyer et al. 1994). During the voluntary rehydration stage, children (aged 9–13 years) who were drinking fluids other than water not only recovered from dehydration but drank enough to increase their body weights above normal (Meyer et al. 1994). Flavour preferences in these children were grape and orange compared with apple. While Canadian children of Caucasian descent tend to prefer grape flavour, children of other cultural backgrounds in other climates may prefer other flavours (Bar-Or & Wilk 1996). Therefore, to encourage adequate hydration practices, children's taste preferences need to be catered for by offering them a variety of different flavoured drinks. While the above study showed adequate consumption of fluid post-exercise, other junior athletes had insufficient fluid intakes during physical activity (Iuliano et al. 1998).

Although children's sweat contains less sodium and chloride than adults' (Meyer et al. 1992), there appears to be no evidence that children's performance improves when given sugary beverages (soft drink, cordial, sports drinks) more diluted than those dilutions currently recommended for adults. More information is needed to identify the optimal electrolyte and CHO content for sports drinks that will specifically meet the needs of young athletes (Bar-Or 1995). In the interim, similar dilutions (~4–8%) to those recommended for adults are used before, during and after training. A guideline for young athletes is to drink periodically 'until you're not thirsty any more, and then another few gulps' (Bar-Or 1995). For a child younger than 10 years, Bar-Or (1995) suggests half a glass (100–125 mL) beyond thirst and for an older child or adolescent a full glass (200–250 mL) beyond thirst.

18.4.3.2 *Dehydration and competition*

Deliberate hypohydration is often practised to achieve weight goals. Rapid weight reduction through deliberate dehydration (e.g. through fluid restriction, diuretic and laxative abuse, excessive sweating in saunas or exercising in plastic clothes, or vomiting) may be practised by young athletes, who compete in weight category sports (e.g. wrestling, weight lifting and sports with specific body-weight demands). It is known that dehydration severely affects performance and can lead to disturbances in thermoregulation, cardiac output, renal function, and electrolyte balance. Hypohydration practices are not recommended at any age because of the adverse consequences of dehydration.

18.5 *FOOD HABITS*

Data on food consumption behaviour and influences on food choice in children and adolescent athletes is scarce. Most information about food consumption attitudes and behaviour of adolescents comes from selected studies of non-athletic groups. In national dietary surveys of children in Australia, a decrease in reported consumption of total energy and many nutrients occurred in girls but not in boys in early adolescence (English et al. 1987; McLennan & Podger 1997). In contrast, adolescent boys increased energy and nutrient intakes at levels comparable with their increased requirements (English et al. 1987). Several studies suggest that adolescent girls involved in elite or recreational sports also reported similar or even lower energy intakes compared to population data, despite extra energy requirements needed to support training programs (see Chapter 6, Section 6.4.2.3 and Table 6.1).

Adolescents, generally, have eating habits distinct from children and adults. Adolescents are regular breakfast eaters with 78.9% of 12–15-year-olds and 67.6% of 16–18-year-olds eating breakfast five or more times per week (McLennan & Podger 1997). With increasing age, however, there is an apparent increase in the number of breakfast skippers, particularly with girls (McLennan & Podger 1997).

Children and young adolescents rely heavily on snacking, which contributes substantially to the nutrient density of their daily intakes. Data from the 1995 NNS of Australia indicated that 63.2% of young adolescents aged 12–15 years ate five to six times per day. Older adolescents snacked less often, with only 47.8% of 16–18-year-olds snacking this frequently, and only 37% snacking between two to four times per day. Boys ate the most frequently, with 20% of 16–18-year-olds eating seven or more times a day compared with only 7% of girls. Forty-four per cent of girls at this age ate only two to four times per day compared with only 3% of boys (McLennan & Podger 1997).

Food consumption patterns from the Australian NNS indicated that cereals and cereal products were the major source of energy for adolescents. Males tended to eat larger quantities than females and had a higher mean daily intake of food from all food groups, with the exception of fruit (McLennan & Podger 1997). In another study, adolescent girls were more likely to try to eat well, had better nutrition knowledge and ate fewer high-fat and sugary foods as well as more fruits and vegetables than boys (Nowak & Speare 1996). Older children were more likely to obtain and consume food and beverages away from home. Take-away and other pre-prepared foods formed a larger proportion of their diet than they did for younger children (McLennan & Podger 1997).

In educating and counselling young athletes, it is important to understand their eating habits and attitudes and factors that influence their food choices. Table 18.5 summarises the main factors influencing food choices of adolescents. Convenience and time considerations are major influences, as adolescents want foods that are easy to access, easy to carry and require little preparation time. Taste and appearance are also priorities (Neumark-Sztainer et al. 1999).

As is the case with adults, emotional factors affect eating habits of children and adolescents. Nowak and Speare (1996) found that half the boys (n = 412, 12–15 years) in their study and two thirds of the girls (n = 379, 12–15 years) sometimes ate from boredom. One in four children reported eating more when depressed. Attitudes also have an impact on food choice and eating patterns. In another study of 791 year-eight students in Australia, more than 65% believed that the food they ate was important, and more than 80% felt food was important for health (Nowak & Speare 1996). Adolescents recognise the importance of food in the prevention of future illness, but attach more importance on the relationship between nutrition and appearance (Nowak & Crawford 1998). Gender differences also start to become apparent during adolescence, with girls more concerned about the nutritional content of foods than boys (Nowak & Speare 1996).

Table 18.5	Factors affecting adolescent food choice
Hunger	Parental influence
Food cravings	Health beliefs
Appeal of food	Mood
Time considerations	Body image
Convenience	Habit
Food availability	Cost
Peer influence	Media

Adapted from Neumark-Sztainer et al. 1999

18.6 PERCEPTION OF BODY IMAGE

Body image is an important issue for many adolescents (Gibbons et al. 1995; O'Dea 1995). With the physical and emotional changes that occur with pubertal maturation, a self-consciousness about the body is accentuated (Baum 1998). Concerns about body image start early in both boys and girls. The adolescent male is vulnerable to pressure to attain a masculine muscular physique (the perceived ideal body image) (McKay Parks & Read 1997), while female adolescents prefer to be small and lean and thin (O'Dea 1995).

These concerns about body image often translate to poor eating practices and disordered eating (O'Dea 1995; Neumark-Sztainer et al. 1999). As many as 63% of girls and 16% of boys had dieted at least once, and many claimed to have used extreme dieting methods (Gibbons et al. 1995). For adolescent athletes, although body-image concerns dominate, other factors also contribute to the development of disordered eating patterns. These include: pressure to optimise performance; pressure to meet unrealistic body-weight and fat goals; societal expectations; and established norms for certain sports, which may influence athletes to attain a certain body shape (Van de Loo & Johnson 1995).

In addition, athletes who are not overweight often seek to lose weight and resort to weight-loss techniques that can have deleterious effects on their health and performance. For instance, of 487 female elite swimmers aged 9–18 years, 60.5% of those who were of average weight and 17.9% of those underweight reported trying to lose weight (Van de Loo & Johnson 1995). The swimmers used various methods of weight loss, including skipping meals (62%), eating smaller meals (77%), vomiting (12.7%), using laxatives (2.5%) and using diuretics (1.5%) (Van de Loo & Johnson 1995).

18.7 SOURCES OF NUTRITION INFORMATION FOR ADOLESCENTS

Adolescents appear to obtain the majority of their food and nutrition information from parents, television and the school environment. There is a significant gender difference in information sources derived from their parents and their friends. Twice as many girls as boys obtained nutrition information from magazines, and five times more girls than boys obtain their weight-loss information from magazines (Nowak & Speare 1996). Teachers and doctors were twice as likely to be information sources than dietitians (Nowak & Speare 1996). Therefore, it is important that these sources of information are reliable. Athletes are unlikely to be different from their non-athletic peers in their sources of nutrition information except that coaches, sports dietitians and other athletes also have a major influence on athletes' attitudes and food behaviour.

Healthy eating habits should be promoted early in life, as the habits acquired and established in childhood are more likely to persist in later life (National Health & Medical Research Council 1995; Tuttle & Truswell 1998; Koivisto Hursti 1999). Parents, carers, siblings, peers and coaches act as role models and are the main influences of young children's food choices (Thompson 1995; Koivisto Hursti 1999).

18.8 SUMMARY

Children and adolescent athletes may enhance sporting performance by ensuring that their nutrition complements their training schedules and growth requirements. No specific dietary recommendation for energy, protein, CHO and fat for children of different ages and stage of maturation participating in different sports have been published. Population dietary goals and targets for children and adolescents serve as guidelines for nutrient and energy intakes. Since young athletes expend more energy than their less active peers, their nutrition needs are slightly higher, especially with respect to energy and CHO, but should still fit within recommended daily allowances. Further research needs to be conducted to determine definitive minimum nutrient intakes that would be estimated to meet the nutrient requirements for young athletes involved in elite sports. Further studies are needed to determine protein needs, glycogen resynthesis rates, fat requirements and specific energy needs in children and adolescent athletes.

Micronutrient intake in young athletes appears to be varied, with sub-optimal intakes for calcium, iron and zinc often well below daily recommended allowances for both athlete and non-athlete populations. Young athletes who severely restrict their energy intake (for example, gymnasts and ballet dancers) are those at greatest risk of inadequate intakes of these micronutrients and delaying onset of maturation and growth. Long-term energy deprivation may be irreversible, although to date it is not possible to detect an individual's susceptibility to permanent effects. Sports dietitians should ensure that these at-risk athletes have well-balanced, nutrient-dense diets and are not in chronic negative energy balance. In most cases, specific vitamin and/or mineral supplements should not be recommended routinely for young athletes, without a clinical diagnosis of depletion or deficiency. Emphasis should be placed on obtaining nutritional requirements from food before advocating the use of vitamin and/or mineral supplements.

Ergogenic aids are probably not suitable because of the unknown efficacy, mechanisms of action and potential long-term harmful effects in this age group.

Since children and adolescents are at increased risk of developing heat stress during exercise, practising appropriate prevention strategies, including fluid replacement during training, is essential. Deliberate dehydration to 'make weight' should be actively discouraged. During hot weather, modifications to training sessions or competitions may be required, or in some situations cancellation may be more appropriate.

External pressure placed on young athletes to conform to stringent body weights and body-fat levels is a concern. The importance of understanding the food habits and factors that influence the dietary practices of adolescent athletes cannot be underestimated. Ideally, improved nutrition knowledge, understanding and practice will result in better sporting performance and recovery as well as better overall health. The nutritional requirements of young athletes have largely been ignored in the scientific literature. With advancing technology and increased political interest in developing young athletes from an early age, specific guidelines for nutrient intakes for young athletes may be developed. It is important to remember that sports dietitians need to be concerned not only with the implications of diet for optimal sporting performance, but also for the growth and maturation and short- and long-term health outcomes of the young athlete. A team approach to management of the young athletes is important—the athlete, parent, coach, dietitian and other members of the health-care team should work together to ensure the young athlete has the best possible care.

18.9 *PRACTICE TIPS*

Kylie Andrew

Getting started

- Children and adolescents are generally unaware of the role of diet in enhancing athletic performance. It can not be assumed that their nutrition knowledge is at any particular level, as they may know very little or be misinformed.

- Children and adolescents should be encouraged at an early age by parents and coaches to adopt healthy dietary practices so that adequate nutritional requirements for growth, maturation and sporting performance are attained. It is easier to establish healthy habits during childhood than later in life.

- Children and adolescents don't usually present to a dietitian of their own accord. If brought in by parents or coaches they often hide their true feeling for fear of being judged or reprimanded. Follow-up sessions on a one-to-one basis without a parent or coach present make it easier to build rapport and assess the problem from the athlete's perspective.

Assessment

- Growth should be assessed at regular intervals. Anthropometric measures including height, weight, skinfolds and circumferences are used. Evaluation is best based on relative changes in these variables in the individual, although comparison with population growth charts are useful in children. Any substantial change in skinfolds or deviation from the normal growth curve should be evaluated and the reasons for these changes should be investigated. For example, illness, an increase or decrease in training intensity, and physiological, medical or psychological problems can alter food intake. The outcome could potentially be growth retardation or a delay in maturation. Pubertal stage and bone age can also be used to assess growth and maturation and should be assessed annually in high risk athletes.

- Investigation of all forms of physical activity undertaken by the young athlete is important to determine an estimate of energy expenditure as well as lifestyle issues. Young athletes are often involved in many different sports including school, club and national or representative sport. Sports involvement varies considerably between seasons.

- Diet history is the usual method for assessing dietary intakes in young athletes in a clinical situation. This method quickly reveals if there are erratic or inconsistent eating patterns and gives a comprehensive insight into lifestyle, health and social issues affecting food behaviour. Alternatively, for those young athletes who are erratic eaters, food records can be used. Food records, however, require extensive training and substantially distort usual eating behaviour (see Chapter 3), but at least provide a starting point, especially for those who are vague or forgetful. Food intake checklists and 24-hour recalls of food are useful for young athletes as they provide a window into eating habits. Short-term recall techniques are likely to be more accurate and revealing about food and lifestyle habits than food records for this age group.

- A thorough assessment also includes gathering information about medical history, medication and supplement usage and dosage (including use of sports products and foods), relevant information on who shops and prepares meals, and the family situation. This information is important in planning and educating young athletes on dietary strategies. Young athletes may have trouble remembering the names of the supplements they take (or are given) so it is worthwhile requesting to see all supplements. Some may be banned and others may have adverse side-effects if misused (see Chapter 12 and Chapter

17). Refer to the Australian Drug Advisory Service for a handbook of banned medications (ASDA 1998).

- Young athletes, especially adolescent girls, are at high risk of iron depletion and deficiency. Blood counts and iron status screening are routinely conducted on elite athletes in sports institutes and national squads as preventive measures. Such tests may be warranted in any young athlete with symptoms of fatigue and lethargy who habitually consumes a poor quality diet (see Chapter 11).

- Any cessation of menses for more than three months should be cause for concern, and referred to a sports physician for further assessment.

- Alcohol intakes by adolescents are of concern in the general population, and young athletes, especially those involved in team sports, are likely to be exposed to alcohol and to peer pressure to consume alcohol at an early age, even under-age.

- Changes in eating behaviour frequently occur during competition and need to be assessed at interview.

- Asking an athlete to define their sporting, weight and nutrition goals (if any) helps you to provide effective behavioural strategies that are specific to the individual's attitudes and beliefs.

Counselling and education

- Repeated advice or regular practical information sessions about how to choose food in different situations and the reasons these choices are made, are effective in young athletes. Communal cooking nights have also been popular with young athletes in teams and have been used extensively as an education vector at the Australian Institute of Sport and state institutes of sport around Australia. Guidelines for organising cooking sessions are found in Chapter 26. Use of appropriate language and an understanding of the differences in the eating habits and culture between girls and boys at different ages is invaluable in conducting these sessions and in individual counselling. Dietary strategies and suggestions for change need to be realistic and acceptable. Lunch boxes at high school are 'not cool'.

- Education of other members in the family, particularly the person responsible for cooking, helps improve compliance, and promotes permanent changes in habits and food choices in children. Cooking nights for parents of young athletes are also welcomed as an opportunity for a social event for the parent and a platform for the dietitian to address key concerns and issues.

- Most young athletes, especially adolescents, are focussed on their body image and weight. A counselling approach that emphasises sporting performance, but also recognises and addresses the importance of weight and body image issues, even at very young ages, is critical. Children and adolescents are likely to be more receptive to your advice.

- A positive approach and positive reinforcement is recommended when counselling children and adolescents. Praise for changes made, rather than constant criticism about existing poor practices, and policing food intake have better results.

- Children should be encouraged to take some responsibility for their food choices and eating behaviour. It is well accepted that children can influence parents' food choice and change food purchasing patterns of their parents. Food providers, parents and coaches should be discouraged from dictating what children (and adolescents) should and shouldn't be eating. Self-reliance should be encouraged; athletes seem to benefit from direct involvement in assessing their own diets, identifying problems, setting goals and developing their own strategies.

Meeting nutritional needs

- Specific recommendations for energy requirements in young athletes do not exist and there appears to be a large variation in young athletes' energy intakes that is specific to age, sport and gender. Therefore, each child or adolescent athlete needs to be treated as an individual and monitored closely to see that their energy intake matches their needs.

- Chronic negative energy balance is contraindicated in young athletes and, if prolonged, increases the risk of short stature, delayed puberty, menstrual irregularities, poor bone health, increased incidence of injuries and risk of developing eating disorders. At-risk athletes, including gymnasts, dancers and distance runners, whose sports place an emphasis on being lean, should be regularly assessed.

- To meet energy and nutrient needs, children and adolescents need to eat at least three nutritious meals per day in addition to between-meal snacks (preferably low in fat). Providing specific examples of suitable between-meal snacks that are convenient, portable and accessible to their living or education environment is essential, including appropriate food choices at school canteens or local take-away shops. Suggesting that high-fat, sugary foods should be avoided is too restrictive and promotes cravings for these foods. If large quantities of these foods that particularly appeal to adolescents and children (e.g. soft drink, ice-cream, confectionery, crisps and hot chips) are consumed every day or in place of meals and a well balanced diet, some limitations need to be implemented.

- For children with high energy needs, who find it difficult to maintain energy balance, food high in energy but low in bulk may be required. These include white breads and cereal products, dried and stewed fruits, high-energy muesli and fruit bars, smoothies and milkshakes. Adding extra sugar to foods is a better alternative than fat to help increase energy intakes. In contrast, for children and adolescent athletes who put on weight easily and usually need to follow lower energy intakes, ensure that they are not in chronic negative energy balance and that their diet meets daily nutrient recommendations.

- Protein recommendations are easily met in a mixed diet, but may be a problem with vegetarians, especially those avoiding dairy products.

- Currently there are no published specific recommendations for CHO intakes to support training and recovery (glycogen resynthesis) in young athletes. This age group is generally too young to participate in the sort of events that require CHO loading. If energy requirements are met, an every-day training diet providing 55% of energy intake from CHO (the same recommendation for adult athletes) is likely to be adequate to support training and recovery. A higher relative CHO intake, mainly from consuming lots of bread and cereals that are high in fibre and phytates, may make it difficult to meet energy needs and decrease mineral absorption (see Chapter 11).

- Tips for increasing CHO intakes include:
  — base all meals on CHO-rich foods;
  — snack on high-CHO foods between meals;
  — pack CHO-rich foods to take to school and training;
  — enjoy a high-CHO recovery snack as soon as possible after training; and
  — make use of CHO-containing fluids such as sports drinks, milk smoothies and fruit juices.

- The following tips for improving dental hygiene should be encouraged:
  — brush and floss teeth frequently;
  — drink high-CHO drinks from a squeeze bottle or use a straw;
  — drink plenty of milk and other casein-containing foods;
  — drink water after eating between meals to rinse the mouth;
  — chew sugar-free gum; and
  — drink fluids chilled.

- Practical suggestions for low-fat snack foods and take-aways should also be provided.

- Currently RDIs/RDAs can be used for young athletes. Children and adolescents should be encouraged to include at least three to four serves of calcium-rich dairy products in their daily diet or equivalent in other foods rich in calcium. Supplements may be warranted in those who are lactose intolerant or are allergic to or dislike milk and milk products.

- Early detection and intervention of iron depletion is important to prevent the Strategies to increase iron intakes and bioavailability are outlined in Chapter 11.

- Indiscriminate use of vitamin supplements should be discouraged, although they may be necessary in some situations, such as for vegetarians, amenorrheic athletes, iron deficient athletes and those on restricted-energy diets.

- Ergogenic aids are not recommended for young athletes as the efficacy and safety of these products have not been investigated in children.

Fluid

- Young athletes often begin training after school already hypohydrated. A guideline for young athletes is to drink periodically 'until you're not thirsty any more, and then another few gulps' (Bar-Or 1995). For a child younger than ten years old, Bar-Or (1995) suggests half a glass (100–125 mL) beyond thirst; and for an older child or adolescent, a full glass (200–250 mL) beyond thirst. Weighing before and after training determines the extent of fluid loss. As a crude guideline 500 g of weight lost is equivalent to 500 mL fluid.

- Water, diluted fruit juice (by 50%) or very dilute cordial are suitable beverages during training and competition. Sports drinks are suitable for children and adolescent athletes. Usually flavoured drinks encourage greater fluid consumption.

- Guidelines for the pre-competition meal, eating between events and recovery should be provided. Young athletes are reticent to try new foods and eat in strange environments when travelling away from home for competition. A supply of familiar foods packed for such emergencies is good advice and well received.

- Eating immediately or as soon as possible after training and competition (especially when competing on consecutive days or more than once in the one day) facilitates recovery.

Follow-up

- A series of consultations are usually needed. One visit is insufficient to fully develop a rapport and influence change in food choice. Any behavioural change is a learned response and needs encouragement and support. Shorter, more frequent consultations provide the opportunity to do this, as the concentration spans of children and adolescents may be short, and information retention may not be as good as that of adults.

- Children and adolescents respond well to take-home tasks or activities, such as keeping a fluid balance chart or using a CHO counter to calculate intake. This helps them focus their goals and practise suggested strategies, as well as providing encouragement and positive reinforcement.

Multidisciplinary approach

- A multidisciplinary, team approach has advantages in clinical counselling and education of young athletes. Other members of the medical team, including the sports physician and psychologist, may be involved, and regular communication is essential for the best management of the athlete to occur. Coaches are often present at the interview and can either inhibit or enhance communication. It is important that coaches are informed and kept involved, as they are also an important member of the support team. When counselling and educating children and adolescents, parental involvement is essential for support but should not interfere with your communication with the individual athlete.

Specific issues

- Where there is evidence of an eating disorder, a multidisciplinary approach is essential.

- Rapid weight loss is discouraged. Weight maintenance or gradual weight loss (where required) is recommended. Both the child and parents need to understand the dangers of rapid weight loss. Regular monitoring is essential.

- Children and adolescents who have difficulty maintaining their weight may find commercial liquid meal supplements, such as Sustagen Sport™, useful to help meet their energy needs.

- Young athletes wanting to bulk-up should be encouraged to eat five to six meals per day high in CHO with adequate protein. They will also benefit from energy-dense snacks, high-energy milkshakes and smoothies made with fortified milk (a mixture of skim milk powder and regular milk) and high-energy supplements like sports drinks, bars and liquid meal supplements.

- Vegetarian athletes should be educated about the at-risk nutrients when following a vegetarian diet and should be taught how to meet these nutrient needs.

- Fussy eaters should be encouraged to try new foods. Lists of new foods to try can be made up at each consultation and checked at the next consultation. The child or adolescent should be involved in deciding what foods to try. A list can then be constructed of what foods they like and added to as new ones are discovered.

REFERENCES

Alaimo K, McDowell M, Briefel R, et al. Dietary intake of vitamins, minerals, and fiber of persons ages 2 months and over in the United States. Third National Health and Nutrition Examination Survey, Phase 1, 1988–1991. Adv Data 1994;14:1–28.

American Dietetic Association. Position of the American Dietetic Association: oral health and nutrition. J Am Diet Assoc 1996a;96:184–9.

American Dietetic Association. Position of the American Dietetic Association: vitamin and mineral supplementation. J Am Diet Assoc 1996b;96:73–7.

American Dietetic Association. Timely statement of the American Dietetic Association: nutrition guidance for adolescent athletes in organised sports. J Am Diet Assoc 1996c;96:611–12.

American Dietetic Association. Timely statement of the American Dietetic Association: nutrition guidance for child athletes in organised sports. J Am Diet Assoc 1996d;96:610–11.

American Heart Association. Dietary recommendations: fighting heart disease and stroke. http//www.deliciousdecisions.org/ee/wbd_easy_main.html 1998.

Astrand P. Experimental studies of physical working capacity in relation to sex and age. Copenhagen: Munskgaard, 1952.

Bachrach LK, Katzman DK, Litt IF, Guido D, Marcus R. Recovery from osteopenia in adolescent girls with anorexia nervosa. J Clin Endocrinol Metab 1991;72:602–6.

Bailey DA, Wedge JH, McCulloch RG, Martin AD, Bernhardson SC. Epidemiology of fractures of the distal end of the radius in children as associated with growth. J Bone Joint Surg 1989;71A:1225–31.

Bar-Or O. Temperature regulation during exercise in children and adolescents. In: Gisolfi C, Lamb D, eds. Perspectives in exercise science and sports medicine: youth, exercise and sport. Indianapolis: Benchmark Press, 1989:335–67.

Bar-Or O. The young athlete: some physiological considerations. J Sports Sci 1995;13:S31–S3.

Bar-Or O. Personal communication—regarding nutritional requirements for young athletes, 1999.

Bar-Or O, Barr S, Bergeron M, et al. Youth in sport: nutritional needs. Sports Science Exchange Roundtable 1997;8:4.

Bar-Or O, Daton R, Inbar O, Rotshtein A, Zonder H. Voluntary hypohydration in 10–12 year-old boys. J App Phys 1980;48:104–8.

Bar-Or O, Unnithan V. Nutritional requirements of young soccer players. J Sports Sci 1994;12:S39–S42.

Bar-Or O, Wilk B. Water and electrolyte replenishment in the exercising child. Int J Sport Nutr 1996;6:93–9.

Bass S, Bradney M, Pearce G, et al. Short stature and delayed puberty in gymnasts: influence of selection bias on leg length and the duration of training on trunk length. J Paediatrics 2000;136:149–55.

Bass S, Delmas PD, Pearce G, et al. The differing tempo of growth in bone size, mass and density in girls is region-specific. J Clin Invest 1999;104:795–804.

Bass S, Pearce G, Bradney M, et al. Exercise before puberty may confer residual benefits in bone density in adulthood: studies in active prepubertal and retired female gymnasts. J Bone Miner Res 1998;13:500–7.

Baum A. Young females in the athletic arena. Child and Adolescent Psychiatric Clinics of North America 1998;7:745–55.

Benardot D, Schwarz M, Weitzenfeld-Heller D. Nutrient intake in young, highly competitive gymnasts. J Am Diet Assoc 1989;89:401–3.

Benson J, Allemann Y, Thientz G, Howald H. Eating problems and calorie intake levels in Swiss adolescent athletes. Int J Sports Med 1990;11:249–52.

Benson J, Gillian D, Bourdet K, Loosli A. Inadequate nutrition and chronic calorie restriction in adolescent ballerinas. Phys Sports Med 1985;13:79–90.

Bergstrom E, Hernell O, Lonnerdal B, Persson L. Sex differences in iron stores of adolescents: what is normal? J Ped Gastroenterol Nutr 1995;20:215–24.

Blethen SL, Gaines S, Weldon V. Comparisons of predicted and adult height in short boys: effect of androgen therapy. Pediatr Rev 1984;18:467–9.

Blimkie CJR, Lefevre J, Beunen GP, et al. Fractures, physical activity, and growth velocity in adolescent Belgian boys. Med Sci Sports Exerc 1993;25:801–8.

Boersma B, Rikken B, Wit JM. Catch-up growth in early treated patients with growth hormone deficiency. Arch Dis Child 1995;72:427–31.

Borer KT. The effects of exercise on growth. Sports Med 1995;20:375–97.

Borms J. The child and exercise: an overview. J Sports Sci 1986;4:3–20.

Bourguignon JP. Linear growth as a function of age at onset of puberty and sex steroid dosage: therapeutic implications. Endoc Rev 1988;9:467–88.

Brookes-Gunn J, Warren MP. Mother–daughter differences in menarcheal age in adolescent girls attending national dance company schools and non-dancers. Ann Human Biol 1988;15:35–43.

Brooks-Gunn J, Warren MP, Hamilton LH. The relation of eating problems and amenorrhoea in ballet dancers. Med Sci Sports Exerc 1987;19:41–4.

Buckler JM. A longitudinal study of adolescent growth. London: Springer-Verlag, 1990.

Burke L. Dietary CHOs. In: Maughan R, ed. IOC encyclopaedia of sports medicine: nutrition in sports. Chapter 5. Oxford: Blackwell Science, 1998.

Caine D, Cochrane B, Caine C, Zemper E. An epidemiological investigation of injuries affecting young competitive female gymnasts. Am J Sports Med 1989;17:811–20.

Caine D, Lewis R, O'Connor P, Howe W. The effect of diet and intensive training on the growth and maturation of female gymnasts. 2000 (in review).

Caine D, Roy S, Singer K, Broekhoff J. Stress changes of the distal radial growth plate: a radiographic survey and review of the literature. Am J Sports Med 1992;20:290–8.

Cara JF. Growth hormone in adolescence, normal and abnormal. Endocrine and metabolic clinics of North America 1993;22:533–53.

Cobiac L, Dreosti I, Baghurst K. Australia's RDIs and those of other countries: should we harmonise? In: Draft background and discussion paper (4). Canberra: CSIRO Division of Human Nutrition, for the Commonwealth Department of Health and Family Services, 1997.

Constantini NW, Brautber C, Manny N, et al. Differences in growth and maturation in twin althletes. Med Sci Sports Exerc 1997;29:S150.

Cooper C, Cawley M, Bhalla A, et al. Childhood growth, physical activity, and peak bone mass in women. J Bone Miner Res 1995;10:940–7.

Costill D. CHOs for exercise: dietary demands for optimal performance. Int J Sports Med 1988;9:1–18.

Cowart V. Dietary supplements: alternatives to anabolic steroids? Phys Sports Med 1992;20:189–98.

Daniels J. Differences and changes in VO_2 among runners 10–18 years of age. Med Sci Sports Exerc 1978;10:200–3.

Davies PSW, Feng JY, Crisp JA, et al. Total energy expenditure and physical activity in young chinese gymnasts. Pediatric Exer Sci 1997;9:243–52.

Dawson EB, Albers J, McGarrity W. Serum zinc changes due to iron supplementation in teenage pregnancy. Am J Clin Nutr 1989;50:848–52.

Delamarche P, Monnier M, Gratas-Delamarche A, et al. Glucose and free fatty acid utilisation during prolonged exercise in prepubertal boys in relation to catecholamine responses. Eur J Appl Physiol 1992;65:66–72.

Eichner E, King D, Myhal M, Prentice B, Ziegenfuss T. Muscle builder supplements. Sports Science Exchange Roundtable 1999;10:1–5.

English R, Cahsel K, Lewis J, Waters A, Bennett S. National dietary survey of school children (aged 10–15 years): 1985. No. 2: Nutrient intakes. Canberra: Australian Government Publishing Service, 1987.

Falk B. Effects of thermal stress during rest and exercise in the pediatric population. Sports Med 1998;25:221–40.

Falk B, Bar-Or O, Calvert R, MacDougall J. Sweat gland response to exercise in the heat among pre-, mid-, and late-pubertal boys. Med Sci Sports Exerc 1992;24:313–19.

Faulkner RA, Bailey DA, Drinkwater DT, et al. Regional and total body bone mineral content, bone mineral density, and total body tissue composition in children 8–16 years of age. Calcif Tissue Int 1993;53:7–12.

Fournier P-E, Rizzoli R, Slosman D-O, Theintz G, Bonjour J-P. Asynchrony between the rates of standing height gain and bone mass accumulation during puberty. Osteoporosis Int 1997;7:525–32.

Friedl KE, Moore RJ, Marchitelli LJ. Steroid replacers: let the athlete beware. NSCA J 1992;14:14–19.

Frisch RE, Gotz-Welbergen AV, McArthur JW, et al. Delayed menarche and amenorrhoea of college athletes in relation to age of onset of training. JAMA 1981;246:1559–63.

Georgopoulos N, Markou K, Theodoropoulou A, et al. Growth and pubertal development in elite female rhythmic gymnasts. J Clin Endocrinol Metab 1999;84:4525–30.

Gertner JM. Childhood and adolescence. In: Favus MJ, ed. Primer on the metabolic bone diseases and disorders of mineral metabolism. Philadelphia: Lippincott, Williams & Wilkins, 1999:45–9.

Gibbons K, Wertheim E, Paxton S, Petrovich J, Szmukler G. Nutrient intake of adolescents and its relationship to desire for thinness, weight loss behaviours, and bulimic tendencies. Aust J Nutr Diet 1995;52:69–74.

Girandola R, Wuiswell R, Frisch F, Wood K. Metabolic differences during exercise in pre- and post-pubescent girls. Med Sci Sports Exerc 1981;13:110–12.

Gluckman PD. Foetal growth: an endocrine perspective. Acta Paediatr Scand 1989;349(suppl):21–5.

Gluckman PD. The endocrine regulation of foetal growth in late gestation: the role of insulin-like growth factors. J Clin Endocrinol Metab 1996;80:1047–50.

Gordon C, Halton J, Atkinson S, Webber C. The contribution of growth and puberty to peak bone mass. Growth Dev Aging 1991;55:257–62.

Greulich WW, Pyle SI. Radiographic atlas of skeletal development of the hand and wrist, 2nd edn. Palo Alto, CA: Stanford University Press, 1959.

Grimston SK, Ensberg JR, Kloiber R. Menstrual, calcium, and training history: relationship to bone health in female runners. Clin Sports Med 1990;2:119–28.

Guilland J, Penaranda T, Gallet C, et al. Vitamin status of young athletes including the effects of supplementation. Med Sci Sports Exerc 1989;21:441–9.

Haymes E. Vitamin and mineral supplementation to athletes. Int J Sport Nutr 1991;1:146–69.

Haymes E, Buskirk E, Hodgson J, Lundergren H, Nicholas W. Heat tolerance of exercising lean and heavy prepubertal girls. J App Phys 1974;36:566–71.

Iuliano S, Naughton G, Collier G, Carlson J. Examination of the self-selected fluid intake practices by junior athletes during a simulated duathlon event. Int J Sport Nutr 1998;8:10–23.

Jahreis G. Influence of intensive exercise on insulin-like growth factor I, thyroid and steroid hormones in female gymnasts. Growth Regulation 1991;1:95–9.

Karlberg J. On the construction of the infancy–childhood–puberty growth standard. Acta Paediatr Scand 1989a;356(suppl):26–37.

Karlberg J. A biologically-oriented mathematical model (ICP) for human growth. Acta Paediatr 1989b;350(suppl):70–94.

Karlberg J. The infancy-childhood growth spurt. Acta Paediatr Scand 1990;367(suppl):111–18.

Katzman D, Bachrach L, Carter D, Marcus R. Clinical and anthropometric correlates of bone mineral acquisition in healthy adolescent girls. J Clin Endocrinol Metab 1991;73:1332–9.

Keen AD, Drinkwater BL. Irreversible bone loss in former amenorrheic athletes. Osteoporosis Int 1997;7:311–15.

Koivisto Hursti U. Factors influencing children's food choice. Ann Med 1999;31(suppl1):26–32.

Kopp-Woodroffe S, Manore M, Dueck C, Skinner J, Matt K. Energy and nutrient status of amenorrheic athletes participating in a diet and exercise training intervention program. Int J Sport Nutr 1999;9:70–88.

Largo RH. Catch-up growth during adolescence. Horm Res 1993;39(suppl3):41–8.

Laron Z. Paediatric endocrinology. Oxford: Blackwell Scientific Publications, 1969.

Laron Z, Arie B, Dende S. Endocrinology 1963;72:470–5.

Laron Z, Klinger B. Does intensive sport endanger normal growth and development? New York: Serono Symposia Publications from Raven Press Book Ltd, 1989.

Lemon PW. Effects of exercise on dietary protein requirements. Int J Sport Nutr 1998;8:426–47.

Lindholm C, Hagenfeldt K, Ringertz BM. Pubertal development in elite juvenile gymnasts: effects of physical training. Acta Obstet Gynecol Scand 1994;73:269–73.

Lindholm C, Hagenfeldt K, Ringertz H. Bone mineral content of young female former gymnasts. Acta Paediatr 1995;84:1109–12.

Loosli A, Benson J, Gillien D, Bourdet K. Nutritional habits and knowledge in competitive adolescent female gymnasts. Phys Sports Med 1986;14:118–30.

MacDoughall J, Roche P, Bar-Or O, Moroz J. Oxygen cost of running in children of different ages: maximal aerobic power of Canadian school children. Can J Appl Sports Sci 1979;4(abs):237.

Macek M, Vavra J. Prolonged exercise in 14-year-old girls. Int J Sports Med 1981;2:228–30.

Maffulli N, King JB. Effects of physical activity on some parts of the skeletal system. Sports Med 1992;13:393–407.

Malina RM. Physical growth and biological maturation of young athletes. Ex Sport Sci Rev 1994;22:389–433.

Malina RM. Growth, maturation and performance. In: Exercise and sport science. Garrett W, Kirkendall DT, eds. Philadelphia: Lippincott, Williams & Wilkins, 2000.

Malina RM, Bouchard C. Growth, maturation and physical activity. Champaign, Illinois: Human Kinetics, 1991.

Malina RM, Ryan RC, Bonci CM. Age at menarche in athletes and their mothers and sisters. Ann Human Biol 1994;21:417–22.

Mandelbaum BR, Bartolozzi AR, Davis CA, Teurlings L, Bragonier B. Wrist pain syndrome in the gymnast. Am J Sports Med 1989;15:305–17.

Mansfield JM, Emans SJ. Editor's Column: Growth in female gymnastics: should training decrease during puberty? J Paediatrics 1993;122:237–40.

Maresh MM. Linear growth of long bones of extremities from infancy through adolescence. Am J Dis Child 1955;89:725–42.

Marshall WA. Puberty. New York: Plenum Press, 1978.

Martinez L, Haymes E. Substrate utilization during treadmill running in prepubertal girls and women. Med Sci Sports Exerc 1992;24:975–83.

Massad S, Shier N, Koceja D, Ellis N. High school athletes and nutritional supplements: a study of knowledge and use. Int J Sport Nutr 1995;5:232–45.

McKay Parks P, Read M. Adolescent male athletes: body image, diet and exercise. Adol 1997;32:593–602.

McLennan W, Podger A, eds. National Nutrition Survey, selected highlights, Australia 1995. ABS Catalogue No. 4802.0. Canberra: Australian Bureau of Statistics and the Department of Health and Family Services, 1997.

Meeussen R, Borms J. Gymnastic injuries. Sports Med 1992;13:337–56.

Meyer F, Bar-Or O, MacDougall D, Heigenhauser G. Sweat electrolyte loss during exercise in the heat: effects of gender and maturation. Med Sci Sports Exerc 1992;24:776–81.

Meyer F, Bar-Or O, Salsberg A, Passe D. Hypohydration during exercise in children: effect on thirst, drink preferences and rehydration. Int J Sport Nutr 1994;4:22–35.

Micheli LJ. Overuse injuries in children's sports: the growth factor. Orthop Clin North Am 1983;14:337–60.

Micklesfield LK, Reyneke L, Fataar A, Myburgh KH. Long-term restoration of deficits in bone mineral density is inadequate in premenopausal women with prior menstrual irregularity. Clin J Sports Med 1998;8:155–3.

Milesovic A. Sports drinks hazard to teeth. Br J Sports Med 1997;31:28–30.

Moen S, Sanborn C, Dimarco N. Dietary habits and body composition in adolescent female runners. Women in Sport and Physical Activity Journal 1992;1:85–95.

Moffatt R. Dietary status of elite female high school gymnasts: inadequacy of vitamin and mineral intake. J Am Diet Assoc 1984;84:1361–3.

Mosier HD, Jr. The control of catch-up growth. Acta Endocrinology (Copenh) 1986;113:1–8.

Mosier HD. Set point for target size in catch-up growth: auxology 88. In: Tanner JM, ed. Perspectives in the science of growth and development. London: Smith-Gordon, 1989:343–51.

Murray R, Drummond B. Are there risks to dental health with frequent use of CHO foods and beverages? Aust J Nutr Diet 1996;53(suppl4):S47.

National Health & Medical Research Council. Dietary guidelines for children and adolescents. Canberra: Australian Government Publishing Service, 1995:85–96, 61–6, 103–10.

Neinstein LS. Menstrual dysfunction in pathological states. West J Med 1985;143:476–84.

Neumark-Sztainer D, Story M, Perry C, Casey M. Factors influencing food choices of adolescents: findings from focus-group discussions with adolescents. J Am Diet Assoc 1999;99:929–34, 937.

Nickerson H, Holubets M, Weiler B, et al. Causes of iron deficiency in adolescent athletes. J Pediatr 1989;114:657–63.

Niewoehner CB. Endocrine pathophysiology. Connecticut: Fence Creek Publishing, 1998.

Nowak M, Crawford D. Getting the message across: adolescents' health and concerns and views about the importance of food. Aust J Nutr Diet 1998;55:3–8.

Nowak M, Speare R. Gender differences in food-related concerns, beliefs and behaviours of North Queensland adolescents. J Paediatr Child Health 1996;32:424–7.

O'Connor H. Special needs: children and adolescents in sport. In: Burke L, Deakin V, eds. Clinical sports nutrition. Sydney: McGraw-Hill, 1994:390–414.

O'Dea J. Body image and nutritional status among adolescents and adults—a review of the literature. Aust J Nutr Diet 1995;52:56–67.

Oski F. The nonhematologic manifestations of iron deficiency. Am J Dis Child 1979;133:315–22.

Peltenburg AI, Erich WBM, Zonderland MJE, et al. A retrospective growth study of female gymnasts and girl swimmers. Int J Sports Med 1984;5:262–7.

Perron M, Endres J. Knowledge, attitudes, and dietary practices of female athletes. J Am Diet Assoc 1985;85:573–6.

Prader A. Pubertal growth. Acta Paediatr J 1992;34:222–35.

Prasad A, Miale A, Farid A, Sandstead H, Schulert A. Biochemical studies of dwarfism, hypogonadism and anemia. Arch Intern Med 1963;111:426–30.

Preece M. The development of skeletal sex differences at adolescence. In: Russo P, Gass G, eds. Human adaptation: a workshop on growth and physical activity. Sydney: Department of Biological Sciences, Cumberland College of Health Sciences, 1982:1–13.

Preece MA, Ratcliffe SG. Auxological aspects of male and female puberty. Acta Paediatr 1992;383(suppl):11–13.

Pugliese MT, Lifshitz F, Grad G, et al. Fear of obesity: a cause of short stature and delayed puberty. N Eng J Med 1983;309:513–18.

Rankinen T, Fogelholm M, Kujala U, Rauramaa R, Uusitupa M. Dietary intake and nutritional status of athletic and non-athletic children in early puberty. Int J Sport Nutr 1995;5:136–50.

Rees JM. Management of obesity in adolescence. Med Clin North Am 1990;74:1275–92.

Rees M. Menarche when and why? Lancet 1993;342:1375–6.

Riddell M. Personal communication—substrate utilisation and CHO requirements of young athletes, 1999.

Robinson TL, Snow-Harter C, Taaffee DR, et al. Gymnasts exhibit higher bone mass than runners despite similar prevalence of amenorrhoea and oligomenorrhoea. J Bone Miner Res 1995;10:26–35.

Roche AF. The final phase of growth in stature. Growth, genetics and hormones 1989;5:4–6.

Roche AF, Chumlea WC, Thissen D. Assessing the skeletal maturation of the hand-wrist: Fels method. Springfield, Illinois: Charles C Thomas, 1988.

Roche AF, Davila GH. Late adolescent growth in stature. Pediatrics 1972;50:874–80.

Rogol AD. Growth and growth hormone secretion at puberty in males. In: Blimkie CJR, Bar-Or O. New Horizons in pediatric exercise science. Australia: Human Kinetics, 1995:53.

Rowland T. Iron deficiency in the young athlete. Sports Med 1990;37:1153–63.

Rowland TW. The 'trigger hypothesis' for aerobic trainability: a 14-year follow-up. Pediatr Exerc Science 1997;9:1–9.

Rowland T, Black S, Kelleher J. Iron deficiency in adolescent endurance athletes. J Adol Health Care 1987;8:322–6.

Sandstead H. Requirement of zinc in human subjects. J Am Coll Nutr 1985;4:73–82.

Sank L. Dental nutrition. Nutrition Issues and Abstracts 1999;19:1–2.

Siimes M, Addiego J, Dallman P. Ferritin in serum: diagnosis of iron deficiency and iron overload in infants and children. Blood 1974;43:581–90.

Sirota L. Vitamin and mineral toxicities: issues related to supplementation practices of athletes. J Health Ed 1994;25:82–8.

Smith DW, Truog W, Rogers JE, et al. Shifting linear growth during infancy: illustration of genetic factors in growth from foetal life through infancy. J Paediatrics 1976;89:225–30.

Smith WJ, Underwood L, Clemmons D. Effects of caloric or protein restriction on insulin-like growth factor-1 (IGF-1) and IGF-1 binding proteins in children and adults. J Clin Endocrinol Metab 1995;80:443–9.

Smolander J, Bar-Or O, Korhonen O, Ilmarinen J. Thermoregulation during rest and exercise in the cold in pre- and early pubescent boys and in young men. J App Phys 1992;72:1589-94.

Sobal J, Marquart L. Vitamin/mineral supplement use among high school athletes. Adol 1994;29:835–43.

Sports Dietitians Australia. Consensus statement on fluid and energy replacement for exercise and sports activities. Victoria: Sports Dietitians Australia, 1998:1–3.

Sports Medicine Australia. Safety guidelines for children in sport and recreation. Canberra: Sports Medicine Australia, 1997.

Steen S, McKinney S. Nutrition assessment of college wrestlers. Phys Sports Med 1986;14:100–16.

Swissa-Sivan A, Simkin A, Leichter I, et al. Effect of swimming on bone growth and development in young rats. Bone Miner 1989;7:91–105.

Tanner JM. Growth at adolescence. London: Blackwell Scientific Publications and Springfield Thomas, 1962.

Tanner JM, Whitehouse RH, Marshall WA, et al. Assessment of skeletal maturity and prediction of adult height. London: Academic Press, 1975.

Tanner JM, Whitehouse RH, et al. Assessment of skeletal maturity and prediction of adult height, 2nd edn. New York: Academic Press, 1983.

Tarnopolsky M. Personal communication—protein requirements and young athletes, 1999.

Theintz G, Howald H, Weiss U, Sizonenko P. Evidence for a reduction of growth potential in adolescent female gymnasts. J Paediatrics 1993;122:306–13.

Theintz GE. Endocrine adaptation to intensive physical training during growth. Clin Endocrinol 1994;41:267–72.

Thompson JL. Energy balance in young athletes. Int J Sport Nutr 1998;8:160–74.

Thompson S. A healthy start for kids: building good eating patterns for life. Sydney: Simon & Schuster, 1995.

Tonz O, Stronski SM, Gmeiner CYK. Wachstum und Pubertat be 7-bis 16 jahrigen Kunstturnerinnen: eine prospektive studie. Schweiz Med Wochenschr 1990;120:10–19.

Tuttle C, Truswell S. Childhood and adolescence. In: Mann J, Truswell S. Essentials of human nutrition. Oxford: Oxford University Press, 1998:481–90.

Tveit-Milligan P, Spindler AA, Nichols JE. Genes and gymnastics: a case study of triplets. Sports Med Training Rehab 1993;4:47–52.

Van de Loo D, Johnson M. The young female athlete. Clin Sport Med 1995;14:687–707.

Van den Brande JL. Catch-up growth: possible mechanisms. Acta Endocrinol (Copenh) 1986;113:13–24.

Van Erp-Baart M, Fredrix L, Binkhorst RA, et al. Energy intake and energy expenditure in top female gymnasts. In: Binkhorst RA, Kemper HCG, Saris WMH, eds. Children and Exercise. Champaign, Illinois: Human Kinetics, 1985:218–23.

Warren MP. The effects of exercise and pubertal progression and reproductive function in girls. J Clin Endocrinol Metab 1980;51:1150–7.

Warren M. The effects of under-nutrition on reproductive function in the human. Endocr Rev 1983;1983:4.

Warren MP, Brooks-Gunn J. Delayed menarche in athletes: the role of low energy intake and eating disorders and their relation to bone density. New York: Serona Symposia Publications from Raven Books Ltd, 1989.

Warren MP, Stiehl AL. Exercise and female adolescents: effects on the reproductive and skeletal systems. J Am Med Ass 1999;53:115–20.

Wiita B, Stomabaugh I. Nutrition knowledge, eating practices and health of adolescent female runners: a 3-year longtitudinal study. Int J Sport Nutr 1996;6:414–25.

Wollmann HA, Ranke MB. GH treatment in neonates. Acta Paediatr 1996;85:398–400.

World Health Organisation. Energy and protein requirements. Switzerland: World Health Organisation, 1985.

Zonderland ML, Claessons AL, Lefevre J, et al. Delayed growth and decreased energy intake in female gymnasts. In: Armstrong N, Kirby B. Welsman J. Children and Exercise XIX. London: E & FN Spon, 1997:533–6.

Nutrition and the ageing athlete

Peter Reaburn

19.1 INTRODUCTION

During the last two decades there has been an enormous increase in the number of older individuals engaging in regular exercise for the health benefits of decreasing all-cause mortality and increasing physiologic functioning (Blair & Brodney 1999). Many of these ageing individuals are now becoming recreational or competitive athletes and are focussed on performance. For example, in the late 1980s, 44 Australian sporting organisations had introduced a masters (veterans, seniors, golden oldies) component (Burns 1992). At the beginning of the new millennium, over 70 Australian sporting organisations now cater for the ageing athlete, with many conducting state and national championships and at least 30 hosting world championships and forming their own international federations (Burns 1999).

Recommendations for nutrition in ageing athletes should focus on both the nutritional requirements of the ageing process and the nutrient needs for exercising. However, individuals age at greatly differing rates for genetic, environmental, lifestyle and cultural reasons. Furthermore, ageing athletes participate in sports ranging from lawn bowls to ironman triathlon. These ageing athletes participating in organised masters sport range from the physically dependent to the physically elite and participate for a wide variety of reasons including health, personal challenge, recreation, competition, social and public recognition (Fontane & Hurd 1992; Newton & Fry 1998). Compared to younger athletes, ageing athletes display an age-related decline in training intensity and volume (Walter et al. 1988; Kavanagh & Shephard 1990; Reaburn et al. 1995). Moreover, they may only display functional fitness levels equal to those of non-athletes who live independently

(Shaulis et al. 1996) with many not undertaking any physical training prior to competing in organised sport (Farquharson 1990; Reaburn et al. 1995; Shaulis et al. 1996). For the health professional, consideration of these factors is further complicated by the fact that 85% of the elderly population suffers from some type of chronic degenerative disease requiring medication(s) that may have potential drug-nutrient interactions. Such interaction may affect the intake, digestion, absorption, and utilisation of several nutrients (Jette & Branch 1981; Laukkanen et al. 1997). Indeed, a number of reports have suggested that between 14% and 25% of participants in masters sport have a pre-existing medical condition (primarily hypertension, asthma, coronary heart disease), with up to 34% taking medication (cardiovascular, respiratory, non-steroidal anti-inflammatory) (Farquharson 1990; Reaburn et al. 1995). Thus, the motivations, training practices, chronic illness and medication usage patterns, and variety of sports or activities participated in by ageing athletes, make generic guidelines for nutrition in this group a challenge for the health practitioner.

The ageing process, at least in sedentary individuals, is accompanied by many physiological changes that affect nutritional needs. These include loss of muscle mass, less efficient immune system, gastric atrophy, decreased sensitivity to taste and smell, poor dental health, a loss of thirst sensitivity, decreased cardiovascular health, and decreased bone density. Whether these declines are the result of the ageing process *per se* or the inactivity that accompanies the ageing process remains to be conclusively evaluated. However, a number of empirical studies appear to suggest that a number of these factors do decline with age, even in ageing athletes. For example, several studies have shown that muscle mass declines with age in ageing endurance athletes (Klitgaard et al. 1990; Proctor & Joyner 1997), even in those with a lifetime of involvement in sprint and power events (Reaburn 1994). Furthermore, bone mineral density in postmenopausal athletic women has been shown to be lower than in younger athletic women (Nelson et al. 1991). Thus, the health practitioner must be aware that ageing athletes present with a wide range of motivations, training backgrounds, physiology, medical conditions and dietary practices that must be considered together when giving individualised advice.

Recommended Dietary Allowances (RDAs) and Recommended Dietary Intakes (RDIs) define 'the level of intake of essential nutrients that, on the basis of scientific knowledge, are judged by the Food and Nutrition Board to be adequate to meet the known nutrient needs of practically all healthy persons' (National Research Council 1989). However, the data used to determine RDAs/RDIs often did not include athletes or active individuals young or old. Furthermore, the oldest age group for which many recommendations have only recently been developed is 51 to 70 years and, for only several nutrients, greater than 70 years (Institute of Medicine and Food and Nutrition Board 1998; Yates et al. 1998). These age ranges are very large and make little allowance for the metabolic and physiological changes that occur during these years or the activity levels or health status of ageing individuals. Thus, the RDA/RDI may not be a valid means of evaluating the nutritional needs of the ageing athlete in physical training on a regular basis.

A number of previous review papers have been written on nutritional recommendations for an exercising older population (Evans 1992; Kendrick et al. 1994; Evans 1996; Evans & Cyr-Campbell 1997; Sachek & Roubenoff 1999). Furthermore, several investigations have examined the dietary practices of various ageing athletic populations (Rock 1991; Butterworth et al. 1993; Hallfrisch et al. 1994; Sykes 1994; Chatard et al. 1998; Maharam et al. 1999). However, no review to date has examined the nutritional needs of an ageing athletic population. Thus, the purpose of the present chapter is to not only synthesise the available literature examining nutritional practices of the older athlete, but to extrapolate data from studies completed on younger athletes or older sedentary populations in order to make recommendations on the dietary needs of an ageing athletic individual.

19.2 *PHYSIOLOGICAL CHANGES IN AGEING ATHLETES*

A number of physiological changes occur in the ageing athlete that may affect not only training and competition performance, but nutritional recommendations. While it is beyond the scope of this review to examine these changes in detail, Table 19.1 summarises the major changes that may affect the nutritional requirements of ageing athletes. Further reading in the area of ageing athletes can be found by referring to the following papers: Kavanagh & Shephard 1990; Reaburn et al. 1995; Trappe et al. 1996; Pollock et al. 1997; Maharam et al. 1999.

19.3 *ENERGY REQUIREMENTS OF AGEING ATHLETES*

The most important factor that determines energy intake is energy expenditure, even in an ageing population (Durnin 1985). Several longitudinal and cross-sectional studies, including the *Baltimore Longitudinal Study of Ageing*, have suggested that the daily energy requirements of an ageing population decrease due to a decrease in both energy expenditure for physical activity and resting metabolism (Shock 1984; Horber et al. 1996; McLennan & Podger 1998).

An age-related decrease in daily energy expenditure, at least in non-athletes, is primarily due to both age-related decreases in fat-free mass (FFM) and decreases in physical activity levels (Flynn et al. 1992; Rising et al. 1994; Starling et al. 1999). Current RDAs/RDIs suggest that older individuals (> 51 years) have a mean daily energy expenditure, and hence energy requirement, of 1.51 times the resting energy expenditure, which is equal to 9.6 MJ/d (2300 kcal/d) for males and 7.9 MJ/d (1900 kcal/d) for females (National Research Council 1989). However, research evidence from sedentary populations suggests that body composition (fat mass versus FFM) changes dramatically with ageing with an approximate doubling of body fat between 20 and 50–60 years of age and a fall in body fat after 70 years of age

Table 19.1 *Major age-related changes that may influence nutrient requirements of ageing athletes*

Age-related change	Nutritional implication
Decreased muscle mass	Decreased energy requirements
Decreased aerobic capacity	Decreased energy requirements
Decreased muscle glycogen stores	Decreased energy requirements
Decreased bone density	Increased need for calcium and vitamin D
Decreased immune function	Increased need for vitamins B6, E and zinc
Decreased gastric acid	Increased need for vitamin B12, folic acid, calcium, iron and zinc
Decreased skin capacity for cholecalciferol synthesis	Increased need for vitamin D
Decreased calcium bioavailability	Increased need for calcium and vitamin D
Decreased hepatic uptake of retinol	Decreased need for vitamin A
Decreased efficiency in metabolic use of pyridoxal	Increased need for vitamin B6
Increased oxidative stress status	Increased need for carotenoids, vitamins C and E
Increased levels of homocysteine	Increased need for folate and vitamins B6 and B12
Decreased thirst perception	Increased fluid needs
Decreased kidney function	Increased fluid needs

(Steen 1988; Shimokata et al. 1989; Going et al. 1994). Similar observations of decreased FFM are also observed in older male and female endurance runners except that the body fat levels only increase marginally with age (Pollock et al. 1987; Kohrt et al. 1992). These data suggest that the current RDAs/RDIs need to be updated to account for these significant changes in body composition that influence the nutritional requirements of an ageing population. In support of this suggestion, recent methods of measuring energy expenditure, including the doubly-labelled water method, have suggested that the present RDAs/RDIs for older persons are too low except in persons 75 years of age or greater (Pannemans & Westerterp 1995; Roberts & Dallal 1998).

Athletes of all ages require energy to maintain normal metabolic functioning and provide substrates for working muscles when training or competing. Physical training (aerobic and/or resistance training) has been shown to effectively increase energy requirements and maintain metabolically active muscle mass in healthy, previously sedentary ageing individuals (Fiatarone et al. 1993; Campbell et al. 1994).

A number of studies examining the energy intakes of older athletes suggested that older athletes undertaking regular physical training have higher energy intakes than those of age-matched sedentary but healthy controls (Butterworth et al. 1993; Hall-frisch et al. 1994). Furthermore, a number of these studies have also found that the energy intakes of these older athletes are higher than those suggested for their respective age groups or gender in the RDAs/RDIs (Butterworth et al. 1993; Hall-frisch et al. 1994; Chatard et al. 1998). For example, energy intakes ranging between 10 336 kJ/d (Hallfrisch et al. 1994) and 11 549 kJ/d (Chatard et al. 1998) have been reported by older (55–75 years) male endurance athletes, with a mean intake of 8663 kJ/d reported by 65–84-year-old female endurance athletes undertaking physical training of at least one hour per day (Butterworth et al. 1993).

The reported energy intakes of older athletes are lower than those observed in similarly-trained younger athletes (van Erp-Baart et al. 1989; Burke et al. 1991; Hawley et al. 1995; Niekamp & Baer 1995). This may be due to an age-related decrease in active muscle mass previously observed in ageing athletes (Klitgaard et al. 1990; Reaburn 1994; Proctor & Joyner 1997), reduced training volumes (frequency, intensity, duration) that has previously been observed in older athletes (Walter et al. 1988; Kavanagh & Shephard 1990; Reaburn et al. 1995), or reduced leisure time activity levels commonly reported in older populations (McLennan & Podger 1998).

19.4 MACRONUTRIENTS

Carbohydrate (CHO), fat and protein intakes are essential for meeting not only the energy requirements of an individual, but to ensure normal bodily functioning through the associated intake of fibre, vitamins and minerals. Age-related decreases in the intakes of these macronutrients have been observed in a sedentary ageing population (Flynn et al. 1992; Ruiz-Torres et al. 1995). However, to the author's knowledge, no studies on ageing athletes have compared the percentage contributions of these macronutrients to those of younger, similarly trained athletes. The purpose of the following section is to examine the evidence available on the macronutrient nutritional needs of ageing athletes.

19.4.1 Carbohydrate

Nutritionally, CHOs have numerous physiological functions within the body, including energy provision, effects on satiety and gastric emptying, effects on blood glucose and insulin metabolism, effects on protein glycosylation, short-chain fatty acid production, and effects on bowel activity (WHO 1997). Importantly for athletes, CHO is the primary fuel source for working muscles and is stored within the liver and muscle as glycogen (Wilmore & Costill 1999). During high intensity or prolonged endurance exercise, low muscle glycogen levels have been linked to exhaustion (Gollnick et al. 1974).

In older endurance athletes, glycogen storage per unit of muscle is lower than in similarly trained younger runners, while glycogen utilisation per unit of energy expenditure is higher during sub-maximal exercise (Meredith et al. 1989). However, following regular endurance training, older individuals are able to increase muscle glycogen storage and restore glycogen stores post-exercise at rates similar to younger athletes (Meredith et al. 1989; Tarnopolsky et al. 1997). Previous studies have also observed that healthy, previously sedentary older individuals who undertake aerobic exercise training are able to improve glucose tolerance, the rate of insulin-mediated glucose disposal, and increase skeletal muscle glucose transporter (GLUT-4) activity (Seals et al. 1984; Hughes et al. 1993; Kirwan et al. 1993).

The recommended CHO intake for athletes is similar to that of the general population, and therefore is similar for older athletes since CHO absorption and utilisation remains intact with ageing (Saltzman & Russell 1998). Thus, the older athlete should consume at least 55% of caloric intake as CHO obtained from a variety of food sources and the bulk of the CHO-containing foods consumed should be those rich in complex CHOs and with a low glycaemic index (FAO 1998). A high percentage of this intake should be starchy CHO (bread, cereals, rice, pasta, potato) which also provides protein, vitamin, mineral and fibre intake. However, too high a level of fibre (> 35 g/d) in these foods (e.g. wholegrain products, bran, wheatgerm) may not be advantageous to older athletes due to the associated gastrointestinal discomfort or mineral imbalances that may arise (Council on Scientific Affairs 1989).

The recently introduced *Dietary Guidelines for Older Australians* (National Health & Medical Research Council 1999) suggests to 'Eat plenty of cereals, bread and pastas' which differs from the 1992 dietary guidelines which read 'Eat plenty of breads and cereals (preferably wholegrain), vegetables (including legumes) and fruits'. For older Australians, the recommendation for fruit and vegetables has been separated and the word wholegrain removed due to problems an ageing population, including older athletes, may have with poor dentition. The revised guideline places cereals, cereal grains, cereal products and grain-based foods ahead of bread in order to highlight the lower salt content of cereals compared to most breads and emphasises cereals that are high in fibre and have a low glycaemic index. In an ageing population, a diet high in cereals and fibre is important to:

- assist with obesity prevention by increasing eating time, decreasing energy density, slowing gastric emptying rates, and affecting some gastrointestinal hormones that influence food intake (Rimm et al. 1996);
- lower the risk of developing non-insulin-dependent diabetes mellitus by helping maintain lower blood glucose, insulin and blood lipid levels through the relatively low glycaemic index of cereals and other high fibre CHOs (Salmoren et al. 1997a, 1997b);

- reduce the risk of cardiovascular disease by lowering plasma cholesterol, lowering the activity of plasminogen activator inhibitor type 1, slowing macronutrient absorption, and providing nutrients such as vitamin E and folic acid (National Heart Foundation 1997);
- play a role in cancer prevention (World Cancer Research Fund and American Institute for Cancer Research 1997);
- reduce the rates of constipation and diverticular disease (Aldoori et al. 1998);
- protect against hypertension by reducing salt intake and increasing dietary fibre and magnesium (Ascherio et al. 1996); and
- help prevent the age-related decline in immune function by increasing dietary vitamin E and zinc, both of which have been shown to enhance immune function in older adults (Duchateau et al. 1981; Meydani et al. 1990a).

Thus, apart from the physical benefits (enhanced performance and recovery) gained by a high CHO diet of 5 g/kg body mass (BM)/d (Hawley et al. 1995), an older athlete can also derive great health benefits that may lower all-cause mortality and morbidity.

19.4.2 *Fat*

Dietary fat is essential as a source of essential fatty acids, fat-soluble vitamins (A, D, E and K), and as an energy source during low intensity or prolonged exercise at below 70% of maximal aerobic power (Hurley et al. 1986; Romijn et al. 1993). The optimal daily intake of fat need only be 25–30% of kilojoule intake in both a young and older sedentary or exercising population (National Research Council 1989; National Health & Medical Research Council 1992). It appears that older populations are meeting this recommendation as the 1995 Australian National Nutrition Survey (NNS) showed that the mean per cent energy intake for persons aged 25–65 years and over was approximately 32% for males and 33% for females, with no difference between young and older groups (McLennan & Podger 1998). The consensus of scientific data suggests that saturated fats be less than 10% of kilojoule intake with no more than 10% as polyunsaturated fatty acids and 10–15% as mono-unsaturated fatty acids (National Health and Medical Research Council 1992).

An ageing population retains the ability to digest, absorb and utilise fat (Arora et al. 1989; Saltzman & Russell 1998) and older athletes appear to consume more fat relative to total energy than the recommended population targets or than healthy sedentary age-matched controls (Butterworth et al. 1993; Reaburn & Le Bon 1995; Chatard et al. 1998). This might suggest that older athletes consume greater daily energy intakes, the RDA/RDI are not specific enough for older age groups, or more likely that an older population may not be as informed about the benefits of a low-fat diet. Moreover, older athletes consuming greater than 30% of daily energy intake as fat may compromise cardiovascular health. As in younger athletes, older athletes on a low-energy diet should consume between 20–25% of daily energy intake from fat sources for more energy to be derived from CHO and protein (Economos et al. 1993). A daily energy intake containing less than 20% fat may compromise the absorption of fat-soluble vitamins (A, D, E, K) and decrease satiety between meals.

19.4.3 *Protein*

Protein is continually being degraded and synthesised within the human body so that a dietary supply of amino acids is necessary to offset protein losses. Amino acids are used in the synthesis of structural proteins (e.g. connective tissue, muscle tissue), functional proteins (e.g. enzymes, antibodies, haemoglobin), and as an energy source in the absence of adequate glucose or fatty acids (Marieb 1998).

The current United States RDA for protein for adults of all ages is 0.8 g/kg/d (National Research Council 1989) and the Australian RDI is 0.75 g/kg/d. However, Gersovitz and others (1982) examined the adequacy of the United States RDA in seven men between 71 and 99 years of age and found that supplementation with 0.8 g of egg protein per kilogram of BM per day was inadequate to maintain a positive energy balance. This suggests the RDAs/RDIs for older populations may need to be revisited.

An athlete's protein needs are even greater than those of a non-athlete because of increased use of protein during physical activity for gluconeogenesis, amino acid oxidation, and the tissue breakdown accompanying both training and competing (Tarnopolsky et al. 1988; Friedman & Lemon 1989; Meredith et al. 1989). Furthermore, within an athletic population, the Recommended Dietary Intakes for protein may vary depending upon exercise intensity, CHO availability, exercise mode, energy balance, gender, training age, timing of macronutrient intake and age (see Lemon 1998 for review).

Insufficient energy intakes are also associated with a negative nitrogen balance and protein loss, given that there is a well-defined interaction between total energy intake and protein need (Cheng et al. 1978). Moreover, increased protein requirements have been observed with high- versus low-intensity exercise (Lemon et al. 1982) and long- versus short-duration exercise (Haralambie & Berg 1976). Thus, it has been suggested that younger endurance-trained athletes in regular training consume about 1.2–1.4 g/kg BM/d (150% of current United States RDA) and young strength-trained athletes consume about 1.6–1.7 g/kg BM/d (200% of current United States RDA) (Lemon 1998).

Older endurance or power athletes may have lower protein requirements than suggested above for a number of reasons. First, the ageing process is accompanied by a decline in muscle mass in both healthy active individuals (Lexell et al. 1988; Evans & Campbell 1993) and older athletes (Klitgaard et al. 1990; Reaburn 1994; Proctor & Joyner 1997) secondary to an age-related decrease in both whole-body protein turnover and protein synthesis (Nair 1995; Morais et al. 1997). Second, older athletes appear not to train with the same intensity and/or volume as younger athletes (Walter et al. 1988; Kavanagh & Shephard 1990; Reaburn et al. 1995; Trappe et al. 1995). Third, although not conclusively investigated, there may be an age-related reduction in the absorptive capacity of the gut for amino acids and peptides (Saltzman & Russell 1998). Fourth, due to a number of underlying problems (dietary recall problems, inadequate equilibration periods or inadequate energy intakes given by researchers in nitrogen-balance studies), the protein requirements suggested in the RDIs/RDAs may have been over-estimated (Sachek & Roubenoff 1999). Taken together, the above factors suggest that older athletes may require a lower daily protein intake than those suggested above by Lemon (1998).

Thus, although the protein needs of different aged athletic populations is not considered, it has recently been suggested that ageing exercisers may require 0.8–1.0 g/kg BM/d (Sachek & Roubenoff 1999), with Evans (1995) suggesting older exercisers may require 1.0–1.25 g/kg BM/d in order to maintain or promote a positive nitrogen balance. Adjustments may have to be made for illness, chronic disease, or sub-optimal total energy intakes. This figure approximates the reported protein intakes of 1.25–1.45 g/kg BM/d observed in older athletes and regular exercisers from a variety of training backgrounds (Chatard et al. 1998; Starling et al. 1999). However, older athletes in heavy training, particularly those involved with strength and power sports, may require increased intakes (Lemon 1998) since resistance exercise increases muscle protein synthesis in both elderly and young individuals (Yarasheski et al. 1993).

Recent data suggests that exogenous amino acids may stimulate protein synthesis in an elderly male population (Volpi et al. 1998). However, other studies have observed either no anabolic effect of high-protein diets (Welle & Thornton 1998) or no relationship between protein intake (adjusted for BM and physical activity) and appendicular muscle mass. These data suggest that protein intake above the RDA/RDI is not linked to preservation of muscle mass in older populations (Starling et al. 1999).

There appear to be a number of possible negative side-effects associated with very high protein intakes in susceptible people. These include impaired kidney function, increased calcium loss and atherogenic effects. While it is acknowledged that older individuals with impaired kidney function should not consume high-protein diets (Brenner et al. 1982), there appears to be no convincing evidence that the additional nitrogen excretion that accompanies a high-protein diet cannot be handled by a normally functioning kidney (Lemon 1998). High-protein diets may also increase calcium loss (Allen et al. 1979) and therefore be hazardous for older athletes, who have an increased risk of osteoporosis. However, it appears that the observed calcium loss may be associated with use of protein supplements rather than excess dietary protein. The presence of phosphate in some protein foods can help negate the side effects. Finally, it has also been recently suggested that diets containing protein in the ranges 1.2–1.7 g/kg BM/d will not adversely affect cardiovascular health (Lemon 1998).

19.5 *MICRONUTRIENTS*

Vitamins and minerals are essential for efficient nutrient metabolism and numerous bodily functions affecting sports performance. Research has shown that a linear relationship exists between overall energy intake and vitamin and mineral intake (van Erp-Baart et al. 1989). High energy intakes are required by both younger (Burke et al. 1991; Hawley et al. 1995) and older athletes (Butterworth et al. 1993; Hallfrisch et al. 1994; Chatard et al. 1998) in order to meet the energy demands of physical training and competition. It would thus be expected that the micronutrient intake in these groups should be in excess of the RDIs/RDAs, assuming that a well-balanced diet is chosen. However, numerous studies examining the dietary practices of younger athletes have shown that dietary intakes of the minerals zinc, iron, magnesium, copper and calcium, together with the vitamins B6, B12, and D are below the RDI/RDA (Burke et al. 1991; Economos et al. 1993; Hawley et al. 1995). The few studies that have examined nutritional intakes of older endurance athletes suggest low intakes of the minerals calcium, iron, zinc, and magnesium and vitamin D, despite consuming energy intakes that were well above the RDIs/RDAs (Butterworth et al. 1993; Hallfrisch et al. 1994; Reaburn & Le Bon 1995; Chatard et al. 1998) (see Table 19.2).

Athletes, in general, have increased losses of many micronutrients, especially minerals, compared to non-athletes, as a result of losses through sweat and urine (Haymes 1989), especially during endurance activities (Lukaski 1995). When associated with low dietary intakes, the body stores of these micronutrients can be reduced (Clarkson & Haymes 1994), resulting in a deficiency state which negatively affects performance (Campbell & Anderson 1987; McDonald & Keen 1988). Furthermore, the risk of micronutrient deficiency may be higher in athletes who have very low energy intakes, or who have chronic medical conditions that may impair micronutrient absorption or utilisation.

Older athletes may be at a greater risk of micronutrient deficiencies than younger athletes. Possible reasons for this increased risk are age-related gut impairment associated with reduced nutrient absorption (Saltzmann & Russell 1998), different nutrient requirements between individuals (National Research Council 1989; National Health & Medical Research Council 1991), use of medication (Farquharson 1990; Reaburn et al. 1995), and the presence of chronic disease states (Webster 1990). The following sections examine the available evidence on dietary intakes of micronutrients in ageing athletes, and extrapolate information from studies of ageing sedentary populations to allow recommendations to be made on micronutrient needs of the ageing athlete.

Table 19.2 Summary table of studies examining dietary intakes of ageing athletes

Study sample	Age (years)		Compared to	Results
Butterworth et al. (1993)	72.5±1.8	Female endurance (n=12)	RDA	↓ Calcium (Ca) ↑ Energy intake
Butterworth et al. (1993)	72.5±1.8	Female endurance (n=12)	Age-matched Healthy controls	↑ Energy intake ↑ CHO, fat, protein ↑ Fibre ↑ Vit B6, E, folate ↑ Riboflavin, thiamin, niacin ↑ Ca, Ph, Mg, Fe, Zn, Na, K, Cu
Chatard et al. (1998)	63±4.5	Male endurance (n=18)	RDA	↓ Mg, Vit D, Ca ↑ Energy intake ↑ CHO, fat, protein ↑ Fe, vit A, B1, B12, C, E
Hallfrisch et al. (1994)	66.6±1.3	Male endurance (n=16)	Age-matched Healthy controls	↑ Energy intake ↑ CHO, protein
Reaburn & Le Bon (1995)	50.6±4.2	Male runners (n=14) Female runners (n=15)	RDA	↑ Protein (M & F), fat (M & F) ↑ Riboflavin, niacin, thiamin (M & F) ↑ Vit A, C (M & F) ↑ Na, K (M & F) ↓ Ca (F), Fe (F), Zn (M & F), Mg (M&F)

M = male, F = female, CHO = carbohydrate

19.5.1 *Vitamins*

19.5.1.1 *Vitamin A*

Vitamin A (retinol) is essential for vision, growth, maintenance of epithelial tissues and the integrity of the immune system (McArdle et al. 1999). Together with ß-carotene, vitamin A's precursor, this vitamin has been suggested as an antioxidant and thus helps prevent tissue damage and facilitate tissue repair (McArdle et al. 1999). In a healthy ageing population, the clearance of vitamin A is decreased by about 50% compared to younger adults. This suggests that the current RDIs/RDAs for retinol, of 1000 and 800 µg/d for older males and females respectively, may be too high. In support of this finding, a number of international nutritional surveys have observed both adequate dietary intakes and high serum retinol values in elderly populations (Kivela et al. 1989; Saito & Itoh 1991).

Supplementation of vitamin A may lead to vitamin A toxicity (skin peeling, headaches, vomiting) or decreased cell-mediated immune response, if consumed in large amounts (Krasinski et al. 1990; Fortes et al. 1998). Thus, ageing athletes should focus on consuming vitamin A precursors, the carotenoids from food sources, as suggested in the *Dietary Guidelines for Older Australians* (National Health & Medical Research Council 1999), to take advantage of the antioxidant and immune system benefits of vitamin A.

19.5.1.2 *Vitamin B6*

Vitamin B6 is a coenzyme involved in amino acid and glycogen metabolism. It aids in the formation of haemoglobin and myoglobin and thus plays an important role in an athlete's diet (McArdle et al. 1999). The requirement for vitamin B6 increases as the intake of protein increases because of vitamin B6's role in amino acid metabolism (Miller & Linkswiler 1967). Since vitamin B6 and protein tend to occur together in foods (meat, fish, poultry, cereals, vegetables, wholegrains), dietary adequacy of this vitamin is usually satisfactory in younger individuals eating the normal Western diet (National Research Council 1989).

The current United States RDA for vitamin B6 is 1.7 and 1.5 mg/d for elderly (> 51 years) males and females respectively, and does not differ from the recommendation for younger adults (National Research Council 1989). However, most dietary intake surveys have confirmed that the intake of vitamin B6 in elderly persons is inadequate to meet the RDIs/RDAs (Russell & Suter 1993; CSIRO 1996). Furthermore, evidence from depletion and repletion studies suggests that the amount of vitamin B6 needed to obtain balance in older persons is greater than the United States RDA (Ribaya-Mercado et al. 1991).

In an ageing population, the serum concentrations of vitamin B6 appear to decrease and there appears to be a greater amount of the vitamin needed to ensure immune system functioning in elderly individuals (Meydani et al. 1990b, 1991). Furthermore, vitamin B6 plays a crucial role in converting homocysteine to cystathionine. High levels of homocysteine are a risk factor for cardiovascular disease (Selhub et al. 1993). Thus, for health and physical performance reasons, it has recently been suggested that the RDA/RDI for vitamin B6 be increased in ageing athletes to 2.0 mg/d (Sachek & Roubenoff 1999).

19.5.1.3 *Vitamin B12*

Vitamin B12 is required for haematopoiesis and acts as a coenzyme in nucleic acid metabolism. It thus plays an important role in an athlete's diet (McArdle et al. 1999). The major dietary intakes of vitamin B12 come from red and organ meats. However, older people may eat less red meat in an attempt to keep cholesterol and fat intakes down, but in doing so they may limit their intake of B12. Moreover, strict vegetarians may not meet the RDA for vitamin B12 of 2.4 µg/d (National Research Council 1989) as B12 is only found in animal food sources. Furthermore, a 1996 Australian study by the CSIRO observed a decreased vitamin B12 intake over a five-year period in Australians with 3–10% of adult men and 10–17% of women consuming less than the RDI (CSIRO 1996).

A decrease in the overall energy intake of older athletes relative to younger athletes (Butterworth et al. 1993; Hallfrisch et al. 1994; Reaburn & Le Bon 1995; Chatard et al. 1998) might suggest a decrease in the need for thiamin and niacin. The incidence of pernicious anaemia, as a result of malabsorption and deficiency of B12, increases in ageing individuals. This type of anaemia is linked to an age-related atrophic gastritis seen in approximately 30% of those over 60 years of age (Krasinski et al. 1986) and the subsequent decrease in stomach acid and intrinsic factor secretion (Russell 1992).

Despite the suggestion that older athletes may have an increased need for vitamin B12 for haemopoiesis, the only published study to date that has examined vitamin B12 intakes in older endurance athletes on a mixed diet showed intake of this vitamin was above the French RDA (Chatard et al. 1998). However, it has been suggested that the vitamin B12 and folate requirements necessary to prevent anaemia in older persons may be less than that required to maintain low homocysteine levels necessary for cardiovascular health (Ubbbink et al. 1993). Thus, Russell and Suter (1993) have suggested that the RDA for vitamin B12 be increased in older people to 150% of the current United States RDA (2.4 µg/d) in order to prevent deficiency symptoms. Sachek and Roubenoff (1999) have recently suggested that a further increase of the RDA to 2.8 µg B12 per day may be needed for older persons undertaking regular exercise, particularly those who are vegetarians or have atrophic gastritis.

19.5.1.4 *Vitamin C*

The antioxidant properties of vitamin C play a role in the protection of connective tissue damage, enhancing tissue repair, and may, therefore, enhance recovery from physical training and competition (Jakeman & Maxwell 1993; Kanter 1998).

Moreover, vitamin C enhances iron absorption from foods and acts as a cofactor in some hydroxylation reactions such as converting dopamine to noradrenaline (McArdle et al. 1999). Importantly, for an older population more at risk of chronic disease, diets rich in antioxidants have also been linked to reduced risk of cancer, cardiovascular disease and cataracts (Frei 1991; Jacques & Chylack 1991; Simon et al. 1998). Major sources of vitamin C include citrus fruits, tomatoes, green peppers and salad greens.

At present, there is no evidence to suggest that vitamin C absorption or utilisation is impaired with ageing (Blanchard et al. 1990) or that dietary intakes in an ageing sedentary population (Garry et al. 1982) or ageing athletes (Butterworth et al. 1993; Hallfrisch et al. 1994; Reaburn & Le Bon 1995; Chatard et al. 1998) are lower than the current United States RDA of 60 mg/d. While vitamin C requirements may be increased in hot climates, by smoking cigarettes or heavy pollution, there appears to be no suggestion to encourage supplementation of vitamin C in older athletes (Russell & Suter 1993; Sachek & Roubenoff 1999). Importantly, for an older population with increased prevalences of chronic disease, megadoses of vitamin C (> 1000 mg/d) have been shown to cause side effects. Kidney stone formation, gout (in those predisposed to this disease), impairment of copper absorption, and destruction of B12 have been reported with megadoses of vitamin C (Herbert et al. 1977; Alhadeff et al. 1984). Vitamin C supplements in megadoses have also been associated with 'runners diarrhoea' (Hoyt 1980).

19.5.1.5 *Vitamin D*

Vitamin D, together with calcium, phosphorus and protein, is widely regarded as promoting growth and mineralisation of bones, as well as enhancing the absorption of calcium (McArdle et al. 1999). Importantly for athletes undertaking heavy training loads, vitamin D is also a modulator of mononuclear phagocyte and lymphocyte functioning (Manolagas et al. 1990), which is important to the body's immune response. Apart from dietary intake of vitamin D (fortified cereals and margarines, and eggs), most vitamin D is manufactured in the liver and, to a lesser extent in the kidney, by the action of UV light on a vitamin D precursor in the skin.

Adequate intakes of vitamin D appear crucial for older individuals given its importance in maintenance of bone integrity. However, there appears to be an age-related decrease in the capacity of ageing skin to synthesise vitamin D precursors (MacLaughlin & Holick 1985). Vitamin D production may also be compromised by seasonal variations in light, latitude, clothing, and sunscreens (Hollick 1995). Moreover, there appears to be an age-related reduction in the renal production of activated vitamin D3 (Tsai et al. 1984) and a decreased dietary intake and absorption of vitamin D in healthy but sedentary ageing populations (Barragry et al. 1978; Saltzmann & Russell 1998).

The United States National Research Council (1989) reported that about 75% of elderly Americans (> 51 years) met two-thirds of the RDA of 5 μg/d. Moreover, the

Australian NNS of 1995 also showed that the dietary intakes of vitamin D on the day of the survey were inadequate in ageing Australians, an observation confirmed in other studies of free-living North Americans and Europeans (Krall et al. 1989). In light of the importance of vitamin D in calcium absorption and bone mineralisation and thus osteoporosis prevention, these findings suggested that the United States RDA increase to 10 µg/d in persons over 51 years of age and 15 µg/d in those over 70 years of age (Institute of Medicine and Food and Nutrition Board 1998). Thus, vitamin D supplementation may be warranted in older persons including athletes who have difficulty meeting recommendations by dietary means or have little exposure to sunlight.

19.5.1.6 *Vitamin E*

Vitamin E is another antioxidant that has a protective role similar to vitamin C and vitamin A. Vitamin E is thought to protect tissues against lipid peroxidation that can result from prolonged or eccentric exercise (e.g. running, cycling, weight training) (Packer 1991; Rokitzki et al. 1994). Elderly populations have been shown to benefit from vitamin E supplementation through improved immune function (Meydani et al. 1990a), and reduced incidence of cataracts (Robertson et al. 1989), cancers (Knekt et al. 1991) and cardiovascular disease (Rimm et al. 1993).

No evidence of vitamin E deficiency has been observed in older athletes (Butterworth et al. 1993; Hallfrisch et al. 1994; Chatard et al. 1998), with a recent study of 18 older male endurance athletes suggesting a more than adequate intake of vitamin E (Chatard et al. 1998). The current United States RDA for vitamin E is 10 and 8 mg of tocopherol equivalents (TE) per day for males and females, respectively (National Research Council 1989). This requirement may increase with increasing intakes of polyunsaturated fat in the diet which are more susceptible to lipid peroxidation than diets higher in saturated fat.

Vitamin E is found in vegetable oils, nuts and seeds, green leafy vegetables and wheatgerm and no negative side effects have been observed with supplementation of up to and over 700 mg TE/d (Meydani et al. 1998). Sachek and Roubenoff (1999), in a recent review of nutrition for elderly exercisers, suggested that older individuals undertaking endurance training who were concerned about cardiovascular problems may consider a vitamin E supplement of 100–200 mg TE/d.

19.5.1.7 *Riboflavin*

Riboflavin or vitamin B2 is a major constituent of two flavin nucleotide coenzymes involved with energy metabolism (FAD and FMN) and as such is of importance to athletes (McArdle et al. 1999), particularly those embarking on a new training program or increasing the intensity of physical activity (Belko et al. 1983). The current United States RDA for riboflavin is 1.4 and 1.2 mg/d for elderly males and females, respectively (National Research Council 1989). In Australia, depending upon the age group concerned, 14–26% of men and 4–11% of women reported intakes of riboflavin below the RDI (CSIRO 1996). Low riboflavin intakes have been reported in countries with low dairy product consumption (Russell & Suter 1993).

Older athletes may have a greater need for riboflavin than the present RDI/RDA. A 1992 study identified that 14 older women (aged 50–67 years) undertaking an exercise program and having a riboflavin intake equal to the United States RDA, had a decrease in urinary riboflavin excretion which may be indicative of riboflavin depletion (Winters et al. 1992). Russell & Suter (1993), in their classic paper examining the vitamin needs of the elderly, suggest that the nutrient recommendation for riboflavin for older persons be the same as for younger persons (1.7 mg/d for males and 1.3 mg/d for females).

19.5.1.8 *Folate*

Folate is a coenzyme for both nucleic acid and amino acid metabolism and red blood cell formation (McArdle et al. 1999). Results from the 1995 NNS of Australians suggested that older persons consuming a Western diet are not likely to be at risk of folate deficiency (McLennan & Podger 1997). In Australia in 1995, folate was allowed to be added to some commercial foods, for example, breakfast cereal, bread and fruit juice. Folate-rich foods include nuts, seeds, dark green leafy vegetables, legumes, meats, milk products and now the fortified products. However, in older athletes with gastric atrophy so common in elderly persons (Krasinski et al. 1986), the associated decrease in stomach acid production may lead to decreased folate absorption (Rosenberg & Miller 1992). Sachek and Roubenoff (1999) have recently suggested that ageing athletes consume at least 200 µg/d of folate, as long as vitamin B12 intake is adequate, since high levels of folate can mask vitamin B12 deficiency.

19.5.2 *Minerals*

19.5.2.1 *Calcium*

Calcium is essential for neuromuscular transmission, blood coagulation, muscular contraction, and bone health (Marieb 1998). Calcium becomes even more important with ageing given that there is an age-related loss of bone minerals in both males and females as a result of bone resorption predominating over bone formation, particularly postmenopause (Arnaud 1988; Lewis & Modlesky 1998). Although weight-bearing exercise promotes bone density, older athletes who already have low bone density and poor dietary intakes of calcium are likely to be at high risk of stress fractures when undertaking repetitive impact activities (Myburgh et al. 1990). Moreover, such repetitive impact activities (e.g. running), particularly in a hot and/or humid environment, may lead to significant calcium loss via sweating (Krebs et al. 1988). Thus, calcium is an important dietary mineral in older athletes, particularly peri-menopausal/postmenopausal women, to help maintain long-term bone health.

The 1996 study by the CSIRO in Australia showed that 18–32% of men and 32–58% of women had calcium intakes below the RDI (CSIRO 1996). Ageing is accompanied by an overall decrease in calcium absorption, particularly in post-menopausal women. This decrease, together with sub-optimal calcium intakes reported in some older athletes (Butterworth et al. 1993; Reaburn & Le Bon 1995; Chatard et al. 1998), increases the requirements for calcium (see Table 19.2). This increase is reflected by the higher RDI in Australia for postmenopausal women compared to younger women.

Calcium bioavailability is also affected by atrophic gastritis, which is common in older persons as a result of decreased stomach acid decreasing the dissociation of calcium from food complexes (Eastell et al. 1991). Calcium absorption is dependent on activated vitamin D. Vitamin D status as suggested earlier, may be sub-optimal in older people (see Section 19.5.1.5). A deterioration in renal function, where active vitamin C is manufactured, has been attributed to the age-related decrease in circulating active vitamin D and thus the decreases in calcium absorption.

The RDI for calcium in Australia is 800 mg/d for males over 64 years and 1000 mg/d for females over 54 years (NHMRC 1991). In older (> 65 years) healthy females, mean calcium intakes from the Australian NNS (1995) were only 68% of the RDI (McLennan & Podger 1998), a major concern given the aetiology of osteoporosis, risks of fall fractures, and the role of calcium in bone mineralisation. In the United States, the current RDA for calcium is higher: 1200 mg/d for both men and women over 51 years of age (National Research Council 1989). However, calcium balance studies have suggested intakes of 1000 mg/d for oestrogen-treated post-menopausal females and as high as 1500 mg/d for untreated females (Heaney et al. 1978; Dawson-Hughes et al. 1990). On the other hand, the National Institute of Health Consensus Development Panel on Optimal Calcium Intake (1994) recommended 1000 mg/d for males and oestrogen-sufficient females less than 65 years of age and 1500 mg/d for males and females older than 65 years of age. It would appear prudent to suggest calcium intakes at the higher end of these recommended ranges for older athletes who lose sweat profusely, as substantial amounts of calcium can be lost through sweat (Krebs et al. 1988).

In older athletes, both exercise and calcium-enriched diets have been shown to have independent effects on bone mineral density in postmenopausal women (Nelson et al. 1991; Nelson et al. 1994; Lewis & Modlesky 1998). The majority of available evidence from studies of older athletes suggests that older persons in regular physical training are not consuming enough calcium in the diet (Butterworth et al. 1993; Reaburn & Le Bon 1995; Chatard et al. 1998) (see Table 19.2). Calcium supplements may be warranted in those people who are lactose intolerant, dislike milks and dairy products, are allergic to milk, or cannot meet these calcium requirements through other dietary means. Supplements of calcium citrate malate are better absorbed than calcium carbonate supplements in postmenopausal women with low dietary intakes of calcium and appear more effective than calcium carbonate in reducing bone demineralisation and lowering bone fracture rates (Dawson-Hughes et al. 1990; Reid et al. 1995). Indeed, it has recently been suggested that calcium supplementation (~1000 mg/d) can reduce bone loss in premenopausal and late postmenopausal women consuming 700 to 1000 mg calcium/d (see Lewis & Modlesky 1998 for review).

Kulak and Bilezikian (1998) and Anderson and others (1996) have suggested that the following strategies are major components in preventing osteoporosis in ageing men and women:

1. ensure optimal bone mass through childhood, adolescence and early adulthood;
2. ensure adequate dietary calcium and vitamin K intake throughout life;
3. high load exercise;
4. avoid tobacco and excessive alcohol;
5. avoid steroids and anticonvulsants;
6. avoid excess phosphorus consumption;
7. avoid excess dietary protein, sodium and caffeine;
8. ensure adequate calcium and vitamin D throughout the lifetime; and
9. hormone replacement therapy.

19.5.2.2 *Iron*

In athletes of any age, particularly those involved with endurance exercise, iron is an integral component of the oxygen carrying capacity of both haemoglobin in the blood and myoglobin within muscle. Moreover, iron is also found within the mitochondrial cytochrome complex and thus is crucial for aerobic metabolism (Wilmore & Costill 1999).

Iron deficiency anaemia has been shown to reduce performance capacity and maximal aerobic power in younger athletes (Celsing et al. 1986) and is commonly observed in both younger endurance athletes, particularly those who are females and vegetarians (Spodaryk et al. 1996; Chatard et al. 1998). It also appears that weight-bearing endurance athletes such as runners are more prone to iron deficiency since iron losses occur with excessive sweating (Waller & Haymes 1996), gastrointestinal bleeding (Stewart et al. 1984) and haemolysis (Hunding et al. 1981). While the iron losses of older athletes have not been examined, our unpublished observations are that the dietary intakes of older male and female endurance athletes are below the Australian RDI for Australians (Reaburn & Le Bon 1995). These observations are in contrast to the average reported iron intake of 14–15 and 11–12 mg/d in 65–80-plus-year-old males and females in the NNS in Australia in 1995 (McLennan & Podger 1997).

Although losses of iron in younger endurance athletes may be as high as 18 mg/d (Haymes & Lamanca 1989), iron losses have not been studied in older athletes undertaking similar levels of physical activity. Iron stores usually increase with ageing in both males and females (Casale et al. 1981). Older people, therefore, usually need less dietary iron than younger people. In a male sedentary older population, nutritional iron deficiency is rare and any observed anaemia is most commonly associated with chronic illness that may decrease or interfere with iron absorption (Yip & Dallman 1988). However, an Australian survey has suggested that up to 30–45% of adult females had estimated dietary intakes of iron below the RDI (CSIRO 1996). The United States RDA for both elderly males and females is 10 mg/d and should be adequate for ageing athletes adhering to the *Dietary Guidelines for Older Australians* (National Health & Medical Research Council 1999) (see Table 19.3). However, older athletes who are female and/or vegetarians involved with intense endurance running in thermally stressful environments might benefit by consuming up to 15 mg iron/d (Sachek & Roubenoff 1999).

Table 19.3 *Dietary Guidelines for Older Australians*
1. Enjoy a wide variety of nutritious foods
2. Keep active to maintain muscle strength and a healthy body weight
3. Eat plenty of vegetables (including legumes) and fruit
4. Eat plenty of cereals, breads and pastas
5. Eat a diet low in saturated fat
6. Drink adequate amounts of water and/or other fluids
7. If you drink alcohol, limit your intake
8. Choose foods low in salt and use salt sparingly
9. Include foods high in calcium
10. Use added sugars in moderation
11. Eat at least three meals every day
12. Care for your food: prepare and store it correctly

Source: National Health & Medical Research Council

19.5.2.3 *Zinc*

Dietary zinc is an important mineral in older individuals because of its role in tissue repair and immune function (Mann & Truswell 1998). Zinc is also an essential component of a large number of enzymes that synthesise and degrade CHOs, fats, proteins, and nucleic acids (Sandstrom 1997). Zinc is primarily lost through urine, faeces and sweating (Anderson et al. 1984; Couzy et al. 1990) and may be high in athletes training in hot, humid climates or environments. There is also a suggestion that zinc has a higher turnover in anaerobic exercise (Krotkiewski et al. 1982; Lukaski 1995). These investigators suggested that zinc may be required during muscular work that predominantly depends on glycolysis with a high production of lactate. This might suggest increased zinc requirements for older power athletes, team players, or endurance athletes undertaking high-intensity interval training. However, there is no evidence to suggest that the zinc balance is different between young and older populations on a similar type of diet. While there is evidence of decreased zinc absorption in elderly persons, there is evidence that zinc excretion is also diminished, thus zinc balance is better maintained (Turnland et al. 1986).

The 1995 Australian NNS revealed that the average zinc intake for older males (> 65 years) was borderline but was below the RDI of 12 mg/d for the same cohort of women (McLennan & Podger 1998). A further Australian study has observed poor dietary zinc intakes with the finding that 30–69% of Australian adults had intakes less than the RDI (CSIRO 1996). Sub-optimal dietary intakes of zinc are also reported in both younger (Economos et al. 1993; Hawley et al. 1995; Nuviala et al. 1999) and older (Reaburn & Le Bon 1995) athletes. High intake of foods containing phytates (e.g. cereals and grains) reduces the bioavailability of zinc from these and other zinc-rich foods (Solomons & Cousins 1984). Moreover, the bioavailability of zinc can be further compromised in athletes taking calcium or iron supplements with food (Wood & Zheng 1997). Thus, athletes on high-CHO diets (e.g. vegetarians), who have small amounts of meat or seafood (good sources of zinc) and are on iron or calcium supplements, may be at risk of zinc deficiency. These athletes may warrant supplementation.

In summary, zinc depletion may be a problem in an ageing population or for older endurance athletes with high sweat rates and high-CHO diets with a high phytate content (see Chapter 11, Table 11.6 for phytate content of foods). It may be of benefit to increase dietary zinc intake to 15 mg/d for both males and females in this cohort.

19.6 WATER

Fluids are lost from the body via respiratory loss, faeces, urine and sweating (McArdle et al. 1999). In young adult athletes, particularly those involved in endurance sports, sweat losses of up to 2 L/h have been reported during long-duration, high-intensity exercise in hot and humid conditions (Sawka & Pandolf 1990).

The ageing process is associated with a number of age-related changes that may make the older athlete more susceptible than younger athletes to hydration problems. First, the commonly observed decrease in total body protein leads to an age-related decrease in total body water (Schoeller 1989). Second, it appears that renal antidiuretic hormone receptors lose their efficiency, leading to increased water excretion by the kidneys (Rolls & Phillips 1990). Third, an age-related reduction in thirst sensation is caused by a decrease in osmoreceptors that are sensitive to blood concentrations of fluid-regulating hormones and electrolytes (Rolls & Phillips 1990). When older 'average, fit' males (~60 years) and younger (~20 years) males were systematically dehydrated for three hours, the older men rated themselves less thirsty, despite reducing blood volume and increasing blood osmolality to a greater extent than the younger men (Meischer & Fortney 1989). Fourth, during exercise in the heat, aged skin exhibits decreased blood flow (25–40%) due to a reduced ability to vasodilate (Kenney et al. 1990; Ho et al. 1997). Finally, there appears to be an age-related decrease in sweat production (Kenney & Fowler 1988), together with a delay in the onset of the sweat response (Silver et al. 1964; Catania et al. 1980). However, Buono (1991) reported that lifelong aerobic exercise may retard the decrease in peripheral sweat production reported in earlier studies. Taken together, these age-related changes strongly suggest that ageing athletes may have problems with heat exchange and fluid balance, and should be cautious about fluid intake during exercise, particularly during prolonged endurance exercise in thermally stressful environments.

The following fluid intake guidelines (Horswill 1998) have been suggested for both young and older athletes (American College of Sports Medicine 1996; Shirreffs et al. 1996):

- Before exercise: drink 500 mL (17 oz).
- During exercise: drink 600–1200 mL (20–40 oz) per hour with 150–300 mL (5–10 oz) every 15–20 minutes.
- After exercise: based on BM lost, drink 150% of fluid lost, to account for urine losses.

19.7 NUTRIENTS, HEALTH AND CHRONIC DISEASE

A wide variety of nutrients have been associated with a variety of diseases or health states, often with varying degrees of association. The association between nutrients, health and chronic diseases are reviewed elsewhere. (Vessby et al. 1995; Bradley & Xu 1996; Rimm et al. 1996; Giacosa et al. 1997; Halliwell 1997; Cobiac et al. 1998).

19.8 MEDICATIONS: NUTRIENT INTERACTIONS

There are many nutrient–nutrient interactions, such as the relationship between calcium intake, protein intake, vitamin D and sodium intake in the prevention or cause of osteoporosis. With up to 85% of older persons having at least one chronic medical condition (Webster 1990), the aged population uses more medications compared to younger persons. There also appears to be a high rate of chronic illness in masters athletes (primarily hypertension, asthma and coronary heart disease) and thus it is not surprising that up to 34% of masters athletes take medication (primarily cardiovascular, respiratory and non-steroidal anti-inflammatory) (Farquharson 1990; Reaburn et al. 1995). The following section provides an overview of some of the important medication–nutrient interactions that may affect the health or performance of the older athlete.

The number of medications used is an important predictor of the adverse nutrient interactions which may occur, since the number of reactions increases exponentially with the number of drugs used (Stewart & Cooper 1994). These interactions are further complicated by an age-related decrease in endocrine function, prescriptive dietary restrictions and the pathophysiologic changes that occur with ageing. While prescribing drugs with a meal is an effective means of reminding older persons to take their medication, the interaction of food and drug may not maximise ingestion of either (Thomas 1995). For example, anticholinergics may change gastrointestinal tract motility, and antacids may alter the pH within the same tract (Thomas 1995).

Certain drugs can affect nutritional status and may lead to over- or undernutrition. Table 19.4 summarises the major medication–nutrient interactions that may affect older athletes. In summary, the mechanisms by which nutritional status can be affected is by a decrease or increase in appetite, malabsorption of nutrients, stimulation of basal metabolic rate, and changes in the glycaemic level of food (Binns 1999). Given the complexity of the drug–nutrient interaction, it is important that the health professional work closely with a sports physician in maximising both nutrient and drug effectiveness.

19.9 *SUPPLEMENTATION*

It is well recognised that physically active persons eating well-balanced diets and following the recommended dietary guidelines (see Table 19.3) may not need to take vitamin supplements. Moreover, most experts agree there is little harm in taking multivitamin/multimineral capsule(s) containing the recommended quantity of each vitamin or mineral, particularly in those with marginal intakes. However, it is important to recognise that a number of negative side-effects, including adverse effects on the immune system, can present, not only by deficiencies but also excessive intakes of certain nutrients (Shephard & Shek 1998).

Athletes in physical training tend to increase food and energy intake and thus meet macronutrient and micronutrient recommendations. Moreover, vitamin and mineral supplementation appears to have no effect on performance when standard dietary guidelines for older persons, such as those in Table 19.3, are met. However, supplementation may be recommended in older athletes with low energy intakes, high energy outputs or excessive sweat losses, specific diseases affecting micronutrient requirements, a diagnosed micronutrient deficiency, or with poor dietary practices.

Research suggests that up to 60% of older persons have been reported to use supplements on a daily basis (Stewart 1989; Houston et al. 1997). It also appears that the majority of elderly supplement users are more health conscious and physically active than non-users (Kato et al. 1992; Houston et al. 1997), and that more active individuals aged 68–90 years were vitamin supplement users (Kato et al. 1992). These findings are similar to those observed in studies examining supplement use in younger athletes (van Erp-Baart et al. 1989; Sobal & Marqhart 1994).

It has recently been suggested that a daily multivitamin/mineral supplement that provides no more than 100% of the United States RDA may be recommended for

Table 19.4 Drug–nutrient interactions

Drug	Effect	Nutrients affected
Diuretics (e.g. Aldactone, Chlotoride, Lasix)	Alterations in renal tubular function	Loss of sodium, potassium and magnesium
Antipsychotic/psychoactives	Disinterest in food	Protein and calories intake reduced
Cardiac glycosides (e.g. Digoxin)	Anorexia, nausea, vomiting, disinterest in food	Protein and calories intake reduced
Anticonvulsants (e.g. Phenytoin, Dilantin, Phenobarbitone)	Induction of liver enzymes	Altered vitamin D metabolism
Salicylate (e.g. Aspirin, Voltaren, Nurofen, Orudis)	Gastrointestinal blood loss	Iron deficiency
Corticosteroids (e.g. Prednisone, Prednisolone, Cortisone)	Inhibition of calcium absorption, alterations in glucose metabolism and electrolyte imbalance	Calcium imbalance (osteoporosis), hyperglycaemia, sodium retention and potassium deficiency
Mineral oil laxatives (e.g. Agarol)	Inhibition of fat-soluble vitamin absorption	Vitamins A, D, E and K malabsorption

ageing exercisers involved in regular physical training. Furthermore, the same authors suggested that single-nutrient supplements should be limited to calcium and vitamins B6, B12, D and E, depending on an individual's risk for certain diseases and food consumption patterns (Sachek & Roubenoff 1999).

19.10 SUMMARY

Nutritional recommendations for older athletes must consider the following important factors:

1. age-related changes in physiology;
2. dietary changes that occur with exercise;
3. the type of exercise (power, endurance);
4. training volumes (frequency, intensity, duration);
5. the presence of chronic illness or disease;
6. nutrient–medication interactions; and
7. the goals of the older athlete (competitive, health and fitness or recreational).

In summary, it appears the small amount of available research examining the nutritional practices of older athletes or exercising older adults suggests the need for older athletes to monitor vitamins B6, B12, D and E and the minerals calcium, iron and zinc. Moreover, older athletes should become aware of guidelines such as the *Dietary Guidelines for Older Australians* that emphasise the need for maintaining energy balance through selection of a wide variety of foods high in vegetables (including legumes) and fruit, cereals, breads and pastas and low in saturated fat (National Health and Medical Research Council 1999). Finally, and as suggested by a number of previous investigators (Blumberg 1994; Russell 1997; Cobiac et al. 1998), it appears that it may be appropriate to revisit the available RDAs/RDIs for ageing populations to account for differing levels of physical activity, illnesses, medication usage and smaller age cohorts.

19.11 PRACTICE TIPS

Glenn Cardwell

Introduction

- Most veteran athletes are involved in sport for fun, camaraderie, socialising, fitness and the pure pleasure of being active. Some have a competitive spirit and will seek specific nutrition advice to enhance their sports performance. In many cases, they are as healthy as younger athletes, just a little slower and less flexible. Fortunately, veteran athletes are likely to be people with a greater than average interest in all aspects of their health, including their nutritional health. Generally the sports dietitian will be offering healthy eating advice, including tips to improve carbohydrate and protein intake, and tips to avoid dehydration.

Thirst and fluid intake

- There is a reduced sensation of thirst as one ages. This could result in too few fluids being consumed during and after exercise, especially in hot conditions, compromising thermoregulation. The athlete must be aware that hypohydration will severely affect performance, and they should not rely on thirst as an indication of fluid needs, especially in the recovery period. The older a person is, the older might be their ideas on fluids and sport. For example, fluids may be avoided due to an outdated belief that dehydration toughens the body or that too much fluid causes cramp. Fluid may be purposefully restricted to minimise night-time toileting (although this is probably not effective, as concentrated urine irritates the bladder and encourages frequent urination). This, in turn increases the risk of long-term hypohydration in the active person. A simple check is the colour of the urine. Pale urine suggests adequate hydration and darker coloured urine suggests inadequate fluids (although this may not be a good indication of hydration when vitamin supplements are taken as these will make the urine darker in a well-hydrated person).

- The following fluid intake guidelines have been suggested by the American College of Sports Medicine (1996) for both young and older athletes:
  1. Just before exercise: drink 500 mL (17 oz).
  2. During exercise: drink 600–1200 mL/h (20–40 oz) with 150–300 mL (5–10 oz) every 15–20 minutes.
  3. After exercise: based on body mass lost, drink 150% of fluid lost, to account for urine losses.

Bone problems

- Activity will help minimise bone loss, but the sports dietitian will also need to ensure an adequate calcium and vitamin D intake. The calcium requirement for older men is 800 mg/d and for older women 1000 mg/d (see also Chapter 10 for information on strategies to meet calcium recommendations). Vitamin D status is mainly determined by exposure to sunlight; 15–30 minutes of sunlight on the hands and face daily is enough for adequate endogenous production of vitamin D. For some people, it might be difficult to get out of the house in daylight hours, or they may live in a part of the world where there is very little daylight in winter months. In such cases, a vitamin D supplement might be suggested (7.5–10 µg/d, although 15–20 µg/d may be required in the absence of any sunlight). Good food sources of vitamin D include oily fish (e.g. tuna, sardines and mackerel), cod liver oil, liver, eggs, cheese and margarine. Some foods are fortified with vitamin D (e.g. margarine in Australia and the UK, and milk in the United States).

Older athletes with other chronic diseases

- A veteran athlete may be at a higher risk of diabetes, hyperlipidaemia, hypertension and arthritic conditions than younger athletes, because these problems increase with ageing. A medical history will reveal whether your dietary advice is influenced by concurrent medical concerns. Some people may have received outdated nutritional advice for their condition, or may avoid entire food groups in the belief that this action will forestall disease, e.g. avoiding all dairy foods to lower blood cholesterol levels.

- People with age-related conditions, such as cancer, heart disease, arthritis, failing eyesight, and short-term memory loss, may desire to seek food products and supplements claiming to alleviate symptoms. You will need to assess the value of the product, inform the client of the current thinking, then allow them to make the decision to buy the product. Much of the advice given in Chapter 17 on nutrition supplements applies in this case. (Note: The Arthritis Foundation of Australia, National Heart Foundation of Australia and cancer authorities provide advice on proven and unproven remedies.) Your advice will need to consider that some supplements may be used purely for sports performance, for example, creatine, and others (multivitamins and herbal supplements) will be for general use.

- Arthritis may make food preparation more difficult. Discuss the athlete's manual capabilities and from there discuss:
  1. Meals that can be prepared by those people with reduced dexterity and mobility.
  2. Healthy meals and snacks that can be purchased at the supermarket.
  3. Simple and nutritious meals that don't require cooking.
  4. Suitable take-away and frozen meals.
  5. Suitable home delivered meals.

- Check to see if the dentition is adequate for chewing, as a poor fit may influence food choice and possibly contribute to constipation if good sources of fibre are being deliberately avoided. The overuse of unprocessed bran is not recommended as a constipation cure as this may reduce zinc, iron and calcium absorption. Note that acidic drinks such as sports drinks, soft drinks, fruit juice and wine have the potential to cause tooth enamel erosion and tooth enamel may already be compromised in an older person.

Social factors influencing food choice in older athletes

- A veteran athlete may live alone and have very few social support systems. Discuss food preparation for one person, such as the value of making more than needed for one meal and freezing the extra serves for later. There are cookbooks with recipes for one or two people, although cooking four serves at a time and freezing the remainder may be more useful. Be aware that poor choices can be common in people living alone, especially if they have difficulty shopping, shop infrequently, or don't see nutrition as a priority.

- Veteran athletes may be overly concerned about nutrition issues and avoid too many foods in the belief that this will enhance health and longevity. Some unproven diet regimes for preventing arthritis and Alzheimer's disease can dramatically reduce the range of foods available to the athlete and possibly compromise good nutrition. Ask if, and why, any foods or food groups are being avoided and discuss the potential health implications.

Changes in taste and smell in older people

- The sensations of taste and smell diminish with age, possibly leading to a reduced appetite and loss of enjoyment of food. Loss of appetite is also common after hard exercise and can last a long time. It becomes important that energy dense foods are consumed if the appetite is diminished, e.g. nuts, peanut butter, dried fruit, avocado, milkshakes, or adding skim milk powder to foods like mashed potato. Eating with others often improves the appetite and personal interest in food. Small amounts of alcohol can also stimulate appetite, but only one or two standard drinks daily are recommended for those who enjoy alcohol.

Nutrient requirements in older people

- As a person ages, their nutrient requirements remain the same or higher, while their energy intake usually decreases. Hence, nutrient dense foods are a very important part of healthy eating, and there may be less room for 'indulgence' foods.

Guidelines for commencing exercise in older athletes

- The dietitian may be asked for exercise advice. If the athlete is starting an exercise program after previously being sedentary, recommend that they first consult their physician. General advice can be given:
  — Choose an exercise that is enjoyable and sustainable.
  — Begin at an easy level and gradually increase the effort as fitness improves.
  — Weight training with lightweights will improve muscle strength and bone density.
  — The ultimate goal is for a minimum of 30 minutes activity each day.
  — Walking and gardening are the most popular activities in older people. Weight bearing activities such as swimming, aquarobics and cycling are popular also, especially in those who are overweight or have arthritis.

- As always, treat each person as an individual. The older a person becomes, the more dissimilar they are from others in their age group, so expect a great variety of fitness levels, personal goals and nutrition knowledge.

- For the more competitive older athlete, suggest they contact their state or national sporting organisation for contacts in masters sport.

Resources

A useful booklet on nutrition in the older person is: *Eat Well for Life: A practical guide to the Dietary Guidelines for Older Australians* by the National Health and Medical Research Council, 1999. It is available free of charge through:

Mail order sales
Ausinfo
GPO Box 84
Canberra
Australian Capital Territory 2601

Ph: 1800 020 103 (extn 8654)
Fax: 02 6289 8360
Email: phd.publications@health.gov.au
Website: http://www.nhmrc.health.gov.au

REFERENCES

Aldoori W, Giovannuci EL, Rockett HRH, et al. A prospective study of dietary fibre types and symptomatic diverticular disease in men. J Nutr 1998;128:714–19.

Alhadeff L, Gualtiery CT, Lipton M. Toxic effects of water-soluble vitamins. Nutr Rev 1984;42:33–40.

Allen LH, Oddoye EA, Margen S. Protein-induced hypercalciuria: a longer term study. Am J Clin Nutr 1979;32:741–9.

American College of Sports Medicine. Position stand on exercise and fluid replacement. Med Sci Sports Exerc 1996;28:i–vii.

Anderson JJ, Rondano P, Holmes A. Roles of diet and physical activity in the prevention of osteoporosis. Scand J Rheumatol 1996;103(suppl):65–74.

Anderson RA, Polansky MM, Bryden NA. Strenuous running: acute effects on chromium, copper, zinc, and selected clinical variables in urine and serum of male runners. Biol Trace Elem Res 1984;6:327–36.

Arnaud CD. Mineral and bone homeostasis. In: Wyngaarden JB, Smith LH, Plum F, eds. Cecil textbook of medicine, 18th edn. Philadelphia: WB Saunders, 1988:1469–79.

Arora S, Kassarjian Z, Krasinski SD, et al. Effect of age on tests of intestinal and hepatic function in healthy humans. Gastroenterology 1989;96:1560–5.

Ascherio A, Hennekens D, Willett WC, et al. Prospective study of nutritional factors, blood pressure and hypertension among United States women. Hypertension 1996;27:1065–72.

Barragry JM, France MW, Corles D, et al. Intestinal choleacalciferol absorption in the elderly and in younger adults. Clin Sci 1978;55:213–20.

Belko AZ, Miller D, Haas JD, et al. Effects of exercise on riboflavin requirements of young women. Am J Clin Nutr 1983;37:509–17.

Blair SN, Brodney S. Effects of physical inactivity and obesity on morbidity and mortality: current evidence and research issues. Med Sci Sports Exerc 1999;31(suppl):S646–S62.

Blanchard J, Conrad KA, Mead RA, Garry PJ. Vitamin C disposition in young and elderly men. Am J Clin Nutr 1990;51:837–45.

Blumberg J. Nutrient requirements of the healthy elderly—should there be specific RDAs? Nutr Rev 1994;52:S15–S18.

Bradley J, Xu X. Diet, age, and the immune system. Nutr Rev 1996;54:S43–S50.

Brenner BM, Meyer TW, Hostetter TH. Dietary protein intake and the progressive nature of kidney disease: the role of hemodynamically mediated glomerular injury in the pathogenesis of progressive glomerular sclerosis in aging, renal ablation, and intrinsic renal disease. N Engl J Med 1982;307:652–9.

Buono MJ, McKenzie BK, Kasch FW. Effects of ageing and physical training on the peripheral sweat production of the human eccrine sweat gland. Age Ageing 1991;20:439–41.

Burke LM, Gollan RA, Read RS. Dietary intakes and food use of groups of elite Australian male athletes. Int J Sport Nutr 1991;1:378–94.

Burns R. Play on: report of the Masters Sport Project on mature aged sport in Australia. Canberra: Australian Sports Commission and Confederation of Australian Sport, 1992.

Burns R. Master Power. Sports Australia 1999;2:120–2.

Butterworth DE, Nieman DC, Perkins R, et al. Exercise training and nutrient intake in elderly women. J Am Diet Assoc 1993;93:653–7.

Campbell WW, Anderson RA. Effect of aerobic exercise and training on the trace minerals chromium, zinc, and copper. Sport Med 1987;4:9–18.

Campbell WW, Crim MC, Dallal GE, et al. Increased protein requirements in the elderly: new data and retrospective reassessments. Am J Clin Nutr 1994;60:501–9.

Casale G, Bonora C, Migliavacca A, et al. Serum ferritin and ageing. Age Ageing 1981;10:119–22.

Catania J, Thompson JW, Michalewski HA, et al. Comparison of sweat gland counts, electrodermal activity and habituation behavior in young and old groups of subjects. Psychophysiology 1980;17:146–52.

Celsing F, Blomstrand W, Werner B, et al. Effects of iron deficiency on endurance and muscle enzyme activity in man. Med Sci Sports Exerc 1986;18:156–61.

Charlton RW, Bothwell TH. Iron absorption. Ann Rev Med 1983;34:55–68.

Chatard JC, Boutet C, Tourny C, et al. Nutritional status and physical fitness of elderly sportsmen. Eur J Appl Physiol 1998;77:157–63.

Cheng AHR, Gomez A, Bergan JG, et al. Comparative nitrogen balance study between young and aged adults using three levels of protein intake from a combination wheat–soy–milk mixture. Am J Clin Nutr 1978;31:12.

Clarkson PM, Haymes EM. Trace mineral requirements for athletes. Int J Sport Nutr 1994;4:104–19.

Cobiac L, Dreosti I, Baghurst K. Recommended Dietary Intakes—is it time for a change? Canberra: Commonwealth Department of Health and Family Services, 1998.

Council on Scientific Affairs. Dietary fiber and health. JAMA 1989;262:542.

Couzy F, Lafargue P, Guezennec CY. Zinc metabolism in the athlete: influence of training nutrition and other factors. Int J Sports Med 1990;11:263–6.

CSIRO Division of Human Nutrition. Food and nutrition in Australia–does five years make a difference? Results from the CSIRO Australian Food and Nutrition Surveys 1988 and 1993. Adelaide: CSIRO Division of Food and Nutrition, 1996.

Dawson-Hughes B, Dallal GE, Kraall EA, et al. A controlled trial of the effect of calcium supplementation on bone density in post-menopausal women. N Engl J Med 1990;323:878–83.

Devine A, Criddle RA, Dick IM, et al. A longitudinal study of the effect of sodium and calcium intakes on regional bone density in postmenopausal women. Am J Clin Nutr 1995;62:740–5.

Duchateau J, Delespresse G, Vrigens R, et al. Beneficial effects of oral zinc supplementation on the immune response of older people. Am J Med 1981;70:1001–4.

Durnin JVGA. Energy intake, energy expenditure, and body composition in the elderly. In: Nutrition, immunity and illness in the elderly. Chandra RK, ed. New York: Pergamon, 1985:19–33.

Eastell R, Yergey AL, Vieira NE, et al. Interrelationship among vitamin D metabolism, true calcium absorption, parathyroid function, and age in women: evidence of an age-related intestinal resistance to 1-25-dihydroxyvitamin D action. J Bone Miner Res 1991;6:125–32.

Economos CD, Bortz SS, Nelson ME. Nutritional practices of elite athletes: practical recommendations. Sports Med 1993;16:381–99.

Evans WJ. Exercise, nutrition and aging. J Nutr 1992;122:796–801.

Evans WJ. Exercise, nutrition, and aging. Clin Geriatr Med 1995;11:725–34.

Evans WJ. Effects of aging and exercise on nutrition needs of the elderly. Nutr Rev 1996;54:S35–S9.

Evans WJ, Campbell WW. Sarcopenia and age-related changes in body composition and functional capacity. J Nutr 1993;123(suppl2):465–8.

Evans WJ, Cyr-Campbell D. Nutrition, exercise, and healthy aging. J Am Diet Assoc 1997;97:632–8.

FAO. Carbohydrate in human nutrition. Report of a joint FAO/WHO expert consultation. FAO Food and Nutrition Paper No. 66. Rome: FAO, 1998.

Farquharson T. Masters medicine—SA style. Report to Sports Medicine Australia, Canberra: 1990.

Fiatarone MA, O'Neill EF, Doyle ND, et al. High-intensity strength training and nutritional supplementation on physical frailty in the oldest old. J Am Geriatr Soc 1993;41:333–7.

Flynn MA, Nolph GB, Sherqood Baker A, Krause G. Aging in humans: a continuous 20-year study of physiologic and dietary parameters. J Am College Nutr 1992;11:660–72.

Fontane PE, Hurd PD. Self-perceptions of national senior Olympians. Behavior, Health, and Aging 1992;2:101–9.

Fortes C, Forastiere F, Agabiti N, et al. The effect of zinc and vitamin A supplementation on immune response in an older population. J Am Geriatr Soc 1998;46:19–26.

Frei B. Ascorbic acid protects lipids in human plasma and low-density lipoprotein against oxidative damage. Am J Clin Nutr 1991;54:S1113–S18.

Friedman JE, Lemon PW. Effect of chronic endurance exercise on retention of dietary protein. Int J Sports Med 1989;10:118–23.

Garry PJ, Goodwin JS, Hunt WC, et al. Nutritional status in a healthy elderly population: vitamin C. Am J Clin Nutr 1982;36:332–9.

Gersovitz M, Motil K, Munro HN, et al. Human protein requirements: assessment of the adequacy of the current recommended dietary allowance for protein in elderly men and women. Am J Clin Nutr 1982;35:6–14.

Giacosa A, Filiberti R, Hill MJ, Faivre J. Vitamins and cancer chemoprevention. Eur J Cancer Prev 1997;6(suppl1):S47–S54.

Going SB, Williams DP, Lohman TG, Hewitt MJ. Aging, body composition, and physical activity: a review. J Aging Phys Activ 1994;2:38–66.

Gollnick PD, Piehl K, Saltin B. Selective glycogen depletion patterns in human muscle fibers after exercise of varying intensity and at varying pedalling rates. J Physiol (London) 1974;241:45–57.

Hallfrisch J, Drinkwater DT, Muler DC, et al. Physical conditioning status and dietary intake in active and sedentary older men. Nutr Res 1994;14:817–27.

Halliwell B. Antioxidants and human disease: a general introduction. Nutr Rev 1997;55(1 Pt 2):S44–S9;discussion S49–S52.

Haralambie G, Berg A. Serum urea and amino nitrogen changes with exercise duration. Eur J Appl Physiol 1976;36:39–48.

Hawley JA, Dennis SC, Lindsay FH, Noakes TD. Nutritional practices of athletes: are they suboptimal? J Sports Sci 1995;13:S75–S81.

Haymes EM, Lamanca JJ. Iron loss in runners during exercise: implications and recommendations made for athletes. Sports Med 1989;7:277.

Heaney RP, Recker RR, Saville PD. Menopausal changes in calcium balance performance. J Lab Clin Med 1987;92:953.

Herbert V, Jacob E, Wong KT. Destruction of vitamin B12 by vitamin C (letter). Am J Clin Nutr 1977;30:297–9.

Ho CW, Beard JL, Farrell PA, Minson CT, Kenney WL. Age, fitness, and regional blood flow during exercise in the heat. J Appl Physiol 1997;82:1126–35.

Hoffman N. Diet in the elderly: needs and risks. Med Clin North Am 1993;77:745–56.

Hollick MF. Environmental factors that influence the cutaneous production of vitamin D. Am J Clin Nutr 1995;61(suppl):638–45.

Horber FF, Kohler SA, Lippuner K, Jaeger P. Effect of regular physical training on age-associated alteration of body composition in men. Eur J Clin Invest 1996;26:279–85.

Horswill CA. Effective fluid replacement. Int J Sport Nutr 1998;8:175–95.

Houston DK, Johnson M, Daniel TD, et al. Health and dietary characteristics of supplement users in an elderly population. Int J Vitam Nutr Res 1997;67:183–91.

Hoyt CJ. Diarrhea from vitamin C. JAMA 1980;244:1674.

Hughes VA, Fiatarone MA, Fielding RA, et al. Exercise increases muscle glut 4 levels and insulin action in subjects with impaired glucose tolerance. Am J Physiol 1993;264:E855–E62.

Hunding A, Jordal R, Paulev PE. Runner's anemia and iron deficiency. Acta Med Scand 1981;209:315–18.

Hurley B, Nemeth P, Martin W, et al. Muscle triglyceride utilization during exercise: effect of training. J Appl Physiol 1986;60:582–7.

Institute of Medicine and Food and Nutrition Board. Dietary reference intakes for thiamine, riboflavin, niacin, vitamin B-6, folate, vitamin B-12, pantothenic acid, biotin, and choline. Washington, DC: National Academy Press, 1998.

Jacques PF, Chylack LT. Epidemiologic evidence of a role for the antioxidant vitamins and carotenoids in cataract prevention. Am J Clin Nutr 1991;53(suppl):352–5.

Jakeman P, Maxwell S. Effect of antioxidant vitamin supplementation on muscle function after eccentric exercise. Eur J Appl Physiol 1993;67:426–30.

Jette AM, Branch LG. The Framingham disability study: II. Am J Pub Health 1981;71:1211–16.

Kanter M. Antioxidant supplementation for persons who are physically active. In: Berning JR, Steen SN, eds. Nutrition for Sport and Exercise, 2nd edn. Gaithersburg: Aspen Publishers, 1998:109–18.

Kato I, Nomura AM, Stemmerman GN, Chyou PH. Vitamin supplement use and its correlates among elderly Japanese men residing in Oahu, Hi. Pub Health Report 1992;6:712–17.

Kavanagh T, Shephard RJ. Can regular sports participation slow the aging process? Data on masters athletes. Phys Sportsmed 1990;18:6:94–104.

Kendrick ZV, Nelson-Steen S, Scafidi K. Exercise, aging and nutrition. South Med J 1994;87:5:S50–S60.

Kenney WL. Control of heat-induced cutaneous vasodilation in relation to age. Eur J Appl Physiol 1988;57:120–5.

Kenney WL, Fowler SR. Methylcholine-activated eccrine sweat gland density and output as a function of age. J Appl Physiol 1988;65:1082–6.

Kenney WL, Tankersley CG, Newswanger DL, et al. Age and hypohydration independently influence the peripheral vascular response to heat stress. J Appl Physiol 1990;68:1902–8.

Kirwan JP, Kohrt WM, Wojta DM, et al. Endurance exercise training reduces glucose-stimulated insulin levels in 60- to 70-year-old men and women. J Gerontol 1993;48:M84–M90.

Kivela SL, Maenpaa P, Nissinen A, et al. Vitamin A, vitamin E and selenium status in an aged Finnish male population. Int J Vit Nutr Res 1989;59:373–80.

Klitgaard H, Mantoni M, Schiaffino S, et al. Function, morphology and protein expression of ageing skeletal muscle: a cross-sectional study of elderly men with different training backgrounds. Acta Physiol Scand 1990;140:41–54.

Knekt P, Aromaa A, Maatela J, et al. Vitamin E and cancer prevention. Am J Clin Nutr 1991;53(suppl):283–6.

Kohrt WM, Malley MT, Dalsky GP, Holloszy JO. Body composition of healthy sedentary and trained, young and older men and women. Med Sci Sports Exerc 1992;24:7:832–7.

Krall EA, Sahyoun N, Tannenbaum S, et al. Effect of vitamin D intake on seasonal variations in parathyroid hormone secretion in postmenopausal women. N Engl J Med 1989;321:1777–83.

Krasinski SD, Cohn JS, Schaefer EJ, et al. Postprandial plasma retinyl ester response is greater in older subjects compared with younger subjects. J Clin Invest 1990;85:883.

Krasinski SD, Russell RM, Samloff IM, et al. Fundic atrophic gastritis in an elderly population: effect on hemoglobin and several serum nutritional indicators. J Am Geriatr Soc 1986;34:800–6.

Krebs J, Schneider V, Smith J, et al. Sweat calcium loss during running. FASEB J 1988;2:A1099.

Krotkiewski M, Gudmundsson M, Backstrom P, Mandroukas K. Zinc and muscle strength and endurance. Acta Physiol Scand 1982;116:309–11.

Kulak CA, Bilezikian JP. Osteoporosis: preventive strategies. Int J Fertil Womens Med 1998;43:56–64.

Laukkanen P, Sakari-Rantala R, Kauppinen M, Heikkinen E. Morbidity and disability in 75- and 80-year-old men and women: a five-year follow-up. Scan J Soc Med 1997;53(suppl):79–106.

Lemon PWR. Effects of exercise on dietary protein requirements. Int J Sport Nutr 1998;8:426–47.

Lemon PWR, Nagle FJ, Mullin JP, Benevenga NJ. In vivo leucine oxidation at rest and during two intensities of exercise. J Appl Physiol 1982;53:947–54.

Lewis RD, Modlesky CM. Nutrition, physical activity, and bone health in women. Int J of Sport Nutr 1998;8:250–84.

Lexell J, Taylor CC, Sjostrom M. What is the cause of the ageing atrophy? Total number, size and proportion of different fiber types studied in whole vastus lateralis muscle from 15- to 83-year-old men. J Neurol Sci 1988;84:275–94.

Lukaski HC. Micronutrients (magnesium, zinc, and copper): are mineral supplements needed for athletes? Int J Sport Nutr 1995;5(suppl):S74–S83.

MacLaughlin J, Holick MF. Aging decreased the capacity of human skin to produce vitamin D3. J Clin Invest 1985;76:1536.

Maharam LG, Bauman PA, Kalman D, et al. Masters athletes—factors affecting performance. Sports Med 1999;28:273–85.

Mann J, Truswell AS, eds. Essentials of human nutrition. Oxford: Oxford University Press, 1998.

Manolagas SC, Hustmyer FG, Yu XP. Immunomodulating properties of 1,25-dihydroxyvitamin D3. Kidney Int Suppl 1990;29:S9–S16.

Marieb EN. Human anatomy & physiology, 4th edn. New York: Benjamin Cumming, 1998.

McArdle WD, Katch FI, Katch VL. Sport and exercise nutrition. New York: Lippincott, Williams & Wilkin, 1999.

McDonald R, Keen CL. Iron, zinc and magnesium nutrition and athletic performance. Sports Med 1988;5:171–84.

McLennan W, Podger A, eds. National Nutrition Survey: selected highlights Australia, Catalogue No. 4802.0. Canberra: Australian Bureau of Statistics and Department of Health and Family Services, 1997.

McLennan W, Podger A, eds. National Nutrition Survey: nutrient intakes and physical measurements Australia, Catalogue No. 4805.0. Canberra: Australian Bureau of Statistics and Department of Health and Family Services, 1998.

Meischer E, Fortney SM. Responses to dehydration and rehydration during heat exposure in young and older men. Am J Physiol 1989;257:R1050–R6.

Meredith CN, Frontera WR, Fisher EC, et al. Peripheral effects of endurance training in young and old subjects. J Appl Physiol 1989;66:2844–9.

Meydani SN, Barklund MP, Liu S, et al. Vitamin E supplementation enhances cell-mediated immunity in healthy elderly subjects. Am J Clin Nutr 1990a;52:557–63.

Meydani SN, Meydani M, Blumbery JB, et al. Assessment of the safety of supplementation with different amounts of vitamin E in healthy older adults. Am J Clin Nutr 1998;68:311–18.

Meydani SN, Ribaya-Meracdo JD, Russell RM, et al. Vitamin B-6 deficiency impairs interleukin 2 production and lymphocyte proliferation in elderly adults. Am J Clin Nutr 1991;53:1275–80.

Meydani SN, Ribaya-Mercado JD, Russell RM, et al. The effect of vitamin B6 on immune response in healthy elderly. Ann N Y Acad Sci 1990b;587:303–6.

Miller LT, Linkswiler H. Effect of protein intake on the development of abnormal tryptophan metabolism by men during vitamin B6 depletion. J Nutr 1967;93:53–9.

Morais JA, Gougeon R, Pencharz PB, et al. Whole-body protein turnover in the healthy elderly. Am J Clin Nutr 1997;66:880–9.

Myburgh KH, Hutchins J, Fataar AB, et al. Low bone density is an etiologic factor for stress fractures in athletes. Ann Intern Med 1990;113:754–9.

Nair KS. Muscle protein turnover: methodological issues and the effect of aging. J Germ Series A 1995;50A(special issue):107–12.

National Health & Medical Research Council. Recommended Dietary Intakes for use in Australia. Canberra: Australian Government Publishing Service, 1991.

National Health & Medical Research Council. The role of polyunsaturated fats in the Australian diet. Report of the NHMRC working party. Canberra: Australian Government Publishing Service, 1992.

National Health & Medical Research Council. Binns C, ed. Dietary guidelines for older Australians. Canberra: National Health and Medical Research Council, 1999.

National Heart Foundation. Dietary fibre. A policy statement prepared by the Diet and Heart Disease Advisory Committee for the National Heart Foundation. Canberra: National Heart Foundation, 1997.

National Research Council. Recommended Dietary Allowances, 10th edn. Washington, DC: National Academy Press, 1989.

Nelson ME, Fiatarone MA, Morganti CM, et al. Effects of high-intensity strength training on multiple risk factors for osteoporotic fractures. JAMA 1994;272:1909–14.

Nelson ME, Fisher EC, Dilmanian RA, et al. A 1 year walking program and increased dietary calcium in postmenopausal women: effects on bone. Am J Clin Nutr 1991;53:1304–11.

Newton M, Fry MD. Senior Olympians' achievement goals and motivational responses. J Aging Phys Act 1998;6:256–70.

Niekamp RA, Baer JT. In-season dietary adequacy of trained male cross-country runners. Int J Sport Nutr 1995;5:45–55.

NIH Consensus Development Panel. Optimal calcium intake—NIH Consensus Conference. JAMA 1994;272:1942–8.

Nuviala RJ, Lapieza MG, Bernal E. Magnesium, zinc and copper status in women involved in different sports. Int J Sport Nutr 1999;9:295–309.

Packer L. Protective role of vitamin E in biological systems. Am J Clin Nutr 1991;53 (suppl):S1050–S5.

Pannemans DL, Westerterp KR. Energy expenditure, physical activity and basal metabolic rate of elderly subjects. Br J Nutr 1995;73:571–81.

Pollock ML, Foster C, Knapp D, et al. Effect of age and training on aerobic capacity and body composition of masters athletes. J Appl Physiol 1987;62:725–31.

Pollock ML, Mengelkoch LJ, Graves JE, et al. Twenty-year follow-up of aerobic power and body composition of older track athletes. J Appl Physiol 1997;82:1508–16.

Proctor DN, Joyner MJ. Skeletal muscle mass and the reduction of $VO_{2\,max}$ in trained older subjects. Am Physiol Soc 1997;1411.

Reaburn PRJ. The lifetime athlete—physical work capacities and skeletal muscle characteristics. Unpublished PhD thesis. University of Queensland, 1994.

Reaburn PRJ, Gillespie A, Lowe J, Balanda K. The World Masters Games (1994) injury study. Report to Australian Sports Commission, 1995.

Reaburn PRJ, Le Bon C. Unpublished observations. 1995.

Reid IR, Ames RW, Evans MC, et al. Long-term effects of calcium supplementation on bone loss and fractures in postmenopausal women: a randomized controlled trial. Am J Med 1995;98:331–5.

Ribaya-Mercado JD, Russell RM, Sahyoun N, et al. Vitamin B6 requirements of elderly men and women. J Nutr 1991;121:1062–74.

Rimm E, Ascherio A, Giovannucci E, et al. Vegetable, fruit and cereal fiber intake and risk of coronary heart disease in men. JAMA 1996;275:447–51.

Rimm E, Stampfer M, Ascherio A, et al. Vitamin E consumption and the risk of coronary heart disease in men. N Engl J Med 1993;328:1450–6.

Rising R, Harper IT, Fontvielle AM, Ferraro RT, et al. Determinants of total daily energy expenditure: variability in physical activity. Am J Clin Nutr 1994;59:800–4.

Roberts SB, Dallal GE. Effects of age on energy balance. Am J Clin Nutr 1998;68(suppl):S975–S9.

Robertson JM, Donner AP, Trevithick JR. Vitamin E intake and risk of cataracts in humans. Ann NY Acad Sci 1989;570:372–82.

Rock CL. Nutrition of the older athlete. Clin Sports Med 1991;10:445–57.

Rokitzki L, Logemann E, Sagredos AN, et al. Lipid peroxidation and antioxidative vitamins under extreme endurance stress. Acta Physiol Scand 1994;151:149–58.

Rolls BJ, Phillips RA. Aging and disturbances of thirst and fluid balance. Nutr Rev 1990;48:137–44.

Romijn JA, Coyle EF, Sidossis LS, et al. Regulation of endogenous fat and carbohydrate metabolism in relation to exercise intensity. Am J Physiol 1993;265:E380–E91.

Rosenberg IH, Miller JW. Nutritional factors in physical and cognitive functions of elderly people. Am J Clin Nutr 1992;55(suppl6):S1237–S43.

Ruiz-Torres A, Gimeno A, Munoz FJ, Vicent D. Are anthropometric changes in healthy adults caused by modifications in dietary habits or by aging? Gerontol 1995;41:243–51.

Russell RM. Micronutrient requirements of the elderly. Nutr Rev 1992;50:463–6.

Russell RM. New views on the RDAs for older adults. J Am Diet Assoc 1997;97:515–18.

Russell RM, Suter PM. Vitamin requirements of elderly people: an update. Am J Clin Nutr 1993;58:4–14.

Sacheck JM, Roubenoff R. Nutrition in the exercising elderly. Clin Sports Med 1999;18:3:565–77.

Saito, M, Itoh R. Nutritional status of vitamin A in a healthy elderly population in Japan. Int J Vitam Nutr Res 1991;61:105–9.

Salmoren J, Ascherio EB, Rimm GA, et al. Dietary fiber, glycemic load and risk of NIDDM in men. Diab Care 1997b;20:545–50.

Salmoren J, Manson JE, Stampfer MJ, et al. Dietary fiber, glycemic load and risk of non-insulin-dependent diabetes mellitus in women. JAMA 1997a;277:472–7.

Salonen JT, Nyyssonen K, Korpela H, et al. High stored iron levels are associated with excess risk of myocardial infarction in eastern Finnish men. Circulation 1992;86:803–11.

Saltzman JR, Russell RM. The aging gut: nutritional issues. Gastroenterol Clin North Am 1998;27:309–24.

Sandstrom B. Bioavailability of zinc. Eur J Clin Nutr 1997;51(suppl1):S17–S19.

Sawka MN, Pandolf KB. Effects of water loss on physiological function and exercise performance. In: Gisolfi CV, Lamb DR, eds. Perspectives in exercise science and sports medicine. Vol. 3: Fluid homeostasis during exercise. Carmel, Indiana: Benchmark Press, 1990:1–38.

Schoeller DA. Changes in total body water. Am J Clin Nutr 1989;50:1176–81.

Seals DR, Hagberg JM, Hurley BF, Ehsani AA, Holloszy JO. Effects of endurance training on glucose tolerance and plasma lipid levels in older men and women. JAMA 1984;252:645–9.

Selhub J, Jacques PF, Wilson PWF, et al. Vitamin status and intake as primary determinants of homocysteinemia in an elderly population. JAMA 1993;270:2693–8.

Shaulis D, Golding LA, Tandy RD. Physical characteristics, physical fitness, and lifestyles of senior Olympic athletes and independently living cohorts. J Aging Phys Act 1996;4:1–13.

Shephard RJ, Shek PN. Immunological hazards from nutritional imbalance in athletes. Exerc Immunol Rev 1998;4:22–48.

Shimokata H, Tobin JD, Muller DC, Elahi D, Coon PJ, Andres R. Studies in the distribution of body fat: I. Effects of age, sex, and obesity. J Gerontol 1989;44:M66–M73.

Shirreffs SM, Taylor AJ, Leiper JB, Maughan RJ. Post-exercise rehydration in man: effects of volume consumed and drink sodium content. Med Sci Sports Exerc 1996;28:1260–71.

Shock JW. Energy metabolism, caloric intake and physical activity of the aging. In: Shock JW, ed. Normal human aging: The Baltimore Longitudinal Study of Aging. Washington: NIH Publications, 1984:372–86.

Silver A, Montagna W, Karaean I. Age and sex differences in spontaneous adrenergic and cholinergic human sweating. J Invest Dermatol 1964;43:255–6.

Simon JA, Hudes ES, Browner WS. Serum ascorbic acid and cardiovascular disease prevalence in United States adults. Epidemiol 1998;9:316–21.

Sobal J, Marquart LF. Vitamin/mineral supplement use among athletes: a review of the literature. Int J Sport Nutr 1994;4:320–34.

Solomons NW, Cousins RJ. Zinc. In: Solomons NW, Rosenberg IH, eds. Absorption and malabsorption of mineral nutrients. New York: Alan R. Liss, 1984:125–97.

Spodaryk K, Czekaj J, Sowa W. Relationship among reduced level of stored iron and dietary iron in trained women. Physiol Res 1996;45:393–7.

Starling RD, Ades PA, Poehlman ET. Physical activity, protein intake, and appendicular skeletal muscle mass in older men. Am J Clin Nutr 1999;70:91–6.

Steen B. Body composition and aging. Nutr Rev 1988;46:45–51.

Stewart JG, Ahlquist DA, McGill DB, et al. Gastrointestinal blood loss and anemia in runners. Ann Intern Med 1984;100:843–5.

Stewart RB. Nutritional supplements in the ambulatory elderly population: patterns of use and requirements. Ann Pharmacother 1989;23:490–5.

Stewart R, Cooper J. Polypharmacy in the aged. Drugs Ageing 1994;4:449–61.

Sykes JC. Women, sports, exercise, and nutrition. In: Harris S, Suominen H, Era P, Harris WS, eds. Toward healthy aging—international perspectives. Part I: Physiological and biomedical aspects. New York: Centre for the Study of Aging, 1994:141–5.

Synder AC, Dvorak LL, Roepke JB. Influence of dietary iron source on measures of iron status among female runners. Med Sci Sports Exerc 1989;21:7–10.

Tarnopolsky MA, Bosman M, Macdonald JR, et al. Postexercise protein–carbohydrate and carbohydrate supplements increase muscle glycogen in men and women. J Appl Physiol 1997;83:1877–83.

Tarnopolsky M, MacDougall J, Atkinson S. Influence of protein intake and training status on nitrogen balance and lean body mass. J Appl Physiol 1988;64:187–93.

Thomas J. Drug–nutrient interactions. Nutr Rev 1995;53:271–82.

Trappe SW, Costill DL, Fink WJ, Pearson DR. Skeletal muscle characteristics among distance runners: a 20-year follow-up study. J Appl Physiol 1995;78:823–9.

Trappe SW, Costill DL, Vukovich MD, et al. Aging among elite distance runners: a 22-year longitudinal study. J Appl Physiol 1996;80:285–90.

Tsai KS, Heath H, Kumar R, Riggs BL. Impaired vitamin D metabolism with aging women: possible role in pathogenesis of senile osteoporosis. J Clin Invest 1984;73:1668–72.

Turnland JR, Durkin N, Costa F, et al. Stable isotope studies of zinc absorption and retention in young and elderly men. J Nutr 1986;116:1239–47.

Ubbink JB, Vermaak WJ, van der Merwe A, Becker PJ. Vitamin B-12, vitamin B-6, and folate nutritional status in men with hyperhomocysteinemia. Am J Clin Nutr 1993;57:47–53.

Van Erp-Baart AMJ, Saris WHM, Binkhorst RA, et al. Nationwide survey on nutritional habits in elite athletes. Part II: Mineral and vitamin intake. Int J Sports Med 1989;10(suppl):11–16.

Vessby B. Nutrition, lipids and diabetes mellitus. Curr Opin Lipidol 1995;6:3–7.

Volpi E, Ferrando A, Yedkel C, et al. Exogenous amino acids stimulate net muscle protein synthesis in the elderly. J Clin Invest 1998;101:2000–7.

Waller MF, Haymes EM. The effects of heat and exercise on sweat iron loss. Med Sci Sports Exerc 1996;28:197–203.

Walter SD, Hart LE, Sutton JR, McIntosh JM, Gauld M. Training habits and injury experience in distance runners: age-and sex-related factors. Phys Sportsmed 1988;16:6:101–13.

Weaver CM, Rajaram S. Exercise and iron status. J Nutr 1992;122(suppl3):782–7.

Webster J. Key to healthy aging: exercise. J Gerentol Nurs 1990;14:9–15.

Welle S, Thornton CA. High-protein meals do not enhance myofibrillar synthesis after resistance exercise in 62- to 75-year-old men and women. Am J Physiol 1998;274(4 Part 1):E677–E83.

Wilmore JH, Costill DL. Physiology of sport and exercise, 2nd edn. Champaign, Illinois: Human Kinetics, 1999.

Winters LRT, Yoon JS, Kalkwarf HJ, et al. Riboflavin requirements and exercise adaptation in older women. Am J Clin Nutri 1992;56:526–32.

Wood RJ, Zheng JJ. High dietary calcium intakes reduce zinc absorption and balance in humans. Am J Clin Nutr 1997;65:1803–9.

World Cancer Research Fund and American Institute for Cancer Research. Food, nutrition and prevention of cancer: a global perspective. Washington, DC: AICR, 1997.

World Health Organisation. Carbohydrates in human nutrition. Report of a joint FAO/WHO expert consultation. Rome: World Health Organisation, 1997.

Yarasheski KE, Zachwieja JJ, Bier DM. Acute effects of resistance exercise on muscle protein synthesis rate in young and elderly men and women. Am J Physiol 1993;265(2 Pt 1):E210–E14.

Yates AA, Schlicker SA, Suitor CW. Dietary Reference Intakes: the new basis for recommendations for calcium and related nutrients, B vitamins, and choline. J Am Diet Assoc 1998;98:699–706.

Yip R, Dallman PR. The role of inflammation and iron deficiency as causes of anemia. Am J Clin Nutr 1988;48:1295–300.

CHAPTER 20

Special needs: the athlete with diabetes

Lyn Brown and Dennis Wilson

20.1 INTRODUCTION

Diabetes mellitus is a common condition that affects approximately 150 million people around the world. This number is projected to double in the next 25 years. It is estimated that diabetes affects 900 000 Australians (McCarty et al. 1996). In this condition the body is unable to use glucose properly and an elevated blood glucose level results. This produces the typical symptoms of diabetes such as unusual thirst, increased urination, weight loss, skin infections and, in acute cases, dehydration and diabetic coma.

There are two main types of diabetes. The less common Type I diabetes usually affects young people and may have an abrupt and potentially life-threatening onset of symptoms. Life-long treatment with diet and insulin injections is essential. The more common Type II diabetes usually affects middle-aged and elderly people, who are often overweight, but is increasingly seen in younger, often overweight, people. Diet alone or diet plus tablets may control this form of diabetes, but some of these people eventually require insulin. The exact causes of diabetes are not known, but there is evidence for an inherited susceptibility to both forms of the condition, especially Type II diabetes. External triggering factors such as viral infections are thought to be involved in the development of Type I diabetes, whereas Type II diabetes is often associated with lifestyle factors such as obesity, lack of physical activity, and stress. Both forms of the condition are associated with increased cardiovascular risk, and regular exercise has a role in reducing that risk.

A person with either Type I or Type II diabetes can become an elite athlete or train and compete at a high level of exercise intensity and endurance. Exercise increases insulin sensitivity and predisposes the individual to hypoglycaemia (low blood glucose levels) in the presence of insulin (see Section 20.6.1). Insulin levels fall during exercise (this is a normal physiological response), however for athletes with diabetes, insulin does need adjustment to mimic these falls in insulin associated with exercise. For those athletes with Type II diabetes on oral hypoglycaemic medications, adjustments may also be required. Adjustments vary according to the type, intensity and duration of exercise.

As hypoglycaemia is the most common problem faced by the athlete with Type I diabetes, certain sports (e.g. scuba diving, motor car racing and solo yachting) are contraindicated. Athletes with Type I diabetes involved in endurance sports are advised to train with a companion familiar with the detection and treatment of hypoglycaemia. Regular monitoring of blood glucose levels is crucial because an athlete on insulin must understand their physiological response to exercise when training and competing.

20.2 *PHYSIOLOGICAL EFFECTS OF EXERCISE*

In terms of glucose metabolism, exercise is a potent stimulus for glucose uptake and utilisation by muscle tissue (Ebeling et al. 1993; Kennedy et al. 1999). Plasma insulin levels decrease during exercise and that decrease, along with an increase in plasma glucagon and other counter-regulatory hormones, promotes an increase in glucose production by the liver (gluconeogenesis). The amount of glucose produced by gluconeogenesis matches the amount required by the increased glucose uptake by exercising muscles and by the increased metabolic requirements of other physiological systems (e.g. the neural and cardiovascular systems). As a result, blood glucose levels can remain relatively stable for up to one to two hours of continuous exercise without food intake. With prolonged moderate- to high-intensity exercise of more than 60–90 minutes duration, such as running, cycling and rowing, blood glucose levels tend to fall as hepatic glucose output lags behind glucose utilisation because of depleted hepatic glycogen reserves (Ahlborg et al. 1974). There is some benefit, however, in consuming carbohydrate (CHO) foods during exercise to help maintain blood glucose levels and promote recovery (see Section 17.3.4 and Chapter 7).

Repeated aerobic exercise increases insulin sensitivity throughout the body (Devlin 1993). This effect can be produced for 12–15 hours by a single bout of exercise and for much longer by regular exercise training. During exercise many other hormonal changes that regulate glucose metabolism occur. These changes also regulate cardiovascular response, body temperature, fluid, and electrolyte homeostasis. Regular physical activity also improves lipid profiles by increasing high-density lipoprotein (HDL) cholesterol (Simon 1984).

20.2.1 *Effects of exercise in Type I diabetes*

The metabolic and hormonal response to exercise in Type I diabetes is determined by a number of factors. These include:

- the intensity and duration of exercise;
- the degree of metabolic control before exercise;
- the type and dose of insulin injected before exercise;
- the site of insulin injection;
- the timing of the previous insulin injection; and
- the timing of the previous meal.

The major determinant of the glycaemic response is insulin availability.

20.2.2 *Exercise in the presence of hyperinsulinemia*

In Type I diabetes, plasma insulin levels may not decrease during exercise. This will cause hypoglycaemia, as insulin prevents the appropriate rise in hepatic glucose production, and accelerates the exercise-induced stimulation of glucose uptake into contracting muscle (see Figure 20.1).

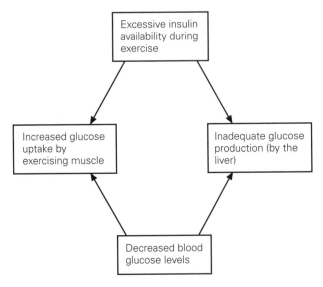

Figure 20.1 *Metabolic response to exercise in diabetes*
Adapted from Franz 1987

Elevated insulin levels also prevent the increase in mobilisation of lipids during exercise, leading to a reduced availability of non-esterified fatty acids as a fuel source (Wasserman et al. 1995). Hyperinsulinemia may occur if a person's normal insulin dose includes short-acting insulin (if injected a few hours before exercise), which reaches its peak action during the exercise. This effect may be exaggerated if the previously injected limb is exercised, promoting an increase in insulin absorption from the injection site (Koivisto & Felig 1978). Abdominal subcutaneous injection is therefore the recommended site for those undertaking exercise. If both dietary intake and insulin are adjusted beforehand in Type I diabetes, hyperinsulinemia can be avoided.

20.2.3 *Exercise in the presence of hypoinsulinemia*

In this situation, the inhibitory effect of insulin on hepatic glucose production and its stimulating effect on glucose uptake are both reduced. In addition, the counter-regulatory hormone response (catecholamines, glucagon, growth hormone and cortisol) to exercise is higher than normal during insulin deficiency. These changes lead to markedly increased hepatic glucose production and diminished glucose utilisation by the exercising muscle, and result in marked hyperglycaemia. During extremely strenuous acute exercise, hyperglycaemia may result from excessive production of counter-regulatory hormones. These hormones may stimulate a surplus of production of hepatic glucose beyond the limits of peripheral utilisation. This can occur in Type I diabetes even in the presence of insulin.

Augmented lipid mobilisation and ketogenesis in the liver also leads to the hypoinsulinemic person becoming hyperketonemic. If both dietary intake and insulin doses are adjusted appropriately in Type I diabetes, this situation can also be avoided.

20.3 NUTRITIONAL MANAGEMENT FOR ATHLETES WITH TYPE I DIABETES

Nutrition goals and guidelines for training and competition recommended for athletes with diabetes are no different to those recommended for athletes without diabetes (see Chapter 2) (American Diabetes Association 1999a, 1999b). A training diet for athletes with diabetes, based on CHO-rich foods with a low glycaemic index (see Chapter 12) and low-fat foods, is compatible with diabetes management and athletic performance. Energy and micronutrient requirements are maintained by selecting a variety of foods according to appetite and activity demands.

Athletes with diabetes should generally be encouraged to adjust their insulin dosage according to their lifestyle and training program rather than distorting their eating patterns to suit the insulin dosage. Although it is not necessary for an athlete with diabetes to follow a rigid pattern of food intake, a reasonably consistent eating routine facilitates diabetic management. Maintaining consistent training and eating routines on a day-to-day basis assists in the establishment of insulin dosage and fine-tuning of food intake. A well-trained athlete who regularly exercises at the same time each day will usually need less adjustment to food and insulin than a person who exercises only occasionally (Franz et al. 1994). For athletes with recently diagnosed Type I diabetes, the stabilisation and adjustment phase should be the first priority and an interruption to training and competition routines may be expected.

The person with Type I diabetes who participates in regular physical exercise needs to consider:

* the macronutrient content and timing of meals and snacks;
* the insulin dose and its predicted peak period of activity in relation to their exercise routine; and
* regular monitoring of blood glucose levels to assist with adjustment of food and insulin to prevent and manage hyperglycaemia and hypoglycaemia.

20.3.1 *Recommended CHO intakes for athletes with diabetes*

The following guidelines are recommendations for CHO intake for exercise of differing intensities and durations. In practice, the recommended CHO intake before, during and after exercise is no different to that recommended for the athlete without diabetes (see Chapters 13, 14 and 15). This assumes that athletes with diabetes have good metabolic control and usually have blood glucose levels between 4 mmol/L and 8 mmol/L. If blood glucose levels are either side of this range, food intake may need to be adjusted or exercise may need to be postponed until the blood glucose level is within the recommended range.

Table 20.1 provides guidelines for amounts of CHO (in grams) recommended for athletes undertaking exercise of varying intensity and duration. Examples of foods containing 50 g of CHO are found in Chapter 15, Table 15.4. The individual will need to monitor blood glucose levels frequently and adapt these CHO recommendations on the basis of their own responses to exercise of differing intensities and duration. The most appropriate method is by trial and error.

20.3.1.1 *Recommendations for CHO intakes for brief, high-intensity sports and light training*

Sprinting, running or swimming less than 1500 m, and other sports involving sudden activity (such as weight lifting) usually require minimal or no adjustment to food intake provided the pre-event blood glucose level is between 5.6 and 10.0 mmol/L (Armstrong 1992; Franz et al. 1994). This is also the case for low-level activity, such as a 30-minute leisurely walk or bike ride.

For a blood glucose level between 10 and 14 mmol/L, there is probably no need for increased food if the exercise is of less than one hour's duration. If the blood glucose level is above 14 mmol/L, the urine should be tested for ketones. The presence of ketones indicates that diabetic control should be improved before the activity is commenced (Armstrong 1992).

20.3.1.2 *Recommendations for CHO intakes for moderate-intensity exercise of short duration (15–30 min)*

A pre-exercise meal of slowly absorbed CHO food (low glycaemic index) one to three hours before the commencement of exercise is recommended according to the

Table 20.1 *Recommended dietary CHO intakes (g) before exercise*

Exercise intensity and duration	Blood glucose (mmol/L)	Dietary CHO (g)
Brief high-intensity (< 30 mins) (e.g. weight lifting, sprints)	6–10	No food required
Light (e.g. walking 30 min, easy-pace aerobics 60 min)	< 6 > 6	15 No food required
Moderate (< 45 min) (e.g. swimming, jogging, tennis, basketball)	< 6 6–10 10–14 14+	30–45 15 No food required Exercise not advised
Moderate (> 60 min) (e.g. football, cycling)	10–14 plus reduced insulin dosage > 13–14 and ketones > 17 (no ketones)	10–15 g/h Exercise contraindicated Exercise not advised
Strenuous (< 60 min) (e.g. triathlon, marathon, canoeing, kayaking, cross-country skiing, cycling)	< 6 6–10 10–14 14+	45 30–45 15–30 Exercise not advised
Strenuous (> 60 min) (e.g. triathlon, marathon, canoeing, kayaking, cross-country skiing, cycling)	< 6 6–10 10–14	50 g/h 25–30 g/h 10–15 g/h

Exercise at any level is contraindicated if ketones are present

principles of preparation for exercise (see Chapter 12). If insulin action is likely to peak at the time of the event, an additional 10–15 g CHO taken 20–30 minutes before the event should be sufficient to maintain blood glucose levels, provided the blood glucose level is between 5.6 and 10.0 mmol/L (Armstrong 1992; Franz et al. 1994). If the blood glucose level is more than 14 mmol/L, postponement of exercise is recommended.

After exercise, 15–30 g CHO food may be required to maintain adequate blood glucose levels, prevent hypoglycaemia and promote recovery (see Chapter 15, Table 15.4).

20.3.1.3 *Recommendations for CHO intakes for moderate- to strenuous-intensity exercise of medium to long duration (> 30 min)*

A pre-exercise meal of an additional 15 g CHO from foods with a high to moderate glycaemic index for each 20 minutes of planned activity should be tried initially. This should be eaten one to three hours before exercise, with the support of an additional 15 g CHO from high–glycaemic index foods taken just before competition.

Dietary CHO eaten at around 60–90 minutes into a prolonged bout of physical activity helps prevent hypoglycaemia during exercise and maintain exercise capacity (Kahn & Vinik 1988; Armstrong 1992). In practice, the form of CHO (i.e. solid or liquid) consumed makes no difference to performance outcomes and depends on individual preferences and opportunities for consumption during the activity.

The previously held belief that a sugar solution or quickly absorbed CHO food consumed 30–60 minutes before the activity would reduce exercise tolerance is not justified (Maynard 1992; Franz et al. 1994), and a fluid containing 5–7% CHO is recommended instead (see Chapter 14).

20.3.1.4 *Pre-event CHO loading*

Adequate diabetic control is required before an athlete with diabetes should attempt any form of CHO loading.

Dietary and training techniques for CHO loading of glycogen stores for competition are considered in detail in Chapter 13. As CHO loading is dependent on the availability of insulin to store muscle glycogen, this technique should be used with caution in an athlete requiring insulin. The insulin dose should be adjusted to match the changes in diet and the tapering effects of exercise before competition. For the athlete on insulin who has poor diabetic control, stabilising blood glucose is already difficult and CHO loading can lead to further deterioration in diabetic control. It is important to regularly monitor diabetes control.

20.3.1.5 *Post-exercise refeeding*

For the athlete undertaking physical activity on repeated days, a CHO-rich diet with an increased proportion of easily absorbed CHO may be required to minimise the cumulative effect of glycogen depletion, chronic fatigue and fluctuating diabetes control (Franz et al. 1994).

CHO should be eaten soon after the completion of exercise (where possible) to promote muscle glycogen resynthesis (see Chapter 15). An amount of 1.0–1.5 g CHO per kilogram of body weight shortly after exercise and again at 60 minutes is recommended to aid recovery (Armstrong 1992).

20.3.2 *Fluids*

Athletes with Type I diabetes tend to become preoccupied with replacing CHO and forget their requirements for fluid. Adequate hydration is essential for optimum performance. Because the thirst mechanism is less sensitive during exercise, it is important to drink water before becoming thirsty. Conversely, for an athlete with Type I diabetes, excessive thirst may be a sign of hypoglycaemia and fluid intakes are likely to be higher if hyperglycaemia is present. Guidelines for the composition and volume of suitable fluids for everyday training and specific competition are included in Chapter 13. These guidelines are also applicable for athletes with diabetes.

20.3.3 *Alcohol*

Alcohol is a potent inhibitor of hepatic glucose production and may precipitate late and severe hypoglycaemia in a person with diabetes on insulin. It may also impair the recognition of symptoms of the condition. Alcohol intake should therefore be moderate and always accompanied by food. Alcoholic drinks may precipitate hyper-glycaemia in the short term if soft drinks are used as mixers, or if sweet wines or liqueurs are consumed.

20.4 *INSULIN ADJUSTMENTS FOR ATHLETES WITH TYPE I DIABETES*

As mentioned in Section 20.2.1, the major determinant of the glycaemic response to exercise is insulin availability.

20.4.1 *Available insulins*

Most insulins in common usage are human preparations produced by recombinant DNA technology. A few people continue to use bovine or porcine preparations. In recent years insulin analogues have become available. The short-acting analogue, insulin lispro is already in clinical use and others, such as insulin arspart, are expected to become available in the near future. Long-acting insulin analogues are also under development. The short-acting analogues have an onset of action within minutes after subcutaneous injection, peak at one to two hours and have a duration of approximately four hours. The commonly used regular or neutral (clear) insulins have an onset of action about 30 minutes after subcutaneous injection, peak at two to three hours and have a duration of approximately seven hours. Both these kinds of insulin may be given alone, before each meal, using a syringe or a pen injector, or in combination with an intermediate- or long-acting insulin before breakfast and the evening meal. If given alone, they are combined with an injection of an intermediate- or long-acting insulin before bed. The intermediate-acting insulins (Isophane™ or Lente MC™) have an onset of action after one to two hours, peak at six to ten hours and have a duration of 16–20 hours. The long-acting insulin (Ultralente MC™) has an onset of action after two to three hours, peaks at eight to 14 hours and has a duration of approximately 24 hours. Pre-mixed preparations of neutral and isophane insulins are also available. The amount of neutral insulin in these preparations varies from 20–50% insulin with the remainder being iso-phane insulin.

20.4.2 *Insulin adjustment*

Less total daily insulin dosages are required in athletes with Type I diabetes, under-taking regular physical activity, largely because of an increase in insulin sensitivity associated with exercise. If physical activity is of less than 30 minutes duration it is usually not necessary to reduce insulin dosage. For more prolonged physical activity, the insulin is adjusted to reduce the insulin operating at the time of the exercise by 15–40%. The exact reduction depends on the intensity and duration of exercise and varies considerably between individuals. For physical activity undertaken in the morning, the short-acting insulin dose should be reduced before breakfast by 15–40%. If physical activity is undertaken in the afternoon, intermediate-acting insulin (if used before breakfast) should be reduced. If an athlete is on a combination of short-acting insulin before each meal, and intermediate-acting insulin at night, the pre-lunch short-acting dose is reduced for afternoon exercise.

If physical activity is continuous over several hours (e.g. a three- to four-hour cycle, or a two-hour run), then a more substantial reduction in insulin doses will be required. In this situation, reducing both morning short-acting (clear) and intermediate-acting (cloudy) doses by up to 50% could be indicated. For some events, such as a marathon or triathlon, insulin has been omitted completely, without adverse effects on the athlete (Meinders et al. 1988). However, although it is important to avoid the development of hypoglycaemia during exercise, an excessive reduction in insulin doses can lead to hypoinsulinemia and result in hyperglycaemia, leading to increased fluid loss, possible ketosis and a high risk of dehydration and heat stress.

20.5 *MONITORING BLOOD GLUCOSE LEVELS*

Individuals vary considerably in their metabolic response to physical activity and their diabetic control. It is important to take into account what type of sporting situation the athlete is participating in (e.g. training or competition) when making decisions about appropriate insulin dosage and how frequently blood glucose is monitored. A management plan based on food requirements after physical activity and corresponding insulin requirement can then be formulated. Once a response pattern is established for a particular individual to a particular type of exercise, it is likely to be similar on future occasions and, therefore, appropriate adjustments can be predicted.

If physical activity is unplanned and insulin has already been administered, then adjustments to CHO intake during or prior to exercise will be needed. Adjustments to insulin doses and food intake after the exercise may still be warranted if low blood sugar levels are evident.

20.6 *SPECIAL PROBLEMS FOR THE ATHLETE WITH TYPE I DIABETES*

20.6.1 *Hypoglycaemia*

The most common problem for the athlete with Type I diabetes is hypoglycaemia. This may lead to increased sweating, signs of anxiety, often nausea and disorientation and may be confused with effects simply produced by exercise. If symptoms of hypoglycaemia are not recognised or masked by alcohol misuse, then severe hypoglycaemia will develop. Untreated hypoglycaemia, associated with too much insulin or too little food, eventually leads to hypoglycaemic coma. It is, therefore, most important for an athlete with Type I diabetes to undertake vigorous or prolonged exercise in the company of a friend or a coach who is aware of hypoglycaemic symptoms and is able to treat the condition appropriately. This is particularly important for athletes involved in sporting pursuits such as distance running, long-distance swimming, and cross-country skiing.

20.6.1.1 *Late hypoglycaemia after exercise*

A further problem affecting an athlete on insulin is the occurrence of late hypoglycaemia after exercise. It has already been pointed out that exercise increases insulin sensitivity for several hours afterwards (see Section 20.2). The athlete is at risk of hypoglycaemia during that time and may need to reduce the next insulin dose to avoid this. Alcohol is also a precipitating factor for late hypoglycaemia, as it blocks gluconeogenesis (see Section 20.3.1.7). The effects of too much alcohol also mask the early symptoms of hypoglycaemia and, therefore increase the risk of hypoglycaemic coma.

20.6.1.2 *Dietary treatment of hypoglycaemia*

While foods containing 15 g of quickly absorbed CHO (with a high glycaemic index) such as sugar may relieve the early symptoms of hypoglycaemia under normal circumstances, it may be necessary to have two or three times this amount to relieve hypoglycaemia induced after strenuous exercise (Franz 1992). Dietary treatment must be continued until stable blood glucose levels are achieved.

CHO loading prior to competition involving CHO restriction is not recommended. The resulting low glycogen stores will markedly increase any risk of severe hypoglycaemia.

20.6.1.3 *Hypoglycaemic coma*

A 50% dextrose solution is injected intravenously to treat hypoglycaemic coma. Fluid or food must not be administered by mouth. If intravenous glucose cannot be given, the alternative approach is an intramuscular injection of 1 mg glucagon which induces glucose release from glycogen stores in the liver. However, this alternative approach may not work after prolonged exercise if hepatic glycogen stores are depleted. Rapid medical assistance is crucial for anyone in a diabetic coma.

20.6.1.4 *Impaired temperature regulation*

A further risk associated with hypoglycaemia is impaired temperature regulation. If there is risk of hypothermia (in sports such as cross-country skiing) or hyperthermia (in marathon events), then particular care should be taken to prevent hypoglycaemia.

20.6.2 *Hyperglycaemia*

The usual causes of hyperglycaemia (high blood glucose levels) are infection, overconsumption of food, inadequate insulin and, in some cases, alcohol consumption (if sweet wines, liqueurs or soft drinks are consumed). Exercise is not recommended in individuals with hyperglycaemia (see Section 20.2.3) as it may lead to even higher blood glucose levels and ketosis. An athlete who exercises with very high blood sugar levels can become confused and disoriented and is at high risk of dehydration. Hyperglycaemia following exercise is usually due to over-consumption of food, frequently in an attempt to avoid post-exercise hypoglycaemia. Often athletes with diabetes who fear the onset of hypoglycaemia during exercise consume excess food before or during exercise as a preventive measure. Frequent monitoring of blood glucose levels in this situation is again important (Franz 1994; Monk et al. 1995).

20.6.3 *Long-term complications*

20.6.3.1 *Cardiovascular disease*

Type I diabetes is associated with a number of long-term complications which include an increase in cardiovascular disease risk. This is related to increasing age and increasing duration of diabetes. It is also related to the presence of microvascular disease, peripheral vascular disease, autonomic neuropathy and any additional risk factors for coronary artery disease, especially smoking. Any athlete with established Type I diabetes contemplating a vigorous training program should have a detailed cardiovascular assessment prior to initiating a program. With the increasing tendency of older people to undertake athletic activities, there is an even stronger case in these individuals for formal cardiac assessment before commencing an exercise program. For most people, however, the cardiovascular and psychological benefits of regular physical activity far exceed the risks (Norris et al. 1990).

20.6.3.2 *Retinopathy*

Another complication of Type I diabetes which develops over time is retinopathy. If this is of a proliferative type, vigorous physical activity and especially nonaerobic activity involving sudden stress, such as weight lifting, should be avoided as the associated rise in blood pressure could increase the chance of a vitreous haemorrhage or traction retinal detachment.

20.6.3.3 *Peripheral neuropathy*

Many people with Type I diabetes also develop peripheral neuropathy (damage to nerves in the extremities) over time. This results in loss of sensation in the feet and, in older individuals is often associated with peripheral vascular disease. This increases the risk of damage to the feet, which is not recognised by the usual symptoms of soreness and pain, but the feet can become ulcerated. Foot ulcers are particularly difficult to heal and often require long hospital admission. Appropriate choice of footwear and advice from a podiatrist is important for all athletes involved in weight-bearing exercise.

20.6.3.4 *Autonomic neuropathy*

Autonomic neuropathy is an abnormality of the autonomic nervous system, which may be induced by long-standing, poorly controlled diabetes and may result in loss of ability to control heart rate, blood pressure, sweating and bladder function. This complication of diabetes may limit exercise capacity and increase the risk of an adverse cardiovascular event during exercise. Disturbances in blood pressure control that are linked to autonomic neuropathy are more common at the start of an exercise program than in a person who exercises regularly. A medical assessment to determine the extent of damage from autonomic neuropathy is strongly recommended prior to embarking on an exercise program.

20.7 *PHYSICAL ACTIVITY FOR PEOPLE WITH TYPE II DIABETES*

As described in Section 20.1, the prevalence of Type II diabetes has reached pandemic proportions. Physical activity has an important role in primary prevention of this condition by improving blood glucose control and reducing cardiovascular mortality risk (Helmrich et al. 1994). Unfortunately, long-term adherence to lifestyle interventions, particularly modification in physical activity, is poor. In addition, Type II diabetes often occurs in older people who have a variety of age-related disabilities which limit the feasibility of exercise. However, increasing numbers of the young elderly are taking part in exercise programs for their own enjoyment and often in competitive situations. For both elderly and young elderly people with Type II diabetes, a cardiac assessment prior to commencing an exercise program is important. This age group is also likely to have peripheral vascular disease, so care of the feet in impact sports should be addressed. Hypoglycaemia can occur in people with Type II diabetes who use insulin or one of the sulfonylureas medications (which enhance insulin secretion). The dosage of these drugs is reduced in people who undertake regular physical activity. Hypoglycaemia is unlikely to occur in individuals using biguanides (e.g. metformin) or insulin-sensitising agents (e.g. glitazones) or glucosidase inhibitors (e.g. acerbose). As many individuals with Type II diabetes are overweight, it is usually appropriate to encourage weight reduction and emphasise medication reduction during exercise rather than increased CHO intake.

20.8 *HIGH-RISK SPORTS*

Individuals with diabetes on treatment with insulin or sulfonylureas are at risk of hypoglycaemia and disorientation. Sporting activities that would pose a risk to themselves or to those around them are best avoided. Hypoglycaemia may occur in any sporting situation where the individual is alone and does not recognise the symptoms, or in a situation where glucose cannot be readily administered as treatment. These situations include hang-gliding, scuba diving, solo yachting or motor car racing. Other activities where there is a lesser element of risk—such as cross-country skiing, surfboard riding or long-distance running—should only be undertaken if the individual is accompanied by someone who is able to recognise and treat hypoglycaemia.

20.9 INTERNATIONAL DIABETIC ATHLETES ASSOCIATION

This association was founded in 1985 to educate people with diabetes about the benefits of regular physical activity (Thurm et al. 1992). Regular meetings are arranged and a quarterly newsletter is published. The headquarters are in Phoenix, Arizona with chapters and interest groups in many parts of the world, including North and South America, Europe and Australia.

20.10 INSULIN ABUSE AND SPORT

Insulin is an anabolic agent, which promotes protein synthesis and inhibits protein breakdown in muscle (Fryburg et al. 1995). It also transports electrolytes and fluid into muscle cells which makes them swell and gives the muscle a better definition. The misuse and abuse of insulin was reported twenty years ago in body builders and is still happening today. Use of insulin as an anabolic agent has been claimed in other sports, including cross-country skiing. Deliberately using insulin to produce hypoglycaemia to initiate the physiological release of growth hormone has also been claimed. These practices are not without risk, as evident in a body builder who developed severe and permanent brain damage after inducing hypoglycaemia from using intravenous insulin (Elkin et al. 1997). There are also risks associated with sharing of needles to give insulin. The forms of insulin used for injection can be detected from blood tests. Athletes with diabetes who are prescribed insulin or other diabetic drugs need medical clearance in case of drug testing. Insulin, its analogues and other anabolic agents are banned substances.

20.11 SUMMARY

Athletes with diabetes are able to participate in virtually all sports, apart from a few exceptions that pose a risk because of hypoglycaemia. The dietary recommendations for training and competition for athletes with diabetes are similar to those for athletes without diabetes, provided the blood glucose range is within acceptable levels at the commencement of exercise. Older athletes, and those with long-standing diabetes, need to be screened for complications of the condition, such as cardiovascular disease, retinopathy and neuropathy. All athletes need to be properly instructed on strategies to avoid and treat exercise-induced hypoglycaemia. Frequent monitoring of blood glucose levels should be encouraged. Exercise should not be undertaken in the presence of hyperglycaemia and ketosis. Sports coaches of athletes with diabetes should be conversant with the effect of diabetes on athletic performance and, in particular, should be able to recognise and adequately treat hypoglycaemia.

20.12 *PRACTICE TIPS*

Elizabeth Broad

- People with diabetes come in many ages, shapes and forms. People with diabetes can train at high levels of intensity and endurance. Diabetes, if well controlled, will not prevent an athlete from achieving the highest level in their sport. However, some precautions may need to be taken, such as training with a partner who is aware of the problem, who can recognise symptoms of hypoglycaemia and who knows how to treat it.

- It is important for the sports dietitian to liaise or establish a good working relationship with the doctor and diabetes educator who are working with the athlete to provide a coordinated approach to management.

- Hyperinsulinemia is a risk in athletes with Type I diabetes. To avoid this, athletes will need to reduce their insulin dosage, timing and injection site according to their training/competition type and duration. Similarly, athletes with Type II diabetes, who are on medication, may also need to reduce their medication. Early in the training program, such adjustments are best made under the supervision of a diabetes specialist to accurately predict and interpret results.

- It is important to encourage athletes to monitor blood glucose levels and corresponding insulin dosage, especially during the training season, and to keep these records for tracking responses to physical activity and other external factors (e.g. injury or sickness) where insulin adjustments were made. It must be emphasised that maintaining relatively even blood glucose levels will maximise the benefits of training as opposed to large fluctuations in levels or regularly high blood glucose levels. Blood glucose responses to exercise vary substantially between individuals, so alterations to treatments need to be made on a case-by-case basis.

- If blood glucose levels are greater than 14 mmol/L (especially if ketones are present in urine), exercise should be postponed until better control is achieved. Exercising with high blood glucose levels disrupts normal metabolic responses and will elevate these levels even further, which can be damaging. The recommended diet for an athlete with diabetes is no different to that of a non-diabetic person. Athletes with diabetes should be encouraged to adjust insulin or other medication according to the response to exercise rather than distorting their food intake to suit insulin or medication doses.

- As with all athletes, those with diabetes should try to maintain a consistent food intake over the day with regular intake of food, preferably CHO-rich food sources, in between meals.

- Consuming CHO during exercise is strongly advised for those undertaking endurance events. CHO loading, particularly involving a depletion phase, should not be attempted unless good diabetic control has been regularly maintained. Insulin doses require careful adjusting depending on the method of loading used and the style of exercise tapering practised before a competition. Even for a diabetic who has their diabetes well controlled, this adjustment is difficult and the glucose response is often erratic. CHO loading is not recommended for children with diabetes on insulin. Children are unlikely to be competing in the sort of events that benefit from CHO loading (e.g. marathon or even half marathon events).

- Athletes with Type I diabetes need to be cautious with alcohol consumption. Too much alcohol inhibits gluconeogenesis and is associated with delayed hypoglycaemia, which is responsible for the hangover effect of nausea, and light headedness observed after a drinking binge. This is a normal physiological response to alcohol and the reaction is the same in a person without diabetes. In a person with diabetes on insulin, the 'morning-after' effects of alcohol, in combination with insulin, however, can accelerate a hypoglycaemic state into a potentially life-threatening coma.

- Athletes with diabetes should be strongly encouraged to take full responsibility for managing their diabetes. This includes always having food readily available, including emergency food in case of hypoglycaemia, eating regularly, and being responsible for changes to insulin levels during times of physical activity, illness or infection.

REFERENCES

Ahlborg G, Felig P, Hagenfelt L, Hendler R, Wahren JB. Substrate turnover during exercise in man: splanchic and leg metabolism of glucose, free fatty acids and amino acids. J Clin Invest 1974;53:1080–90.

American Diabetes Association. Nutrition recommendations and principles for people with diabetes mellitus. Diab Care 1999a;22(suppl):S42–S45.

American Diabetes Association. Diabetes mellitus and exercise. Diab Care 1999b;22(suppl):S49–S53.

Armstrong JJ. Overview of diabetes mellitus and exercise. Diab Educ 1992;17:1750–8.

Devlin JT. Effects of exercise on insulin sensitivity in humans. Diabetes Care 1992;11:1690–3.

Ebeling P, Bourney R, Koranyi L, et al. Mechanism of enhanced insulin sensitivity in athletes: increased blood flow, muscle glucose transport protein (GLUT-4) concentration and glycogen synthetase activity. J Clin Invest 1993;92:1623–31.

Elkin SL, Brady S, Williams JP. Bodybuilders find it easy to obtain insulin to help them in training. BMJ 1997;314:1280.

Franz MJ. Exchanges for all occasions. Minnesota: International Diabetes Centre, 1987.

Franz MJ. Nutrition: can it give athletes with diabetes a boost? Diab Educ 1991;17:163–4, 166, 168.

Franz MJ, Horton ES Sr, Bantle JP, et al. Nutrition principles for the management of diabetes and related complications. Diab Care 1994;17:490–518.

Fryburg DA, Jahn LA, Hill SA, Oliveras DM, Barrett EJ. Insulin and insulin-like growth factor 1 enhance human skeletal muscle protein anabolism during hyperaminoacidemia by different mechanisms. J Clin Invest 1995;96:1722–9.

Helmrich SP, Ragland DR, Paffenbarger RS. Prevention of non-insulin dependent diabetes mellitus with physical activity. Med Sci Sports Exerc 1994;26:824–30.

Kahn J, Vinik A. Exercise training in the diabetic patient. Intern Med 1988;9:117–25.

Kennedy JW, Hirshman MF, Gervino EV, et al, Acute exercise induced GLUT-4 translocation in skeletal muscle of normal human subjects and subjects with Type ll diabetes. Diabetes 1999;48:1192–7.

Koivisto VA, Felig P. Effects of leg exercise on insulin absorption in diabetic patients. N Eng J Med 1978;298:79–83.

Maynard T. Physiological responses to exercise. Diab Educ 1992;17:19–200.

McCarty CA, Keeffe JE, Livingston PM, Taylor HR. The importance and state of medical and public health research related to vision in Australia. Aust NZ J Opthal 1996;24:3–5.

Meinders A, Willekens FLA, Heere LP. Metabolic and hormonal changes in IDDM during a long distance run. Diab Care 1988;11:1–7.

Monk A, Barry B, McClark K, Weaver T, Coopa N, Franz MJ. Exercise and the managememnt of diabetes mellitus. J Am Diet Assoc 1995;95:999–1006.

Norris R, Carroll D, Cochran R. The effects of aerobic and anaerobic training on fitness, blood pressure, and psychological stress and well-being. Psychosom Res 1990;34:367–75.

Simon HB. Sports medicine. In: Rubenstein E, Federman D, eds. Current topics in medicine. New York: Scientific American Medicine, 1984:1–26.

Thurm U, Harper PN. I'm running on insulin: summary of the history of the International Diabetic Athletes Association. Diab Care 1992;15:1811–13.

Wasserman DH, O'Doherty RM, Zinker BA. Role of the endocrine pancreas in control of fuel metabolism by the liver during exercise. Int J Obes Relat Metab Disord 1995;19(suppl):S22–S30.

Special needs: the vegetarian athlete

Greg Cox

21.1 INTRODUCTION

Vegetarian diets are now part of mainstream eating in Western countries. A number of studies have reported both short- and long-term health benefits of vegetarian eating. To date, most studies investigating food intakes of vegetarians have investigated groups following such diets for religious reasons, or groups who differed from non-vegetarians in other lifestyle habits. Vegetarians do not represent a homogeneous group of people. Individuals choose to adopt a vegetarian diet for a number of different reasons. Cultural and religious nominations, moral beliefs concerning animal rights, health implications and environmental issues are all motivating factors.

In a national survey of 9242 American runners, researchers found that 8.2% of female runners and 2.7% of male runners self-reported following a vegetarian diet (Williams 1997). Barr (1986) reported 37% of 209 Canadian recreational female athletes followed a 'semi-vegetarian' diet (no red meat), with 1.9% following a lacto-ovo-vegetarian diet. Reasons for adopting a vegetarian diet may differ between athletes and untrained individuals. In order to meet increased carbohydrate (CHO) requirements for training or to assist in weight control, some athletes may adopt a vegetarian diet. Vegetarian or near-vegetarian eating patterns are more likely to be found in endurance athletes such as runners, cyclists and triathletes, that is, those athletes continually striving to consume a high-CHO diet and maintain a low BM.

This chapter describes various categories of vegetarian diets and discusses the impact of vegetarian eating on meeting current dietary goals and guidelines for optimal sports performance. Studies investigating the benefit of consuming a vegetarian diet on sports performance are reviewed. Potential nutritional concerns of different categories of vegetarian diets in an athletic population are also discussed. Practical guidelines for health professionals to ensure appropriate nutritional strategies are used to assist vegetarian athletes in meeting daily nutritional requirements are outlined.

21.2 CATEGORIES OF VEGETARIAN DIETS

According to the *Little Oxford Dictionary of Current English* (1980), 'vegetarian' refers to 'one who eats no animal food or none obtained by destruction of animal life'. In daily use, the term vegetarian is used more broadly than this strict definition, describing diets based exclusively on plant-based foods, to diets including some flesh foods. Table 21.1 defines numerous vegetarian diets. The fruitarian diet is the most restrictive form of vegetarian diet, with individuals relying solely on raw fruits, nuts and seeds. The lacto-ovo-vegetarian diet is more commonly followed and is the most liberal form of vegetarian diet.

Table 21.1 *Classification of vegetarian diets*

Type	Comments
Fruitarian	Diet consists of raw or dried fruits, nuts, seeds, honey and vegetable oil.
Macrobiotic	Excludes all animal foods, dairy products and eggs. Uses only unprocessed, unrefined, 'natural' and 'organic' cereals, grains and condiments such as miso and seaweed.
Vegan	Excludes all animal foods, dairy products and eggs. In the purest sense, excludes all animal products including honey, gelatine, silk, wool, leather and animal-derived food additives.
Lacto-vegetarian	Excludes all animal foods and eggs. Does, however, include milk and milk products.
Lacto-ovo-vegetarian	Excludes all animal foods, however, includes milk, milk products and eggs.

The term 'vegetarian' has also been incorrectly used to describe a diet where red meat is excluded, with chicken, cheese and fish included as staple meat alternatives. Many people, athletes included, regard themselves as vegetarians simply because they avoid eating red meat. Some individuals avoid eating red meat because they don't like the taste, the smell or the appearance. Others, typically endurance athletes, exclude red meat from their diet as they believe it is high in fat and/or cholesterol (Burke & Read 1987). These individuals rarely explore suitable alternatives to red meat and simply replace red meat with chicken, fish and/or cheese. This eating plan has been referred to as 'quasi-', 'semi-', or 'part-time' vegetarian. Rather than defining this style of eating as vegetarian, which it is not, perhaps it is more correctly referred to as 'fussy meat-eating'. Many health professionals, dietitians included, are quick to misclassify this group as vegetarians. This chapter describes the nutrient composition and examines nutritional concerns relevant to each category of vegetarian eating as well as 'fussy meat-eating'.

21.3 *EFFECT OF A VEGETARIAN DIET ON EXERCISE PERFORMANCE*

Vegetarian dietary practices appear to have a protective effect from lifestyle diseases seen in many affluent countries. Lower mortality rates from coronary artery disease and certain forms of cancer, and lower risks of obesity and diabetes are typical among vegetarian populations (Snowdon & Phillips 1985; Levin et al. 1986; Burr & Butland 1988; Burr & Sweetnam 1994; Giovannucci et al. 1994). Lifestyle factors other than diet may partially account for the observed health differences seen between vegetarians and non-vegetarians (Phillips & Snowdon 1985; Dwyer 1988; Thorogood et al. 1994).

To date, the majority of dietary surveys of vegetarians have been on females of various ages. The perceived nutritional concerns of vegetarian diets are more relevant to females than males (i.e. inadequate iron and calcium intakes), which explains to some extent the reason for the focus. Overall, a vegetarian diet appears conducive to maximising exercise performance for athletes during training and competition (American Dietetic Association 1997). Vegetarians' reported intakes are usually higher in CHO than non-vegetarians, containing adequate protein, iron, and calcium (see Table 21.2). Nieman (1988) suggests that athletes who practise a near-vegetarian diet are more likely to meet current recommendations for CHO. Fat intakes appear similar to those of meat eaters, however, some studies have reported lower total fat intakes in female vegetarians (Tylavsky & Anderson 1988; Nieman et al. 1989; Haddad et al. 1999). Not surprisingly, numerous studies report lower saturated fat and cholesterol intakes in female lacto-ovo-vegetarians and vegans compared with non-vegetarians (Janelle & Barr 1995; Ball & Bartlett 1999; Haddad et al. 1999).

Despite numerous studies investigating the health benefits of a vegetarian diet, few studies have examined exercise performance differences between vegetarians and non-vegetarians. Hanne et al. (1986) reported no differences in aerobic or anaerobic capacities of 49 (29 male; 20 female) lacto-ovo-vegetarian and lacto-vegetarian athletes, compared with 49 (29 male; 20 female) matched (for age, body size, and type of physical activity) non-vegetarian athletic controls. Synder and colleagues (1989) reported similar results, finding no differences in maximal oxygen uptake between nine female athletes following a modified vegetarian diet (< 100 g of red meat per week) and nine female athletes following a mixed diet.

Nieman and colleagues (1989) compared haematologic, anthropometric and metabolic factors of 19 elderly female vegetarians with 12 elderly non-vegetarians (mean ages 72.3 ± 1.4 and 69.5 ± 1.0 years, respectively). Vegetarian subjects had significantly lower blood glucose and cholesterol levels, and tended to have less body fat than non-vegetarians. No electrocardiographic differences were observed between groups at sub-maximal or maximal exercise workloads. Also, no differences were observed between groups for maximal oxygen uptake.

In another study, Nagel et al. (1989) noted no difference in performance between 50 runners consuming a lacto-ovo-vegetarian diet or 60 runners consuming a conventional Western diet during a 1000 km stage foot-race. Researchers formulated the diets to contain CHOs, fats and protein in the ratio 60 : 30 : 10 for both dietary groups. Half of each group completed the race, with the order of finishers and total running time no different between groups.

In a series of studies, using a crossover design, researchers investigated the effect of a six-week lacto-ovo-vegetarian diet and a six-week mixed diet on immune parameters, serum sex hormones and exercise performance in eight well-trained male endurance athletes (mean $VO_{2\,max}$ = 68 mL/min/kg) (Richter et al. 1991; Raben et al. 1992). Diets were isocaloric and formulated to contain similar macronutrient contents (57% and 58% of energy from CHOs, 28% and 29% of energy from fats, and 15% and 13% of energy from protein for the lacto-ovo-vegetarian diet and mixed diet, respectively). Researchers concluded that measures of immune function, endurance performance to exhaustion, isometric strength and muscle glycogen levels were not different between the two diet periods. However, testosterone levels decreased significantly following the lacto-ovo-vegetarian diet. Reasons for this reduction in testosterone were unclear and may have been indirectly related to diet. Researchers suggested that the higher fibre intake during the vegetarian dietary treatment or the sudden change in dietary intake may explain the observed reduction in testosterone levels.

Studies have not directly examined the effect, if any, of a vegetarian diet on exercise performance. Studies have controlled for inherent differences between vegetarian diets and non-vegetarian diets, used populations that are not representative of athletes or failed to accurately assess training and competition performance. The training and competition benefits of consuming a high-CHO diet, which is achieved more easily with a vegetarian diet than a mixed diet, have been well researched (Simonsen et al. 1991). Future research is required to determine any possible benefits of consuming a vegetarian diet on exercise performance.

21.4 NUTRITION CONSIDERATIONS FOR VEGETARIAN ATHLETES

21.4.1 *Energy*

Table 21.2 summarises dietary surveys of females following vegetarian diets compared with non-vegetarian controls. Only one study in Table 21.2 reports dietary data for female vegetarians who are athletes. It is difficult to collect dietary intake information on vegetarian athletes, particularly elite-level athletes, due to small numbers of athletes choosing a vegetarian diet.

As can be seen from Table 21.2, vegetarian diets are often higher in fibre, raising concern about the ability of vegetarian athletes to consume adequate kilojoules to meet daily energy requirements (Grandjean 1987; Ruud 1990). Meat alternatives for vegetarians, such as legumes, dried beans and dried peas, are high-fibre foods. Incorporating vegetarian meat alternatives such as nuts, tofu, tempeh, textured vegetable protein and commercially prepared meat analogues, helps increase energy density. Pritikin (1984) suggested that vegetarian athletes could consume sufficient kilojoules, even when daily energy requirements are high.

21.4.2 *Protein*

Daily protein requirements are slightly higher for athletes (1.2–1.5 g/kg BM/d) than for sedentary people (see Chapter 5). Concern has been raised regarding the ability of vegetarian athletes, in particular vegan athletes, to meet these added demands (Grandjean 1987; Ruud 1990). Although vegetarians often consume less protein than non-vegetarians, the Australian Recommended Dietary Intake (RDI) for protein of 0.75 g/kg BM/d (National Health & Medical Research Council 1991) is easily met (see Table 21.2).

Plant food sources of protein often contain low levels of one of the essential amino acids and may (certainly not exclusively) have low digestibility compared to animal sources of protein. Some concern currently exists, at least at the consumer level, that insufficient levels of amino acids in plant foods will result in inadequate protein intake. In a recent review, Young and Pellett (1994) state that mixtures of plant proteins can serve as a complete source of amino acids, providing that the daily total protein intake met daily recommendations. It was thought that complementing plant sources of protein at individual meals was necessary to provide all essential amino acids. The American Dietetic Association (1997) stated that combining plant sources of protein in such a way as to meet all the essential amino acids is unnecessary. Vegetarian diets can provide adequate protein without the use of supplements or special foods, if daily energy demands of the athlete are met (American Dietetic Association 1997).

21.4.3 *Iron*

Athletes, particularly female endurance athletes, are at greater risk of low iron stores than non-athletes (Fogelholm 1995). Iron requirements are usually higher in athletes (especially endurance and adolescent athletes) than in untrained people. The American Dietetic Association (1993), in a position statement on vegetarian diets, concluded that vegetarians in developed countries were not at greater risk of iron deficiency than non-vegetarians. However, recent studies have reported low iron status in male and female vegetarians compared with omnivores, despite similar or

Table 21.2 Average daily nutrient and energy intakes from dietary surveys comparing female vegetarians to non-vegetarians

Reference	Type of diet	Diet assessment	Age (yr)	N	Energy (MJ/d)	CHO (g/d)	P (g/d)	P (g/kg/d)	Fat (g/d)	Ca++ (mg/d)	Fe++ (mg/d)	Fibre (g/d)	Vit C (mg/d)
Non-athletes													
Marsh et al. (1988)	LOV	7 d weighed FR	66.8	10	6.74	-	56	-	65	898	12.3	5.2	92
	NV		64.4	10	6.86	-	68	-	77	712	13.3	4.7	105
Tylavsky & Anderson (1988)	LOV	QFFQ	73.0	88	6.41	216	55	0.87	56	823	10.7	5.6	184
	NV		78.8	287	6.83	188**	70***	1.16	88***	902	10.2	4.2**	157***
Nieman et al. (1989)	LOV	7 d FR	72.3	19	5.95	228	44	0.75	49	-	-	23.2	-
	NV		69.5	12	6.09	186***	56	0.88	61*	-	-	13.3**	-
Pedersen et al. (1991)	LOV	3 d FR	35.5	34	7.64	264	63	1.08	67	931	20.0	26.0	316
	NV		29.4	41	7.14	218*	75*	1.26	61	873	22.0	15.0**	184
Tesar et al. (1992)	LOV	6 d semi-weighed FR + 24 hr DH	62.9	28	6.91	242	63	1.02	56	820	13.0	10.3	143
	NV		62.9	28	6.94	199**	77*	1.22	62	863	15.5	7.6**	118*
Janelle & Barr (1995)	V	3 d FR	28.0	8	8.04	300	51	0.87	64	578²	17.7	35.01*	186¹*
	LOV		25.8	15	8.46	288	57	0.97	76	875	13.7	24.7	141
	NV		27.9	22	8.72	284	77*	1.24	75	950	15.3	22.4	116
Ball & Bartlett (1999)	LOV	12 d weighed FR	25.3	50	6.9	211	54	-	60	-	10.7	24.4	150
	NV		25.2	24	6.9	183	67**	-	65	-	9.9	17.3**	111**
Haddad et al. (1999)	V	3 d FR + 24hr DH	36.0	15	7.09	-	52	-	52	590	17.6	38.0	275
	NV		33.5	10	8.24	-	74***	-	76*	830	15.3	15.0³	125*
Athletes													
Synder et al. (1989)	MV	3 d FR	37.8	9	7.46	229	59	1.05	71	-	14.7	-	-
	NV		39.2	9	6.99	186*	73*	1.22	71	-	14.0	-	-

Diet: V = vegan, LOV = lacto-ovo-vegetarian, MV = modified vegetarian, NV = control,
FR = food record, QFFQ = quantitative food frequency questionnaire, DH = dietary history
*, **, ***, Mean intake of NV differed from means of V, LOV and MV at P < 0.05; P < 0.01, P < 0.001
¹ Significant at P < 0.05 compared to LOV and NV
² Significant at P < 0.05 compared to NV only
³ Significant at P < 0.001 compared to NV and V

higher iron intakes (Ball & Bartlett 1999; Haddad et al. 1999). Among athlete populations, where iron requirements are increased, it is still unclear whether vegetarian diets can provide adequate bioavailable iron.

In a review on vegetarianism in athletes, Ruud (1990) concluded that poor absorption of non-haem iron from plant-based foods increased risk of iron deficiency in vegetarian athletes. One case study reported iron deficiency anaemia in a strict vegetarian male long-distance runner with an estimated intake of 16.8 mg/d of iron (Jacobs & Wilson 1984). The cause of iron deficiency was impossible to determine and may have been related to poor iron bioavailability which was not directly assessed, and/or high iron requirements which are likely in endurance running (Siegal et al. 1979).

Synder and colleagues (1989) investigated dietary iron intakes and haematological parameters in nine female endurance runners consuming a modified vegetarian diet (MV) (< 100 g per week of red meat) with nine controls consuming a mixed diet (RM) (including red meat). No significant difference in total iron intake between groups was noted (see Table 21.2), yet serum ferritin levels were significantly lower for athletes in the MV group. The low bioavailability of iron of MV was suspected to account for these differences. Seiler et al. (1989) also reported lower serum ferritin levels in 39 male and 11 female ultra-endurance runners who followed a lacto-ovo-vegetarian diet compared with 52 male and eight female non-vegetarian controls. However, no impairment in running performance between the two dietary groups was observed.

Vegan and lacto-ovo-vegetarian diets rely predominantly on non-haem iron sources. Sources of iron are similar in vegan and lacto-ovo-vegetarian diets, as milk and other dairy products are poor iron sources. Absorption of non-haem iron from plant foods is poor (2%–20%) compared to absorption of haem iron from animal foods (15%–35%) (Hallberg 1981). In a vegetarian diet, the abundance of naturally occurring iron inhibitors in plant foods, including phytates, polyphenols and tannins, may further inhibit iron absorption (see Chapter 11, Section 11.5.2.2). Of benefit, however, is that vegetarian diets are usually high in vitamin C and citric acid, which helps negate the effects of iron inhibitors and increases absorption of non-haem iron from food (American Dietetic Association 1997).

21.4.4 *Calcium*

Lacto-ovo-vegetarians usually report similar calcium intakes to omnivores. Pederson et al. (1991) used three-day food records to compare dietary intakes of pre-menopausal lacto-ovo-vegetarian women to non-vegetarian controls. Calcium intakes of 34 vegetarians were not significantly different to that of the 41 non-vegetarians (931 ± 69 mg/d versus 873 ± 78 mg/d). Other studies report similar or even higher calcium intakes for lacto-ovo-vegetarians compared with non-vegetarian controls (Marsh et al. 1988; Tylavsky & Anderson 1988; Slattery et al. 1991; Tesar et al. 1992).

In most dietary studies of vegetarians, vegans are combined with lacto-ovo-vegetarians, making it difficult to determine differences in calcium intakes between these groups. In one study, Janelle and Barr (1995) found that vegan females had lower calcium intakes compared to lacto-ovo-vegetarians and ominvores. Using three-day food records, reported calcium intakes were 578 mg/d, 875 mg/d and 950 mg/d, for the vegan, lacto-ovo-vegetarian and non-vegetarian groups, respectively. In contrast, Haddad and colleagues (1999) found no difference in daily calcium intakes between vegan males and females compared with matched non-vegetarian controls.

Apart from dairy products, relatively few foods provide concentrated sources of calcium (Baghurst et al. 1993). Cereal foods were the second supplier of calcium in the diet of respondents to the Australian National Nutrition Survey (McLennan & Podger 1998). Until recently, individuals who limited or excluded dairy foods had few other alternatives, relying heavily on calcium-rich green leafy vegetables, calcium-fortified tofu and cereals to assist in increasing daily calcium intake. Weaver et al. (1999) suggested that individuals who avoid eating dairy products should include calcium-fortified foods or supplements in their diet to meet daily calcium requirements. Recently, calcium-fortified soy milks, yoghurts and custards have been made available in major supermarkets in response to the growing number of people choosing to use these products.

To assess the full impact of a vegetarian diet on daily calcium balance, it is prudent to consider factors that alter absorption and retention of calcium in the body. Calcium bioavailability from plant foods is reduced in the presence of phytates and oxalates, known inhibitors of calcium absorption (Weaver & Plawecki 1994; Weaver et al. 1999). Calcium-rich plant foods such as spinach and rhubarb have high oxalate contents and provide negligible absorbable calcium. However, low-oxalate vegetables such as kale, broccoli and bok choy can provide rich sources of calcium in diets based solely on plant foods. Factors such as sodium and protein content of the diet should also be considered, as these factors significantly influence calcium urinary excretion rates (Weaver et al. 1999).

21.4.5 *Vitamin B12*

Clinical vitamin B12 deficiency is rare and is more probably associated with an absence or defect in secretion of Intrinsic Factor than inadequate intake of vitamin B12 in the diet (American Dietetic Association 1988). However, a dietary deficiency of vitamin B12 can develop in a strict vegan, fruitarian or macrobiotic diet (Herbert 1994). People consuming a mixed or lacto-ovo-vegetarian diet easily meet daily vitamin B12 requirements. Active vitamin B12 is found exclusively in animal foods and products. No active vitamin B12 is naturally found in any plant foods, including meat analogues or fermented soy products such as tempeh (Herbert 1988). For vegans, fruitarians or individuals following a macrobiotic diet, a reliable, fortified source of vitamin B12 should be included in the diet (American Dietetic

Association 1988). Dairy products and eggs provide sufficient vitamin B12 for lacto-ovo-vegetarians. Vegans should consume vitamin B12-fortified soy milks or consider vitamin B12 supplementation, or risk the possibility of vitamin B12 deficiency disease (Herbert 1988).

21.4.6 *Zinc*

Meat, meat-based dishes and dairy products provide roughly 50% of the zinc in the diet of respondents to the Australian National Nutrition Survey (McLennan & Podger 1998). Cereals are the primary zinc source in the vegetarian diet; vegetarian meat alternatives (legumes, nuts, soya products and eggs) and dairy foods are secondary sources (Gibson 1994). Studies report similar or lower zinc intakes in vegetarians compared to non-vegetarians (Haddad et al. 1999; Janelle & Barr 1995). Haddad et al. (1999) found no difference in zinc intake or zinc status of ten male and 15 female vegans compared to non-vegetarian controls. Higher intakes of dietary fibre are regularly reported in vegetarian diets which may negatively impact on zinc status (Latta & Liebman 1984).

21.4.7 *Riboflavin*

The major source of riboflavin in the diet of respondents in the Australian National Nutrition Survey was milk and milk products (McLennan & Podger 1998). For the vegan athlete who excludes soy milk and soy-milk products, consuming adequate riboflavin may be difficult as soy is a good source of riboflavin. Janelle and Barr (1995) reported lower intakes of riboflavin in eight female vegans compared with 15 lacto-ovo-vegetarians and 22 non-vegetarian controls.

21.4.8 *Creatine*

It has been demonstrated that vegetarians have lower body creatine pools than non-vegetarians (Maughan 1995). Creatine supplementation is likely to increase muscle creatine stores significantly in vegetarians if muscle creatine stores are initially low (see Chapter 17, Section 17.6.1). For vegetarian athletes competing in sports involving repeated bouts of short-term activity, creatine supplementation may therefore be beneficial (see Chapter 17, Section 17.6.1).

21.5 *VEGETARIAN EATING AND AMENORRHOEA*

Pedersen et al. (1991) found that the frequency of menstrual irregularity in vegetarian non-athletes was five times that of controls. In this study, no differences were observed in total energy intake between the vegetarians and controls, although fibre intake was significantly higher in the vegetarians than controls. In a study investigating 26 female runners, Brooks and colleagues (1984) reported a higher incidence of secondary amenorrhoea in athletes following a modified vegetarian diet (< 200 g red meat per week). Interestingly, the fat intake was significantly less for the amenorrheic runners (68 ± 8 g/d) compared with regularly menstruating runners (98 ± 11 g/d). Slavin et al. (1984) found similar results in 89 females engaging in physical activity at least twice per week. Researchers reported a higher prevalence of secondary amenorrhoea in vegetarians (31%) compared to non-vegetarians (4%). However, other studies reported no difference in menstrual irregularities between female vegetarian and non-vegetarian athletes (Hanne et al. 1986). In a recent review, Barr (1999) suggested that no single dietary or lifestyle factor solely accounted for menstrual irregularities. Further studies are required to understand the effects of vegetarian diets on menstrual status in athletes.

21.6 SUMMARY

As dietary surveys of vegetarian athletes are scarce, this chapter has reported nutrient intakes of non-athletic adult populations following lact-ovo-vegetarian and vegan diets. Many of these dietary survey studies have focussed on elderly female populations, hardly representative of athletes. Further dietary survey studies on athletic populations are required to fully understand the influence of a long-term vegetarian diet on exercise performance. Minimal information is available on the nutrient adequacy of restrictive vegetarian diets such as fruitarian and macrobiotic diets, particularly among athletic populations. The high-CHO content usually consumed in vegetarian diets is conducive to restoring and maintaining adequate glycogen stores in athletes in hard training programs. A well-planned lacto-ovo-vegetarian diet and vegan diet will meet the nutrient requirements of most athletes. However, meeting energy requirements of athletes with high energy expenditures may be difficult. Although animal foods are good sources of protein, iron, zinc and vitamin B12, and dairy products are rich sources of calcium, alternative sources are available in most vegetarian diets. Energy-dense plant foods high in protein should be encouraged for athletes with high energy and protein requirements. Food sources fortified with vitamin B12 should be included in a vegan diet to ensure adequate amounts are consumed. Further research is required to gain a better understanding of the influence of a long-term vegetarian diet on menstrual status in female athletes. Athletes following a 'fussy meat-eating diet' appear to face similar nutrient concerns to vegetarians and may be at greater risk of nutritional inadequacies as they often fail to replace red meat with suitable alternatives.

21.7 PRACTICE TIPS

Greg Cox

Dietary assessment

• Clarify why an athlete chooses a vegetarian diet early in the interview process. Cultural, moral, environmental and religious reasons for choosing a vegetarian diet should always be respected. Fussy meat eaters often avoid eating red meat or limit intake of dairy foods for fear of them being high in fat and/or cholesterol. For these athletes, addressing issues regarding the nutritional composition of red meat and dairy foods, and providing suitable, convenient plant or meat alternatives warrants discussion.

- Determine the style of vegetarian diet followed and assess potentially limiting nutrients. Diets of vegan athletes should be assessed for usual daily energy, calcium, vitamin B12, iron and zinc intake. Assess the athlete's nutrition knowledge, and whether efforts are made to plan well-balanced meals.

Key nutrient concerns for vegetarian athletes, including dietary strategies to address these concerns

- If an athlete has recently converted to a vegetarian diet, assess usual daily energy intake and weight history. It may be difficult for newly converted vegetarian athletes to maintain their previous energy intake if their diet contains bulky, high-fibre, wholesome CHO foods. Increasing consumption of high-fibre meat alternatives such as legumes and beans may make it difficult to meet daily energy requirements and cause an increase in flatulence. Encourage the use of energy-dense, low-bulk foods to assist in increasing energy intake. Examples of such foods include gluten meat alternatives, textured vegetable protein, tempeh, tofu, fruit juices, dried fruits, nuts, peanut or nut butter, honey and jams. For lacto-ovo-vegetarians, low-fat milk, reduced-fat cheese and other low-fat dairy products are also low in bulk and energy dense.

- Examine sources of protein, especially at the midday meal. Many lacto-ovo-vegetarians will use cheese as a convenient meat alternative, whereas vegans may fail to use suitable protein alternatives. As athletes often have limited time for meal preparation, providing examples of suitable, convenient meat alternatives for lunch is crucial. Ready-prepared beans (e.g. baked beans) are an excellent choice, along with nut and seed spreads, such as peanut butter, tahini and almond spread. Ready-made luncheon meats, derived from wheat gluten, are also an excellent sandwich meat alternative.

- Many dietitians are quick to encourage legumes or tofu as meat alternatives, failing to realise the diverse array of semi-prepared, vegetarian meat alternatives available in supermarkets. Encouraging more regular use of lentils or other dried beans or peas automatically increases the bulkiness and satiety of meals. This is a concern for athletes with high energy requirements, and those who lose their appetite after exercise. Numerous products, derived from soy, nut or vegetable protein are an energy-dense alternative. Becoming familiar with these foods will facilitate more effective counselling when dealing with vegetarian athletes.

- Assess calcium intake, particularly in a vegan diet. Determine the types of soy milk consumed, if any, and recommend calcium-fortified varieties. Other suitable non-dairy calcium-rich alternatives include tofu, soy yoghurts, soy custards, cereals and low oxalate green vegetables such as broccoli, bok choy and kale.

- Dietary intake of riboflavin may be limited in vegan athletes, particularly those who avoid consuming soy milk and soy-milk products. Rich sources of riboflavin for the vegan athlete include fortified breakfast cereals, grains, textured vegetable protein, soy milks, soy yoghurts, soy custards, soy cheeses and yeast extract spreads such as Marmite™ and Vegemite™.

- Assess sources of vitamin B12 in athletes following a vegan diet. Dairy foods and eggs provide sufficient vitamin B12 in athletes following a lacto-ovo-vegetarian diet. Vegan athletes should include a known source of vitamin B12 such as fortified soy milks.

- Assessment of iron status is warranted in all athletes following a vegetarian diet. Be sure to assess total dietary iron and factors likely to promote or inhibit iron bioavailability. Significant sources of iron for vegetarians include breakfast cereals (especially those commercially fortified with iron), bread, textured vegetable protein, legumes, dried beans, gluten-based vegetarian meat alternatives, nuts, dried fruits and green leafy vegetables. Chapter 11 describes strategies for improving total dietary iron and optimising iron bioavailablity. Iron supplements are only warranted where iron depletion or iron deficiency anaemia has been diagnosed.

- Vegetarian diets usually provide macronutrients in amounts similar to those recommended for optimal sports performance. Generally, studies show that vegetarian diets contain adequate protein, are high in CHO and low in fat. Certain athletes following a vegetarian diet, however, may have a high fat intake by consuming large amounts of full-fat dairy products and excess amounts of added fats, oils and salad dressings. Where necessary, recommend low-fat dairy foods and soy alternatives, low-fat cooking methods and meat alternatives to ensure recommended levels of fat in the diet are more easily met.

- Some female adolescent athletes following a vegetarian diet may simply be restricting dietary intake and masking disordered eating behaviour. Female adolescent athletes are sensitive to issues regarding BM and body-fat levels, and may disguise a restricted eating pattern by describing their intake as vegetarian.

- Encourage variety in food choice and consumption of protein-rich and CHO-rich foods at each meal. Vegetarian meat alternatives include lentils, dried beans and peas (ready-to-use products are available), tofu, tempeh, textured vegetable (or soy) protein, and ready-made nut, soy or wheat-derived alternatives. Encourage athletes to experiment with new foods and direct them to suitable cookbooks specialising in vegetarian cuisine. Sanitarium Health Food Company is the largest vegetarian company within Australia and New Zealand, and produces numerous nutrition resources including cookbooks, nutritional product analysis brochures and newsletters. Their current web page address is: http//:www.sanitarium.com.au.

Problems in nutrient analysis of vegetarian diets

- Nutrient analysis of a vegetarian diet can be difficult, as many commercially available vegetarian meat alternatives are not included in food composition databases. To obtain an accurate nutrient analysis, it may be necessary to obtain nutrient information for food labels or approach the company for nutrient composition of the food. For instance, Sanitarium Health Food Company produces a range of nutrition analysis brochures for their products. However, food labels do not include a comprehensive nutrient analysis of the product and are not valid for research purposes.

Resources for vegetarians

- Refer the athlete to credible sources in vegetarianism. The Australia Vegetarian Society produces a quarterly journal (*New Vegetarian and Natural Health*) which contains reliable nutrition education messages, suitable vegetarian recipes, details of vegetarian meeting groups and restaurants throughout Australia. The current website address for the Australian Vegetarian Society is: http//:www.moreinfo.com.au/avs.

- Other recommended vegetarian website addresses include the following:
  — The International Vegetarian Union (http//:www.ivu.org) have a comprehensive website providing website addresses for the various vegetarian societies throughout the world.
  — The Vegetarian Resource Group's current website address is: http//:www.vrg.org.
  — The current website address of the Vegan Society, based in the United Kingdom, is: http//:www.vegansociety.com.

REFERENCES

American Dietetic Association. Position of The American Dietetic Association: vegetarian diets—technical support paper. J Am Diet Assoc 1988;88:352–5.

American Dietetic Association. Position of the American Dietetic Association: vegetarian diets. J Am Diet Assoc 1993;93:1317–19.

American Dietetic Association. Position of The American Dietetic Association: vegetarian diets. J Am Diet Assoc 1997;97:1317–21.

Baghurst K, Record S, Syrette J, et al. What are Australians eating? Results from the 1985 and 1990 Victorian nutrition surveys. Adelaide, Australia: CSIRO Division of Human Nutrition, 1993.

Ball MJ, Bartlett MA. Dietary intake and iron status of Australian vegetarian women. Am J Clin Nutr 1999;70:353–8.

Barr SI. Nutrition knowledge and selected nutritional practices of female recreational athletes. J Nutr Ed 1986;18:167–74.

Barr SI. Vegetarianism and menstrual cycle disturbances: is there an association? Am J Clin Nutr 1999;70:S549–S54.

Brooks SM, Sanborn CF, Albrecht BH, Wagner WW Jr. Diet in athletic amenorrhoea. Lancet 1984;1:559–60.

Burke LM, Read RSD. Diet patterns of elite Australian male triathletes. Phys Sportsmed 1987;15:140–55.

Burr ML, Butland BK. Heart disease in British vegetarians. Am J Clin Nutr 1988;48:830–2.

Burr ML, Sweetnam PM. Vegetarianism, dietary fiber, and mortality. Am J Clin Nutr 1982;36:873–7.

Dwyer JT. Health aspects of vegetarian diets. Am J Clin Nutr 1988;48:712–38.

Fogelholm M. Indicators of vitamin and mineral status in athletes' blood: a review. Int J Sport Nutr 1995;5:267–84.

Gibson, RS. Content and bioavailability of trace elements in vegetarian diets. Am J Clin Nutr 1994;59:S1223–S32.

Giovannucci E, Rimm EB, Stampfer MJ, Colditz GA, Ascherio A, Willett WC. Intake of fat, meat and fiber in relation to risk of colon cancer in men. Cancer Res 1994;54:2390–7.

Grandjean AC. The vegetarian athlete. Phys Sportsmed 1987;15:191–4.

Haddad EH, Berk LS, Kettering JD, Hubbard RW, Peters WR. Dietary intake and biochemical, hematologic and immune status of vegans compared with non-vegetarians. Am J Clin Nutr 1999;70:S586–S93.

Hallberg L. Bioavailability of dietary iron in man. Annu Rev Nutr 1981;1:123–47.

Hanne N, Dlin R, Rotstein A. Physical fitness, anthropometric and metabolic parameters in vegetarian athletes. J Sports Med 1986;26:180–5.

Herbert V. Vitamin B-12: plant sources, requirements and assay. Am J Clin Nutr 1988;48:852–8.

Herbert V. Staging vitamin B-12 (cobalamin) status in vegetarians. Am J Clin Nutr 1994;59:S1213–S22.

Jacobs MB, Wilson W. Iron deficiency anemia in a vegetarian runner. JAMA 1984;252:481–2.

Janelle KC, Barr SI. Nutrient intakes and eating behaviour scores of vegetarian and non-vegetarian women. J Am Diet Assoc 1995;95:180–6, 189.

Latta D, Liebman M. Iron and zinc status of vegetarian and non-vegetarian males. Nutr Rep Int 1984;30:141–9.

Levin N, Rattan J, Gilat T. Energy intake and body weight in ovo-lacto-vegetarians. J Clin Gastroenterol 1986;8:451–3.

McLennan W, Podger A, eds. National Nutrition Survey: nutrient intakes and physical measurements, Australia 1995. ABS Catalogue No. 4805.0. Canberra, Australia: Australian Bureau of Statistics, 1998.

Marsh AG, Sanchez TV, Michelsen O, Chaffee FL, Fagal SM. Vegetarian lifestyle and bone mineral density. Am J Clin Nutr 1988;48:837–41.

Maughan RJ. Creatine supplementation and exercise performance. Int J Sport Nutr 1995;5:S39–S61.

Nagel D, Seiler D, Franz H, Leitzmann C, Jung K. Effects of an ultra-long-distance (1000 km) race on lipid metabolism. Eur J Appl Physiol 1989;59:16–20.

National Health & Medical Research Council. Recommended Dietary Intakes for use in Australia. Canberra, Australia: Australian Government Publishing Service, 1991.

Nieman DC. Vegetarian dietary practices and endurance performance. Am J Clin Nutr 1988;48:754–61.

Nieman DC, Sherman KM, Arabatzis K, et al. Hematological, anthropometric and metabolic comparisons between vegetarian and non-vegetarian elderly women. Int J Sport Med 1989;10:243–50.

Pedersen AB, Bartholomew MJ, Dolence LA, Aljadir LP, Netteburg KL, Lloyd T. Menstrual differences due to vegetarian and non-vegetarian diets. Am J Clin Nutr 1991;53:879–85.

Phillips RL, Snowdon DA. Dietary relationships with fatal colorectal cancer among Seventh-Day Adventists. J Natl Cancer Inst 1985;74:307–17.

Pritikin N. The brave soldiers in the ironman army travel on their stomachs. Runner's World 1984;Feb:129.

Raben A, Kiens B, Richter EA, et al. Serum sex hormones and endurance performance after a lacto-ovo-vegetarian and a mixed diet. Med Sci Sports Exerc 1992;24:1290–7.

Richter EA, Kiens B, Raben A, Tvede N, Pedersen BK. Immune parameters in male athletes after a lacto-ovo-vegetarian diet and a mixed Western diet. Med Sci Sports Exerc 1991;23:517–21.

Ruud, JS. Vegetarianism—implications for athletes. Omaha: International Center for Sports Nutrition, 1990.

Siegel AJ, Hennekens CH, Solomon HS, Van Boeckel B. Exercise-related hematuria: findings in a group of marathon runners. JAMA 1979;241:391–2.

Seiler D, Nagel D, Franz H, Hellstern P, Leitzmann C, Jung K. Effects of long-distance running on iron metabolism and hematological parameters. Int J Sports Med 1989;10:357–62.

Simonsen JC, Sherman WM, Lamb DR, Dernbach AR, Doyle JA, Strauss R. Dietary CHO, muscle glycogen, and power output during rowing training. J Appl Physiol 1991;70:1500–5.

Slattery ML, Jacobs DR, Hilner JE Jr, et al. Meat consumption and its associations with other diet and health factors in young adults: the Cardia study. Am J Clin Nutr 1991;54:930–5.

Slavin J, Lutter J, Cushman S. Amenorrhoea in vegetarian athletes. Lancet 1984;1:1474–5.

Snowdon DA, Phillips RL. Does a vegetarian diet reduce the occurrence of diabetes? Am J Public Health 1985;75:507–12.

Synder AC, Dvorak LL, Roepke JB. Influence of dietary iron source on measures of iron status among female runners. Med Sci Sports Exerc 1989;21:7–10.

Tesar R, Notelovitz M, Shim E, Kauwell G, Brown J. Axial and peripheral bone density and nutrient intakes of postmenopausal vegetarian and omnivorous women. Am J Clin Nutr 1992;56:699–704.

The Little Oxford Dictionary of Current English. Oxford: Oxford University Press, 1980.

Thorogood M, Mann J, Appleby P, McPherson K. Risk of death from cancer and ischaemic heart disease in meat and non-meat eaters. BMJ 1994;308:1667–70.

Tylavsky FA, Anderson JJB. Dietary factors in bone health of elderly lacto-ovo-vegetarian and omnivorous women. Am J Clin Nutr 1988;48:842–9.

Weaver CM, Plawecki KL. Dietary calcium: adequacy of a vegetarian diet. Am J Clin Nutr 1994;59:S1238–S41.

Weaver CM, Proulx WR, Heaney R. Choices for achieving adequate dietary calcium with a vegetarian diet. Am J Clin Nutr 1999;70:S543–S8.

Williams PT. Interactive effects of exercise, alcohol and vegetarian diet on coronary artery disease risk factors in 9242 runners: the national runners' health study. Am J Clin Nutr 1997;66:1197–206.

Young VR, Pellett PL. Plant proteins in relation to human protein and amino acid nutrition. Am J Clin Nutr 1994;59:S1203–S12.

Athletes with gastrointestinal disorders

Kieran Fallon

22.1 INTRODUCTION

Gastrointestinal (GI) problems are common reasons for presentation to medical practitioners, but very little is known about their prevalence in the athletic population. A number of studies have reported both upper- and lower-GI symptoms during exercise (Brouns et al. 1987; Riddoch & Trinnick 1998), however, there is little to no investigation of the cause of these symptoms, or confirmation of similar symptoms at rest. It is recognised that exercise, particularly at high intensities, leads to GI symptoms and may exacerbate existing GI conditions.

22.2 UPPER-GI TRACT

Major upper-GI problems include gastro-oesophageal reflux disease, gastritis and peptic ulcer, and functional dyspepsia.

22.2.1 Gastro-oesophageal reflux disease

Gastro-oesophageal reflux disease (GERD) is a common disorder with about one-third of adults experiencing heartburn once a month and 5–10% of adults experiencing heartburn each day. Many patients experience accompanying reflux of gastric contents into the mouth. The majority of cases are recurrent but overeating may induce an acute, isolated episode.

The major factor preventing GERD is normal functioning of the lower-oesophageal sphincter; however, delayed gastric emptying, with its attendant maintenance of an elevated gastric volume, and the presence of a sliding hiatus hernia, are also important in the pathogenesis of this condition (de Carle 1998). High pressure in the gut lumen keeps the oesophageal sphincter closed, preventing stomach contents from entering the oesophagus. Until recently, it was thought that the pressure holding the oesophageal sphincter closed was persistently low in GERD sufferers, but it now appears that most patients have frequent transient relaxations of the sphincter muscle at inappropriate times, such as after a meal. This relaxation allows acid to enter the oesophagus and induce a chemical burn. The primary cause of abnormal function of the lower-oesophageal sphincter is unknown, but adult-onset GERD may be a familial condition. Fortunately, only about 10% of cases of GERD are associated with chronic inflammation of the oesophagus.

Several forms of exercise can induce gastro-oesophageal reflux (GOR), which may be asymptomatic. Yazaki et al. (1996) compared the incidence of GOR in normally asymptomatic athletes involved in rowing and running, by measurement of intra-oesophageal pH, before, during and after rowing, fasted running and postprandial running. While GOR was demonstrated in two out of 17 athletes prior to exercise, it was induced by exercise in 70% of rowers, in 45% of fasted runners and in 90% of runners who had just eaten. This study indicated that athletes with a history of GOR should avoid even small meals close to the time of exercise.

Fortunately, GOR and GERD are easily treated in the majority of cases. Medical management generally involves:

- avoidance of aggravating factors, some of which may be specific to the individual;
- weight loss, if overweight;
- antacids or medications to reduce acid secretion (e.g. H_2 receptor antagonists, proton pump inhibitors); and
- prokinetic agents which increase the rate of gastric emptying.

Factors that reduce the muscle tone in the lower-oesophageal sphincter, and hence lower-oesophageal sphincter pressure, include cigarette smoking and the use of various classes of medication including anticholinergics, theophylline, progesterone, calcium channel blockers, diazepam, $beta_2$ agonists and alpha adrenergic antagonists (Hughes 1997). In addition, athletes with established reflux oesophagitis should avoid drugs which are directly damaging to the oesophageal mucosa, including non-steroidal anti-inflammatory drugs (NSAIDs) and iron supplements.

Specific dietary factors which decrease lower-oesophageal sphincter pressure and/or increase gastric acid secretion include caffeine, fat, chocolate, alcohol and peppermint. Although the effectiveness of avoiding these foods is not evidence-based, avoidance, especially on an empty stomach, does provide relief for some people. When compared with caffeinated coffee, decaffeinated coffee has been demonstrated to reduce the period of abnormally low oesophageal pH in reflux patients (Pehl et al. 1997). Decaffeinated coffee, therefore, may be a useful alternative for coffee drinkers. Tomatoes, citrus juices and spicy foods have been implicated as direct oesophageal mucosal irritants. However, some people experience no symptoms eating these foods. Often patients can identify their own problem foods, which give them symptoms. Ingestion of large meals and eating just before going to bed also give many people symptoms. Large meals stimulate a corresponding high secretion of gastric acid.

22.2.2 *Functional dyspepsia*

Functional dyspepsia is defined as chronic or recurrent pain or discomfort in the upper abdomen, with no clinical or endoscopic evidence of known organic disease. It is a common but poorly understood condition.

The symptomology is varied, but four subgroups have been identified as seen in Table 22.1.

Table 22.1 *Subgroups of the condition functional dyspepsia, including symptoms*

Subgroups of functional dyspepsia	Symptoms
Ulcer-like dyspepsia	Nausea, vomiting, epigastric pain. More severe cases may be accompanied by severe pain and haematemesis.
Reflux-like dyspepsia	Heartburn, reflux of stomach contents into the mouth.
Dysmotility-like dyspepsia	Early satiety, post-prandial fullness, nausea, retching and/or vomiting that is recurrent, bloating in the upper abdomen (not accompanied by visible distension), upper-abdominal discomfort, often aggravated by food.
Unspecified dyspepsia	Symptoms do not fill the criteria of other categories.

Adapted from Talley et al. 1991

The diagnosis of functional dyspepsia should only be made following clinical evaluation and, ideally, an upper-gastrointestinal endoscopy. This excludes other disorders, including peptic ulceration, reflux oesophagitis, and malignancy.

In view of the uncertain aetiology of this condition, management is difficult. The placebo response in dyspepsia is between 30% and 60% and only a few of the large number of drugs tested for this condition have shown benefit in properly conducted clinical trials (Hu & Talley 1998). Despite this poor response, medications used to reduce acid secretion and enhance motility are commonly tried in clinical practice. As up to 50% of patients with functional dyspepsia have delayed gastric emptying and antral dysmotility (Waldron et al. 1991), it is appropriate to advise avoidance of foods known to retard gastric emptying (e.g. fatty meals). As in GERD, specific foods may be related to symptoms in some patients, and a formal diet diary recording the relationship of food ingestion to symptoms is useful. Small low-fat meals may be useful in some patients (Talley 1996).

Despite the high incidence of this condition in the general population, its incidence in the athletic population has not been studied, but is often seen in sports medicine practice.

22.2.3 *Gastritis and peptic ulcer*

Gastritis refers to inflammation of the mucosa of the stomach, which may be acute or chronic. Acute gastritis is associated with severe illness when it is termed 'acute erosive' or 'stress-induced gastritis'. In the athletic population or those suffering from rheumatological disorders, direct irritants such as aspirin, NSAIDs and alcohol can induce gastritis. Acute gastritis is also associated with infection by the bacteria Helicobacter pylori. In milder cases, which occur most frequently, symptoms include nausea, vomiting and epigastric pain. Severe pain and haematemesis occur in more advanced cases. Chronic gastritis is most often associated with Helicobacter pylori infection with active inflammation apparent in about 30–50% of Helicobacter pylori infections.

Management of most acute cases involves avoidance of further irritation and prescription of antacids or medications which inhibit acid secretion. Those cases associated with Helicobacter pylori infection are treated with the addition of antibiotics to the above-mentioned measures.

Peptic ulcer is a generic term for a common condition, which includes both duodenal and gastric ulcers. The aetiology is multifactorial but involves the action of acid and digestive enzymes, reduction of mucosal defenses and infection by Helicobacter pylori. Helicobacter pylori infection is found in 95% of cases of duodenal ulcer and 70% of gastric ulcers. NSAIDs are responsible for large numbers of gastric ulcers. Diagnosis is based on clinical history and examination and is usually confirmed by endoscopy. The typical symptom is recurrent epigastric pain, commonly described as sharp burning or gnawing, which may be relieved by eating food or ingestion of antacids. The pain recurs several hours after eating and is common at night. Complications include perforation, peritonitis and haematemesis (bleeding and vomiting blood).

Treatment involves eradication of Helicobacter pylori (Dev & Lambert 1998), if present, through the use of antibiotics and the use of medications which inhibit acid secretion. NSAIDs, aspirin and smoking should also be avoided. There is no evidence that bland diets reduce gastric acid secretion, promote healing or relieve symptoms of duodenal ulcer (McGuigan 1994). Although milk and other dairy products are often tried for early symptomatic relief, they do not assist in healing. The relatively low acidity of milk can actually lead to large production of gastric acid which promotes more pain and discomfort later on. Caffeine also increases gastric acid secretion and should be avoided, especially on an empty stomach. Otherwise, sufferers can eat the diet of their choice.

22.2.4 *Gastroenteritis*

Probably the most common gastrointestinal disease in athletes, and indeed in the general population, is acute viral gastroenteritis. While rotavirus is the most common causative agent in children, adults are more likely to develop symptoms following infection by Norwalk and related enteric caliciviruses. Such infections alter small intestinal microarchitecture and function and are associated with mild steatorrhoea, carbohydrate (CHO) malabsorption and decreased levels of enzymes in the brush border of the intestinal villi (Greenberg 1994).

The symptoms are well known and include nausea, vomiting, diarrhoea and abdominal pain in some cases, accompanied by headache, mild fever and malaise. No laboratory investigations are usually required, however, bloody diarrhoea suggests an invasive pathogen. A stool culture and microscopy is warranted if this occurs.

Treatment for uncomplicated viral cases is usually by oral rehydration therapy as well as anti-emetic and antidiarrhoeal medications. When a specific bacterial pathogen is suspected or identified, antibiotics are useful and, in these cases, anti-diarrhoeal medications are usually avoided.

Adequate volumes of fluids, which contain optimum amounts of sodium and CHO, are recommended for management of chronic and acute cases. Sports drinks may be useful in this situation but need to be sipped. In case of the possibility of transient lactose intolerance, a short period of abstinence from milk and dairy products is often advisable. Conventional advice suggests avoidance of fatty or fried foods for a short period.

22.3 LOWER-GI TRACT

22.3.1 *Inflammatory bowel disease*

The term inflammatory bowel disease includes ulcerative colitis and Crohn's disease, both of which are chronic relapsing diseases of the intestine. The main relevance to the sporting population lies in the age distribution of both diseases. While the prevalence is low in the general population, (5–8 per 100 000 for ulcerative colitis and 2–4 per 100 000 for Crohn's disease), the peak incidence for both diseases occurs between the ages of 15 and 35 years (Glickman 1994). The prevalence in the athletic population is not known.

The cause of inflammatory bowel disease is unknown but both genetic and environmental factors are implicated. Tobacco smokers are twice as likely to develop Crohn's disease as non-smokers but only half as likely to develop ulcerative colitis. Users of the oral contraceptive pill have about double the risk of development of Crohn's disease (Timmer et al. 1998).

Crohn's disease has multiple presentations, including prolonged intermittent abdominal discomfort with periods of diarrhoea and constipation, an appendicitis-like illness with right-sided abdominal pain, low-grade fever and tenderness, bloody diarrhoea, chronic diarrhoea or perianal disease. Management usually involves corticosteroids, immunosuppressive agents, and mesalazine-delivering drugs and antibiotics for perianal disease. More than 50% of patients require surgery at some time.

Ulcerative colitis most commonly presents as proctitis with rectal bleeding with mild diarrhoea; as colitis of mild to moderate degree with bloody diarrhoea; or as severe colitis with severe bloody diarrhoea, abdominal pain, fever, weight loss and anaemia. Pharmacological management is similar to that for Crohn's disease.

Dietary management involves correction of nutrient deficiencies, which are common when the disease is active. These are usually due to reduced food intake, but extensive involvement of the terminal ileum in Crohn's disease may significantly impair vitamin B12 absorption. The most commonly encountered nutrient deficiencies in moderate to severe cases are protein-energy, zinc, magnesium, selenium and a number of vitamins. In the acute phase, a low-residue diet is recommended. Seeds, skins, corn and large intakes of fibre may lead to complications in cases where small bowel stenosis is present, and should be avoided. If fat malabsorption is present, high oxalate foods may lead to the production of oxalate stones (Gibson & Anderson 1998). The meticulous use of elemental and polymeric diets has been shown to be as effective as oral prednisone in leading to remissions of small bowel Crohn's disease (Ferguson et al. 1998). Problems with long-term compliance, cost and acceptability preclude the use of elemental diets, except in severe cases.

22.3.2 *Irritable colon syndrome*

Irritable colon syndrome (ICS) is a condition characterised by abdominal pain and altered bowel habit in the absence of any abnormality on radiological, endoscopic or laboratory investigations. Approximately one-third of patients have constipation, one-third diarrhoea and one-third alternate between these symptoms. All have abdominal pain. ICS is the most common chronic gastroenterological disorder and has a prevalence of 15–25% in females and 5–20% in males in the general population (Malcolm & Kellow 1998). It is more common in the young and, therefore, may be frequently found in the young active population, although the prevalence in this age group has not been studied.

The cause is unknown but involves abnormalities in intestinal motor function, intestinal sensory function and central nervous system–enteric nervous system regulation. Infection and psychological factors have been implicated in triggering ICS and also in determining which patients present for treatment. True allergic or immunologically mediated responses to foods have little role in the aetiology of ICS. Food intolerance, however, may play a role, with dairy products and grains implicated as the most common precipitants of symptoms (Nanda et al. 1989).

Management involves exclusion of serious intestinal disease, and education—particularly in relation to trigger factors and reassurance. Medication choice depends on current symptoms and includes antidiarrhoeals, laxatives, antispasmodics and anticholinergics.

Possible dietary interventions include gradual increases in fibre intake and reduction of intake of caffeine, alcohol and cigarettes, which may contribute to loose bowel motions. Some patients complain of bloating and flatulence, and, for these people, lentils, beans, broccoli and leafy vegetables, carbonated drinks, large amounts of simple sugars and complex CHOs may need to be limited. Limiting intakes of CHO will be difficult in most athletes, so any restriction of these foods should be done on an individual basis in response to offending foods. Bloating and flatulence are also linked to swallowing air and advice on methods to reduce aerophagy including eating slowly, avoidance of gulping fluid and food (a commonly observed behaviour in athletes), and abstinence from chewing gum is often useful.

22.3.3 *Coeliac disease*

Coeliac disease, also known as gluten-sensitive enteropathy, is an inflammatory disease of the small intestine. It is caused by the ingestion of a specific protein (gliadin) found in oats, barley, wheat, rye and hybrid grains of these cereals. Most frequently seen in those of Celtic extraction, the prevalence in Australia is estimated to be one in 2000–3000 adults and in twice as many females to males (Pham & Barr 1996). Many patients have minimal to no symptoms so the prevalence may be much greater than estimated figures demonstrate.

The common clinical features in adults are abdominal pain, bloating, fatigue, weight loss, mild diarrhoea and steatorrhoea. Mouth ulcers, glossitis and stomatitis may also be present and, in more chronic cases, osteomalacia, osteoporosis, anaemia due to iron and/or folate deficiency, and hypoalbuminaemia are also seen.

Screening for this disease is through measurement of anti-endomysial antibodies. This is more sensitive and specific than the previously used antigliadin antibody test. A positive anti-endomysial antibody test should be followed by small-bowel biopsy, which generally reveals variable inflammation, short villi and crypt hyperplasia, which confirms the diagnosis.

Permanent withdrawal of gluten from the diet is standard treatment. Most patients have a rapid response, showing improvement in a few weeks. Wheat, barley and rye cereals and their products are excluded (Feighery 1999) and the assistance of a dietitian and a local coeliac society is invaluable. Oats, which were previously excluded, can be added to the diet of adults with coeliac disease without adverse effects (Janatuinen et al. 1995). Supplements for some nutrients may be required depending on the outcome of nutritional status measures. While withdrawal of gluten is important in terms of alleviating symptoms and general nutrition, it is also important in prevention of malignancy. Coeliac disease is classically associated with

T-cell lymphoma of the small intestine, but also with cancer of the pharynx and oesophagus. A strict gluten-free diet is protective against these malignancies (Holmes et al. 1989).

Dietary adherence to a gluten-free diet can be monitored by serial tests for anti-endomysial and antigliadin antibodies as well as by nutritional status measurements (see Chapter 3).

22.3.4 *Lactose intolerance*

Lactose intolerance is caused by lactase deficiency. Lactose is the principal CHO contained in milk and milk products, therefore, the typical symptoms of abdominal cramps (e.g. bloating and perhaps diarrhoea) follow the ingestion of milk and some dairy products. Lactose is not digested or absorbed and its presence in the gut leads to fluid shift into the intestinal lumen. Osmotic diarrhoea can occur after ingestion of large quantities of milk. Primary lactose intolerance, while having a hereditary basis, often does not become clinically apparent until adolescence, and is irreversible. Secondary lactase deficiency, which is transitory and associated with loss of enzyme function following mucosal damage, is usually associated with intestinal mucosal damage. It is most commonly seen following viral gastroenteritis, but may also be present in association with giardiasis, coeliac disease or inflammatory bowel disease.

Management is simple. Avoidance of products containing lactose leads to absence of symptoms. Most people with lactose intolerance can consume small amounts of milk at a time (around 100 mL) with no adverse effects.

22.3.5 *Haemochromatosis*

Haemochromatosis, an iron storage disease characterised by excessive mucosal absorption of iron, is an autosomal recessive disorder, which is symptomatic in one in 300 Caucasians. Deposition of excess iron occurs in the liver, heart, pancreas, joints and other organs. The most common clinical manifestations are skin pigmentation, diabetes and arthropathy. Presenting symptoms include lethargy, polyuria and excessive thirst, arthralgia and loss of libido.

Very commonly the diagnosis is suggested from routine screening of iron status measures, or during investigation of persistent fatigue in athletes. If the transferrin saturation is above 50%, and/or the serum ferritin is above the normal range and the athlete is not on iron supplementation, the test should be repeated (see Chapter 11, Section 11.6.1.4). If these iron status measures remain at high levels, a nucleic acid amplification gene test is required. It should be remembered that serum ferritin is an acute phase reactant and may be elevated following prolonged endurance exercise (Fallon et al. 1999). If such an elevation is suspected, the repeat test should be conducted 48–72 hours after exercise.

Management of early cases involves low dietary iron intake and measures to decrease iron absorption. More established cases, characterised by very high ferritin levels, require repeated phlebotomy.

Haemochromatosis highlights the need for correct diagnosis of iron deficiency in athletes prior to recommendation of iron supplementation (which would clearly be contraindicated should this condition be present).

22.4 *THE EFFECT OF EXERCISE ON THE GASTROINTESTINAL SYSTEM: DISORDERS SPECIFICALLY RELATED TO EXERCISE*

22.4.1 *Gastrointestinal motility and blood-flow*

Exercise is associated with a decrease in lower-oesophageal sphincter pressure (Peters et al. 1988). A reduction in duration, frequency and amplitude of oesophageal contractions is also observed with exercise intensities above 60% $VO_{2\,max}$ (Soffer et al. 1993).

The effect of exercise on gastric emptying has been addressed elsewhere (see Chapter 14). At exercise intensities up to 70% $VO_{2\,max}$, the gastric emptying rate is usually not influenced by exercise, but is controlled by other physiological, neural factors and nutrient composition of foods present (Fordtran & Salting 1967).

The majority of studies indicate that physical activity delays the transit time of food in the small bowel, most likely the result of decreased propulsion (Brouns & Beckers 1993). In contrast, hard physical activity speeds up transit time of faecal contents in the colon; probably because of increased mucosal secretion, which dilutes colonic contents. As the majority of intestinal transit time of faecal waste occurs in the colon, the overall effect of physical activity on total gastrointestinal transit time is a reduction.

Disturbances of gastrointestinal function may be related to reduction in local blood-flow. During exercise, splanchnic vasoconstriction occurs, allowing increased blood to be shunted to muscle and skin for oxygen and substrate transport, and thermoregulation, respectively. Both the splanchnic and coeliac circulations experience decreased blood-flow. Rowell et al. (1964) studied subjects working at 70% $VO_{2\,max}$ and observed a 60–70% decrease in splanchnic blood-flow. This suggested a relationship between increasing exercise intensity and reduction in blood-flow. At $VO_{2\,max}$ splanchnic flow has been shown to be reduced by as much as 70–80%. The reductions in blood-flow are worsened by concomitant dehydration. Blood-flow improves in the trained athlete and when exercise intensity is reduced (Clausen 1977). There may be some adaptation operating in highly trained athletes.

22.4.2 *Diarrhoea and other gastrointestinal disturbances during competition*

Gastrointestinal symptoms are common in athletes and have been extensively studied in marathon runners and triathletes (Sullivan 1981, 1986; Keeffe et al. 1984; Worobetz & Gerrard 1985; Halvorsen et al. 1990). Riddoch and Trinick (1988) summarised the findings of four surveys of recreational and competitive runners, marathon runners, quadrathletes and triathletes and presented their own survey data from marathon runners. They reported the incidence of the following gastrointestinal symptoms during or immediately after running: loss of appetite 28–50%, heartburn 9.5–24%, nausea 6–20%, vomiting 4–6%, abdominal cramps 19.3–39%, urge for a bowel movement 30–42% and diarrhoea 14–27%.

These authors found that both upper- and lower-gastrointestinal symptoms were more likely to occur during a hard run than an easy run and were as frequent during as after running. Lower-gastrointestinal symptoms were more common than upper-tract symptoms and this is consistent with previous surveys. The most common strategies used to minimise symptoms were to run in a fasted state and to have a bowel movement prior to running.

Rehrer et al. (1992) studied dietary intake in relation to gastrointestinal complaints in 55 male triathletes in a half-ironman distance triathlon. In these athletes, hyperosmotic beverage consumption during competition was associated with increased incidence of severe gastrointestinal symptoms. Dietary fibre ingestion before competition increased the likelihood of GI symptoms. The ingestion of fat and protein in a pre-race meal was thought to increase the risk of upper-GI distress in some athletes.

Brouns and colleagues (1987), based on an extensive review of the literature, suggested the recommendations in Table 22.2 for minimisation of exercise-related GI symptoms.

Table 22.2 *Recommendations for minimising exercise-related GI symptoms during training or competition*

- Solid food should be avoided during the last three hours prior to exercise.
- Liquid foods can be taken as a pre-competition meal and also during exercise.
- Whenever fluid is of first priority, drinks should be low in CHO.
- When maximum intakes of both CHO and water are desired, the optimal concentration should be in the range of isotonicity (e.g. sports drinks).
- Athletes suffering frequently from diarrhoea or the urge to defecate during exercise may benefit from liquid meal supplements (low in fibre content) during the last day preceding competition.
- Drinking during exercise should be part of the training program.
- In addition, high-fibre foods and caffeine should be avoided prior to exercise.

Adapted from Brouns et al. 1987

22.4.3 *Gastrointestinal blood loss*

Gastrointestinal bleeding, although fairly uncommon, is a dramatic gastrointestinal symptom, which may occur in response to hard physical activity. It is most frequently described in long-distance runners (Sullivan 1986). In one study, up to 22% of runners had evidence of GI bleeding based on a positive test for faecal occult blood following a marathon (Schwartz et al. 1990) and almost 85% showed a positive test following an ultra-marathon (Baska et al. 1990). Bleeding, again based on the same test, has also been reported in 12 competitive cyclists with 8.4% of 310 stool samples collected intermittently over one year being positive (Dobbs et al. 1988). Yet other studies have reported much lower incidences of blood in the stools of athletes. None out of 63 runners reported blood in the stool following a marathon (Halvorsen et al. 1990) and only 6% out of 125 runners reported blood in the stool in another marathon (McCabe 1986). These reports were based on self-observation rather than laboratory testing and may have been under-estimations, as the presence of blood in the stool may not be readily apparent by visual examination.

Bleeding is most likely related to gastrointestinal ischaemia, but early studies suggested that mechanical trauma to the gut could be the cause (Porter 1982). The site of bleeding has been assessed by endoscopy in two studies. Gaudin et al. (1990) assessed seven runners by upper-GI endoscopy before and after training runs of between 12 and 30 miles. All had gastric mucosal lesions consistent with ischaemia following the run, but only four had normal examinations prior to exercise. All had previous GI symptoms, which make conclusions from this study uncertain. Schwartz et al. (1990) examined seven runners who had occult blood loss following a marathon by oesophago-gastro-duodenoscopy and colonoscopy. Three runners were examined within 48 hours of the race; two of these runners had gastric antral erosions. The third had erosion of the mucosa at the splenic flexure. The other four runners, examined between four and 30 days following the run, had normal examinations. The authors concluded that ischaemia was the causative factor in mucosal lesions. Risk of bleeding correlates well with intensity of exercise but not with use of aspirin or NSAIDs (McMahon et al. 1984).

The cause of macroscopic bleeding should be elucidated by thorough investigation, even in young athletes. The extent of investigation required for microscopic bleeding associated with exercise is age-dependent, with those over 40 requiring full investigation.

Preventative strategies include gradual increases in training, careful hydration and, in cases of recurrent upper-gastrointestinal bleeding, medication is warranted. Use of H_2 receptor antagonists has been shown to significantly lower the rate of bleeding (Baska et al. 1990).

22.5 PRACTICE TIPS

Julie Tatnell

- Before any dietary modification is recommended, it is important that the sports dietitian checks if a medical diagnosis of the cause of gastrointestinal symptoms has been made. If no examination has been undertaken, the athlete should be referred for a medical assessment.

- Once a medical diagnosis is obtained, specific dietary modifications can then be made.

Gastro-oesophageal reflux disease

- Athletes experiencing this condition usually benefit from eating smaller meals (not over-eating) and frequent snacks throughout the day to meet energy demands. It is important for these athletes to be given advice about planning their shopping to ensure that appropriate between-meal snacks may be organised. Reducing caffeine and alcohol consumption and avoiding known mucosal irritants specific to each individual helps reduce the symptoms of gastro-oesophageal disease. Foods typically reported to be irritant foods are spicy foods, citrus juices, tomatoes and pineapple. Some people, however, have no symptoms when they eat these foods. Reducing the volume of food consumed immediately prior to exercise may also be of benefit.

Functional dyspepsia

- Symptoms of this condition may be reduced by minimising intake of foods that retard gastric motility, for example, fatty foods. Once again, the athlete must be aware of the need to have food available at all times to ensure energy needs are met.

Gastritis

- Inflammation of stomach mucosa is likely to be attributable to chronic or inappropriate use of anti-inflammatory drugs for the treatment of soft tissue or joint injury in athletes. The dietary management of gastritis is usually individual, but it is generally recommended that irritants such as spicy foods be avoided.

Peptic ulcer

- This includes either gastric or duodenal ulcers and the dietary management for both is again based on individual responses to foods. However, a reduction in caffeine and fat intake may be of benefit for some athletes. Drinking milk to soothe the pain works immediately or very quickly but is associated with a marked increase in gastric acid secretion later on, thereby exacerbating the pain and discomfort (see Section 22.2.3). Bland foods are no longer recommended or necessary.

Gastroenteritis

- In the acute phase, anti-emetic and antidiarrhoeal medications are commonly prescribed. The immediate dietary issue is rehydration. The most suitable rehydrating agents are iso-osmolar solutions containing both sodium and CHO, which are available over the counter at pharmacies. Athletes should be encouraged to sip a rehydrating solution intermittently rather than drink a large bolus, which often causes further pain, diarrhoea and emesis. Food should be introduced as soon as possible with small frequent feedings of low-fat foods that empty quickly from the stomach. CHO-rich foods should remain the focus to ensure glycogen levels are more quickly restored in the liver and muscle. There may also be transient lactose intolerance associated with gastroenteritis, so lactose-containing foods should be avoided until bowel symptoms subside.

Inflammatory bowel diseases: ulcerative colitis and Crohn's disease

- When these conditions are not active, specific dietary intervention is not warranted. When active, however, dietary modification helps to alleviate the symptoms. In some severe cases, elemental and polymeric diets are required. In less severe cases, low-fibre, low-fat, bland diets may be necessary for short-term use. In sufferers with small-bowel stenosis, large amounts of fibre should be avoided, along with irritants such as seeds and skins which can become trapped and accumulate into an out-pouching of the intestine, resulting in diverticulitis. Once the inflammation has subsided, high-fibre and high-fluid intakes are the cornerstone for treatment and prevention. Nutrient deficiencies are more likely to occur when the diseases are active, because of impairment of nutrient absorption and often loss of appetite resulting in a reduction in food intake. Weight loss therefore often occurs during active stages. Weight gain advice may be required once symptoms improve.

Irritable colon syndrome

- This condition usually requires some modification of fibre and fluid intake in sufferers. Too little fibre and fluid can cause constipation, while excessive fibre is associated with bloating and flatulence. Some sufferers benefit from reducing caffeine and alcohol consumption.

Coeliac disease

- Avoidance of wheat, barley, rye and hybrids of these cereals, including commercial foods using these foods as ingredients (e.g. flour and its products), is important to treat and prevent the recurrence of coeliac disease. Avoidance of oats may not be necessary, as the gliadin content (the implicated allergen) of oats is very low. However, many endocrinologists prudently advise avoidance of oats in case of a reaction. Foods derived from these grains are all excellent sources of CHO and the staple food in many Western countries. Rice, legumes, fruit, corn and starchy vegetables and other grains and their manufactured products are an alternative CHO source. Support groups in the community, including the Coeliac Society of Australia and local groups of coeliac sufferers, are invaluable for the newly diagnosed person with coeliac disease. These groups supply safe-food lists, often provide special products, swap recipes, share problems and assist in adjustment to the ensuing lifestyle. We have found these groups invaluable in providing practical advice about the problems and pitfalls of eating a gluten-free diet away from home and on trips overseas. Carrying a supply of gluten-free foods and snacks as well as a meal replacement formula is essential for the travelling athlete with coeliac disease.

Lactose intolerance

- Athletes with this condition need to avoid or limit lactose intake to prevent symptoms such as diarrhoea, bloating, nausea, flatulence and general abdominal discomfort. Instructions on how to read labels and detect hidden sources of lactose in commercial foods are necessary. Advice on food sources low in lactose (e.g. hard cheese) and alternative sources of calcium-rich foods in place of animal milks and their high-lactose products also need to be addressed. It is difficult to meet calcium recommendations in people who are lactose intolerant, dislike milk or milk products or are allergic to milk. Strategies for meeting the calcium recommendation for these people can be found in any clinical nutrition textbook.

Gastrointestinal symptoms with no known cause

- Should medical examination reveal no known cause of gastrointestinal symptoms, the sports dietitian must take a detailed dietary and symptom history to determine any association between particular foods and symptoms. A detailed food and symptom diary completed by the athlete can also be very useful. Other potential causes of gastrointestinal disturbances should not be discounted, for example, stress or anxiety. Stress management advice is of assistance to many athletes. It should also be considered whether non-specific symptoms and reported difficulty with food is masking an eating disorder.

- Diarrhoea and gastrointestinal disturbances occur more commonly during physical activity. Dietary suggestions to help reduce the occurrence and severity of these symptoms are listed in Table 22.3.

Table 22.3 *Suggestions for dietary intervention to help avoid GI disturbances before and during physical activity*

Problems	Solutions
Any GI pain or discomfort, nausea	Avoid hyperosmolar (e.g. fruit juice, milk) and carbonated beverages (e.g. lemonade) and alcohol. Drink water, sports drinks—preferably sipped not guzzled. Avoid foods known to irritate, fatty foods, caffeine, chocolate, peppermint. Eat a snack during or before physical activity that is known to be emptied quickly from the stomach and well tolerated (e.g. low-fat, light). Practice eating during training. For short events allow sufficient time between eating and commencement of physical activity (where food intake during physical activity is not necessary).

(continues)

(*continued*)

Problems	Solutions
Urge to defecate during physical activity	Establish a routine of emptying the bowel before physical activity; so that most of the stomach contents are gone at the start of activity consume a low-fibre, low-residue diet before competition.
Diarrhoea induced by exercise or loose bowel motions during physical activity	Low-fibre, low-residue diet or diet high in soluble fibre depending on Individual response and nature of the problem AND/OR antidiarrhoeal drug therapy.
Diarrhoea or vomiting from an infective agent (e.g. bacteria, virus, parasite)	Cease physical activity. Practise safe eating and drinking habits (see Chapter 14, Table 14.4). Rehydration strategies crucial (see Chapter 14, Table 14.5). Seek medical advice, if prolonged. Drug therapy may be warranted.

REFERENCES

Baska RS, Moses FM, Graeber G, Kearney G. Gastrointestinal bleeding during an ultramarathon. Dig Dis Sci 1990;35:276–9.

Brouns F, Beckers E. Is the gut an athletic organ? Digestion, absorption and exercise. Sports Med 1993;15:242–57.

Brouns F, Saris WHM, Rehrer NJ. Abdominal complaints and gastrointestinal function during long-lasting exercise. Int J Sports Med 1987;8:175–98.

Clausen JP. Effect of physical training on cardiovascular adjustments to exercise in man. Physiol Rev 1977;57:779–815.

de Carle DJ. Gastro-oesophageal reflux disease. Med J Aust 1998;169:549–54.

Dev AT, Lambert JR. Diseases associated with Helicobacter pylori. Med J Aust 1998;169:220–5.

Dobbs TW, Atkins M, Ratliff R, Eichner ER. Gastrointestinal bleeding in competitive cyclists. Med Sci Sports Exerc 1988;20:S78.

Fallon KE, Robinson EN. The travelling athlete. In: Fields KB, Fricker PA, eds. Medical problems in athletes. Malden: Blackwell Science, 1997:70–6.

Fallon KE, Sivyer G, Sivyer K, Dare A. The biochemistry of runners in a 1 600 km ultramarathon. Br J Sports Med 1999;33:264–9.

Feighery C. Coeliac disease. BMJ 1999;319:236–9.

Ferguson A, Glen M, Ghosh S. Crohn's disease: nutrition and nutritional therapy. Balliere's Clin Gastroenterol 1998;12:93–114.

Fordtran JS, Salting B. Gastric emptying and intestinal absorption during prolonged severe exercise. J Appl Physiol 1967;23:331–5.

Gaudin C, Zerath E, Guezennac CY. Gastric lesions secondary to long distance running. Dig Dis Sci 1990;35:1239–43.

Gibson PR, Anderson RP. Inflammatory bowel disease. Med J Aust 1998;169:387–94.

Glickman RM. Inflammatory bowel disease. In: Isselbacher KJ, Braunwald E, Wilson JD, et al, eds. Harrison's principles of internal medicine. New York: McGraw-Hill, 1994:1738–52.

Greenberg HB. Viral gastroenteritis. In: Isselbacher KJ, Braunwald E, Wilson JD, et al, eds. Harrison's principles of internal medicine. New York: McGraw-Hill, 1994:819–21.

Halvorsen FA, Lyng J, Ritland S. Gastrointestinal bleeding in marathon runners. Scand J Gastroenterol 1986;21:493–7.

Halvorsen FA, Lyng J, Glomsaker T, Ritland S. Gastrointestinal disturbances in marathon runners. Br J Sports Med 1990;24:266–8.

Holmes GKT, Prior P, Lane MR, Pope D, Allan RN. Malignancy and coeliac disease—effect of a gluten-free diet. Gut 1989;30:333–8.

Hu WH, Talley NJ. Functional (non-ulcer) dyspepsia: unexplained but not unmanageable. Med J Aust 1998;168:507–12.

Hudson B. Developing-country travel and endemic diseases. Aust Fam Phys 1994;23:1666–77.

Hughes D. Gastroenterology and Sport. In: Fields KB , Fricker PA, eds. Medical Problems in Athletes. Malden: Blackwell Science, 1997:151–69.

Janatiunen EK, Pikkarainen PH, Kamppainen TA, et al. A comparison of diets with and without oats in adults with coeliac disease. N Eng J Med 1995;333:1033–7.

Keeffe E, Lowe D, Goss J, Wayne R. Gastrointestinal symptoms of marathon runners. West J Med 1984;141:481–4.

McCabe ME, Peura DA, Kadakia SC, Bocek Z, Johnson LF. Gastrointestinal blood loss associated with running a marathon. Dig Dis Sci 1986;31:1229–32.

McGuigan JE. Peptic ulcer and gastritis. In: Isselbacher KJ, Braunwald E, Wilson JD, et al, eds. Harrison's principles of internal medicine. New York: McGraw-Hill, 1994:1363–82

McMahon LF, Ryan MJ, Larson D, Fisher RL. Occult gastrointestinal blood loss in marathon runners. Ann Intern Med 1984;101:846–7.

Malcolm A, Kellow J. Irritable bowel syndrome. Med J Aust 1998;169:274–9.

Nanda R, James R, Smith H, Dudley CR, Jewell DP. Food intolerance and the irritable bowel syndrome. Gut 1989;30:1099–104.

Pehl C, Pfeiffer A, Wendl B, Kaess H. The effect of decaffeination of coffee on gastro-oesophageal reflux in patients with reflux disease. Alimentary Pharmacol Ther 1997;11:483–6.

Peters O, Peters P, Clarys JP, et al. Oesophageal motility and exercise. Gastroenterol 1988;94:A351.

Pham TH, Barr GD. Coeliac disease in adults: presentation and management. Aust Fam Phys 1996;25:62–5.

Porter AMW. Marathon running and the caecal slap syndrome. Br J Sports Med 1982;16:178.

Rehrer NJ, van-Kemenade M, Meester W, Brouns F, Saris WHM. Gastrointestinal complaints in relation to dietary intake in triathletes. Int J Sport Nutr 1992;2:48–59.

Riddoch C, Trinick T. Gastrointestinal disturbances in marathon runners. Brit J Sports Med 1988;22:71–4.

Rowell LB, Blackman JR, Bruce RA. Indocyanine green clearance and hepatic blood flow during mild exercise to maximal exercise in upright man. J Clin Invest 1964;43:1766–90.

Ruff T. Illness in returned travellers. Aust Fam Phys 1994;23:1711–21.

Schwartz AE, Vanagunas A, Kamel PL. Endoscopy to evaluate gastrointestinal bleeding in marathon runners. Ann Intern Med 1990;113:632–4.

Soffer EE, Merchant RK, Duethman G, et al. Effect of graded exercise on oesophageal motility and gastro-oesophageal reflux in trained subjects. Dig Dis Sci 1993;38:220–4.

Sullivan S. The gastrointestinal symptoms of running. N Eng J Med 1981;304,5:915.

Sullivan SN. Gastrointestinal bleeding in distance runners. Sports Med 1986;3:1–3.

Talley NJ. Modern management of dyspepsia. Aust Fam Phys 1996;25:47–52.

Talley NJ, Colin-Jones D, Koch KL, Nyren O, Stanghellini V. Functional dyspepsia: a classification with guidelines for diagnosis and management. Gastroenterol Int 1991;4:145–60.

Timmer A, Sutherland LR, Bryant HE, Fick G. Oral contraceptive use and smoking are risk factors for relapse in Crohn's disease. Gastroenterol 1998;114:1143–50.

Waldron B, Cullen PT, Kumar R, et al. Evidence for hypomotility in non-ulcer dyspepsia: a prospective multifactorial study. Gut 1991;32:246–51.

Worobetz L, Gerrard D. Exercise associated symptoms in triathletes. Phys Sportsmed 1985;15:105–10.

Yazaki E, Shawdon A, Beasley I, Evans DF. The effect of different types of exercise on gastro-oesophageal reflux. Aust J Sci Med Sport 1996;28:93–6.

CHAPTER 23

Special needs: athletes with disabilities

Elizabeth Broad

23.1 INTRODUCTION

Sport and exercise have long been recognised as important components in the therapy and rehabilitation of people with disabilities. Since the inception of the Summer Paralympic Games in 1960, and the Winter Paralympics in 1992, the number of individuals with disabilities training and competing at high levels has increased dramatically. Competitions are held locally, nationally and internationally, in summer and winter disciplines, throughout the world. Performance standards vary considerably between classes of disabilities, but all are improving at a rapid rate, such that world records are frequently broken. Even in non-Paralympic sports, athletes with disabilities are accomplishing amazing feats, such as paraplegics swimming the English Channel and completing the Hawaii Ironman Triathlon well within the maximum time period allowed.

While the participation of athletes with disabilities is large and in many different sports, scientific research about athletes with disabilities and physical activity has mostly been ignored. This chapter will limit the discussion to current knowledge of the particular differences between athletes with disabilities and able-bodied athletes.

23.2 CLASSIFICATION OF DISABILITIES

Athletes with disabilities are classified into six primary classes as shown in Table 23.1.

Cerebral palsy (CP) is a group of permanent disabling symptoms primarily affecting voluntary control musculature. CP results from non-progressive damage to the motor control areas of the brain (Winnick 1995). The most common symptoms include impaired muscle coordination, reduced capacity to maintain posture and

Table 23.1 *Classes of disabilities and number of sub-classes*

Amputees	9 sub-classes
Cerebral palsy	8 sub-classes
Wheelchair / spinal injured	8 sub-classes
Visually impaired	3 sub-classes
Intellectual disability	0 sub-classes
Les autres (others)	6 sub-classes

balance, and reduced ability to perform normal movements and skills. Some athletes with CP will use a wheelchair because their functional ability to walk is so impaired that walking and general daily activities are greatly limited without it. Encouraging these athletes to walk for short periods of time remains important for improving circulation, bladder control and metabolism. The CP category also includes athletes with acquired non-progressive brain lesions (e.g. head injury).

'Wheelchair/spinal injured' incorporates athletes with traumatic spinal cord (SC) lesions, poliomyelitis and spina bifida. Figure 23.1 explains the spinal cord segments and likely effects of a disruption along the cord. Traumatic SC lesions generally result from an accident (e.g. sporting or motor vehicle), so the duration of disability will vary between individuals. Spina bifida is a congenital developmental defect of the spinal column in which vertebral arches have failed to fuse, resulting in an abnormal gap in the spinal column (Winnick 1995; Goodman et al. 1996). Since nerve tissue can protrude through this gap, it can become damaged, resulting in varying degrees of paralysis and loss of sensation in the legs and lower trunk. As with traumatic spinal cord injuries, the degree of damage depends on the location of the deformity and the amount of damage done to the spinal cord (Winnick 1995). Hence, the physiological response of individuals with spina bifida and traumatic spinal lesions are very similar, and for the purposes of this chapter will be grouped as spinal cord injuries (SCI).

The class 'Les Autres' currently includes multiple sclerosis, Freidrichs ataxia, osteoporosis, severe burns, muscular dystrophies, musculo-skeletal or neural pathway damage, and lower-limb deformities. In addition, people with organ transplants and hearing impairments will be included in some events.

Within the major classes there are subclassifications relating to a medical classification of severity of disability. Many sports have now developed their own classification system, which categorises athletes according to their potential physical ability (Goodman et al. 1996). This system helps to ensure that athletes compete at the highest functional level. All athletes with disabilities must hold an internationally authorised classification to participate in competition. Those athletes whose disability is progressive are reclassified each year. Hence, the running of a competition for athletes with disabilities is far more complex than that for able-bodied athletes as athletes may only compete against similarly classified individuals.

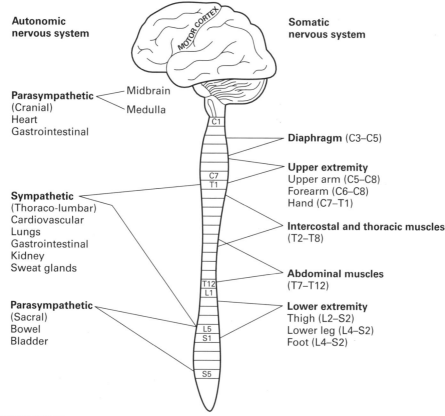

Autonomic nervous system

Parasympathetic — Midbrain
(Cranial) — Medulla
Heart
Gastrointestinal

Sympathetic
(Thoraco-lumbar)
Cardiovascular
Lungs
Gastrointestinal
Kidney
Sweat glands

Parasympathetic
(Sacral)
Bowel
Bladder

Somatic nervous system

Diaphragm (C3–C5)

Upper extremity
Upper arm (C5–C8)
Forearm (C6–C8)
Hand (C7–T1)

Intercostal and thoracic muscles
(T2–T8)

Abdominal muscles
(T7–T12)

Lower extremity
Thigh (L2–S2)
Lower leg (L4–S2)
Foot (L4–S2)

Figure 23.1 *Spinal cord injury innervation*
Adapted from Glaser 1985, p. 269 with permission

23.3 COMPETITIVE SPORTING OPPORTUNITIES FOR ATHLETES WITH DISABILITIES

There are few sports or activities in which an athlete with a disability cannot compete. At the Paralympic Games, athletes compete in the disciplines outlined in Table 23.2. Not all classes of disability will be able to compete in each sport. For example, wheelchair rugby is limited to only those athletes who mobilise in a wheelchair and have a disability involving all four limbs and trunk, usually tetraplegia.

In order for a person with a disability to compete in their chosen sport, some rule modifications may be required. For the most popular sports, a rules manual is available entitled 'International Stoke Mandeville Wheelchair Sports Federation: Officials Rules 1992–1996'. A summary of these rules is outlined by Goodman et al. (1996).

Table 23.2	Current Paralympic sports	
Archery	Fencing	Swimming
Athletics (all forms)	Football	Table tennis
Basketball	Goalball	Tennis
Boccia	Judo	Volleyball
Cycling	Powerlifting	Wheelchair rugby
Equestrian events	Sailing	Skiing (downhill, cross-country,
	Shooting	Slalom) – winter Paralympics

23.4 PHYSIOLOGICAL DIFFERENCES BETWEEN ATHLETES WITH DISABILITIES AND ABLE-BODIED ATHLETES

Despite the ever-increasing participation rate of athletes with disabilities in competitive sport, the extent of scientific information available remains limited. The majority of existing research about disabled athletes' responses to exercise presented in this section is focussed on the physical capabilities of paraplegic and tetraplegic individuals.

23.4.1 Medical and health-related differences

As a group, athletes with disabilities have higher incidences of medical problems than other athletes. For example, persons confined to wheelchairs have a high risk of pressure sores or infections as a result of wounds, and may have other medical complications depending on the cause of their disability. A person who became paraplegic as a result of a vehicle accident may have also suffered internal injuries and therefore have a colostomy, ileostomy or other internal problems. Individuals with CP have a higher incidence of epileptic seizures, especially under stress, due to the neurological effects of the disorder (Buckley 2000, personal communication). They may also have more feeding difficulties.

Disabilities seen in older athletes may be a direct result of a pre-existing medical problem, such as diabetes (which can lead to visual impairment or amputation if untreated). Existing medical issues present an additional consideration when working with these athletes.

23.4.2 Physiological differences

While athletes with disabilities may have impaired functional abilities compared to their able-bodied counterparts, there is little evidence to suggest that their physiological capabilities differ. The exceptions to this rule are athletes with SCI.

It is logical to assume that there is a reduced capacity in SCI athletes to undertake high-intensity exercise, particularly for long periods of time, due to their smaller active muscle mass. The 'normal' physiological response to exercise may also be disrupted in persons with SCI through a number of mechanisms: ineffective vasoregulation below the SC lesion, increased total peripheral resistance, and the inability to increase stroke volume (the amount of blood pumped per heart beat) because of blood pooling through the absence of a musculo-skeletal pump from lower limbs. Hence, individuals with paraplegia, poliomyelitis or spina bifida tend to have dampened maximal/peak oxygen uptakes (Shephard 1988). As Figure 23.2 indicates, tetraplegics are unable to raise their maximal heart rates above 120–130 bpm due to the disruption of their sympathetic nervous system (Wicks et al. 1983; Hjeltnes 1984; Coutts and Stogryn 1987; Bhambhani et al. 1994, 1995). Similarly, their peak oxygen uptake and lactate levels will fall well below those of other athletes undertaking similar work. Even athletes with SC lesions between T1 and T6 may have a more restricted heart rate peak relative to able-bodied persons (Wicks et al. 1983; Hopman et al. 1993). Research findings are often confusing because of the limited numbers of individuals tested, the large individual variation in functional capacity, and the different levels of training between individual athletes. In other words, each athlete has an individual response to exercise.

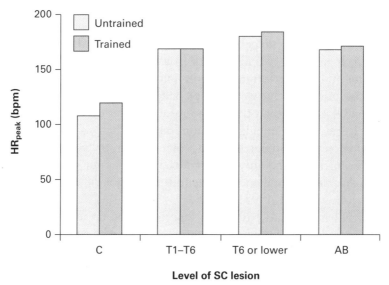

Figure 23.2 *Comparative peak heart rates in SCI and able-bodied athletes Adapted from data in Wicks et al (1983); Hjeltnes (1984); Coutts & Stogryn (1987); Bhambhani et al (1994, 1995)*

Whether SCI athletes use a different fuel mix to able-bodied athletes during exercise remains unknown. Only one study has investigated muscle glycogen status in SCI persons. Skrinar et al. (1982) took muscle glycogen samples from the deltoid muscle before and after one hour of sub-maximal exercise in four subjects. Although the authors did not control for effects of pre-exercise diet and used the deltoid muscle (which is not the primary muscle used in wheelchair ambulation), it was interesting to note that the mean pre-exercise glycogen level in the deltoid muscle (92 mmol/kg wet weight) was lower than reported resting glycogen in able-bodied athletes (120–140 mmol/kg wet weight). The mean change over the one hour of exercise was 30 mmol/kg wet weight (Skrinar et al. 1981). This change was comparable to leg muscle glycogen losses in able-bodied athletes at the same relative exercise intensity (Karlsson & Saltin 1971). The researchers suggested that the lower pre-exercise glycogen levels in the wheelchair athletes compared to able-bodied athletes could be attributed to a greater dependence on glycogen stores for simple daily ambulation in this population. An alternative explanation could be that upper-body musculature may have smaller muscle glycogen stores *per se*. Irrespective of the small sample size and limitations of the experimental methodology (e.g. no control group), it appears that large glycogen losses occur during physical activity, even in muscle with a secondary use. Clearly, high carbohydrate (CHO) intakes are required for SCI athletes training hard to support glycogen resynthesis.

23.4.3 *Differences in metabolism*

The typical daily energy expenditure of persons with CP varies substantially depending on their mode of ambulation. In a study of non-athletes using doubly-labelled water (used to determine energy expenditure) (see Chapter 6, Section 6.4.2.2), those athletes who were wheelchair-dependent had lower total energy expenditures (8430 kJ/d) than those who were ambulating (10 360 kJ/d) (Johnson et al. 1997). Regardless of ambulatory status, having athetosis (uncontrollable, jerky movements) increased estimated resting metabolic rate (RMR) (Johnson et al. 1996), however, this immobility also reduced the amount of day-to-day activity undertaken. As a result, total energy expenditure did not differ to non-athetotic CP individuals (Johnson et al. 1997).

RMRs of SCI individuals have been reported to be up to 30% lower than the able-bodied population, primarily because of the reduced active muscle mass (Noreau & Shephard 1995). Hence, the reduction in metabolism increases with higher levels of SC lesion. As with the able-bodied population, metabolic rates tend to be higher in people who regularly participate in physical activity compared to non-participants. There have, however, not been any reported cases with SCI who have RMRs higher than 9500 kJ/d (Noreau & Shephard 1995).

23.4.4 *Differences in bladder and bowel control*

A common result of SCI is incontinence (lack of bladder and/or bowel control) (Goodman et al. 1996). Therefore, many athletes with SCI must consciously schedule visits to the toilet, and generally require greater control over these bodily functions. Limited mobility as a result of CP, lower-limb amputations, or other disorders may also affect normal bowel function. The management of toileting is almost always carefully controlled by the athlete to coincide with the needs of their sport, and may be acutely affected by dietary changes, especially fluid intake.

23.4.5 *Differences in thermoregulation*

Due to the neurological interruption of a spinal cord (SC) lesion, evaporative cooling from sweating in athletes with SCI is diminished as non-innervated areas cease to release sweat (Hopman et al. 1993). The potential surface area available for cooling (through sweating) is related to the level and completeness of the SC lesion—the higher the lesion, the smaller the surface area (Normell 1974). Although lower sweat rates may appear to be advantageous for minimising dehydration and slowing the decline in stroke volume in the SCI, such a decrease actually presents a disadvantage for controlling body temperature. In addition, some medications, such as anticholinergics (used to control muscle spasms), can also impair thermoregulatory abilities (Kennedy 1995). Finally, the unique body positioning and movements in a wheelchair further limit heat dissipation (Sawka et al. 1984).

In hot conditions, the SCI individual will effectively gain heat from the environment (Petrofsky 1992; Broad 1997). Consequently, the body temperature of an individual with a SCI is more difficult to regulate effectively, even when they are not actively exercising (such as in archery and shooting events). Active cooling is often required, by keeping athletes in the shade as much as possible, spraying them with water and applying cooling devices (head pieces, neck wraps, cooling jackets). These methods need to be applied regularly, especially when exercising in the heat, as the metabolic heat produced may exceed the cooling potential of the mechanism used (Armstrong et al. 1995; Broad 1997).

In cold environments, active heating and heat loss prevention is necessary since the ability to vasoconstrict peripheral blood vessels is usually impaired (Petrofsky 1992), resulting in rapid heat loss in an SCI athlete.

23.5 *USE OF MEDICATIONS IN ATHLETES WITH DISABILITIES*

The use of medications in SCI athletes is higher than in other athletes with disabilities. Many medications, although necessary for maintaining quality of life and functionality, have potential side-effects (see Table 23.3). It is important for the sports dietitian to be familiar with the medications used, the reason for their use, and their potential side-effects as these factors can have an impact on dietary recommendations.

23.6 *BODY COMPOSITION*

In general, the measurement and modification of body composition (i.e. appropriate weight and skinfold) remains as relevant to athletes with disabilities as it does to any able-bodied athlete. Traditional approaches to measuring body composition may need to be modified for some athletes. For example, the measurement of body mass needs to allow for muscle atrophy and bone resorption in individuals with SCI, spina

Table 23.3 Frequently used medications among athletes with disabilities

Primary classification	Common medications used
Bowel management/stool softeners and laxatives	Docusate, sodium (Coloxyl™) Sennoside (Senekot™) Enemas (Bisalax™)
Bladder control/antiseptics	Hydrochloride oxybutynin (Ditropan™) Hexamine hippurate (Hiprex™) Cranberry juice or tablets
Antispasmodics/muscle relaxants	Diazepam (Valium™) Dantrolene sodium (Dantrium™) Baclofen (Clofen™, Lioresal™)
Pain relief/antidepressants	Amitriptyline hydrochloride (Tryptanol™, Tryptine™) Carbamazepine (Tegretol™) Medications containing codeine

Adapted from MIMS Australia 1999

bifida and severe cases of CP. Furthermore, where muscle atrophy is present, it can be difficult to differentiate the body-fat component of skinfold thicknesses (Gass 1988). Hence, regression equations that were once used in able-bodied athletes to estimate percentage body fat from skinfold thicknesses and underwater weighing are also inappropriate for athletes with disabilities (see Chapter 4).

Despite these concerns, it is believed that body mass (weight) and sum of skin-folds remains the best practice for assessing and tracking body composition changes for most individual athletes with disabilities (Gass 1988). No normative data have been reported, presumably because of the larger within-sport variability in body shape and size for athletes with disabilities compared with able-bodied athletes.

23.7 DIETARY ISSUES FOR ATHLETES WITH DISABILITIES

Unfortunately, the shortage of information specific to athletes with disabilities means that we can only assume the general dietary recommendations should be the same as for able-bodied athletes. Perhaps the main differences will be in lower daily energy requirements and specific competition recommendations.

23.7.1 Current dietary intakes

Dietary intakes of athletes with disabilities have not been reported in the literature. Some papers have reported dietary intakes of non-athletic SCI individuals with reference to their increased risk of cardiovascular disease. Levine et al. (1992) reported that healthy SCI persons ate less energy than the average population (7065 kJ for males, 5385 kJ for females). Dietary intakes were relatively higher in fat and lower in CHO than the dietary goals and targets, and were not unlike dietary intakes of the general population. Even considering the extent of under-reporting of energy intake in any dietary survey, low energy intakes, if valid, make it more difficult to achieve adequate nutrient intakes (see Chapter 3, Section 3.3).

23.7.2 *Fibre, timing of food intake and bowel control*

Large bowel (and sometimes small bowel) function can be impaired if mobility is limited and gastrointestinal tract damage has occurred. As a result, frequency of bowel movement and stool formation and consistency in some athletes with disabilities can be affected. Some individuals may have a colostomy or ileostomy. Constipation is very common. The use of bowel softeners is frequent among immobile athletes. Timing and frequency of bowel motions need to be fairly well controlled to occur at a convenient time. To achieve this control, a fairly consistent diet and fluid intake, in addition to routine training of bowel habits is important.

Dietary fibre intake and regularity of food intake are important issues for disabled athletes to help control bowel movements and therefore avoid embarrassment and discomfort. The effects of changing these routines can have practical implications, and can therefore require careful consideration, discussion and practice to achieve these changes with the individual athlete. Modifications should be made gradually and at a time and place where access to bathroom facilities is relatively easy.

23.7.3 *Fluid intake*

While maintaining hydration levels is important for all athletes, the practical consequences of consuming adequate fluid require more attention for those athletes with disabilities. Proximity to appropriate toilet and water facilities and use of urine collection bags require consideration, especially in wheelchair athletes. It is also important to remember that for SCI athletes, heat illness is not necessarily a result of insufficient fluid intake or dehydration, but can be associated with hot and humid weather conditions. The volume, frequency and types of fluids recommended in Chapter 14 remain appropriate for athletes with disabilities, provided their gastrointestinal tract is competent. For example, an athlete with an ileostomy may not tolerate the usual prescribed volumes of fluid pre-exercise and during exercise. Large volumes can dump into and fill the ileostomy bag too rapidly.

23.7.4 *Weight control*

Weight control issues at extremes of underweight and overweight are evident in athletes with disabilities. While some weight issues are related to the disability itself, the genetic background of the athletes is also a contributing factor. Each athlete will need to be considered on an individual basis according to the nature of their disability and any impact their disability may have on their metabolism.

People with intellectual disabilities often have body-mass control problems for a wide variety of reasons including: poor food choices from lack of insight, food used as a comforter, either limited or excess voluntary activity, and genetic disorders (such as Down Syndrome). When working with intellectually disabled athletes, it is imperative to work together with their primary carer(s) in order to manage the foods provided to the athlete. Inclusion of additional forms of activity should be considered for those who are over-fat, while energy-dense foods and fluids are a useful adjunct for those underweight.

Many non–wheelchair-dependent lower-limb amputees or CP athletes appear to have higher energy demands, possibly due to the greater mechanical demand of walking (Buckley 2000). The impact of using poorly fitting prostheses during exercise, and the resultant damage often incurred, leads to high nutrient requirements to facilitate healing.

The lower energy expenditures of people with SCI may be upregulated by functional electrical stimulation (FES) to help muscle activity. If pressure sores are frequent, energy and nutrient requirements will also be increased to assist with healing. In practice, however, SCI athletes cannot consume high energy intakes to the same levels as able-bodied persons without gaining body fat, because of a lower total lean body mass. The focus of their everyday diet should therefore be on nutrient-dense foods (rather than energy-dense foods) that are high in fat and sugar. Additional support and advice is important for athletes with disabilities who travel or eat out frequently, since what may appear to some as being small changes in energy intake can have a larger impact on body mass in this population than in the general community.

23.7.5 *Nutritional supplements*

The need for nutritional supplements in athletes with disabilities is addressed on a case-by-case basis. Vitamin and mineral supplements may be needed if gastrointestinal tract function is disturbed or if athletes have difficulty consuming a balanced diet. Similarly, sports nutrition supplements or sports foods have the potential to improve overall energy intake as well as support performance. However, the potential side-effects also require some thought. For example, the fibre content of a sports bar may stimulate a bowel movement during a wheelchair marathon—an undesirable outcome.

23.7.6 *Eating difficulties and behaviours observed in some athletes with disabilities*

Regardless of whether you are working with an individual or group of athletes with disabilities, you should be aware of various aspects of feeding or eating that differ from able-bodied athletes. Examples include, but are not limited to:

• An amputee or someone with arm deformities may have to eat using their feet, which needs to be accounted for when deciding on accommodation and eating venues.

- Some forms of CP and classes of 'Les Autres' (see Table 23.1 and Section 23.2) will experience general feeding difficulties, with some athletes known to require enteral feeding to supplement their limited oral intake.
- Athletes with visual impairments generally work on a 'clock' system to locate foods on their plates (e.g. meat at 12 o'clock, peas at 6 o'clock). They often eat with their hands and avoid using serving spoons when putting food on plates.
- Athletes with intellectual disabilities can display some 'unusual' responses to food and eating. Examples include: unfounded fears of a specific food due to the way it looks, inability to use eating utensils in the customary manner, and eating excessive quantities of foods but not comprehending why such behaviour is inappropriate. Resolving these issues takes time, patience and understanding, and can challenge a dietitian's imagination. However, even small changes in behaviour can be very rewarding.
- Being aware of, and sensitive to, these differences is important for a sports dietitian.

23.8 *PRACTICE TIPS*

Elizabeth Broad

- Treat athletes with disabilities the same as able-bodied athletes first and foremost. Be aware of the terminology to use with the athlete and specifically understand the effects that inappropriate language can have on individuals with disabilities. Most of their nutritional needs will be the same as an able-bodied person's, however, modification in energy may be needed in athletes with limited mobility or functional limitations.

- Always undertake a medical history to determine other medical issues you may need to consider, including medications. If you are unsure of any aspects of the disability or associated medical conditions, or how their medication works and what its side-effects are, consult a clinical or sports physician.

- Some athletes may have a support person apart from their coach. This support person may perform many functions, such as riding the front of a tandem bike for a visually impaired athlete, to assisting an athlete with CP get into position for a throwing event. It is important to respect the relationship this person has with the athlete and the intimate knowledge they have about the athlete, and to involve them in discussions surrounding diet and food provision.

- Always ask the athlete if they are completely independent or if they require assistance, particularly in lifestyle-management issues; if they do require assistance, ask specifically what they need—they will generally be able to tell you succinctly.

- The energy requirements of some athletes with disabilities may be relatively low, so consuming nutrient-dense foods is a high priority for maintaining nutritional quality.

- When advising about fluid intake, ask the athlete how they manage their bladder control and what effect an increased fluid intake may have on them. Be willing to trial things in conjunction with the athlete to come up with the best scenario and look at additional cooling methods for those with SCI.

- As with able-bodied athletes, when advising about any changes to the diet or use of sports nutrition supplements, discuss openly with the athlete the effect this may have on them and attain a suitable solution in conjunction with them. Athletes with disabilities will experience similar misconceptions over food and diet, concerns about body-fat control, and optimising performance to any other person. However, there are some specific reasons for approaching this topic with consideration, such as the effect it may have on bowel movement frequency or stool consistency, urinary output, and psychological factors.

- If working as part of a team, or in an unfamiliar environment for the athletes, you may be required to provide some assistance. For example, visually impaired athletes will generally require assistance in orientation and locating food and utensils at a dining hall when they first arrive. If operating from self-contained units, it is best to room them with sighted athletes with an understanding of how to explain the presentation of food on a plate (e.g. the clock system). Depending on the disability, some athletes may require soft foods, assistance with carrying food to their table, or may need their food cut up for them.

REFERENCES

Armstrong LE, Maresh CM, Riebe D, et al. Local cooling in wheelchair athletes during exercise—heat stress. Med Sci Sports Exerc 1995;27:211–16.

Bhambhani YN, Burnham RS, Wheeler GD, Eriksson P, Holland LJ, Steadward RD. Physiological correlates of simulated wheelchair racing in trained quadriplegics. Can J Appl Physiol 1995;20:65–77.

Bhambhani YN, Holland LJ, Eriksson P, Steadward RD. Physiological responses during wheelchair racing in quadriplegics and paraplegics. Paraplegia 1994;3:253–60.

Booth DW. Athletes with disabilities. In: Harries M, et al, eds. Oxford textbook of sports medicine. New York: Oxford University Press, 1994.

Broad EM. The effects of heat on performance in wheelchair shooters. Masters thesis. Canberra: University of Canberra, 1997.

Buckley J. Director of medical services for the 2000 Paralympic Games, Gold Coast, Queensland, 2000.

Coutts KD, Stogryn JL. Aerobic and anaerobic power of Canadian wheelchair track athletes. Med Sci Sports Exerc 1987;19:62–5.

De Pauw KP, Gavron SJ. Disability in Sport. Champaign, Illinois: Human Kinetics, 1995.

Gass GC. Physical fitness test procedures for disabled athletes: disabled athlete assessment centre program. Lidcombe, NSW: Cumberland College of Health Sciences, 1988 (unpublished).

Glaser RM. Exercise and locomotion for the spinal cord injured. Ex Sports Sc Rev 1985;13:263–303.

Goodman S, Lee K, Heidt F, eds. Coaching wheelchair athletes. Canberra: Australian Sports Commission, 1996.

Hjeltnes N. Control of medical rehabilitation of paraplegics and tetraplegics by repeated evaluation of endurance capacity. Int J Sports Med 1984;5(suppl):171–4.

Hopman MTE, Oeseburg B, Binkhorst RA. Cardiovascular responses in persons with paraplegia to prolonged arm exercise and thermal stress. Med Sci Sports Exerc 1993;25:577–83.

Johnson RK, Goran MI, Ferrara MS, Poehlman ET. Athetosis increases resting metabolic rate in adults with cerebral palsy. J Am Diet Assoc 1996;96:145–8.

Johnson RK, Hildreth HG, Contompasis SH, Goran MI. Total energy expenditure in adults with cerebral palsy as assessed by doubly-labeled water. J Am Diet Assoc 1997;97:966–70.

Karlsson J, Saltin B. Diet, muscle glycogen and endurance performance. J Appl Physiol 1971;21:203–6.

Kennedy M. The effect of drugs on heat regulation. In: Sutton JR, Thompson MW, Torode ME, eds. Exercise and thermoregulation. Sydney: The University of Sydney, 1995:223–33.

Levine AM, Nash MS, Green BA, Shea JD, Aronica MJ. An examination of dietary intakes and nutritional status of chronic healthy spinal cord-injured individuals. Paraplegia 1992;30:880–9.

MIMS Australia. MIMS Annual 1999. Sydney, NSW: Medi Media, 1999.

Noreau L, Shephard RJ. Spinal cord injury, exercise and quality of life. Sports Med 1995;20:226–50.

Normell LA. Distribution of impaired cutaneous vasomotor and sudomotor function in paraplegic man. Scand J Clin Lab Invest 1974;33(suppl):25–41.

Petrofsky JS. Thermoregulatory stress during rest and exercise in heat in patients with a spinal cord injury. Eur J Appl Physiol 1992;64:503–7.

Sawka MN, Gonzalez RR, Drolet LL, Pandolf KB. Heat exchange during upper- and lower-body exercise. J Appl Physio 1984;57:1050–4.

Shephard RJ. Sports medicine and the wheelchair athlete. Sports Med 1988;4:226–47.

Skrinar GS, Evans WJ, Ornstein LJ, Brown DA. Glycogen utilisation in wheelchair-dependent athletes. Int J Sports Med 1982;3:215–19.

Wicks JR, Oldridge NB, Cameron BJ, Jones NL. Arm cranking and wheelchair ergometry in elite spinal cord–injured athletes. Med Sci Sports Exerc 1983;15:224–31.

Winnick JP, ed. Adapted physical education and sport, 2nd edn. Champaign, Illinois: Human Kinetics, 1995:167–71, 193–212.

www.paralympic.org. Australian Paralympic Federation Website. Provides information on events, class of athletes, history of paralympic sports.

ACKNOWLEDGMENTS

The author would like to acknowledge the assistance of Jane Buckley, Director of Medical Services for the 2000 Australian Paralympic Team, in researching this chapter, and Dr Darren Smith for assisting with editing.

CHAPTER 24

Medical and nutritional issues for the travelling athlete

Mark Young and Peter Fricker

24.1 INTRODUCTION

Today's international athlete is a global traveller, and as a result the sports nutritionist is presented with specific nutritional and medical problems. These problems include an increased risk of illness, particularly food- and water-borne illness, jet lag and environmental stress. Early preparation and education is important for prevention. Well before departure, it is the responsibility of the sports medicine team to identify specific problems at the destination and institute strategies for prevention. Such strategies include the planning of vaccination programs (including malarial prophylaxis) and educating athletes and officials about minimising travel illness and jet lag. This should be done with the help of practitioners who are experienced in the problems of overseas travel, as recommendations vary and are specific to each destination.

24.2 JET LAG AND JET STRESS

International air travel presents the modern phenomena known as jet lag and jet stress. Jet lag refers to problems relating to air travel as a result of the rapid traversal of time zones between countries across the world. It often leads to fatigue, disturbance of the day/night cycle, sleeping difficulties, and mood and bowel disturbances.

A few ways to minimise the symptoms of jet lag are: setting watches to destination time on or before departure; avoiding late-night farewells; careful planning of flights to maximise appropriate sleep time; and the use of hypnotic drugs, during and initially after flight. Adopting destination sleep times before departure can also help decrease the effects of jet lag. On arrival, it is important to establish a new sleep/wake cycle as soon as possible, by early exposure to sunlight, physical activity, and avoiding sleep during the daytime.

Jet lag can hinder performance, so adequate time is needed after arrival and before competition, to adjust to the new time zone. Adjustments vary among individuals, but usually one full day of acclimatisation is required for every (one-hour) time zone crossed (French 1995). Up to three time zones may be crossed, however, before an effect on performance is noticed. Westbound travel tends to cause less jet lag as the body's circadian rhythms are on a 25-hour cycle and travelling west results in a longer day (Manfredini et al. 1998).

Jet stress refers to external problems in transit as a result of air travel and is independent of the number of time zones crossed. The air in the aircraft cabin is relatively dry, so an increased fluid requirement is needed. Drinks that contain caffeine (e.g. coffee) or alcohol, if consumed in excess, also contribute to hypohydration, so these are best avoided. Airlines tend to provide a limited variety of foods during travel, however, special meals can be arranged in advance. Usually a minimum of 24 hours notice is required by most airlines for individual catering requests, but a longer period is advised for teams. In general, during long flights, athletes should be encouraged to make the flight as comfortable as possible (with bulkhead and aisle seats), use music or literature for relaxation, and carry water bottles and small amounts of carbohydrate-rich foods for consumption during the flight. Careful planning and timing of flights to avoid delays or lengthy periods in transit lounges minimises the effects of jet stress.

On arrival, adequate time must be allowed for acclimatisation to environmental conditions as well as to recover from jet lag. As heat acclimatisation may take up to two weeks, many athletes can start acclimatising before departure by exercising in hot environments. However, hypohydration from airline travel itself or from the local climate can negate the adaptive changes of heat acclimatisation accomplished at home prior to the journey. In hot and humid countries and sporting venues, sweat rates during physical activity can exceed 2 L/h. Competing athletes may need to increase fluid consumption by up to 10 L/d in such environments to prevent dehydration (Young et al. 1998). Regular daily body weights of individual athletes are useful to determine hydration status. Fluctuations of more than 1–2 kg weight loss during the day, for example, may indicate hypohydration. Most people put on weight during the day and wake up in a partially hypohydrated condition after a night's sleep. A good indication of adequate hydration is clear, not dark urine. Drinking large volumes of water, especially during hard exercise, may lower the serum sodium concentration and osmolality in susceptible people. Use of a sports drink which contains low levels of sodium and other sugars such that it is iso-osmolar (i.e. the same concentration as solutes in the blood serum) can easily address this potential problem.

24.3 ILLNESSES ASSOCIATED WITH TRAVELLING

All athletes are at risk of acquiring infection from unusual organisms, especially those spread by the faeco-oral route and by insect vectors. Travellers' diarrhoea affects between 20–50% of travellers spending around two weeks in a 'developing' country (O'Kane & Gottlieb 1996). Most travel-related diarrhoea is caused by non-viral pathogens such as enterotoxigenic escherichia coli, salmonella, shigella, campylobacter and giardia lamblia. These pathogens are transmitted in food, water, from other people, from poor sanitary conditions, and from poor personal and food hygiene practices.

24.3.1 Prevention and treatment of diarrhoea, nausea and vomiting

Many of the infections by these pathogens can be prevented by attention to personal hygiene, including washing hands thoroughly with soap before meals, and ensuring that food has been freshly cooked, and that shellfish, unpasteurised milk and unpeeled fruits and vegetables are not consumed. In many countries, the drinking water contains potential pathogenic micro-organisms which can be transmitted in raw food (salads, vegetables) washed in water, in ice cubes and even by brushing the teeth in tap water. Tap water is 'safe' for consumption if boiled for at least five minutes. Water purifying tablets purchased in pharmacies are another alternative but are not always effective.

In countries where the risk of travellers' diarrhoea is high, it may be appropriate to use prophylactic short-term antibiotics, such as ciprofloxacin (500 mg daily), or doxycycline (100 mg/d), or sulphamethoxazole (800 mg/d) with trimethoprim (100 mg/d). If diarrhoeal illness does occur, it is wise to consume a bland diet such as dry toast, biscuits, rice and bananas, and avoid alcohol, fat-rich foods and dairy foods until the diarrhoea settles. When diarrhoea occurs, an increased fluid intake with drinks such as water or electrolyte rehydration salts is required and these should be consumed in small amounts, but often. Antidiarrhoeal drugs can be used if there is no blood or mucus, but since diarrhoea is nature's way of flushing out the pathogens, the illness may be prolonged. If the diarrhoea is associated with fever, blood or mucus, antibiotics may be required and a doctor should prescribe these. If low-grade diarrhoea persists for more than three days, giardia lamblia may be the underlying organism and antibiotics such as metronidazole or tinidazole may be required. Many organisms cause symptoms that may not present until return to the country of origin, and all athletes should be advised to seek medical advice in any case of post-travel illness.

In summary, with careful preparation, education and appropriate management, most travellers' problems can be prevented.

24.4 *PRACTICE TIPS*

Lorna Garden

Prior to departure

- Determining all aspects of the trip (including travel arrangements, accommodation and competition times and venues) well in advance is essential. This information is necessary before appropriate and specific practical advice and education can be provided. Often individual athletes or teams consult you a few days prior to departure, which is insufficient time to re-arrange details that may be better suited to their needs. Table 24.1 provides a checklist of issues to investigate prior to departure.

Table 24.1 *Pre-travel checklist*

- Vaccinations (where necessary).
- Itinerary, including modes of transport, travelling times and likely breaks in the journey (e.g. meal stops, refuelling stops, overnight stopovers).
- Training and competition schedule.
- Type of accommodation and meal arrangements.
- Trip coordinator/team manager's details.
- Familiarity with place of destination (e.g. climate, time zones, food and drink availability).
- Local customs relevant to the athlete (e.g. clothing, language, dietary habits).
- Baggage limits, including equipment.
- Food and fluids provided by team management (where applicable).

- Athletes need help in planning and timing of food and fluid intakes when travelling interstate, overseas or just competing away from home. When an athlete is staying in self-contained accommodation, the sports dietitian should discuss portable foods to carry or purchase, as well as cooking utensils (e.g. hand-held blender for smoothies, rice cooker, electric wok) if appropriate. Chapter 26 provides additional practical suggestions for self-catering and how to choose foods that meet dietary goals when eating out.

- When travelling by private car or hired vehicle, finding appropriate food en route can be difficult and time consuming. Carrying a small esky is a necessity for long trips. Table 24.2 lists suitable snacks for travelling.

- When travelling by train or bus, check availability of food or frequency of food stops, and supplement with suitable snacks where necessary.

- Airlines usually provide special meal options, if requested, when bookings are made. Athletes are advised to ask for a special meal (e.g. sports meal or a low-fat meal) for all flights.

| Table 24.2 | *Suitable snacks for travelling* |

- Grapes, cherries, apples, pears, dates, strawberries, bananas, nectarines, peaches and other seasonal fruit (if travelling locally).
- Canned fruit with flip-top openers.
- Sultanas, raisins, dried apricots, dried apple, nuts.
- Rice crackers, pretzels.
- Popcorn made with minimum fat/oil.
- Muesli bars, breakfast bars, energy bars (low fat).
- Dry cereal (in serve-size boxes).
- Sandwiches, rolls or mini-bagels.
- Low-fat cheese sticks.
- Pikelets.
- Fruit bread or buns.
- Jelly confectionery (in moderation!).
- Low-fat fruit muffins.
- Low-fat flavoured milk.
- Water, fruit juice, sports drinks, liquid meal supplements.

- Athletes travelling to unfamiliar countries benefit by packing food staples in their bags. Meal replacement formulae (e.g. Sports Sustagen™), dried milk powder, breakfast cereal (e.g. wheatflake biscuits), muesli and sports bars are favourites. These foods are invaluable for athletes who have difficulty meeting energy needs and are hesitant to try new and unfamiliar foods. Check customs regulations before taking any food and drink overseas.

- Athletes benefit by eating in local restaurants offering similar cuisine to their destination, thus allowing them to become familiar with likely food choices and common dishes.

Preventing jet lag

- Table 24.3 provides dietary strategies to help minimise jet lag.

Tips for preventing nutrition-related illness when travelling

- Many food- and water-borne illnesses are preventable by paying attention to personal hygiene (i.e. washing hands thoroughly with uncontaminated water before eating), food hygiene (appropriate food handling and storage), and being aware of the main food sources of contamination (see Section 24.3). Raw, uncooked fresh foods (meat, fish, vegetables and eggs), unboiled water and unpasteurised dairy products contain micro-organisms (viruses, bacteria and parasites) that are potential pathogens. Most micro-organisms are destroyed by cooking or when they come into contact with the acid in the human stomach, but grow prolifically in foods improperly cooked, stored and handled (Deakin

Table 24.3	*Dietary strategies to help prevent jet lag*

- Adapt meal and snack times to destination time before and during the flight.
- High-carbohydrate, low-protein meals during transit may help induce drowsiness.
- Hypohydration is a real problem during air travel and it is important to increase fluid intake throughout the flight. Bring a water bottle that can be refilled and sipped continuously.
- Avoid drinks containing caffeine (coffee, tea, cola drinks) and alcoholic beverages, as these can exacerbate fluid losses.
- Pre-arrange special meals that provide carbohydrate and are low in fat.
- Pack portable, high-carbohydrate snacks (including fruit) in hand luggage.
- Keep a food diary to remind you of when you last ate.
- Bring plenty of things to do (books, games, CDs) to prevent boredom eating.
- Adopt regular meal and snack patterns upon arrival and sustain a higher fluid intake until well hydrated.

1998). Sources of contamination are dirty dishes left for hours, food left unrefrigerated or uncovered in the refrigerator, cutting boards, cooking and eating utensils, tea towels and dishcloths. Most young people do not question the safety of food consumed at home or when they eat out and are unaware of sources of food contamination (Deakin 2000, personal communication).

- Table 24.4 lists practical tips for athletes to help increase their awareness of food hygiene and food safety issues and help prevent travel illness, particularly in those athletes travelling overseas. Many of these tips can also be applied to travelling locally or interstate.

Tips for treating diarrhoea and vomiting

- When there is a high risk of travellers' diarrhoea, a low-fat, low-fibre, bland diet should be followed during the acute stage, and solid food should be introduced as appropriate. Table 24.5 details guidelines for dietary treatment of nausea, vomiting and diarrhoea provided to athletes travelling overseas.

Tips for maintaining dietary goals when travelling

- Regular weight and/or skinfold checks are recommended, for athletes who are away for a long time, to prevent dramatic and unwanted changes in body composition. The wide range of foods available at many sporting venues and in athletes' villages, along with a holiday atmosphere, can make it difficult for athletes to adhere to appropriate eating behaviours. These issues should be discussed with athletes prior to departure and strategies should be offered to prevent overeating or other eating problems (see Chapter 26).

Table 24.4 *Tips for preventing nutrition-related illnesses when travelling overseas*

- Wash hands with soap frequently, and for at least 30 seconds, especially before eating. Use a clean towel or air dryer to dry hands.
- If the local water supply is unsafe, boil all drinking water, or preferably drink bottled water. Soft drink is 'safe' but should not be used as a substitute for water.
- Avoid ice in drinks unless you are sure the water is safe for drinking.
- Avoid eating salad or raw vegetables unless the food has been washed in water that is safe for drinking.
- Peel all fruit.
- Avoid other raw foods such as oysters, shellfish and raw fish (as eaten in sushi).
- Avoid buying foods from local stalls and markets, where hygiene may be poor.
- Look for food that is well cooked and served hot (not warm).
- Avoid buffet food that is not served very hot or chilled, or which has been sitting for extended periods of time.
- In countries where food hygiene and safety standards are questionable, select foods that have been cooked to order rather than pre-cooked and re-heated.

Table 24.5 *Diet therapy for nausea, vomiting or diarrhoea*

Nausea/vomiting
- Withhold food in the short term but maintain fluid intake.
- Sip a sports drink or use Gastrolyte™ or other electrolyte replacement drinks if vomiting is frequent and severe; avoid soft drink and fruit juice.
- Avoid fatty foods and high-sugar foods.
- Consume small, frequent meals—e.g. dry crackers, or dry toast at first, then progress to light, low-fat meals as tolerated.
- Elevate the head, eat slowly.

Diarrhoea
- The type of foods listed above are also recommended for diarrhoea.
- Avoid milk, caffeine drinks (e.g. coffee, cola), soft drink and fruit juice and foods associated with abdominal cramping. Foods linked with cramping include gaseous drinks and food that may cause flatulence in certain individuals.

Adapted from Deakin 1998

- Some athletes may find keeping a food diary a useful method of keeping check on their diets, and this will provide a handy resource for future travel and competition eating.

- Where technology permits, arrange regular communication with the athlete via email or fax to encourage and support good dietary habits while they are away.

- Arrange a debriefing when the athlete returns, to assist with planning further events that require travel.

REFERENCES

Deakin V. Prevention and treatment of foodborne illness when travelling. Sports Coach 1998;21:15–16.

French J. Circadian rhythms, jet lag and the athlete. In: Torg JS, Shephard RJ, eds. Current therapeutics in sports medicine. St Louis: Mosby, 1995:596–600.

Manfredini R, Manfredini F, Fersini C, Conconi F. Circadian rhythms, athletic performance, and jet lag. Br J Sports Med 1998;32:101–6.

O'Kane G, Gottlieb T. Travellers' diarrhoea. Curr Therap 1996;Feb:53–60.

Young M, Fricker P, Maughan R, MacAuley D. The travelling athlete: issues relating to the Commonwealth Games, Malaysia, 1998. Br J Sports Med 1998;32:77–81.

CHAPTER 25

Nutritional issues for special environments: training and competing at altitude and in hot climates

Mark Febbraio

25.1 INTRODUCTION

During exercise the conversion of chemical energy into mechanical work is increased several-fold. Given that the origin of most chemical energy is derived from the diet, nutritional supplementation and its effect on exercise performance has been an area of scientific interest since early this century. In the latter half of this century, the popularisation of the muscle biopsy technique, arteriovenous (a-v) balance measurements and, more recently, the use of isotope tracers as metabolic probes during exercise, has made it possible to clearly investigate the role of nutrition in exercise science. Much of the research that has examined the interaction between nutrition and exercise has been conducted at sea level and in comfortable ambient conditions. It is clear, however, that both altitude and environmental temperature are major practical issues one must consider when examining nutrition, training and competition, because athletes inevitably compete in these circumstances. This chapter will examine the altered nutritional requirements for training and competing at high altitude or in extreme temperatures.

25.2 NUTRITIONAL REQUIREMENTS AT HIGH ALTITUDE

25.2.1 *Substrate utilisation at high altitude: acute and chronic exposure*

Acute exposure to high altitude results in an increased dependence on blood glucose as a fuel at rest and during exercise (Brooks et al. 1991a, 1991b, 1992; Roberts et al. 1996b). This increase in glucose utilisation during exercise does not appear to be accompanied by a concomitant decrease in muscle glycogen use (Green et al. 1989), but rather a decreased reliance on fat as a substrate (Roberts et al. 1996a). Interestingly, after chronic exposure to altitude, the increase in blood glucose disposal is augmented rather than attenuated. Brooks et al. (1991b) demonstrated that, upon arrival at altitude (4 300 m), glucose disposal during exercise increased by approximately 25%. However, this increase was markedly augmented after 21 days exposure at this altitude (see Figure 25.1).

This response presents a significant challenge to those exercising at high altitude, particularly those who are exposed to this environment for several days or weeks. The endogenous carbohydrate (CHO) reserves are limited and there is a heavy reliance on CHO during exercise. As subjects become acclimatised to altitude, physical work capacity is increased (Sutton et al. 1988), therefore, the reliance on endogenous CHO stores is increased. Hence, the reliance on CHO as a substrate increases both in relative and absolute terms.

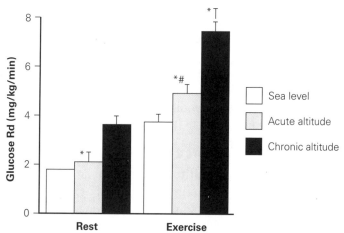

Figure 25.1 *Rate of glucose disappearance (Rd) at rest and after 45 minutes of exercise at sea level, upon arrival at 4 300 m (acute altitude) and after 21 days at 4 300 m (chronic altitude)*
* denotes different (P < 0.05) from rest
\# denotes different (P < 0.05) from sea level
T denotes different (P < 0.05) from sea level and acute altitude
Data expressed as mean ± SE (n = 7)
From Brooks et al. 1991b (with permission)

25.2.2 *Energy requirements at high altitude*

It is clear that upon initial exposure to high altitude, basal metabolic rate (BMR) increases (Kellogg et al. 1957; Moore et al. 1987; Butterfield et al. 1992). This increase may be as high as 28% above that observed at sea level (Butterfield et al. 1992) and although most studies observe an attenuation in the increase in BMR after two to three days of exposure, Butterfield et al. (1992) observed this increase to be maintained for up to three weeks. Although the exact mechanism for the elevation in BMR has not been fully elucidated, it has been suggested that either an increase in stress hormone secretion and/or inadequate energy intake may be responsible (Butterfield 1999). Both acute and chronic exposure to altitude increases the sympatho-adrenal response during exercise (Mazzeo et al. 1991). However, since glucose appears to be the sole contributor to the increased energy turnover at rest, it is unlikely that an increase in adrenaline mediates this response since adrenaline infusion reduces, rather than increases, glucose disposal at rest (Bonen et al. 1992). It is more likely that an inadequate energy intake is responsible for the increase in BMR. High-altitude exposure greater than 3500 m results in appetite suppression and reduced nutritional intake (Consolazio et al. 1968). Interestingly, when weight is maintained during exposure to altitude, the increase in BMR is 7% compared with 28% when subjects ingested food *ad libitum* (Butterfield 1999), suggesting a relationship between BMR and energy balance.

It appears, therefore, that energy intake at high altitude should be greater than that at sea level, even though the appetite is suppressed. Since blood glucose oxidation appears to be increased during exercise at altitude, it would be wise to ingest a diet rich in CHO. In fact, it has been suggested that a CHO-rich diet decreases the symptoms of acute mountain sickness compared with the consumption of a mixed diet (Consolazio et al. 1969). It must be noted, however, that CHO (expressed as a monosaccharide) provides 16 kJ/g compared with 37 kJ/g for fat. Given that appetite is suppressed, it would be wise to ingest CHO-dense food when exercising or competing at altitude.

25.2.3 *Maintaining fluid balance*

One of the major responses to acute altitude exposure is an initial reduction in total body water and plasma volume (Hannon et al. 1969; Pugh 1964). It has been suggested that this fluid loss and resultant haemoconcentration increases the oxygen-carrying capacity of the blood until polycythemia occurs (Grover et al. 1986). In addition, because the air at altitude is dry and cold, water is lost to the environment while breathing. Hence, any fluid loss due to thermoregulation associated with exercise is augmented at altitude. Fluid requirements at rest and during exercise at altitude are thus increased compared with sea level. Given that CHO requirements are increased, it would be practical to ingest a 'sports drink' beverage when exposed to altitude. Importantly, commercially available sports drinks contain sodium, potassium and chloride. Although addition of sodium does not increase glucose or fluid bioavailability during exercise (Hargreaves et al. 1994), such an addition will maintain the drive for drinking, minimise urinary fluid loss during exercise and maintain the extracellular fluid volume space (Nose et al. 1988; Maughan & Leiper 1995; Takamata et al. 1995).

25.2.4 *Summary of altitude nutrition issues*

In summary, when exposed to altitude both acutely and for a period of time, CHO use is increased and BMR is increased. The alterations are accompanied by a reduced appetite, usually energy imbalance and sometimes cachexia. Therefore, CHO intake should be increased. Since the appetite is usually suppressed in this environment, it would be prudent to ingest CHO-dense food. Exposure to altitude also results in a decrease in total body water and, therefore, it is important to increase fluid consumption.

25.3 *EXERCISE IN A HOT ENVIRONMENT*

25.3.1 *Substrate utilisation during exercise in the heat*

Although there is some conflict in the literature, it is generally accepted that exercise in a hot environment results in a substrate shift towards increased CHO utilisation. Muscle glycogenolysis (Fink et al. 1975; Febbraio et al. 1994a, 1994b), liver glucose production (Hargreaves et al. 1996a) and respiratory exchange ratio (Febbraio et al. 1994a, 1994b; Hargreaves et al. 1996a) are higher during exercise in a hot environment. Furthermore, both muscle (Young et al. 1985; Febbraio et al. 1994a, 1994b) and plasma (Fink et al. 1975; Powers et al. 1985; Young et al. 1985; Yaspelkis et al. 1993; Febbraio et al. 1994a) lactate accumulation are increased in humans during exercise in the heat compared with similar exercise in a cool environment. The increase in CHO utilisation appears to coincide with a reduced lipid utilisation during exercise in the heat. Both plasma free fatty acid uptake (Gonzalez-Alonso et al. 1999) and intramuscular triglyceride utilisation (Fink et al. 1975) are reduced during exercise and thermal stress. These data, along with the consistent observation of an increased RER during exercise and heat stress (Febbraio et al. 1994a, 1994b; Hargreaves et al. 1996a), suggest a substrate shift away from lipid and towards CHO use.

Apart from the increase in CHO use during exercise and heat stress, recent data also suggest that protein degradation may increase during exercise in a hot environment. Mittleman et al. (1998) have demonstrated that branched chain amino acid (BCAA) supplementation increased endurance performance during exercise in the heat. This finding is in contrast with studies conducted during exercise in cooler environments (van Hall et al. 1995; Madsen et al. 1996). Of note, studies conducted in our laboratory have observed an increase in ammonia (NH_3) accumulation during exercise and heat stress (Snow et al. 1993; Febbraio et al. 1994a). Although a major pathway for NH_3 production during exercise is via the deamination of adenosine 5'-monophosphate to form NH_3 and inosine 5'-monophosphate (IMP), NH_3 can also be formed in skeletal muscle via the oxidation of BCAA. Accordingly, BCAA supplementation augments muscle NH_3 production during exercise (MacLean et al. 1996). During our more recent study (Febbraio et al. 1994b), the augmented muscle NH_3 accumulation when comparing exercise in the heat with that in a cooler environment was observed in the absence of any difference in IMP accumulation, suggesting that enhanced BCAA oxidation may have accounted for the increase. It appears, therefore, that protein requirements may need to be increased when exercise training is undertaken in a hot environment. It should be noted, however, that few studies have examined the relationship between exercise in the heat and protein requirements and further research is required before defini-tive recommendations can be made.

25.3.2 *Is carbohydrate availability limiting during exercise in the heat?*

During sub-maximal exercise in comfortable ambient temperatures, the rate of energy utilisation is closely matched by rates of energy provision. It is well estab-lished that in these circumstances fatigue is often associated with glycogen depletion and/or hypoglycaemia (Coyle et al. 1986; Sahlin et al. 1990) and endurance can be increased by providing exogenous CHO during exercise (Coyle et al. 1986; Coggan & Coyle 1987). Since CHO utilisation is augmented during exercise in the heat and fatigue often coincides with depletion of this substrate, it is somewhat paradoxical that fatigue during exercise in the heat is often related to factors other than substrate depletion. We (Parkin et al. 1999) and others (Nielsen et al. 1990; Gonzalez-Alonso et al. 1999) have demonstrated that intramuscular glycogen content is approxi-mately 300 mmol/kg dry weight (dw) at fatigue when, during exercise in cooler environments, this figure is usually less than 150 mmol/kg dw (Figure 25.2). This may be because hyperthermia can lead to fatigue prior to CHO stores being com-promised. This hypothesis is supported by the observations that, when exercising in the heat to exhaustion, subjects will fatigue at the same body core temperature even if interventions such as acclimatisation (Nielsen et al. 1993) or fluid/CHO ingestion (Febbraio et al. 1996b) alter the duration of exercise. There may be circumstances, however, where CHO may be limiting during exercise in the heat. If the intensity of exercise is moderate, resulting in a relatively low rate of endogenous heat produc-tion, or the exercise is intermittent in nature allowing for effective heat dissipation, CHO may be limiting. Accordingly, CHO ingestion may (Murray et al. 1987; Davis et al. 1988b; Millard-Stafford et al. 1992) or may not (Davis et al. 1988a; Millard-Stafford et al. 1990; Febbraio et al. 1996b) increase exercise performance in the heat.

25.3.3 *Exercise, heat stress and metabolic perturbations*

As mentioned previously, glycogen content within human skeletal muscle at the point of fatigue during exercise in the heat is often adequate to maintain energy turnover via oxidative phosphorylation. It is somewhat surprising, therefore, that a marked increase in IMP accumulation at fatigue during exercise and heat stress is observed despite glycogen concentration being adequate to maintain the oxidative potential of the contracting skeletal muscle (see Figure 25.2) (Parkin et al. 1999). IMP is a marker of inadequate energy turnover via oxidative phosphorylation and is often observed at fatigue during prolonged exercise (Norman et al. 1987; Sahlin et al. 1990; Baldwin et al. 1999), when glycogen stores can no longer provide substrate to maintain oxidative phosphorylation, but not earlier (Norman et al. 1987; Sahlin et al. 1990) when glycogen stores are adequate.

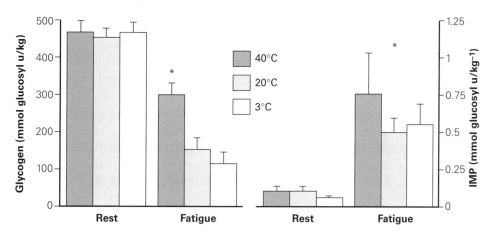

Figure 25.2 *Glycogen content and inosine 5′-monophosphate (IMP) concentration before (Rest) and after (Fatigue) sub-maximal exercise to exhaustion in different ambient temperatures*
Data expressed as mean ± SE (n = 8)
* indicates main effect (P < 0.05) for exercise
From Parkin et al. 1999

These data suggest, therefore, a disruption to mitochondrial function during exercise and heat stress and support recent findings by Mills et al. (1996) who observed an increase in plasma concentrations of lipid hydroperoxides, a marker of oxidative stress, in horses exercising in the heat. In addition, when examining the ratio between ADP production and mitochondrial oxygen consumption (ADP:O ratio) in isolated rat skeletal muscle mitochondria, Brooks et al. (1971) observed a constant ADP:O ratio at temperatures ranging from 25–40°C. Above 40°C, however, the ADP:O ratio declined linearly with an increase in temperature, suggesting that for a given oxygen consumption the increase in ADP rephosphorylation was lower than the rate of ATP degradation. Although the data provide only indirect evidence, they suggest that the combination of exercise and heat stress may disrupt cellular function, resulting in oxyradical formation.

25.3.4 *Benefits of fluid ingestion*

In circumstances where the endogenous heat production and high environmental temperature result in fatigue prior to CHO stores being compromised, fluid ingestion, irrespective of whether it contains CHO, is of major importance in delaying the rise in body core temperature. Exercise-induced dehydration is associated with an increase in core temperature (Hamilton et al. 1991; Montain & Coyle 1992), reduced cardio-vascular function (Hamilton et al. 1991; Montain & Coyle 1992) and impaired exercise performance (Walsh et al. 1994). These effects are reduced, or indeed pre-vented, by fluid ingestion (Costill et al. 1970; Hamilton et al. 1991; Montain & Coyle 1992), which also improves exercise performance (Maughan et al. 1989; Walsh et al. 1994; McConell et al. 1997). Fluid ingestion also reduces muscle glycogen use during prolonged exercise (see Figure 25.3) (Hargreaves et al. 1996b; Gonzalez-Alonso et al. 1999). It is likely that the mechanism/s responsible for the attenuated glycogen use during exercise are the reduced circulating adrenaline and decreased muscle temper-ature that result from fluid ingestion, since muscle temperature (Febbraio et al. 1996a; Starkie et al. 1999) and adrenaline (Febbraio et al. 1998) influence glycogen use. It is clear from these data that fluid ingestion not only attenuates the rise in body core temperature, thereby preventing hyperthermia, but it also reduces the likelihood of CHO depletion. Since sweat rate is augmented during exercise in the heat, dehydra-tion progresses more rapidly and, therefore, the importance of fluid ingestion is

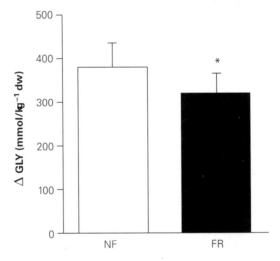

Figure 25.3 *Net muscle glycogen utilisation (Δ GLY; pre-post-exercise) during 120 minutes of exercise in the absence (NF) or presence (FR) of fluid ingestion*
* indicates difference (P < 0.05) compared with NF
Data expressed as mean ± SE (n = 5)
From Hargreaves et al. (1996b)

increased during exercise in extreme heat. Indeed, Below et al. (1995) have demonstrated that fluid ingestion improves exercise performance in a hot environment.

25.3.5 *Nutritional recommendations for exercise in a hot environment*

It is clear that both CHO and fluid are very important when making dietary recommendations for those exercising in the heat. Apart from maintaining a CHO-rich diet and remaining euhydrated in the days leading up to exercise, there are strategies that could be employed during exercise, particularly exercise that lasts for longer than 60 minutes. One should ingest a CHO–electrolyte drink frequently during exercise. Since the relative importance of fluid delivery is increased during exercise in the heat, one may be tempted to ingest water in these circumstances. This practice, however, is not ideal since the ingestion of a CHO–electrolyte drink empties from the gut at the same rate as water (Francis 1979; Owen et al. 1986; Ryan et al. 1989), while it can spare muscle glycogen (Yaspelkis & Ivy 1991), during exercise in the heat. In addition, the relative importance of sodium intake is increased during exercise in the heat, and the addition of sodium in rehydration beverages can replace sweat sodium losses, prevent hyponatraemia, promote the maintenance of plasma volume and enhance intestinal absorption of glucose and fluid (for review see Maughan 1994). The amount of the CHO within a fluid beverage ingested during exercise in the heat appears to have little effect on fluid availability or exercise performance provided the CHO is not too concentrated. The change in plasma volume and exercise performance in the heat is not different when ingesting beverages containing 0%, 4.2% and 7% CHO respectively (Febbraio et al. 1996b). However, when a 14% CHO solution is ingested during exercise in the heat, the maintenance of plasma volume is reduced while the rise in rectal temperature tends to be augmented. Accordingly, exercise performance tends to fall (Figure 25.4) (Febbraio et al. 1996b). It is important, therefore, to keep the concentration of CHO within a fluid beverage < ~10% during exercise in the heat, even though CHO utilisation is augmented in these circumstances. In terms of volume and frequency, a practical recommendation might be 400 ml every 15 min. CHO beverage should also be ingested into recovery to replenish intramuscular glycogen stores and promote rehydration, especially when training in a hot environment.

As previously discussed, there is some evidence to suggest that protein catabolism is increased during exercise in the heat (Snow et al. 1993; Febbraio et al. 1994b; Mittleman et al. 1998), but more research is required before definitive recommendations can be made. Likewise, as discussed, there is some evidence to suggest that oxyradical generation may be increased via the combination of exercise and heat stress (Mills et al. 1996). It may, therefore, be of some benefit to supplement those undertaking repeated exercise in a hot environment with antioxidants such as alpha-tocopherol (vitamin E) and ascorbic acid (vitamin C). This recommendation is speculative, however, since the hypothesis that such supplementation is advantageous during exercise in the heat has not been tested.

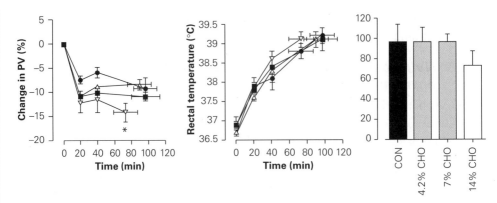

Figure 25.4 *The change in plasma volume (left), rectal temperature (middle) and time to exhaustion (right), while consuming a placebo (CON, –■–), 4.2% CHO (LCHO, –●–), a 7% CHO (–△–) or 14% CHO (HCHO, –▽–) beverage during fatiguing exercise at 70% $VO_{2\,max}$ in 33°C conditions*
* denotes difference (P < 0.05) from other trials
Data expressed as mean ± SE

Data from Febbraio et al. (1996b)

25.4 SPECIAL STRATEGIES FOR EXERCISE IN THE HEAT: GLYCEROL HYPERHYDRATION

Since the deleterious effects of dehydration during exercise (especially that which is conducted in a hot environment) have been well documented, it would be desirable to hyperhydrate prior to exercise in a hot environment. Glycerol, when ingested with a bolus of water, has been widely reported as an effective hyperhydrating agent by most (Lyons et al. 1990; Freund et al. 1995; Montner et al. 1996; Anderson et al. 2001; Hitchen et al. 1999) but not all (Murray et al. 1991; Latzka et al. 1997) previous researchers. While it appears that glycerol is an effective hyperhydrating agent, the exact mechanism of fluid retention remains to be elucidated. It has been suggested that glycerol acts via a renal mechanism, due to changes in circulatory osmotic gradients (Freund et al. 1995). In addition, passive diffusion of glycerol across the renal proximal tubule, due to its lipid solubility, may also cause an osmotic gradient for the reabsorption of water. However, no studies have been sufficiently comprehensive to clearly define the mechanism of action. While most studies observe fluid retention with glycerol ingestion, the consequence of such a change remains equivocal. Glycerol hyperhydration has been demonstrated to reduce thermoregulatory strain and increase sweat rate by some (Lyons et al. 1990) but not all (Latzka et al. 1997) authors. The conflict within the literature may be accounted for by methodological differences such as: environmental conditions;

exercise intensity and duration; subject population; and ingestion protocol. We (Anderson et al. 2000) and others (Hitchens et al. 1999) have recently demonstrated that glycerol ingestion prior to exercise increases fluid retention, reduces thermoregulatory and cardiovascular strain, and enhances exercise performance. However, during our study, subjects exhibited symptoms of gastrointestinal distress. This may have been due to the high osmolality of the glycerol solution (> 600 mosmol/L) resulting in net fluid movement into the gastrointestinal tract. Therefore, athletes must be aware that this practice may have negative repercussions and are advised to test the practice of glycerol hyperhydration in training well before competition. Further discussion of glycerol hyperhydration can be found in Chapter 13, Section 13.4.1.1, and Chapter 17, Section 17.7.3.

25.5 SUMMARY

Both intramuscular glycogen use and glycolysis are augmented, while lipid utilisation appears to decrease during exercise and heat stress. In contrast with sub-maximal exercise in comfortable ambient temperatures, exercise in the heat does not appear to be limited by CHO availability when the heat stress is severe. However, during mild heat stress it is likely that CHO availability is of critical importance.

With respect to diet, athletes should be advised to i) consume a diet rich in CHO and ii) maintain hydration levels when preparing for competition in hot environments. Despite the fact that CHO availability does not always appear to be a major limitation to exercise performance in the heat, it is prudent to ingest a 4–8% CHO beverage throughout exercise since such a beverage empties from the gastrointestinal tract as fast as water, but provides extra glucose and electrolytes which may be required. Importantly, drinking such a beverage may increase *ad libitum* fluid consumption because of increased palatability. Other dietary practices, such as pre-exercise glycerol hyperhydration, BCAA and antioxidant supplementation, might confer some benefit during exercise in the heat.

25.6 PRACTICE TIPS

Louise Burke

- Special nutrition issues arise from living and/or training in stressful environments such as heat or high altitude. To assess special requirements or nutritional strategies that will be important in these conditions, it is important to find out more about the duration of exposure to these environments, the purpose of the exposure, and the training or competition goals during this period. It is useful to differentiate between the following situations.

— The athlete is competing in an important sports competition which has been allocated to a city or country that is at altitude, or experiencing hot or humid weather.

— The athlete is trekking or climbing at high altitude with the goal of completing a route or summiting a peak.

— The athlete is undertaking specialised training in a hot climate or at high altitude in order to 'acclimatise' for competition in a similar environment.

— The athlete is undertaking specialised training in a hot climate or at high altitude to achieve physiological adaptations that may assist performance at sea level or in a cool climate.

— The athlete is using specialised facilities such as a heat chamber or altitude chamber/nitrogen house either to undertake training, or to sleep in this environment. Exposure to this environment will be limited to certain periods during the day, and the athlete will spend the remainder of the day at lower altitudes or in cooler surroundings. These strategies can be used to prepare the athlete for competition in the specialised environment, as well as to achieve desirable physiological adaptations.

- Different nutritional approaches may be appropriate for the various situations listed above. For example, an athlete who is climbing or trekking at very high altitudes (> 5000 m) may expect to experience greater disturbances to energy balance (increased BMR and suppressed appetite) than an athlete who is training at moderate–high altitudes (2000–3000 m). The nutrition strategies for safety and survival over prolonged periods, particularly when the athlete must transport their own food supplies or prepare meals with minimal facilities, will be different to the goals of the athlete who aims to compete at their best at a single event. Similarly, an athlete who is acclimatising to compete in a hot or high-altitude environment should aim to practise and fine tune competition nutrition strategies as an additional requirement to the athlete who is training in such an environment merely for the physiological adaptations. Although athletes should look after fluid and fuel needs in all exercise situations, competition nutrition strategies are more specialised and often more aggressive. The athlete who intends to hyperhydrate with glycerol or consume sports drink according to a pattern provided by aid stations needs to experiment with these practices during training. Such issues may not be important to the athlete who will not be competing in the special environment.

- Fluid losses are increased both in a hot environment and at high altitude. Typically, the athlete will not immediately adjust to increased fluid requirements. Behavioural strategies to increase fluid intake should be implemented to complement physiological factors such as increased thirst. This may be especially important for the athlete who is undertaking intermittent exposure to altitude or heat through specialised chambers. These athletes may incur greater fluid losses during the periods spent at the special environment but miss cues to increase fluid intake when back in their normal environment. The athlete should target drinking patterns related to exercise sessions (drinking before, during and after a prolonged workout) as well as ensure that additional fluid is consumed with meals and between meals. Monitoring body mass in the morning after visiting the toilet provides a crude measure of hydration status. An acute drop in body mass will signal dehydration, but may become confused with the gradual decrease in body fuel stores (glycogen and body fat) that can accompany inadequate CHO and energy intake. Negative energy balance often occurs at high-altitude environments.

• In hot environments, thermoregulation and dehydration play a greater role in determining performance than in a cool environment. Although CHO utilisation is increased in the heat, thermoregulation and dehydration are more likely to be limiting than fuel depletion. Therefore, the athlete should prioritise competition nutrition strategies to promote hydration. Strategies include aggressive rehydration after each workout or event to optimise preparation for the next workout, consideration of hyperhydration strategies such as glycerol loading, and training with fluid intake during exercise to maximise the fluid volume that can be comfortably and practically consumed. Of course, these strategies are not mutually exclusive with practices to promote fuel availability. The athlete should ensure that they have adequately fuelled by consuming a high-CHO diet in association with an exercise taper in the day(s) prior to their event. Athletes who compete in prolonged events should also undertake CHO-loading strategies. It is uncertain whether the water stored with the glycogen within the muscle becomes available as the glycogen is utilised.

• Carbohydrate-containing drinks, especially the commercially produced sports drinks, are suitable for use during exercise in the heat. Although performance during a competitive event undertaken in the heat is more likely to be limited by fluid considerations rather than CHO availability, it is unlikely that a solution of 4–8% CHO will impair fluid delivery. In fact, the taste of such drinks (containing flavour and electrolytes) has been shown to enhance voluntary intake, providing practical advantages over water. In addition, some studies have shown superior performance following the ingestion of CHO intake during exercise in the heat, compared to the intake of water. These situations include high-intensity exercise of about one hour's duration, in addition to the more traditional endurance exercise tasks. Since fluid losses and CHO utilisation during exercise are increased at altitude, sports drinks should also be used during events or workouts in this environment. Again, these drinks offer advantages of promoting additional fluid intake and providing extra fuel.

- Since CHO utilisation is increased at altitude and in hot environments, the total fuel requirements of training and/or competition will be increased. Athletes should plan for this by ensuring adequate CHO intake in meals and snacks. High density CHO foods include dried fruit, grains (rice, noodles, pasta), breakfast cereals, sports bars, sports gels, and powdered versions of sports drink, high carbohydrate sources or liquid meal supplements. These may be useful for athletes who need to carry their own food supplies. These foods may also be appropriate for situations where appetite is suppressed in hot weather or at altitude since they provide a compact source of fuel. Alternatively, CHO-rich foods that have a high fluid content or require minimal chewing may also appeal to an athlete with a depressed appetite. These include fruit smoothies, liquid meal supplements, commercial high carbohydrate source drinks (e.g. concentrated Maxim, Gatorlode), sports gels, flavoured yoghurt, and ice-cream.

- Although there is some evidence that protein requirements are increased at altitude, there is insufficient research to allow definite guidelines to be made. Typically, athletes who increase their total energy intake from a variety of nutritious food choices can expect to meet any additional protein requirements. Athletes who might be identified as 'at risk' for inadequate protein intake include athletes who follow energy-restricted diets (e.g. to 'make weight' or to keep body-fat levels artificially low), or athletes who have limited dietary variety. On occasions, athletes may inadvertently reduce their protein intake by becoming over-reliant on foods that are easy to eat rather than nutritionally sound. Athletes who carry limited food supplies or who struggle to find foods to appeal to a suppressed appetite should remember to include some protein and micronutrient dense foods such as flavoured yoghurts, flavoured milk drinks and smoothies, and liquid meal supplements.

- There is some evidence that oxidative damage arising from exercise is increased by sudden exposure to a hot environment or high altitude. Although there is no evidence to show performance benefits, it may be prudent for athletes who are training hard in these environments to take antioxidant supplementation in the form of vitamins E and C for the first seven to ten days of exposure to the new environment. Equally, it is important that athletes who move to high altitudes have adequate iron status to allow optimal stimulus of red blood cell production. Issues related to iron are summarised in Chapter 11.

REFERENCES

Anderson, MJ, Cotter JD, Garnham AP, Casley DJ, Febbraio MA. Effect of glycerol-induced hyperhydration on thermoregulation and metabolism during exercise in the heat. Int J Sports Med Exerc Metab 2001;11:315–33:in review.

Baldwin J, Snow RJ, Carey MF, Febbraio MA. Muscle IMP accumulation during fatiguing submaximal exercise in endurance trained and untrained men. Am J Physiol 1999;277(1 Pt 2):R295–R300.

Below PR, Mora-Rodriguez R, Gonzalez-Alonso J, Coyle EF. Fluid and carbohydrate ingestion independently improve performance during 1 hour of intense exercise. Med Sci Sports Exerc 1995;27:200–10.

Bonen A, Megeney LA, McCarthy SC, McDermott JC, Tan MH. Epinephrine administration stimulates GLUT-4 translocation but reduces glucose transport in muscle. Biochem Biophys Res Commun 1992 16;187:685–91.

Brooks GA, Butterfield GE, Wolfe RR, Groves BM, Mazzeo RS, Sutton JR, et al. Increased dependence on blood glucose after acclimatization to 4 300 m. J App Physiol 1991a;70:919–27.

Brooks GA, Butterfield GE, Wolfe RR, Groves BM, Mazzeo RS, Sutton JR, et al. Decreased reliance on lactate after acclimatization to 4 300 m. J App Physiol 1991b;71:333–41.

Brooks GA, Hittleman KJ, Faulkner, JA, Beyer RE. Temperature, skeletal muscle mitochondrial functions, and oxygen debt. Am J Physiol 1971;220:1053–9.

Brooks GA, Wolfel EE, Groves BM, Bender PR, Butterfield GE, Cymerman A, et al. Muscle accounts for glucose disposal but not blood lactate appearance during exercise after acclimatization to 4 300 m. J App Physiol 1992;72:2435–45.

Butterfield GE. Nutrient requirements at high altitude. Clin Sports Med 1999;18:607–21.

Butterfield GE, Gates J, Fleming S, Brooks GA, Sutton JR, Wolfel EE, et al. Increased dependence on blood glucose after acclimatization to 4 300 m. J App Physiol 1992;72:1741–8.

Coggan AR, Coyle EF. Reversal of fatigue during prolonged exercise by carbohydrate infusion or ingestion. J Appl Physiol 1987;63:2388–95.

Consolazio CF, Matoush LO, Johnson HL, Krzywicki HJ, Daws TA, Isaac GJ. Effects of high-carbohydrate diets on performance and clinical symptomatology after rapid ascent to high altitude. Fed Proc 1969;28:937–43.

Consolazio CF, Matoush LO, Johnson HL, Krzywicki HJ, Isaac GJ, Witt NF. Metabolic aspects of calorie restriction: nitrogen and mineral balances and vitamin excretion. Am J Clin Nutr 1968;21:803–12.

Costill D, Krammer WF, Fisher A. Fluid ingestion during distance running. Arch Environ Health 1970;21:520–5.

Coyle EF, Coggan AR, Hemmert MK, Ivy JL. Muscle glycogen utilisation during prolonged exercise when fed CHO. J Appl Physiol 1986;61:165–72.

Davis JM, Burgess WA, Slentz CA, Bartoli WP, Pate RR. Effects of ingesting 6% and 12% glucose/electrolyte beverages during prolonged intermittent cycling in the heat. Eur J Appl Physiol 1988a;57:563–9.

Davis JM, Lamb DR, Pate RR, Slentz CA, Burgess WA, Bartoli WP. CHO–electrolyte drinks: effects on endurance cycling in the heat. Am J Clin Nutr 1988b;48:1023–30.

Febbraio MA, Carey MF, Snow RJ, Stathis CG, Hargreaves M. Influence of elevated muscle temperature on metabolism during intense, dynamic exercise. Am J Physiol 1996a;271:R1251–R5.

Febbraio MA, Lambert DL, Starkie RL, Proietto J, Hargreaves M. Effect of epinephrine on muscle glycogenolysis during exercise in trained men. J Appl Physiol 1998;84:465–70.

Febbraio MA, Murton P, Selig SE, Clark SA, Lambert DL, Angus DJ, Carey MF. Effect of CHO ingestion on exercise metabolism and performance in different ambient temperatures. Med Sci Sports Exerc 1996b;28:1380–7.

Febbraio MA, Snow RJ, Hargreaves M, Stathis CG, Martin IK, Carey MF. Muscle metabolism during exercise and heat stress in trained men: effect of acclimation. J Appl Physiol 1994a;76:589–97.

Febbraio MA, Snow RJ, Stathis CG, Hargreaves M, Carey MF. Effect of heat stress on muscle energy metabolism during exercise. J Appl Physiol 1994b;77:2827–31.

Fink WJ, Costill DL, Van Handel PJ. Leg muscle metabolism during exercise in the heat and cold. Eur J Appl Physiol 1975;34:183–90.

Francis KT. Effect of water and electrolyte replacement during exercise in the heat on biochemical indices of stress and performance. Aviat Space Environ Med 1979;50:115–19.

Freund BJ, Montain SJ, Young AJ, Sawka MN, DeLuca J, Pandolf KB, Valeri CR. Glycerol hyperhydration: hormonal, renal and vascular fluid responses. J Appl Physiol 1995;79:2069–77.

Gonzalez-Alonso J, Calbet JA, Nielsen B. Metabolic and thermodynamic responses to dehydration-induced reductions in muscle blood flow in exercising humans. J Physiol Lond 1999;15;520:577–89.

Green HJ, Sutton J, Young P, Cymerman A, Houston CS. Operation Everest II: muscle energetics during maximal exhaustive exercise. J Appl Physiol 1989;66:142–50.

Grover RF, Weil JV, Reeves JT. Cardiovascular adaptations to exercise at high altitude. Exerc Sports Sci Rev 1986;14:269–302.

Hamilton MT, Gonzalez-Alonso J, Montain SJ, Coyle EF. Fluid replacement and glucose infusion during exercise prevent cardiovascular drift. J Appl Physiol 1991;71:871–7.

Hannon JP, Chinn SK, Shields JL. Effects of acute high altitude exposure on body fluids. Fed Proc 1969;28:1178–84.

Hargreaves M, Angus D, Howlett K, Marmy Conus N, Febbraio M. Effect of heat stress on glucose kinetics during exercise. J Appl Physiol 1996a;81:1594–7.

Hargreaves M, Costill D, Burke L, McConell G, Febbraio M. Influence of sodium on glucose bioavailability during exercise. Med Sci Sports Exerc 1994;26:365–8.

Hargreaves M, Dillo P, Angus D, Febbraio M. Effect of fluid ingestion on muscle metabolism during prolonged exercise. J Appl Physiol 1996b;80:363–6.

Hitchen S, Martin DT, Burke L, Yates K, Fallon K, Hahn A, Dobson GP. Glycerol hyperhydration improves cycling time trial performance in hot humid conditions. Eur J Appl Physiol 1999;80:494–501.

Kellogg RH, Pace N, Archibald ER. Respiratory response to inspired CO_2 during acclimatization to an altitude of 12 470 feet. J Appl Physiol 1957;11:665–71.

Latzka WA, Sawka MN, Montain SJ, Skrinar GS, Fielding RA, Matott RP, Pandolf KB. Hyperhydration: thermoregulatory effects during compensable exercise-heat stress. J Appl Physiol 1997;83:860–6.

Lyons TP, Riedesel ML, Meuli LE, Chick TW. Effects of glycerol-induced hyperhydration prior to exercise in the heat on sweating and core temperature. Med Sci Sports Exerc 1990;22:477–83.

McConell GK, Burge CM, Skinner SL, Hargreaves M. Influence of ingested fluid volume on physiological responses during prolonged exercise. Acta Physiol Scand 1997;160:149–56.

MacLean DA, Graham TE, Saltin B. Stimulation of muscle ammonia production during exercise following branched-chain amino acid supplements in human. J Physiol Lond 1996;15;493:909–22.

Madsen K, MacLean DA, Kiens B, Christensen D. Effects of glucose, glucose plus branched chain amino acids, or placebo on bike performance over 100 km. J Appl Physiol 1996;81:2644–50.

Maughan RJ. Fluid and electrolyte loss and replacement in exercise. In: Harries M, Williams C, Stanish WD, Micheli LJ, eds. Oxford textbook of sports medicine. New York: Oxford University Press, 1994:82–93.

Maughan RJ, Fenn CE, Leiper JB. Effects of fluid, electrolyte and substrate ingestion on endurance capacity. Eur J Appl Physiol 1989;58:481–6.

Maughan RJ, Leiper JB. Sodium intake and post-exercise rehydration in man. Eur J Appl Physiol 1995;71:311–19.

Mazzeo RS, Bender PR, Brooks GA, Butterfield GE, Groves BM, Sutton JR, Wolfel EE, Reeves JT. Arterial catecholamine responses during exercise with acute and chronic high-altitude exposure. Am J Physiol 1991;261(4 Pt 1):E419–E24.

Millard-Stafford M, Sparling PB, Rosskopf LB, Dicarlo LJ. CHO–electrolyte replacement improves distance running performance in the heat. Med Sci Sports Exerc 1990;24:934–40.

Millard-Stafford M, Sparling PB, Rosskopf LB, Hinson BT, Dicarlo LJ. CHO–electrolyte replacement during a simulated triathlon in the heat. Med Science Sports Exerc 1992;22:621–8.

Mills PC, Smith NC, Casa I, Harris P, Harris RC, Marlin DJ. Effects of exercise intensity and environmental stress on indices of oxidative stress and iron homeostasis during exercise in the horse. Eur J Appl Physiol 1996;74:60–6.

Mittleman KD, Ricci MR, Bailey SP. Branched-chain amino acids prolong exercise during heat stress in men and women. Med Sci Sports Exerc 1998;30:83–91.

Montain SJ, Coyle EF. Influence of graded dehydration on hyperthermia and cardiovascular drift during exercise. J Appl Physiol 1992;73:1340–50.

Montner P, Stark DM, Riedesel ML, Murata G, Robergs R, Timms M, Chick TW. Pre-exercise glycerol hydration improves cycling endurance time. Int J Sports Med 1996;17:27–33.

Moore LG, Cymerman A, Huang SY, McCullough RE, McCullough RG, Rock PB, Young A, Young P, Weil JV, Reeves JT. Propanolol blocks metabolic rate increase but not ventilatory acclimatization to 4300 m. Respir Physiol 1987;70:95–205.

Murray R, Eddy DE, Murray TW, Paul GL, Seifert JG, Halaby GA. Physiological responses to glycerol ingestion during exercise. J Appl Physiol 1991;71:144–9.

Murray R, Eddy DE, Murray TW, Seifert JG, Paul GL, Halaby GA. The effect of fluid and CHO feedings during intermittent cycling exercise. Med Sci Sports Exerc 1987;19:597–604.

Nielsen B, Savard G, Richter EA, Hargreaves M, Saltin B. Muscle blood flow and muscle metabolism during exercise and heat stress. J Appl Physiol 1990;69:1040–6.

Nielsen B, Hales JRS, Strange S, Juel C, Christensen N, Warberg J, Saltin B. Human circulatory and thermoregulatory adaptations with heat acclimation and exercise in a hot, dry environment. J Physiol Lond 1993;460:467–85.

Norman B, Sollevi A, Kaijser L, Jansson E. ATP breakdown products in human skeletal muscle during prolonged exercise to exhaustion. Clin Physiol 1987;7:503–10.

Nose H, Mack GW, Shi X, Nadel ER. Role of osmolality and plasma volume during rehydration in humans. J Appl Physiol 1988;65:332–6.

Owen MD, Kregel KC, Wall PT, Gisolfi CV. Effects of ingesting CHO beverages during exercise in the heat. Med Sci Sports Exerc 1986;18:568–75.

Parkin JM, Carey MF, Zhao S, Febbraio MA. Effect of ambient temperature on human skeletal muscle metabolism during fatiguing submaximal exercise. J Appl Physiol 1999;86:902–8.

Powers SK, Howley ET, Cox R. A differential catecholamine response during exercise and passive heating. Med Sci Sports Exerc 1985;14:435–9.

Pugh LGCE. Blood volume and haemoglobin concentrations at altitudes above 14 000 feet (5500 m). J Physiol Lond 1964;170:344–54.

Roberts AC, Butterfield GE, Cymerman A, Reeves JT, Wolfel EE, Brooks GA. Acclimatization to 4300 m altitude decreases reliance on fat as a substrate. J Appl Physiol 1996a;81:1762–71.

Roberts, AC, Reeves JT, Butterfield GE, Mazzeo RS, Sutton JR, Wolfel EE, Brooks GA. Altitude and ß-blockade augment glucose utilisation during submaximal exercise. J Appl Physiol 1996b;80:605–15.

Ryan AJ, Bleiler TL, Carter JE, Gisolfi CV. Gastric emptying during prolonged cycling exercise in the heat. Med Sci Sports Exerc 1989;21:51–8.

Sahlin K, Katz A, Broberg S. Tricarboxylic acid cycle intermediates in humans during prolonged exercise. Am J Physiol 1990;259:C834–C41.

Snow RJ, Febbraio MA, Carey MF, Hargreaves M. Heat stress increases ammonia accumulation during exercise. Exp Physiol 1993;78:847–50.

Starkie RL, Hargreaves M, Lambert DL, Proietto J, Febbraio MA. Effect of temperature on muscle metabolism during submaximal exercise in humans. Exp Physiol 1999;84:775–84.

Sutton JR, Reeves JT, Wagner PD, Groves BM, Cymerman A, Malconian MK, Rock PB, Young PM, Walter SD, Houston CS. Operation Everest II: maximum oxygen uptake at extreme altitude. J Appl Physiol 1988;66:1309–28.

Takamata A, Mack GW, Gillen CM, Jozsi AC, Nadel ER. Osmoregulatory modulation of thermal sweating in humans: reflex effects of drinking. Am J Physiol 1995;268(2 Pt 2):R414–R22.

van Hall G, Raaymakers JSH, Saris WHM, Wagenmakers AJM. Ingestion of branched-chain amino acids and tryptophan during sustained exercise in man: failure to affect performance. J Physiol Lond 1995;486:789–94.

Walsh RM, Noakes TD, Hawley JA, Dennis SC. Impaired high-intensity cycling performance time at low levels of dehydration. Int J Sports Med 1994;15:392–8.

Yaspelkis III BB, Ivy JL. Effect of CHO supplements and water on exercise metabolism in the heat. J Appl Physiol 1991;71:680–7.

Yaspelkis III BB, Scroop GC, Wilmore KM, Ivy JL. CHO metabolism during exercise in hot and thermoneutral environments. Int J Sports Med 1993;14:13–19.

Young AJ, Sawka MN, Levine L, Cadarette BS, Pandolf KB. Skeletal muscle metabolism during exercise is influenced by heat acclimation. J Appl Physiol 1985;59:1929–35.

CHAPTER 26

Providing meals for athletic groups

Nicola Cummings

26.1 INTRODUCTION

Catering or providing advice to caterers about feeding athletes is a very exciting and challenging task for a dietitian. A dietitian involved with food service or menu planning is faced with the difficulties of providing for a wide variety of tastes, expectations, and different family/cultural backgrounds. When given the task of menu planning for athletes, a dietitian has the opportunity not only to determine the food that will be available, but also to influence eating behaviour directly. In a dining hall that caters for sportspeople, such as the Australian Institute of Sport (AIS) dining hall in Canberra, the presence of a dietitian working in food service can influence food supply and hence food choices. Most athletes reported consuming an increased carbohydrate (CHO) intake and a greater variety of foods when living at the AIS compared with their usual intakes at home (Cummings, unpublished data 1999). Similar findings were reported in a United States survey, which showed that residential athletes had a higher CHO intake and more optimal training diet than controls living at home. Unfortunately, most sporting venues and catering establishments do not cater adequately for the types of diets recommended for athletes, and the food provided frequently contradicts sports nutrition principles.

This chapter discusses the main considerations in menu planning for athletic groups. Section 26.4 provides tips for improving the food service environment in large-scale residential catering and also for athletes who are self-catering while away from home.

CATERING FOR DIFFERENT ATHLETES

There are many nutritional goals that apply to most athletes, however, large variations in nutrient and energy requirements occur between males and females at different ages, from different backgrounds and between different sports.

26.2.1 *In different sports*

When menu planning for athletes with high energy requirements, such as heavyweight rowers, provision of a much larger meal size than that provided for lightweight rowers is needed. With the trend towards small serve sizes in restaurants, large-energy consumers are at a disadvantage. In contrast, people catering for athletes often serve large meals to all athletes, irrespective of their body mass (BM) or sport. Public perceptions about feeding athletes are often distorted, especially in relation to elite athletes. Despite the apparent intensity and duration of physical activity in some team sports, energy requirements, and hence food intakes, are not that much greater than those in untrained people (see Chapter 6).

In contrast, large meals are quite daunting for many athletes who are watching their BM or skinfolds. For these athletes, foods need to be nutrient-dense so that adequate nutrient intakes can be met from smaller amounts of food. Providing written guidelines to caterers about serve sizes and meal sizes for different athletes helps address these misconceptions. A buffet-style service is best suited to athletes with a wide variety of energy requirements.

26.2.2 *At different ages*

Many young athletes travel both nationally and internationally and are faced with the challenge of eating unfamiliar foods. This situation creates problems for some athletes. Observations at the AIS indicate that adolescent athletes living away from home are quite conservative in their food choices. When menu planning for younger athletes, care should be taken with spicy foods and dishes with unusual flavours. In a large-scale catering establishment, ensure there are sufficient basic or plain menu options available. On a smaller scale, when it is not feasible to serve a wide array of options, meat dishes and their accompanying sauces can be served separately. This strategy caters for the needs of fussy eaters. Adolescent athletes are often reticent to sample unfamiliar foods, especially when away from home.

26.2.3 *Cultural background*

The home and cultural environment has a major influence on eating habits. Traditional Australian eating habits, with the emphasis on meat as the main part of the meal, do not encourage high CHO consumption. This pattern is difficult to change if usually followed at home. Athletes who expect to receive meals that resemble their home cooked meals are often disappointed. In response to this situation, athletes, especially adolescents, will usually only consume familiar foods. Although it is difficult, if not impossible, for a dietitian to present a menu plan that satisfies every individual in a large group setting, it is important to present enough choices to accommodate different types of diets and cultural differences (e.g. vegetarian and non-red-meat eaters). This is paramount with visiting athletes from overseas countries (see Section 26.3.6)

26.2.4 *Gender*

Food choices in athletes are often gender specific. Apart from the obvious requirements of larger serve sizes in males, mixed gender groups have different expectations of the type of meal served. From observations of working with teams, it is evident that male athletes prefer a cooked breakfast and hot meals at lunchtime. Female athletes, in contrast, are satisfied with a breakfast of cereal and/or toast, and sandwiches at lunchtime. These differences were clearly demonstrated in a survey of AIS residential athletes. Most female team athletes (mainly adolescents) stated that they consumed a sandwich for lunch, in contrast to the majority of adolescent male athletes (soccer and basketball) who consumed hot food (Cummings, unpublished data 1999). Adolescent girls appear to be more adventurous in trying new foods than boys of the same age.

To cater for these apparent differences in food choice between males and females, hot items can easily be incorporated into the breakfast menu by using pre-prepared foods (e.g. tinned spaghetti and baked beans). For quick hot lunches, the use of soups, toasted sandwiches or focaccia, or low-fat burgers in crusty rolls will satisfy food preferences for most athletes. The difference in food choices between sexes may be a reflection of the effect of different body perceptions reported between male and female adolescents (see Chapter 18).

26.3 THE MENU

26.3.1 *The menu cycle*

The length of the menu cycle is dependent on the time spent in the dining facilities. If athletes need to be fed for less than a month (e.g. training camps, competition venues), the menu cycle can run on a weekly basis. Athletes staying for such a short term do not have the time to become bored with the menu or even to recognise that there is a menu cycle. Alternatively, to avoid serving the same dishes on the same day of the week, the menu plan can be rotated. When menu planning for athletes living in permanent residences, the menu cycle can be longer. At the AIS, where the athletes are usually in year-long residence, the menu rotation is four weeks, with more popular items served more frequently.

26.3.2 *Variety and nutritional balance*

When designing a menu for large groups of athletes from different sports, a variety of dishes is important. This approach addresses variations in nutrient requirements between individuals and allows a wide range of personal choice. At the AIS, which caters for approximately 250 permanent athletes as well as visiting athletes in training camps, the menu options include four choices of hot meals at dinner (see Appendix 26, Table 26.5 for an example of a weekly menu plan). The meal choices include a high-CHO dish, plain meat, wet dish (e.g. curry or casserole) and a vegetarian dish, as well as a wide selection of salads, fresh fruit and assorted breads. When menu planning for a small group of athletes, it is acceptable to offer only one evening meal choice. Extra CHO-rich foods should be available at each meal time to accompany these dishes. A good option is a selection of novelty breads, such as focaccia, crusty loafs and Italian-style loafs. Individuals with special needs in a small group, including vegetarians, are usually catered for individually. A wide menu choice and variety helps prevent athletes from becoming bored with the food. Suggestions to increase food diversity and to provide well-presented and visually inviting meals include the following:

- Use different meats (for example, if roast meat is served each week in a menu cycle, rotate pork, beef, lamb, turkey, chicken and veal).
- Use a variety of cooking methods (grilled, braised meat, casseroles, stir-fries).
- Try using high-protein plant foods including legumes (incorporated into vegetarian dishes or used to add CHO to meat dishes). Legumes add bulk and therefore have a good satiety value as well as being relatively inexpensive.
- Use a variety of different coloured ingredients in each meal (this improves aesthetic appeal and encourages consumption).
- Enhance flavours of meals (by incorporating flavours from different regions of the world—spicy dishes must be balanced against some plain options).
- Offer a variety of textures (by incorporating dishes with differing 'mouth feel'). For example, if the menu plan has mashed potatoes, the other vegetables can be served 'al dente'.
- Serve a wet dish (e.g. casserole or stew) as well as plain grilled dishes.

In addition to these suggestions, the menu and most recipes should be low in fat and high in CHO to meet the dietary goals of athletes. If modifying recipes from regular cookbooks, an important strategy is to reduce the total amount of fat or oil, either by reducing the total amount of fat added to the recipe or using reduced-fat products, such as low-fat cheese and milk (see Table 26.1, Section 26.6). Alternatively, use one of the many low-fat cookbooks that are widely available on the market. If menu planning for large groups of athletes, a recommended cook book is *Cooking for Champions* (Modulon & Burke 1997).

Although the nutritional message to increase the intake of CHO for athletes is widely used, athletes (and most people) have difficulty translating these messages into actual food choice. Traditionally, food choices in Western diets do not meet the higher CHO diet of athletes in hard training. Some suggested strategies to promote an increase in CHO intake are:

- In a self-serve situation, offer the CHO-rich foods first (e.g. rice, potatoes, pasta and starchy vegetables) in the line up, and offer the meat dishes at the end. This sequence encourages larger serves of CHO, and smaller serves of protein, hence improving the balance.

- Ensure a wide variety of breads and rolls are served at each mealtime and position in strategic places. For example, put baskets of crusty bread rolls next to soup, and have a wide selection of bakery products including muffins, crumpets, pita bread and bagels.
- Maximise CHO content of meals by adding legumes to casseroles and soups, thick layers of pasta to lasagne, noodles to salads and soups, and use thick pizza bases.
- Provide a supply of low-fat snacks including sandwiches, fruits, yoghurts, cereals and cereal bars for in-between meals.
- Encourage athletes to take their own supply of ready-to-eat foods to training.

26.3.3 *Cost*

Food cost is usually a primary concern when designing a menu for a group of athletes. Some cost-cutting measures include:

- Buy food in bulk (try specific wholesale stores).
- Re-use foods leftover from a meal—provided food safety and hygiene have been addressed (see Section 26.3.7).
- Adapt the menu plan to use reduced price items.
- Cook meals in bulk and 're-invent' the dish at a later stage—e.g. Bolognese sauce served with pasta can be turned into a spicy bean-based Mexican dish and served with tortillas, jacket potatoes or rice.
- Bulk-up casseroles and minced meat dishes using cheaper ingredients including legumes and grains.
- Plan the menu on seasonal availability of fruits and vegetables.
- Consider self-catering for a group as an option to eating out.

26.3.4 *Seasonal*

Food preferences vary with season, particularly in countries where there are extremes in temperature. During winter, athletes prefer warming meals including casseroles and soups. Thick hearty soups are an excellent lunchtime option. During summer, athletes prefer lighter dishes including quiches, stir-fries, cold meats and salads. To boost CHO intake to salad dishes, add rice, couscous, bourghul, pasta, potatoes, and corn.

26.3.5 *Timing of meals*

When organising catering for groups of athletes, consider the timing of training and the competition event. In a residential establishment, meal times are usually set within a relatively short time frame. However, there should be enough flexibility to arrange pre- and post-match meals outside of these set times.

When menu planning for athletes who are self-catering, be aware of major competition days and the timing of such events. Organise the menu plan to incorporate high-CHO meals, to be available on competition days, which are quick and easy to prepare rather than relying on eating out. The ease of meal preparation is particularly important if tired, hungry athletes are required to cook for themselves. Suitable snacks need to be provided for the athletes immediately after competition.

If the training or competition schedule is very tight, a post-match meal at a restaurant is a convenient alternative. Phone ahead and notify the restaurant of the group's arrival so that meals are available soon after the team's arrival.

26.3.6   *Cultural and other special dietary requirements*

When menu planning, consider the cultural background of the athletic group. Religious beliefs (Kosher, Halal), medical problems (intolerances, allergies), personal preferences (e.g. vegetarian) or country of origin of the athlete are important considerations. Athletes accustomed to Western diets encounter difficulties when competing in many Asian countries where bread and breakfast cereals are often unavailable. Similarly, difficulties arise when Asians and Africans, for example, experience Western food. If catering on a large scale, it is possible to make special dishes available for a particular group of athletes. At the AIS, because of the popularity of vegetarian-style dishes, there is always a vegetarian option. When designing a menu plan to incorporate vegetarian dishes, it is important to base some of the dishes on meat alternatives and include, for example, pulses, tofu, or tinned nut meat products to cater for true vegetarian athletes. Popular vegetarian choices among athletes are spicy bean burritos, chilli con carne, and vegetable and lentil lasagne. It is easy to disguise the often unpopular lentil in these dishes as well as soups, stews and casseroles.

Athletes who are unadventurous or inflexible in their eating habits can resort to poor food choices in an environment with unfamiliar foods. If this situation continues for a long time, performance and possibly nutritional status is affected. This behaviour has caused many problems when athletes travel both nationally and internationally. For example, an overseas athlete presented to the medical staff with severe stomach pains which was later diagnosed as constipation due to the reliance on consumption of one familiar food: eggs!

26.3.7   *Food safety*

In a large-scale catering facility, all kitchen staff should be trained in food safety and hygiene practices. Although local governments in Australia have encouraged food service staff to be formally trained in food safety and hygiene, it is not yet compulsory. A dietitian involved with menu planning has an excellent opportunity to provide such training, and offer encouragement and adherence to safe food hygiene practices. Food safety issues, including food handling, storage of food, re-use of leftovers, and personal hygiene associated with food, are also important issues for athletes who are self-catering. This is particularly important for athletes who travel overseas where the risk of food-borne illness is high.

26.3.8 *Food service staff and facilities*

An important component of menu planning is to determine whether catering staff has any past experience in feeding athletes. Feeding athletes involves more than simply serving a meal of pasta, as is often encountered. Providing written guidelines to caterers about meal ideas and recommended serve sizes consumed by athletes helps overcome these problems. Suggestions for caterers are: serving pasta, rice, potatoes and vegetables at the start of the service point; serving dishes with accompanying sauces separately; ensuring adequate fluid is available (i.e. carafes or water jugs placed on tables). Numerous recipe books are available for catering for large groups of people (e.g. Modulon & Burke 1997, *Cooking for Champions*). Alternatively, a dietitian can have a positive impact by conducting education sessions for food service staff. The content of these sessions conducted at the AIS is found in Section 26.4.5.

26.4 *FEEDING ATHLETES IN DIFFERENT SITUATIONS*

26.4.1 *Residential catering for athletic groups*

Although foods selected from a menu with a wide selection of choice (i.e à la carte) may be the first preference for most people, it is not feasible or economical when serving large groups of athletes. A buffet-style self-service is more suitable as it:

- provides readily available food for hungry athletes;
- is more cost-effective because of minimal staffing requirements, bulk cooking and low wastage; and
- allows for flexibility in food choice.

Athletes living in residence where buffet-style food is served often complain about boredom and lack of menu variety. These complaints are more often voiced by those athletes who:

- consume food from every dish on the buffet;
- watch what other athletes eat;
- use the dining hall as a social meeting point and linger over meals; and
- eat more than necessary (have two or more meals).

24.4.2 *Overcoming the problems—an operation in practice*

The AIS dining hall was opened in 1987 for resident athletes. In 1995, the catering was tendered to a private contractor with the proviso that a food service dietitian be employed as an adviser and overseer of the menu plan. The mission statement in the dining hall is 'Feeding athletes for today, educating them for tomorrow'. The major tasks of the food service dietitian are to train athletes to choose appropriate foods to meet their nutritional needs, to develop new recipes, to design the menu plan, to check on adherence to recipes, and to train food service staff. Because of the wide range of differences in sports, ages, training schedules, nutritional requirements and personal preferences, the dining hall serves a variety of menu options.

26.4.3 *Recipe modification*

The food service dietitian can assist chefs in recipe modification by adapting traditional higher fat recipes to low- or reduced-fat without compromising flavour, texture or the structure of the finished product. The AIS dining hall prides itself on serving traditional 'popular' menu items such as beef lasagne, chicken schnitzel, and Thai-style curries without the usual high-fat ingredients. For direction on how to modify these recipes, refer to Modulon and Burke (1997).

26.4.4 *Education of athletes*

Dietitians working at the AIS conduct regular education sessions with residential and visiting athletes. The first session for residential athletes is focussed on 'survival in the dining hall', which covers the problems and pitfalls of eating from a buffet-style menu.

All meals have an accompanying nutritional card highlighting ingredients in the dish, and a nutritional analysis per serve. Modulon and Burke (1997) designed a colour-coded system for all meals served in the dining hall, to differentiate between dishes that are high in CHO (excellent choice) and have moderate CHO and fat content (good choice). To emphasise the importance of CHO foods in the athletes' daily diets, dishes that have little or no CHO content (e.g. meat dishes) are highlighted by a blue dot denoting extra CHO needs to be added to the dish. As well as the nutritional cards above the meals, nutritional information about other foods is situated around the dining hall. Figure 26.1 provides an example of a nutrition card.

As an additional educational strategy, groups of athletes are given the opportunity to plan a menu for a specific theme night. With guidance from the team's dietitian, the usual menu planning steps are worked through to ensure a nutritionally balanced menu, with a few of their favourite choices as treats. Examples of theme nights that have been held so far have included AFL (Australian Football League) night, Mexican night, Hawaiian night, an Indian feast and a Turkish night, including entertainment from a belly-dancer.

26.4.5 *Education of catering staff*

Chefs and food service staff are not usually trained to cater for the nutrient requirements of people with specialised nutrient requirements (e.g. hospital patients, people in nursing homes). This task is the role of the clinical dietitian. In addition, clinical dietitians are trained as educators, counsellors and consultants in nutrition education and food service. Therefore, it is a good investment of time and effort for

Singapore Noodles

A dish of lean pork, black beans, vegetables, garlic, chilli and coriander, tossed with Hokkien noodles.

**This dish is low in fat and high in CHO.
Serve with rice for an extra CHO boost.**

Excellent choice

1 serve: 1 heaped cup

Energy	1 000 kJ (238 cal)
CHO	30 g (50% of energy)
Fat	4 g (14% of energy)
Protein	21 g
Iron	2.5 mg

Figure 26.1 *Example of a nutrition card used at the AIS dining hall*

the dietitian to conduct education sessions for food service staff. Because of the unique situation of catering for large numbers of athletes in a live-in environment at the AIS, chefs and food service staff gain additional expertise in the provision of an optimal diet for athletes. Educating food staff at the AIS about healthy food choices and the links between diet, lifestyle and diseases has also encouraged a greater personal interest in healthy eating.

Catering staff are also made aware of the problems and complaints of athletes of a buffet service and present food in a variety of ways to address these problems. For example, serving food in large aluminium dishes in a bain-marie is not always attractive to the eye or palate. Dishes look attractive at the start of service, then deteriorate into a 'mush' once athletes have helped themselves. Pre-portioning dishes can overcome part of this problem, as athletes are encouraged to help themselves to a portion. Section 26.6 provides an outline of education sessions for food service staff.

26.4.6 *Self-catering while away from home*

The advantages of self-catering while away from home are greater flexibility with meal times, provision of familiar foods, and cost effectiveness. It is beneficial to encourage athletes in a team to menu plan and cook for themselves in groups, rather than to rely solely on the coach, team manager, parents or administration staff. Most accompanying personnel on trips away are unpaid volunteers. Some of the large teams provide financial support for these support staff and may also be accompanied by a dietitian. Dietitians who travel with athletes need to be multi-skilled and offer services other than just menu planning, such as shopping and cooking, massage and management of the team. Prior to departure, a dietitian should determine the level of cooking skills of the athletes. Cooking classes with the team just prior to departure are invaluable for instilling confidence in young people with poor cooking skills and for organising a menu plan for the trip.

One of the disadvantages of self-catering away from home is that cooking facilities in self-contained accommodation usually provide equipment for only two to four people. We encourage a communal approach in cooking where one group of four to five athletes takes responsibility for the main meal for the whole group; another group takes responsibility for salad or vegetables and another group for dessert. This pattern rotates every night but fosters a competitive, interactive and fun approach that is fair to everyone. The menu plan is influenced by the equipment available, the type and number of saucepans available, storage facilities (freezers, fridges) and cooking equipment (microwave, cooker, hobs). Any limitation in cooking equipment can easily be overcome by pre-planning the menu, checking the availability of cooking equipment beforehand, and taking only the necessary equipment from home. Because of the small size of saucepans in most self-contained accommodation, we advise athletes to bring their own large-sized pans to cook for the group. Other useful items include a blender, storage containers, plastic film wrap, muffin trays and non-stick pan (or wok). Seasonings that are used in small amounts as ingredients in pre-arranged recipes are best bought from home (e.g. curry powder, stock cubes, dried herbs and spices). Further tips for helping athletes feed themselves by self-catering when away from home are found in Section 26.6.

26.4.7 *Eating out*

Most young athletes have a limited budget and cannot afford the accommodation cost as well as restaurant meals when travelling away from home. However, restaurant dining or take-away foods are a quick convenient meal for athletes who are tired and hungry, and a treat for those who are self-catering. Unfortunately, if food choices are poor, restaurant or take-away meals may not provide a suitable recovery meal. Such meals are usually too high in fat and too low in CHO to meet the needs of athletes preparing for the next bout of competition. Restaurant meals encourage over indulgence and are best visited at the end of competition as a treat or social occasion. In some circumstances, athletes are dependent on restaurants for meals or have accommodation which includes all meals. In these situations, advice about making suitable choices and avoiding meals known to be fatty (e.g. garlic bread and fried or crumbed meat) is warranted.

26.5 SUMMARY

Menu planning and organising food services for athletes is not only challenging, but gives the dietitian an opportunity to directly influence the food supply provided to athletes and to encourage and motivate athletes about food choice. The benefits to athletes of participating in cooking classes and designing their own menus are invaluable in developing much needed cooking skills and confidence in food preparation and selection. Ultimately, the goal of such a hands-on approach is to encourage consumption of the recommended training diet on an everyday basis, and for athletes to take a more active and personal responsibility for feeding themselves.

26.6 PRACTICE TIPS

Nicola Cummings

Introduction

- Menu planning allows the translation of nutrition principles into real food choices for athletes. Helping athletes select food provides an ideal opportunity to raise awareness of food choice, influence existing beliefs and attitudes, and ultimately to improve food selection.

Menu planning for athletic groups

- A menu must cater for the requirements of the team and the characteristics of individuals within that team. In most circumstances, menu planning will be sport-, gender- and age-specific (e.g. all boys or girls, footballers or rowers, under-19 squad or juniors). Menu planning needs to consider catering arrangements and facilities (self-catering or restaurant), climate, cost, timing of competition or training, cultural/special requirements, food safety, staff expertise and equipment.

- When catering for large groups of athletes from differing sports, the preferred option is the buffet-style self-service.

Strategies for providing meals for athletes in residence at the AIS

- The AIS accommodated approximately 250 athletes living in residence in 1999. The dining hall caters for these athletes and hundreds of visiting athletes in training camps, as well as coaches and staff.

- The role of the food service dietitian: a dietitian is employed on a part-time basis (26 hours per week) in food service. Job specifications of this position include:

1. development of the menu plan and the modification and analysis of recipes provided to athletes;
2. education of athletes about nutrition principles for sportspeople and food choice in the dining hall;
3. education and professional development of catering staff; and
4. evaluation of the menu plan by formal surveys and verbal feedback from representative athletes.

Recipe modification for caterers

- Australian cookbooks written specifically for sportspeople are available in bookshops or newsagencies (Burke et al. 1999; Modulon & Burke 1997; Inge & Roberts 1996; O'Connor & Hay 1996). However, any low-fat cookbook or recipe is suitable for athletes, although additional CHO-rich foods may need to be added to the final meal. Modifying existing recipes with lower fat ingredients or alternative ingredients is possible with most recipes, without a large change in texture or flavour. Table 26.1 provides some suggestions for modifying fat content in recipes.

Table 26.1 *Methods to reduce and modify fat in cooking and in recipes*

Oils or fats	Reduce the amount of fat for stir-frying Use spray oils and use water and/or stock for cooking
Butter	Check the amount and reduce if possible Replace with mono- or polyunsaturated margarines. Use moist ingredients such as buttermilk to enhance the taste
Cream	Use evaporated skim milk. For a thickened consistency, heat evaporated skim milk and thicken with corn flour
Salad dressings and mayonnaise	Use fat-free or reduced-fat varieties; skim or low-fat natural yoghurt and herbs
Sour cream	Use skim or low-fat natural yoghurt
Mature cheese (e.g. cheddar)	Use reduced-fat cheese*
Cream cheese	Mix together cottage cheese and low-fat ricotta cheese
Milk	Use skim milk, low- or reduced-fat milk
Curries	Use low-fat coconut milk or evaporated skim milk with a few drops of coconut essence

* For melting purposes, use a mixture of one part full-fat cheddar to four parts reduced-fat cheddar to improve consistency and flavour.

Guidelines for athletes when choosing foods from a buffet

- Most organised meals for athletes at training camps or competition venues are buffet-style.

- Athletes living and eating in a communal environment, and offered a buffet-style service, frequently overeat, miss out or eat sub-optimal amounts of one or more food groups (mostly vegetables), or habitually eat a poorly balanced diet. The advantages of living-in are that they don't have to cook, shop or plan meals. However, the disadvantages are a lack of involvement with food and cooking for themselves, a loss of food and cooking skills and not knowing the ingredients in a recipe.

- At the AIS we address these issues by:
  1. providing education sessions early in the training program on 'survival in the dining hall' and choosing wisely (Table 26.2 provides the written information given to athletes on this topic and summarises the content of this education session);
  2. the use of nutritional cards listing the nutrient composition of meals; and
  3. providing opportunities for teams to organise their own theme night which involves planning the menu, decorating the dining room, dressing up to match the theme and being actively involved in food service.

Nutritional cards

- Nutritional cards accompany the meals in the AIS dining hall. These cards list the ingredients contained in the dish, nutrient analysis (including CHO, fat and protein) and serve size. Calcium, iron and fibre content per serve are also included (if they are good sources). An example of a nutritional card is found in Figure 26.1.

Feeding athletes: an education program for catering staff

- Table 26.3 provides an outline of the content and format of the education sessions for catering staff responsible for feeding athletes at the AIS. The dietitian conducts these sessions. Aspects of this program can easily be adapted or converted into written guidelines to give to caterers who are providing meals for athletes on an ad hoc or one-off basis. Aspects of this information are also useful for the manager of a team who has the responsibility of organising meals or catering staff to feed athletes who are competing away from home.

Menu planning for self-catering

- Prior to departure, the dietitian needs to arrange a meeting with the team, coach and manager to determine the catering requirements, competition or

Table 26.2 *Tips provided to athletes about eating in the dining hall at the AIS*

1. Know clearly your nutritional goals and how to choose foods to achieve these goals most of the time.
   If you are unsure of how to choose foods to achieve these goals, arrange to see a sports dietitian.
2. Be focussed and organised when planning your meal times and snacks.
   Don't leave it to chance. Stick to this plan—don't try anything new or tricky at or around competition.
3. Treat the dining hall like a restaurant.
   Look at the menu or do a lap to check out what is on offer. Make a decision as you wait in the queue. Don't just grab!
4. Don't concern yourself with the amount and type of food that other athletes are consuming.
   The nutritional needs of other athletes may be quite different to your own. Don't be influenced by peer pressure.
5. Don't pile a bit of everything on your plate.
   This type of eating is haphazard and unbalanced, and you'll probably end up eating more than you need.
6. Eat just what you need from a balanced food selection.
   Check your plate for: mostly high-CHO foods, a protein-rich food, some vegetables or fruit—the more colourful, the more vitamins!
7. Read any nutrition information provided to learn more about your meal choice and to help make other food choices.
8. Relax.
   There is plenty of food for everyone and menu items will be repeated. If you decide on one item tonight, you can look forward to another choice the next night. This isn't your last meal.
9. Plan for healthy snacks between meals—especially if you have high-energy needs. *Take what you need from the dining hall—fruit, yoghurt and bread/sandwiches are good choices.*
10. Don't hang around the dining hall once you have finished your meal.
    You'll end up eating things that you don't need and don't remember.

Adapted from Modulon and Burke 1997

training schedules, and food skills of the team and allocated budget. For most local or national competitions where the athletes are not professional, self-catering is usually the preferred option because of financial constraints. Table 26.4 provides an outline of a suggested intervention strategy for a sports dietitian working with such teams.

- Cooking sessions emphasise quick and easy low-fat dishes and basic cooking skills. It is important to discuss food storage, food hygiene and food safety issues at this session.

Table 26.3	*Outline of content of education program for catering staff*

Week 1—Overview of the dining hall, standardisation of recipes, service standards
Week 2—Guidelines for healthy eating
Week 3—Nutrition for athletes: general requirements
Week 4—Nutrition for athletes: specific requirements
Week 5—Menu planning and recipe modification
Week 6 – Menu planning: practical

Table 26.4	*Tips for dietitians to prepare athletes for self-catering*

1. Discuss catering requirements with the athletes/manager/coach
2. Determine the cooking skills of the group
   Plan a pre-camp cooking session(s) if feasible
   Alternatively co-ordinate the cooking session during the camp, if the dietitian is travelling with the team
3. Determine in advance the cooking equipment and facilities available
4. Plan the menu around the length of stay, competition or training program
5. Designate responsibility for shopping and cooking of food among the athletes
6. Develop a list of basic ingredients and cooking equipment that can be taken from home and shared among the team

Planning for dining out

- Book a restaurant in close proximity to the accommodation rather than dropping in unexpectedly.

- Confirm that the menu provides appropriate and suitable foods for the age, budget, and food preferences of the team.

- If a large group of athletes are booked and planning is well in advance, send suitable menu selections (Modulon & Burke 1997).

- For a large group of athletes arrange a set à la carte menu with one of two choices or a buffet-style.

- Inform restaurants of estimated time of arrival.

- Ensure there is plenty of extra bread served with the meal.

- Ensure water and juices are kept well stocked during the meal.

REFERENCES

Burke L, Cox G, Cummings N, et al. Survival for the fittest: The Australian Institute of Sport official cookbook for busy people. Sydney: Murdoch Magazines Pty Ltd, 1999.

Cummings N. Survey—habits and knowledge of team athletes eating in the AIS dining hall. 1999 (unpublished).

Hickson JF, Johnson CW, Schrader JW, et al. Promotion of athletes' nutritional intake by a university foodservice facility. J Am Diet Assoc 1987;87:926–7.

Inge K, Roberts C. Food for sport cookbook, 3rd edn. Melbourne: New Holland Publishers, 1996.

Modulon S, Burke L. Cooking for champions: a guide to healthy large scale cooking for athletes and other active people. Canberra: Australian Sports Commission, 1997.

O'Connor H, Hay D. The taste of fitness, 2nd edn. Australia: JB Fairfax Creative Cooking, 1996.

O'Connor H, Hay D. Nutrition sports basics. Australia: JB Fairfax Creative Cooking, 1998.

APPENDIX 26

Table 26.5 *Weekly menu plan at the AIS dining hall*

	Monday	Tuesday	Wednesday	Thursday	Friday	Saturday
Breakfast	Pancakes Baked beans Tinned spaghetti Grilled mushrooms Boiled eggs	Baked beans Grilled tomatoes Ham/poached egg on English muffin Bircher muesli with tinned berries	Pancakes Tinned spaghetti Stewed fruit Scrambled eggs	Muffins Baked beans Grilled tomatoes French toast Bircher muesli with tinned berries	Pancakes Baked beans Tinned spaghetti Scrambled eggs	Muffins Baked beans Tinned spaghetti Boiled eggs
Lunch Quick hot lunch	Chicken burgers	Pizza supreme Pizza vegetarian	Spicy meatballs with tomato-based sauce and pasta	Felafel with a homemade tomato sauce	Stir-fried vegetables in oyster sauce with rice noodles	Beef burgers, buns and salad
High CHO	Pasta bake	Pork satay with peanut sauce and pasta	Vegetarian fried rice	Pasta with chicken/ aubergine sauce	Pasta Bolognese	Pasta au funghi
Dinner			Barbecue night (served outside)			
Vegetarian	Vegetable strudel	Potato pie	Mexicana sauce with pasta	Vegetable quiche	Spinach and cheese cannelloni	Stir-fried vegetables with rice
High CHO	Pasta carbonara	Chicken stir-fry and noodles	Jacket potatoes with assorted fillings	Alfredo sauce with pasta	Combination chow mien	Tuna pasta
Plain meat	Chicken schnitzel	BBQ pork chops with spicy plum sauce	Tandoori chicken Fish in foil T-bone steaks	Roast lamb and gravy	Steamed fish with grilled calamari	Roast beef with gravy
Other meat	Beef with black bean sauce with rice	Lamb and sun-dried tomato casserole		Stir-fried chicken and vegetable	Minute steaks in plum sauce with rice	Chicken cacciatore
Hot dessert	Stewed fruit	Butterscotch self- saucing pudding	Apple and rhubarb pie	Stewed fruit	Banana nut loaf	Choc self-saucing pudding
Cold dessert	Lemon meringue pie	Jelly & tinned fruit	Fresh fruit	Hazelnut mousse	Fresh fruit salad	Jelly & tinned fruit
Additional	Mango yoghurt Ice-cream Custard	Custard	Chocolate ice-cream Custard	Custard	Vanilla ice-cream Custard	Chocolate custard

Adapted from Australian Institute of Sport Dining Hall—spring/summer menu plan